Male Fertility
and its Regulation

Advances in Reproductive Health Care
Series Editor: **E.S.E. Hafez**

Advances in
Reproductive Health Care

Male Fertility and its Regulation

Editors

T.J. Lobl and E.S.E. Hafez

MTP PRESS LIMITED
a member of the KLUWER ACADEMIC PUBLISHERS GROUP
LANCASTER / BOSTON / THE HAGUE / DORDRECHT

Published in the UK and Europe by
MTP Press Limited
Falcon House
Lancaster, England

British Library Cataloguing in Publication Data

Male fertility and its regulation.—
(Advances in reproductive health care)
1. Fertility, Human   2. Birth control
I. Lobl, T.J.   II. Hafez, E.S.E.   III. Series
612'.61   QP253

Published in the USA by
MTP Press
A division of Kluwer Boston Inc
190 Old Derby Street
Hingham, MA 02043, USA

Library of Congress Cataloging in Publication Data

Main entry under title:

Male fertility and its regulation.

(Advances in reproductive health care)
Based on the proceedings from the Symposium on Male Fertility and Its Regulation
which was held as part of the Reproductive Health Care Congress, 10–15 Oct. 1982 in
Kaanapali, Hawaii.
Includes bibliographies and index.
1. Generative organs, Male—Effect of drugs on—Congresses. 2. Contraceptive
drugs—Congresses.
I. Lobl, T.J.   II. Hafez, E.S.E. (Elsayed Saad Eldin), 1922– . III. Symposium on
Male Fertility and Its Regulation (1982: Kaanapali, Hawaii) IV. Reproductive Health
Care International Symposium (1982: Kaanapali, Hawaii) V. Series. [DNLM:
1. Contraceptive Agents, Male—congresses. 2. Fertility—drug effects—
congresses. 3. Genitalia, Male—physiology—congresses. 4. Gossypol—
pharmacodynamics—congresses.   QV 177 M2455 1982]
RC877.M35   1984   613.9'432   84–23408

ISBN-13: 978-94-010-8667-7   e-ISBN-13: 978-94-009-4894-5
DOI: 10.1007/978-94-009-4894-5

Contents

CONTENTS

CONTENTS

CONTENTS

List of Contributors

M.B. ABOU-DONIA
Department of Pharmacology, Box 3813, Duke University Medical Center, Durham, North Carolina 27710, USA

E.Y. ADASHI
Department of Obstetrics/Gynecology, University of Maryland Hospital and School of Medicine, Room 11-011, Frank Bressler Research Bldg, 655 W. Baltimore Street, Baltimore, Maryland 21201, USA

K.J. ANDERSON
Kettering Medical Center, Kettering, Ohio 45429, USA

P.K. BAJPAI
Department of Biology, University of Dayton, Dayton, Ohio 45469, USA

A. BARTKE
Department of Obstetrics/Gynecology, Southern Illinois University School of Medicine, Southern Illinois University at Carbondale, Carbondale, Illinois, 62901, USA

M.P. BRADLEY
Department of Surgery, Adams Bldg., University of Otogo, Dunedin, New Zealand

J.E. BRAHAM
Agricultural Sciences, Institute of Nutrition of Central America and Panama, P.O. Box 1188, Guatemala City, Guatemala, Central America

R. BRESSANI
Agricultural Sciences, Institute of Nutrition of Central America and Panama, P.O. Box 1188, Guatemala City, Guatemala, Central America

R. BRONSON
Department of Obstetrics/Gynecology, North Shore University Hospital, Cornell University Medical College, 300 Community Drive, Manhasset, New York 11030, USA

A.F. CHEN
Beckman Microbics Operations, 6200 El Camino Real, Carlbad, Canada 92008

V.F. CIOLI
F. Angelini Research Institute, Viale Amelia 70, 00181 Rome, Italy

G. COLAS
INRA, Reproductive Physiology Laboratory, F-37380 Nouzilly, France

G. COOPER
Department of Obstetrics/Gynecology, North Shore University Hospital, Cornell University Medical College, 300 Community Drive, Manhasset, New York 11030, USA

N.J. COSSLER
Department of Obstetrics/Gynecology, Wayne State University, 4707 St. Antoine, Detroit, Michigan 48201, USA

S. DALTERIO
Department of Pharmacology, The University of Texas Health Science Center, 7703 Floyd Curl Drive, San Antonio, Texas 78284, USA

J.R. DANIEL
Department of Food & Nutrition, Purdue University, West Lafayette, Indiana 47907, USA

LIST OF CONTRIBUTORS

S. DELPECH
Reproductive Physiology Laboratory, INRA, F-37380 Nouzilly, France

C. DE MARTINO
Regina Elena Institute for Cancer Research, Viale Regina Elena 291, 00161 Rome, Italy

M.T. de REVIERS
Reproductive Physiology Laboratory, INRA, F-37380 Nouzilly, France

A. DULEBA
Department of Obstetrics/Gynecology, The University of British Columbia, Vancouver, BC, V6T 2B5, Canada

L.C. ELLIS
Department of Biology UMC-53, Utah State University, Logan, Utah 84322, USA

I.T. FORRESTER
Department of Biochemistry, University of Otago, Box 56, Dunedin, New Zealand

V. GOMEL
Department of Obstetrics/Gynecology, New Grace Hospital, 4900 Oak Street, Vancouver, Canada V6H 3V5

E.S.E. HAFEZ
Reproductive Life Center, Medical University of South Carolina, Department of Physiology, 171 Ashley, Charleston, South Carolina 29425, USA

B.F. HALES
Centre for the Study of Reproduction, Department of Pharmacology, McGill University, 3655 Drummond Street, Montreal, Quebec H3G 1Y6, Canada

S.A. HAMDI
Department of Obstetrics/Gynecology, Wayne State University, 275 E. Hancock Avenue, Detroit, Michigan, 48201, USA

J. HARCLERODE
Department of Biology, Bucknell University, Lewisburg, Pennsylvania 17837, USA

B.T. HINTON
Department of Anatomy, Box 439, University of Virginia, School of Medicine, Charlottesville, Virginia 22908, USA

Z.T. HOMONNAI
Institute for the Study of Fertility, Maternity Hospital, Tel Aviv Medical Centre, Tel Aviv University Medical School, P.O. Box 7079, Tel Aviv 61070, Israel

S.S. HOWARDS
Department of Urology, Box 422, University of Virginia, School of Medicine, Charlottesville, Virginia 22908, USA

A.J.W. HSUEH
Department of Reproductive Medicine, M-025, University of California, School of Medicine, San Diego, La Jolla, California 92093, USA

M.E. HULL
Department of Reproductive Endocrinolgy and Infertility, Wayne State University, 275 E. Hancock Avenue, Detroit, Michigan, 48201, USA

L.A. JONES
National Cottonseed Products Association, Inc., P.O. Box 12023, Memphis, Tennessee 38112, USA

K.A. KRISHNAN
Institute for Research in Reproduction, Jehangir Merwanji Street, Parel, Bombay 400 012, India

J.C. LAMB IV
Fertility & Reproduction Group, National Institute of Environmental Health Sciences, National Toxicology Program, P.O. Box 12233, Research Triangle Park, North Carolina 27709, USA

C.-S. LEE
Department of Biochemistry, The Chinese University of Hong Kong, Shatin, N.T., Hong Kong

C.-Y.G. LEE
Department of Obstetrics/Gynecology, The University of British Columbia, Vancouver, British Columbia V6T 2B5, Canada

LIST OF CONTRIBUTORS

I.P. LEE
Laboratory of Reproductive & Developmental Toxicology, National Institute of Environmental Health Sciences, Research Triangle Park, North Carolina 27709, USA

W.M. LEE
Department of Physiology, University of Hong Kong, Li Shu Fan Bldg., Sassoon Road, Hong Kong

A.J. LEVI
Northwich Park Hospital, Clinical Research Centre, Watford Road, Harrow, Middlesex HA1 3UJ, UK

T.J. LOBL
Biotechnology Research, The Upjohn Company, Kalamazoo, Michigan 49001, USA

N.K. LOHIYA
Reproductive Physiology Section, Department of Zoology, University of Rajasthan, Jaipur 302 004, India

T.A. MARKS
Teratology & Reproduction, The Upjohn Company, 301 Henrietta Street, Kalamazoo, Michigan 49001, USA

Y.S. MOON
Department of Obstetrics/Gynecology, The University of British Columbia, Vancouver, BC, V6T 2B5, Canada

J.A. MOORE
Environmental Protection Agency, Rm. 637, East Tower, TS-788, 401 M St., SW, Washington, DC 20460, USA

C. O'MORAIN
Northwich Park Hospital, Clinical Research Centre, Watford Road, Harrow, Middlesex HA1 3UJ, UK

B.R. NEMETALLAH
Department of Physiology, Faculty of Veterinary Medicine, Edfina, Alexandria University, Egypt

A.A. NOMEIR
Department of Pharmacology, Duke University Medical Center, Box 3813, Durham, North Carolina 27710, USA

G.F. PAZ
Institute for the Study of Fertility, Maternity Hospital, Tel Aviv Medical Center, Tel Aviv University Medical School, P.O. Box 7079, Tel Aviv 61070, Israel

G. POTASHNIK
Infertility Clinic, Department of Obstetrics/Gynecology, Soroka University Hospital and Faculty of Health Sciences at the Ben Gurion University of the Negev, Beer-Sheba, Israel Sheva, Israel 84 101

J.I. QUIVY
International Institute of Cellular & Molecular Pathology, UCL 7529, Avenue Hippocrate 75, B-1200 Brussels, Belgium

B. ROBAIRE
Centre for the Study of Reproduction, Department of Pharmacology, McGill University, 3655 Drummond Street, Montreal, Quebec H3G 1Y6, Canada

C.F. ROLIN JACQUEMYNS
International Institute of Cellular & Molecular Pathology, UCL 7529, Avenne Hippocrate 75, B-1200 Brussels, Belgium

D. ROSENFELD
Department of Obstetrics/Gynecology, North Shore University Hospital, Cornell University Medical College, 300 Community Drive, Manhasset, New York 11030, USA

G.G. ROUSSEAU
UCL 7529, Avenue Hippocrate 75, B-1200 Brussels, Belgium

L.L. RUSSELL
Department of Medical Physiology & Pharmacology, Southern Illinois University, School of Medicine, Carbondale, Illinois 62901, USA

B.S. SARVAMANGALA
Institute for Research in Reproduction, Indian Council of Medical Research, Jehangir Merwanji Street, Parel, Bombay 400 012, India

P. SCORZA BARCELLONA
F. Angelini Research Institute, Viale Amelia 70, 00181 Rome, Italy

xi

LIST OF CONTRIBUTORS

O.P. SHARMA
Reproductive Physiology Section, Department of Zoology, University of Rajasthan, Jaipur 302 004, India

A.R. SHETH
Institute for Research in Reproduction, Indian Council of Medical Research, Jehangir Merwanji Street, Parel, Bombay 400 012, India

B. SILVESTRINI
Institute of Pharmacology and Pharmacognosy, University of Rome "La Sapienza", Piazzale Aldo Moro 5, 00185, Rome, Italy

D.A.N. SIRETT
International Institute of Cellular & Molecular Pathology, UCL 7529, Avenue Hippocrate 75, B-1200 Brussels, Belgium

P. SMETHHURST
Northwich Park Hospital, Clinical Research Centre, Watford Road, Harrow, Middlesex HA1 3UJ, UK

C.G. SMITH
Department of Pharmacology, Uniformed Services University of the Health Sciences, 4301 Jones Bridge Road, Bethesda, Maryland 20814, USA

N.J. SPIRTOS
Reproductive Endocrinolgy and Infertility Department, Akron City Hospital, 525 E. Market Street, Akron, Ohio 44309, USA

J.M. TRASLER
Centre for the Study of Reproduction, Department of Pharmacology, McGill University, 3655 Drummond Street, Montreal, Quebec H3G 1Y6, Canada

M.-Y.W. TSO
Radioisotope Unit, Hong Kong University, Pokfulam Road, Hong Kong

W.W. TSO
Department of Biochemistry, The Chinese University of Hong Kong, Shatin, N.T., Hong Kong

T.T. TURNER
Department of Urology, Box 422, University of Virginia, School of Medicine, Charlottesville, Virginia 22908, USA

G.R. VANAGE
Institute for Research in Reproduction, Indian Council of Medical Research, Jehangir Merwanji Street, Parel, Bombay 400 012, India

B.H. VICKERY
Department of Physiology, Syntex Research R2-241, 3401 Hillview Avenue, Palo Alto, California 94304, USA

M.C. VIGUIER-MARTINEZ
Reproductive Physiology Laboratory, INRA, F-37380 Nouzilly, France

R.L. WHISTLER
Department of Biochemistry, Purdue University, West Lafayette, Indiana 47907, USA

P.Y.D. WONG
Department of Physiology, University of Hong Kong, Li Shu Fan Bldg., Sassoon Road, Hong Kong

S-p. XUE (Shieh)
Department of Cell Biology, Institute of Basic Medical Sciences, Chinese Academy of Medical Sciences, 5 Don Dan San Tiao, Beijing, China

Preface

Uncontrolled population growth, a significant problem for many countries, depresses real living standards in all developing areas. As a corollary, uncontrolled population growth also stresses the ability to deliver adequate reproductive health care on both national and individual levels. To focus on this and related problems an International Congress to examine many aspects of male and female Reproductive Health Center Care was held on 10–15 October 1982 in Maui, Hawaii, USA. This volume is a result of the proceedings from the 'Symposium on Male Fertility and its Regulation' which was a part of the Reproductive Health Care Congress.

The organizers of this symposium recognized the need to focus male reproductive understanding on contraceptive development. The ultimate objective was and still is to produce a variety of safe and effective male contraceptives similar to that accomplished in the female. Speakers were invited to review the state of the art in several areas related to male contraception, reproductive toxicity and reproductive biology. The abstracts of these sessions were published as a special issue of *Archives of Andrology* (Vol. 9, No. 1, August, 1982). Subsequently, this volume was assembled from key papers presented at the Symposium. Additionally, invited manuscripts from leaders in specific areas were solicited to provide additional range to the topics covered.

In Section I, Non-hormonal Antifertility Agents, the three chapters cover three different topics. The first reviews the indazole class of antifertility agents. These compounds are attractive antispermatogenic agents and may be safe enough for clinical trials. The second chapter reviews the fertility problems associated with men who undergo chemotherapy for cancer. The third chapter covers 5-thio-D-glucose, another non-hormonal antispermatogenic agent. The indazole carboxylic acid, 5-thio-D-glucose α-chlorohydrin, chlorosugars and gossypol classes of compounds all involve interference with the energy production or metabolism machinery as the activity mechanism.

In the second section, Drug Effects on Male Fertility, we have a general review of therapeutic drug effects and a specific review of sulphasalazine-induced infertility. These are followed by two chapters reviewing the effects of illicit drugs and substances of abuse on the male reproductive system.

The third section, Gossypol, has seven chapters all discussing various aspects of this significant discovery. Although its reproductive activity in the male is a recent observation, it is a well known substance. We have tried to pull together here a wide variety of knowledge about gossypol so that its biology and chemistry can be put into perspective with its contraceptive effects.

The fourth section, Environmental Agents Affecting Fertility, examines several aspects of the increasing recognition that chemicals in the environment or workplace may produce reproductive hazards. The first review of this section covers the methods of identification of various reproductive hazards and gives examples. The second chapter covers the relatively unappreciated area of defects transmitted to progeny by paternal drug exposure. The third chapter compares and contrasts the various US governmental regulations regarding testing for reproductive toxicology and compares the US regulations with those of other countries. The section is concluded with two reviews of specific agents—phenoxy acid herbicides (including Agent Orange-type plant defoliants) and dibromochloropropane (nematocides toxic to farm workers).

Section five covers hormone and hormone antagonists. The first two papers cover the peptide hormone, LHRH, its analogues and other neuropeptides and explores their effects, side-effects and potential for practical utilization. The third chapter of the section reviews the biological activities of non-steroidal competitive binding inhibitors of androgen binding protein and the androgen receptors. This followed by a journal style report on the use of Danazol/testosterone enanthate in monkeys. Finally, there is a lengthy review of inhibin. With the recent successful purification and chemical synthesis of an inhibin, this subject will generate increasing interest.

Section six covers Blood-Testicular and Epididymal Barriers. The subject is reviewed by two scientists experienced in the science of testicular micropuncture. With these techniques they examine the stability, characteristics and biology of these important reproductive barriers.

Section seven covers several specific aspects of sperm physiology. The first chapter reviews mechanisms of sperm maturation and transport. The second chapter explores the effects of various ions on the initiation and quality of sperm motility. The third chapter examines the effects of antisperm antibodies on sperm fertility and function. The fourth chapter reviews the function of calcium ions and the calcium binding proteins, calsemin and calmodulin, on sperm calcium homeostasis. The last chapter of the section reviews the zona-free hamster egg penetration assay as a useful tool in diagnosing male or couple-related infertility.

From the foregoing it is apparent the various subjects were not reviewed comprehensively. Nevertheless, students of andrology will find much useful current information for research and teaching purposes. We trust that by focusing attention on these subjects they will provide a useful stimulus for enquiring minds and progress toward the much needed male contraceptive.

We wish to thank the authors for putting forth the labour of science necessary to complete this book. It is, in fact, their book and their work. We, as editors, only facilitated the organization and publication of this written symposium.

A large amount of work goes into assembling an edited volume and it is not possible to thank everyone who made a contribution suffice it to say we appreciate all the efforts.

Finally, we wish to thank Dr Marks of Upjohn for providing the pictures of deformed fetuses for the section divider for Environmental Agents Affecting Fertility. Dr Anita Hoffer, Department of Anatomy, Harvard Medical School, is thanked for providing photographs of a Sertoli–Sertoli cell tight junction and sperm from gossypol-treated rats for the Blood–Testis and Epididymal Barrier and Sperm Physiology section dividers. Their willingness to provide these pictures has dressed up this volume.

T.J. Lobl
E.S.E. Hafez
July, 1984

Section I
NON-HORMONAL
ANTIFERTILITY AGENTS

1
3-Indazole-carboxylic acids as male antifertility agents

B. SILVESTRINI, V. CIOLI, C. DE MARTINO and P. SCORZA BARCELLONA

Birth control is one of the most pressing problems of the present age, especially in the overpopulated countries, and has encouraged research on chemical agents having the capacity to inhibit the reproductive process. Fertility control is linked to the discovery of chemical agents with a selective inhibiting action on the seminiferous epithelium of man.

Although a variety of non-steroidal drugs with an antispermatogenic activity has been selected, all of them so far have proved to be unsatisfactory for widespread use. In fact, the ideal antispermatogenic agent would be one with a high selectivity on the seminiferous epithelium and no hormonal or systemic toxicity.

Numerous chemical compounds affecting testicular function have been discovered. These include different groups which have been classified according to their specific activity as (a) antispermatogenic agents; (b) substances inducing endocrine changes and (c) chemical agents preventing fertilization (Gomes, 1977). The most promising drugs are included in the first group, comprising many substances which affect the seminiferous epithelium cycle. Among these are the nitrofurans (Nelson and Steinberger, 1952, 1953), thiophenes (Steinberger *et al.*, 1956), dinitropyrroles (Patanelli and Nelson, 1964), bis-(dichloroacetyl)diamines (Drobeck and Coulston, 1962), gossypol (Abou-Donia, 1976), chlorinated sugars (Ford and Waites, 1978) and other chemicals, such as non-alkylating insect chemosterilants, cytostatics, pesticides and fungicides.

Of these different classes of antispermatogenic compounds, only the bis-diamines, gossypol and chlorinated sugars apparently have the characteristics for a potential 'male pill' because of their toxicological profile. The bis-diamines, have an antabuse-like effect, inhibiting alcohol dehydrogenase (Coulston *et al.*, 1975), whereas with gossypol and chlorinated sugars there is insufficient experimental evidence to exclude general toxicity in man.

The antispermatogenic activity of the 3-indazole carboxylic acids was recently discovered during routine pharmacological screening. The first derivative found to be active was 4-chlorobenzyl or AF 1312/TS (Fig. 1.1) (Burberi *et al.*, 1975; Coulston *et al.*, 1975; De Martino *et al.*, 1975;

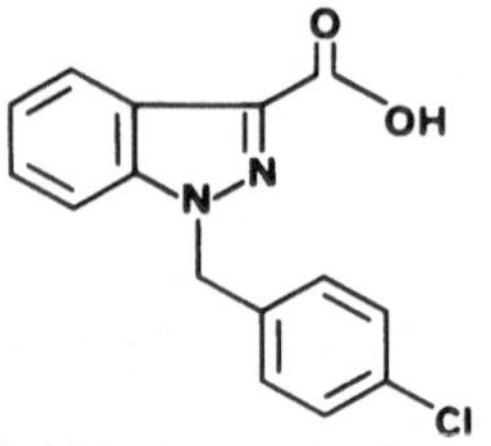

AF 1312/TS

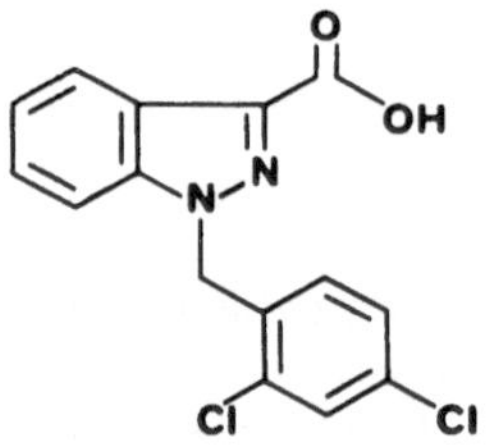

LONIDAMINE 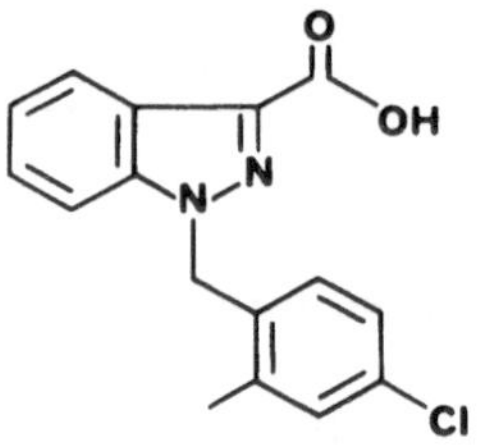   **TOLNIDAMINE**

Fig. 1.1 Structural formulae of AF 1312/TS, lonidamine and tolnidamine

Silvestrini *et al.*, 1975). Small chemical changes considerably increased the activity, without affecting general toxicity (Corsi *et al.*, 1976). Investigations were, therefore, focused on the most active derivatives, namely, 2,4-dichlorobenzyl or lonidamine and 4-chloro-2-methylbenzyl or tolnidamine (Fig. 1.1).

ANTISPERMATOGENIC ACTIVITY

To describe the antispermatogenic effects of these compounds, reference will be made mainly to the activity of lonidamine in the rat which is the

---

Fig. 1.2 (*opposite*) (a) Light microscopy. Rat testis 24 h after a single dose of lonidamine (50 mg/kg p.o.). The early lesions are visible in the Sertoli cells which are characterized by retraction of apical cytoplasmic projections (curved arrows), followed by exfoliation of normal and degenerated (asterisks) spermatids, development of vacuoles in the basal portion (arrow heads) and swelling of Sertoli-germ cell intercellular spaces (double arrow heads). The maturation phase spermatids, typical of this stage (stage III according to Leblond and Clermont), are not visible. (b) Electron microscopy. Rat testis 24 h after a single dose of lonidamine (50 mg/kg p.o.). Spermatids show severe morphological lesions, such as: remarkably dense cytoplasmic matrix, vacuolization of the nucleus (V), anomalies of the acrosomic complex (curved arrows) and numerous elongated mitochondria (asterisks). The apical retraction of Sertoli cells, which induces the sloughing of spermatids in the tubular lumen (TL), is characterized by swelling of the apical cytoplasmic projections (S). (c) Electron microscopy. Rat

4

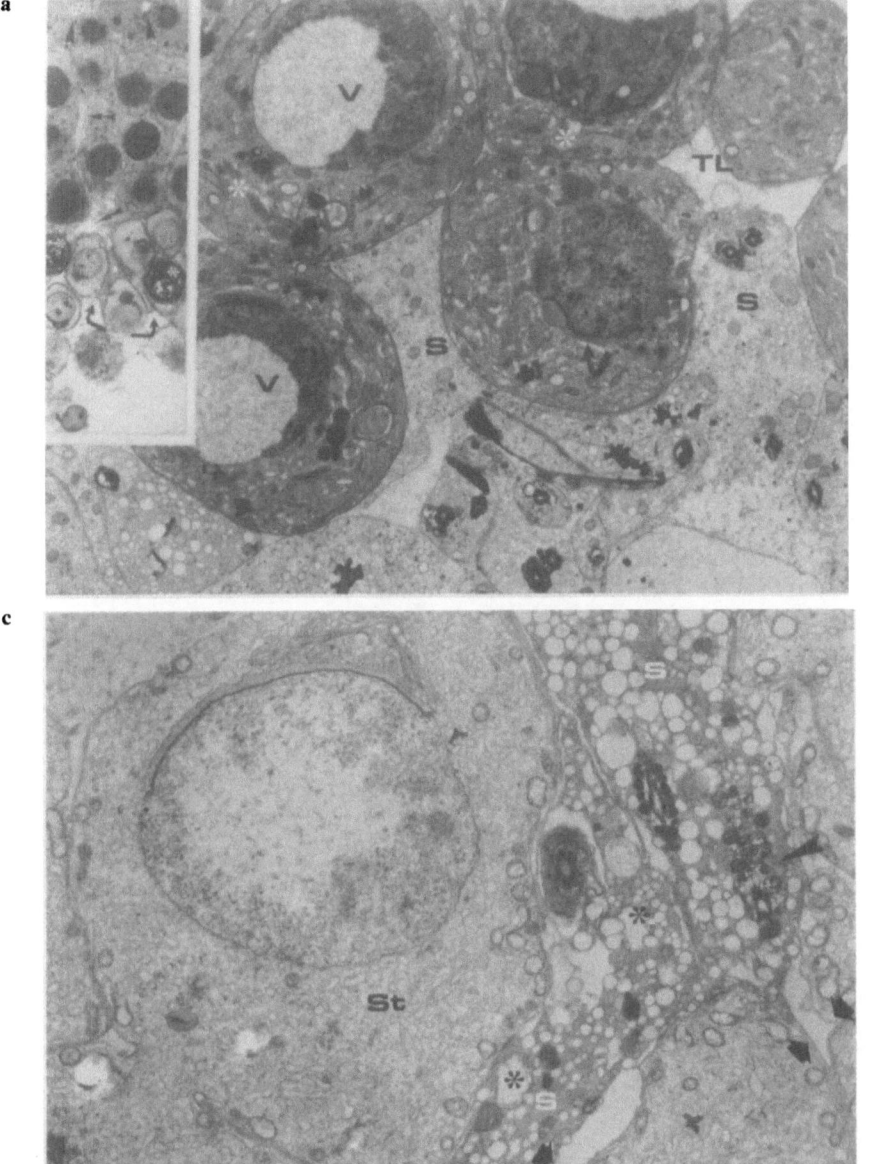

Fig. 1.2 (*continued*)
testis 24h after a single dose of lonidamine (50 mg/kg p.o.). In some tubules, the Sertoli cells (S) are severely damaged: the cytoplasmic matrix increases in electron density; the cisternae of the smooth endoplasmic reticulum are swollen; the mitochondria show rarefaction of the matrix and disruption of the cristae (asterisk), and the virtual intercellular Sertoli-germ cell spaces appear enlarged (arrows). Numerous spermatids in maturation are visible free in the Sertoli cell cytoplasm (arrow head). St: Golgi phase spermatid with chromatin rarefaction

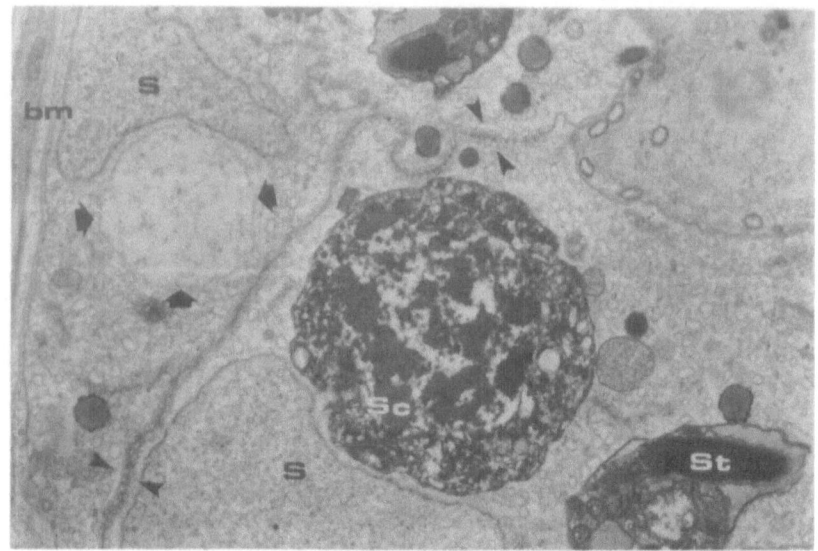

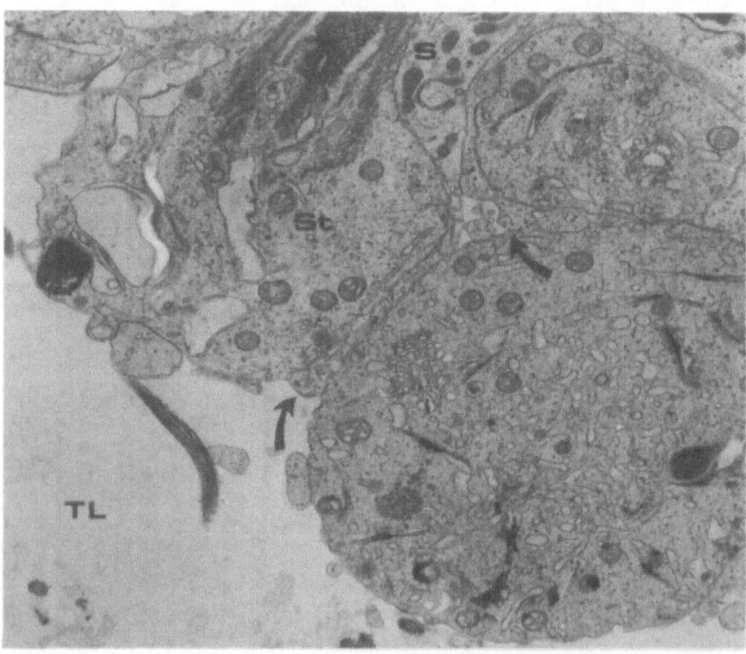

Fig. 1.3 (a) Electron microscopy. Rat testis 24h after a single dose of lonidamine (50mg/kg p.o.). Maturation spermatids (St), partially digested, are engulfed in large phagosomes of Sertoli cells. A spermatocyte (Sc) undergoing degeneration is visible. The basal portion of Sertoli cells (S) shows a large vacuole (arrows), whereas the Sertoli–Sertoli cell junctional complex appears normal (arrow heads). bm: basement membrane. (b) Electron microscopy. Beagle dog testis 24 h after 25 mg/kg/day p.o. of lonidamine for 9 weeks. The lesions consist mainly of apical retraction of Sertoli cell cytoplasm (arrows) with consequent exfoliation of apparently normal spermatids at various stages of maturation. S: Sertoli cells. St: spermatids at acrosomic phase. TL: tubular lumen

most sensitive and, up until now, certainly the best-studied species (Coulston et al., 1975; Silvestrini et al., 1978; Lobl, 1979; De Martino et al., 1981). After a single dose of 50 mg/kg p.o., the first alterations of the seminiferous tubules are observed within 12–24 hours. These changes reach a maximum after 5–10 days, after which there is a gradual recovery of the spermatogenic process. Early lesions are observed in the Sertoli cells which show retraction of the apical cytoplasm, basal vacuolation and swelling of Sertoli-germ cell intercellular spaces (Fig. 1.2a). These alterations cause germ cell exfoliation in the tubular lumen (Figs. 1.2a and b). The altered spermatids show the following changes: nuclear vacuolation, anomalies of the acrosomic complex, dense hyaloplasm, swelling and development of elongated mitochondria (Fig. 1.2b). Moreover, in some tubules the Sertolian lesions involving the smooth endoplasmic reticulum, mitochondria and cytoplasmic matrix are more severe (Fig. 1.2c). Several degenerating spermatocytes are also visible (Fig. 1.3a). Neither the Leydig cells nor the spermatogonia are affected, and the recovery of spermatogenesis is detectable after 15–20 days.

Along with the rat, the mouse, rabbit, dog and monkey were studied (Coulston et al., 1975; Lobl et al., 1979; De Martino et al., 1981; Heywood et al., 1981). Between species, not only quantitative differences exist, in terms of active doses, but also qualitative ones. In the dog, for example, after nine weeks of lonidamine treatment (25 mg/kg p.o.) the only morphological change in the seminiferous epithelium consists of the arrest of spermatogenesis at the latest phases of spermatid maturation (Fig. 1.3b). However, semen analysis shows marked oligospermia after two weeks of treatment. The above observations indicate that in the dog, lonidamine affects a very advanced phase of cell differentiation. Spermatogenesis fully recovers when treatment is discontinued (Heywood et al., 1981).

The antispermatogenic activity of lonidamine in humans appears similar to that observed in the dog. In a preliminary study (Somwini, 1981 personal communication), five healthy volunteers were treated with 150 mg of the drug three times daily for a week and then with 150 mg once a week for 12 weeks. Two weeks after the start of treatment, the ejaculate showed a mean reduction of 83% in the number of spermatozoa and a 45% decrease in their motility. These effects persisted, unaffected by a volumetric reduction of the testes, throughout the treatment period and disappeared within two weeks after treatment had ended.

ENDOCRINOLOGICAL PROFILE

As far as the sex hormonal levels are concerned, in the rat only FSH was increased as a result of lesions to the seminiferous epithelium, while LH and testosterone levels were not appreciably affected (Lobl et al., 1981). The dog and monkey showed no alterations (Heywood et al., 1981; Lobl et al., 1981).

TOXICOLOGICAL EFFECTS

Acute toxicity studies on the 3-indazole carboxylic acids in rats show a wide safety margin between lethal and antispermatogenic doses. Spermatogenesis is inhibited by a single oral administration of about 50–60 mg/kg of lonidamine or tolnidamine (Silvestrini, 1981), whereas the respective LD_{50} values are 1700 and 4000 mg/kg (Heywood et al., 1981). Repeated daily oral doses up to 800 mg/kg of the two compounds to male rats for 30 days strongly affect spermatogenesis and lower the weight of the accessory sex organs without altering their histological appearance with castration-like changes. An increase in pituitary weight can also be observed with the highest doses, presumably due to the feedback effects of blocked spermatogenesis (Heywood et al., 1981). The only severe toxic effect so far detected with lonidamine and tolnidamine is on the kidney. This effect appears species-specific as it is only found in monkeys; in fact, no changes are found in this organ in either rats or dogs nor are there any abnormalities in blood and urine parameters depending on renal function (Heywood et al., 1981). These interspecies differences may be accounted for by the high rate of renal excretion in the monkey, but not in the rat (Segre and Catanese, 1981). The renal excretion of lonidamine in man is similar to that in the rat (Silvestrini, 1981). As to the severity of renal function impairment, tolnidamine is better tolerated than lonidamine since oral doses of 70 mg/kg/day to monkeys for four weeks neither increase urea and creatinine blood levels nor alter renal histology (Heywood et al., 1981).

BIOCHEMICAL TARGET

Physiopharmacological, ultrastructural and biochemical observations would suggest that lonidamine affects the energy metabolism of germ and tumour cells. In both types of cells the drug decreases oxygen consumption. However, in germ cells, lonidamine increases aerobic lactate production, whereas in the tumour cells both aerobic and anaerobic glycolysis are strongly inhibited (Floridi et al., 1981a, b, and 1982). Lonidamine also possesses embryotoxic and antitumour effects which have a close quantitative correlation with the antispermatogenic activity (Scorza Barcellona et al., 1982; Silvestrini, 1981; Silvestrini et al., 1983). This suggests that all these effects may depend on a single mechanism of action. The antispermatogenic action of lonidamine is presumably linked to the structural and functional modification of the 'energy metabolism' of germ cells undergoing maturation. During the differentiation process the germ cell mitochondria undergo a characteristic transformation from the 'orthodox' to the 'condensed' form having a high oxidative capacity coupled with a marked ATP production (De Martino et al., 1979). The condensed appearance of germ cell mitochondria is, therefore, the manifestation of a particular functional state. The condensed mitochondrion is one of the main cell targets for lonidamine (Floridi et al., 1981b, 1982). Following lonidamine treatment or in vitro incubation of isolated germ cells with the drug, a marked reduction of oxygen consumption and an increase of aerobic glycolysis is observed (Floridi *et al.*, 1981b).

AF 1312/TS and lonidamine also induce morphological modifications and functional impairment of the Sertoli cells, besides lesions to the germ cells as demonstrated by the *in vitro* experiments (Marcante *et al.*, 1981). In rat Sertoli cells incubated *in vitro* with AF 1312/TS or lonidamine, oestradiol production was drastically decreased and swelling of the endoplasmic reticulum was observed. These morphological and functional modifications are reversible (Marcante *et al.*, 1981) and are not related to a functional impairment of energy metabolism of the Sertoli cells, since both the oxygen consumption and lactate production of these cells are unaffected by *in vitro* treatment (Floridi *et al.*, 1983). The functional and transitory impairment of Sertoli cells was also demonstrated by *in vivo* inhibition of androgen-binding protein production (Lobl *et al.*, 1981).

In agreement with these data, the 3-indazole carboxylic acids seem to have two cell targets in the seminiferous epithelium: Sertoli cells and germ cells in maturation. The biochemical target in the Sertoli cells, however, remains unclear. Experiments are in progress to elucidate the biochemical mechanisms involved in the temporary and reversible lesions of these cells.

CONCLUDING REMARKS

The 3-indazole carboxylic acids appear promising candidates for a 'male pill' because of the remarkable specificity of their antispermatogenic activity which is exerted at much lower doses than the toxic one. Moreover, in this chemical class there is no correlation between antispermatogenic effects and general toxicity which are two independent variables (Corsi *et al.*, 1976; Heywood *et al.*, 1981).

Acknowledgment

Supported in part by grants from CNR (Consiglio Nazionale delle Ricerche) 'Progetto Finalizzato: Biologia della Riproduzione'.

References

Abou-Donia, M.G. (1976). Physiological effects and metabolism of gossypol. *Residue Rev.*, **61**, 125–60

Burberi, S., Catanese, B., Cioli, V., Scorza Barcellona, P. and Silvestrini, B. (1975). Antispermatogenic activity of 1-*p*-chlorobenzyl-1H-indazole-3-carboxylic acid, AF 1312/TS, in rats. II. A study of treatments of duration between 5 and 180 days. *Exp. Mol. Pathol.*, **23**, 308–20

Corsi, G., Palazzo, G., Germani, C., Scorza Barcellona, P. and Silvestrini, B. (1976). 1-Halobenzyl-1H-indazole-3-carboxylic acids. A new class of antispermatogenic agents. *J. Med. Chem.*, **19**, 778–83

Coulston, F., Dougherty, W.J., LeFevre, R., Abraham, R. and Silvestrini, B. (1975). Reversible inhibition of spermatogenesis in rats and monkeys with a new class of indazole carboxylic acids. *Exp. Mol. Pathol.*, **23**, 357–66

De Martino, C., Floridi, A., Marcante, M.L., Malorni, W., Scorza Barcellona, P., Bellocci,

M. and Silvestrini, B. (1979). Morphological, histochemical and biochemical studies on germ cell mitochondria of normal rats. *Cell Tissue Res.*, **196**, 1-22

De Martino, C., Malorni, W., Bellocci, M., Floridi, A. and Marcante, M.L. (1981). Effects of AF 1312/TS and lonidamine on mammalian testis. A morphological study. *Chemotherapy*, **27** (Suppl. 2), 27-42

De Martino, C., Stefanini, M., Agrestini, A., Cocchia, D., Morelli, M. and Scorza Barcellona, P. (1975). Antispermatogenic activity of 1-*p*-chlororobenzyl-1H-indazole-3-carboxylic acid, AF 1312/TS, in rats. III. A light and electron microscopic study after single oral doses. *Exp. Mol. Pathol.*, **23**, 321-56

Drobeck, H.P. and Coulston, F. (1962). Inhibition and recovery of spermatogenesis in rats, monkeys and dogs medicated with bis-(dichloroacetyl)diamines. *Exp. Mol. Pathol.*, **1**, 251-74

Floridi, A., Bellocci, M., Paggi, M.G., Marcante, M.L. and De Martino, C. (1981a). Changes of energy metabolism in the germ cells and Ehrlich ascites tumor cells. *Chemotherapy*, **27** (Supp. 2), 50-60

Floridi, A., D'Atri, S., Paggi, M.G., Marcante, M.L., De Martino, C., Silvestrini, B., Caputo, A. and Lehninger, A. (1982). Binding of lonidamine to Ehrlich ascites tumor and liver mitochondria. In Galeotti, T., Cittadini, A., Neri, G. and Papa, S. (eds.) *Membranes in Tumor Growth* pp. 559-565. (Amsterdam, New York, Oxford: Elsevier Biomedical)

Floridi, A., De Martino, C., Marcante, M.L., Apollonj, C., Scorza Barcellona, P. and Silvestrini, B. (1981b). Morphological and biochemical modifications of rat germ cell mitochondria induced by new antispermatogenic compounds. Studies 'in vivo' and 'in vitro'. *Exp. Mol. Pathol.*, **35**, 314-31

Floridi, A., Marcante, M.L., D'Atri, S., Feriozzi, R., Menichini, R., Citro, G., Cioli, V. and De Martino, C. (1983). Energy metabolism of normal and lonidamine-treated Sertoli cells of rats. *Exp. Mol. Pathol.*, **38**, 137-47

Ford, W.C.L. and Waites, G.M.H. (1978). A reversible contraceptive action of some 6-chloro-6-deoxy sugars in the male rat. *J. Reprod. Fert.*, **52**, 153-7

Gomes, W.R. (1977). Pharmacological agents and male fertility. In Johnson, A.D. and Gomes, W.R. (eds.) *The Testis*, Vol. 4. pp. 605-628 (New York, San Francisco, London: Academic Press)

Heywood, R., James, R.W., Scorza Barcellona, P., Campana, A. and Cioli, V. (1981). Toxicological studies on 1-substituted-indazole-3-carboxylic acids. *Chemotherapy* **27** (Suppl. 2), 91-7

Lobl, T.J. (1979). 1-(2,4-dichlorobenzyl)-1H-indazole-3-carboxylic acid (DICA), an exfoliative antispermatogenic agent in the rat. *Arch. Androl.*, **2**, 353-63

Lobl, T.J., Bardin, C.W., Gunsalus, G.L. and Musto, N.A. (1981). Effects of lonidamine (AF 1890) and its analogues on follicle-stimulating hormone, luteinizing hormone, testosterone and rat androgen binding protein concentrations in the rat and Rhesus monkey. *Chemotherapy*, **27**, (Supp. 2), 61-76

Lobl, T.J., Forbes, A.D., Kirton, K.T. and Wilks, J.W. (1979). Characterization of the exfoliative antispermatogenic agent (1-(2,4-dichlorobenzyl-1H-indazole-3-carboxylic acid in the Rhesus monkey. *Arch. Androl.*, **3**, 67-77

Marcante, M.L., Natali, P.G., Floridi, A. and De Martino, C. (1981). Effects of AF 1312/TS and lonidamine on cultured Sertoli cells. *Chemotherapy*, **27** (Suppl. 2), 43-9

Nelson, W.O. and Steinberger, E. (1952). Effect of furadoxyl upon the testes of the rat. *Anat. Rec.*, **112**, 367-8

Nelson, W.O. and Steinberger, E. (1953). Effects of nitrofuran compounds on the testis of the rat. *Fed. Proc.*, **12**, 103-4

Patanelli, D.J. and Nelson, W.O. (1964). A quantitative study of inhibition and recovery of spermatogenesis. *Recent Progr. Horm. Res.*, **20**, 491-543

Scorza Barcellona, P., Campana, A., Silvestrini, B. and De Martino, C. (1982). The embryotoxicity of a new class of antispermatogenic agents, the indazole-1H-carboxylic acids. *Arch. Toxicol.* (Suppl. 5), 197-201

Segre, G. and Catanese, B. (1981). Pharmacokinetics of lonidamine. *Chemotherapy*, **27** (Suppl. 2), 77-84

Silvestrini, B. (1981). Basic and applied research in the study of indazole-carboxylic acids. *Chemotherapy*, **27** (Suppl. 2), 9-20

Silvestrini, B., Burberi, S., Cioli, V., Coulston, F., Lisciani, R. and Scorza Barcellona, P. (1975). Antispermatogenic activity of 1-*p*-chlorobenzyl-1H-indazole-3-carboxylic acid, AF 1312/TS, in rats. I. Trials of single and short-term administrations with study of pharmacological and toxicological effects. *Exp. Mol. Pathol.*, **23,** 288-307

Silvestrini, B., De Martino, C., Cioli, V., Campana, A., Malorni, W. and Scorza Barcellona, P. (1978). Antispermatogenic activity of diclondazolic acid in rats. In Fabbrini, A. and Steinberger, E. (eds.) pp. 453-7, *Recent Progress in Andrology.* Vol. 14. (New York: Academic Press)

Silvestrini, B., Hahn, G.M., Cioli, V. and De Martino, C. (1983). Effects of lonidamine, alone or combined with hyperthermia, in some experimental cell and tumor systems. *Br. J. Cancer*, **47,** 221-31

Steinberger, E., Nelson, W.O. and Boccabella, A. (1956). Cytotoxic effects of 5-chloro-2-acetyl thiophen (Ba 11044 Ciba) on testis of the rat. *Anat. Rec.*, **125,** 312

2
Chemotherapeutic agents and male reproduction

P.K. BAJPAI and K.J. ANDERSON

The principal strategy of chemotherapeutic cancer management is to inflict maximal damage to cancerous tissue while causing minimal damage to normal host tissue. Selectivity of anti-cancer drugs is due to their ability to potently inhibit cellular replication. Since cancer cells proliferate more rapidly than host cells, the deleterious effects of chemotherapeutic agents is most profound on cancer cells. However, rapidly dividing host cell systems are also selectively damaged by anti-cancer drugs. The testes are the site of constantly proliferating germinal epithelium. They are damaged by a variety of chemotherapeutic agents (Table 2.1).

Table 2.1 Chemotherapeutic agents which elicit male reproductive damage

Groups	Compounds
Alkylating agents	Busulphan
	Chlorambucil
	Cyclophosphamide
	Nitrogen mustard
Vinca alkyloids	Vincristine
	Vinblastine
Antimetabolites	Methotrexate
	Cystosine arabinoside
	Hydroxyurea
Methyl hydrazines	Procarbazine
Antibiotics	Adriamycin
	Bleomycin

Cytotoxic drugs have been used for 30 years in the management of cancer and other types of diseases. The development of new chemotherapeutic agents and improved treatment modalities has resulted in greatly improved survival rates for cancer victims. Of the approximately 100 different forms of cancer, eleven are now considered curable. These include childhood acute leukemia, Hodgkin's disease, histocytic lymphoma, skin cancer, testicular

13

carcinoma, rhabdomyosarcoma, Ewing sarcoma, retinoblastoma and cho-riocarcinoma. Successful recovery also occurs in many other cancer types (Barber, 1981).

The importance of testicular damage as a function of chemotherapy has been minimized in the past. This may have been due to the non-vital nature of the reproductive system as well as the small population of reproductive age cancer survivors (Schilsky *et al.*, 1980). As the number of long-term cancer survivors increases, reproductive considerations will grow in importance.

The effects of various anti-cancer drugs on the male reproductive system are reviewed here. The discussion includes factors such as clinical fertility, tissue damage, endocrine status and recovery from treatment in both pubertal and prepubertal human and animal subjects.

ALKYLATING AGENTS

Alkylating agents are probably the most commonly used chemotherapeutic drugs (Barber, 1981). As a class, these agents react with amino groups in nucleic acids and other nucleophilic centres in the cell. Cell death is brought about by inhibition of DNA, RNA and protein synthesis (Schwartz and Kanter, 1975). Agents in this class include busulphan, cyclophosphamide, chlorambucil and nitrogen mustard. Since a large proportion of cells in the germinal epithelium of the testes is constantly undergoing cell division, the testes are highly vulnerable to chemotherapeutic agents (Cooke *et al.*, 1978). Azoospermia, germ cell depletion and testicular abnormalities have been reported in men receiving alkylating agents as a part of their chemotherapeutic regimen (Wierzba *et al.*, 1982).

Busulphan

Bulsulphan administration in male rats elicits a progressive depletion of the germinal epithelium. Associated with this tissue damage are elevated levels of luteinizing hormone (LH) and follicle stimulating hormone (FSH) in the pituitary and serum and decreased testes weight. The increased gonadotrophin levels are correlated with decreases in spermatocyte and young spermatid cell counts (Debuljek *et al.*, 1973).

Testicular atrophy (morphological damage to spermatogonia), elevated LH and FSH, and lowered testosterone levels have been observed in men undergoing busulphan therapy for a variety of cancers (Smalley and Wall, 1966; Schoerer *et al.*, 1978). The decrease in testosterone levels suggests that Leydig cells may also be damaged in these patients.

Chlorambucil

Chlorambucil, a nitrogen mustard derivative, elicits a dose-dependent lesion of the germinal epithelium in males treated for malignant lymphoma

(Richter *et al.*, 1970). A dosage of more than 400 mg of chlorambucil causes total depletion of germ cells. Chlorambucil does not have any microscopically apparent effect on Sertoli cells, Leydig cells, or vascular components in the testes. Recovery from an azoospermic state in chlorambucil-treated males is unlikely.

Cyclophosphamide

Cyclophosphamide is a nitrogen mustard derivative used for the control of malignant conditions as well as for the treatment of nephrotic syndrome. Cyclophosphamide crosses the blood–testis barrier in rats (Forrest *et al.*, 1981). In adult patients, the administration of cyclophosphamide results in severe oligospermia or azoospermia. The testes of cyclophosphamide-treated men show seminiferous tubules which contain only Sertoli cells and occasional spermatogonia. Associated with testicular damage are elevated levels of serum FSH with normal serum LH and testosterone levels (Fukutani *et al.*, 1981).

Cyclophosphamide-induced damage to the testes appears to be dose related and prolonged treatment with larger total doses is associated with a higher incidence of spermatogenic inhibition. Shorter duration of treatment with a moderate dose/day regimen can minimize the toxic effects of cyclophosphamide on the germinal epithelium (Hsu *et al.*, 1979).

Cessation of cyclophosphamide therapy does not promote the immediate reversal of these conditions (Rapola *et al.*, 1973). However, reinitiation of spermatogenesis does occur in some men within 15 to 45 months after cyclophosphamide treatment (Buchanan *et al.*, 1975). Cyclophosphamide also restored fertility in a patient who was initially azoospermic (Blake *et al.*, 1976). Caution must be exercised since offspring of cyclophosphamide-treated male and female rats do not develop normally (Adam *et al.*, 1980). Decrease in fertility of cyclphosphamide-treated patients is also associated with decreased acrosomal proteolytic activity of spermatozoa (Ginsberg *et al.*, 1981).

Prepubertal administration of cyclophosphamide may or may not preclude normal reproductive development in treated individuals. Boys, who receive cyclophosphamide before puberty, in general have normal serum FSH, LH and testosterone levels when evaluated prior to puberty (Parra *et al.*, 1978) despite damage to seminiferous elements (Trompter *et al.*, 1981). Whereas some cyclophosphamide-treated boys proceed normally into puberty (Arneil, 1972), spermatic dysfunction occurs in many post-pubertal males treated with cyclophosphamide as children (Lentz *et al.*, 1977). Elevated serum FSH levels correlate with the degree of testicular degeneration (Etteldorf *et al.*, 1976). The increase in serum FSH due to damage to the germinal epithelium increases cell division and exposes the germ cells to further destruction by the chemotherapeutic agents (Glode *et al.*, 1981). Elevated serum LH levels associated with normal levels of serum testosterone have also been observed in cyclophosphamide-treated boys (Etteldorf *et al.*, 1976; Lentz *et al.*, 1977). Thus, compensated failure of Leydig cells in association with depletion of germ cells should be expected in cyclophosphamide-treated boys.

ADRIAMYCIN

Adriamycin is a potent anti-cancer antibiotic which is effective against a wide variety of neoplastic diseases (Carter, 1975). It interrupts DNA replication, transcription and translocation processes by binding to and

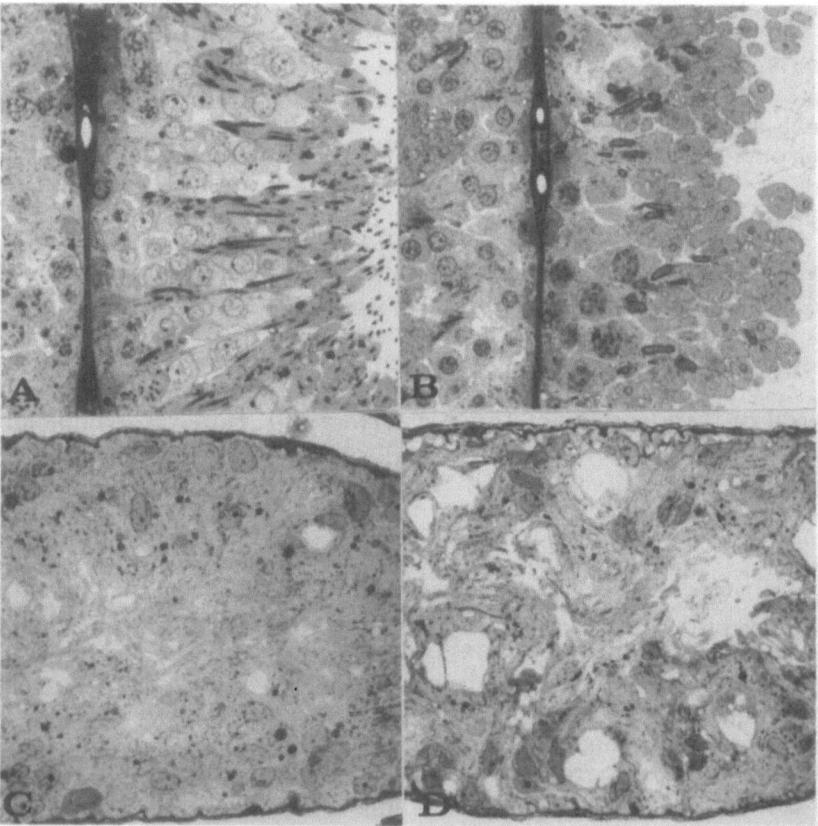

Fig. 2.1 Photomicrographs of testis of adult male rats injected intraperitoneally with physiological saline or adriamycin (3.3 mg/kg body weight weekly). A. Physiological saline for four weeks showing normal basement membrane of seminiferous tubule and spermatogenesis. B. Adriamycin for 4 weeks showing normal tubular basement membrane, Sertoli cells and reduced number of spermatogonia and spermatids. C. Adriamycin for 8 weeks showing reduction in size of seminiferous tubule, irregular tubular basement membrane, vacuolar formation, adherence of spermatogenic cell remnants and questionable spermatogonia and primary spermatocytes. D. Adriamycin for 12 weeks showing collapse of seminiferous tubule, irregular tubular basement membrane with adhering remnants of cells, numerous vacuolar formations, scattered nuclei of degenerated Sertoli cells and cessation of spermatogenesis (× 103)

interfering with the template function of DNA (Schmid and Zbinden, 1979). Adriamycin also exerts toxic effects at the membrane level (Tritton *et al.*, 1983).

Adriamycin is capable of reaching the seminiferous tubule epithelium (Schmid and Zbinden, 1979) and induces severe cellular damage within the seminiferous tubule of the adult male rat (Anderson, 1981). The germinal epithelium progressively deteriorates in proportion to duration of treatment and eventually culminates in total obliteration of germinal cells (Fig. 2.1). Decreased testis weights in adriamycin-treated animals are a reflection of this loss of germinal elements. Sertoli cells are dislocated and abnormal in appearance following long-term treatment of rats with adriamycin (Fig. 2.1D). Adriamycin does not induce detectable damage to Leydig cells, but does retard the growth of seminal vesicles despite adequate amounts of

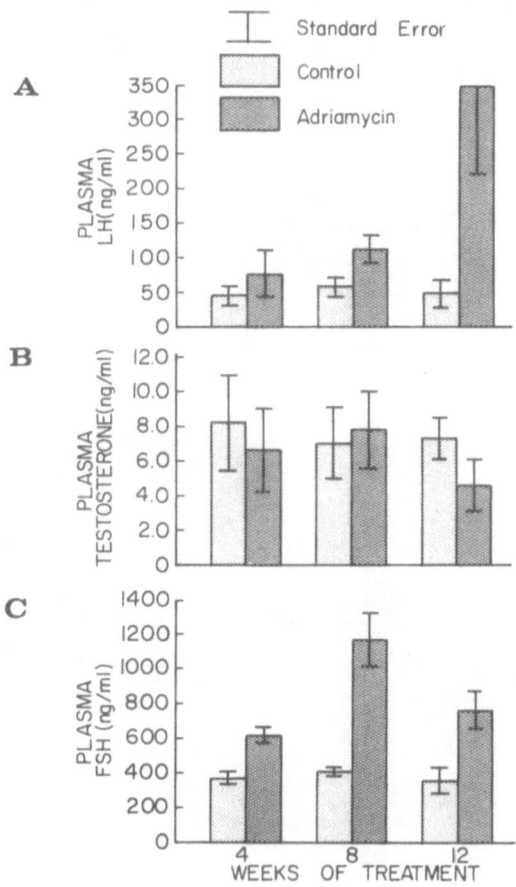

Fig. 2.2 Effect of intraperitoneal injections of physiological saline or adriamycin (3.3 mg/kg body weight weekly) for 12 weeks in adult male rats on the serum levels of: A, luteinizing hormone; B, testosterone; C, follicle stimulating hormone. (Reproduced from Anderson, 1981.)

circulating testosterone. Levels of serum FSH and LH are elevated in adriamycin-treated rats in conjunction with the extent of germinal epithelial injury (Fig. 2.2A, B). Serum testosterone levels are reduced, but not significantly, by long-term adriamycin administration (Fig. 2.2). Ultrastructural examination of adriamycin-treated rat testes indicate that adriamycin causes extensive damage to the basement membrane of the seminiferous tubules (Fig. 2.3) and nuclear components of the Sertoli and germ cells (Bonanni *et al.*, 1983).

In the prepubertal rat, adriamycin significantly depresses spermatogonial cell counts and elevated serum levels of FSH are correlated with seminiferous tubule damage (Fig. 2.4). Levels of LH, prolactin and testosterone in

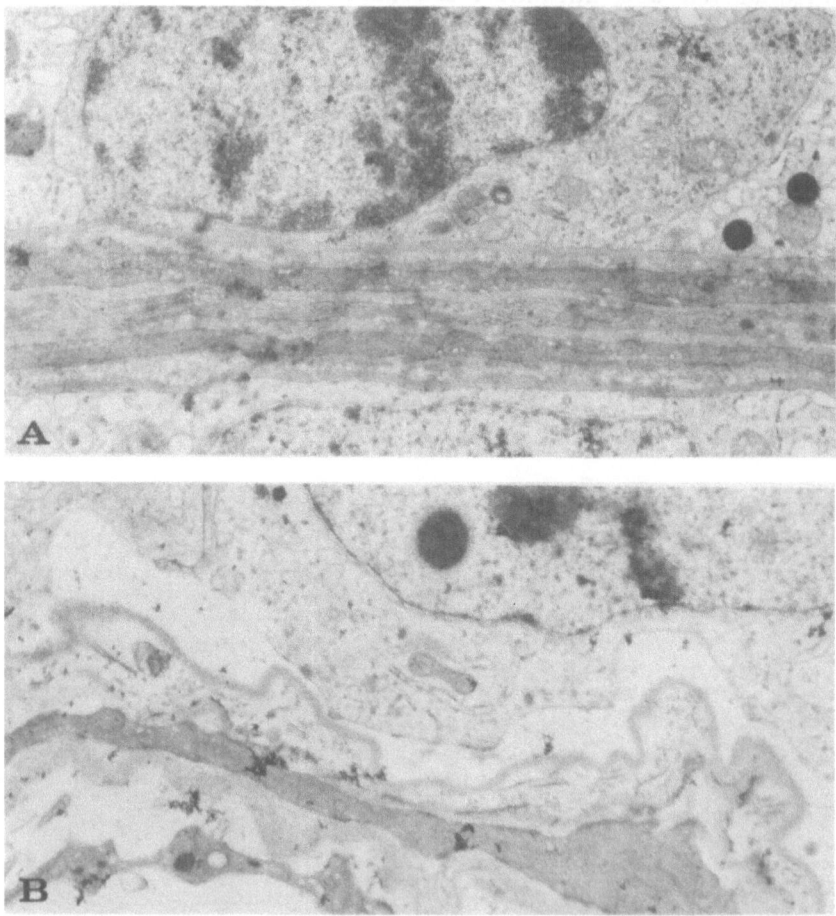

Fig. 2.3 Photomicrographs of the ultrastructure of basement membrane of seminiferous tubule of adult male rats injected intraperitoneally for 12 weeks with: (A) physiological saline showing normal tubular membrane; (B) adriamycin (3.3 mg/kg body weight weekly) showing papillary projections towards the lumen of the tubule and the infolding of the irregular tubular membrane (× 2990)

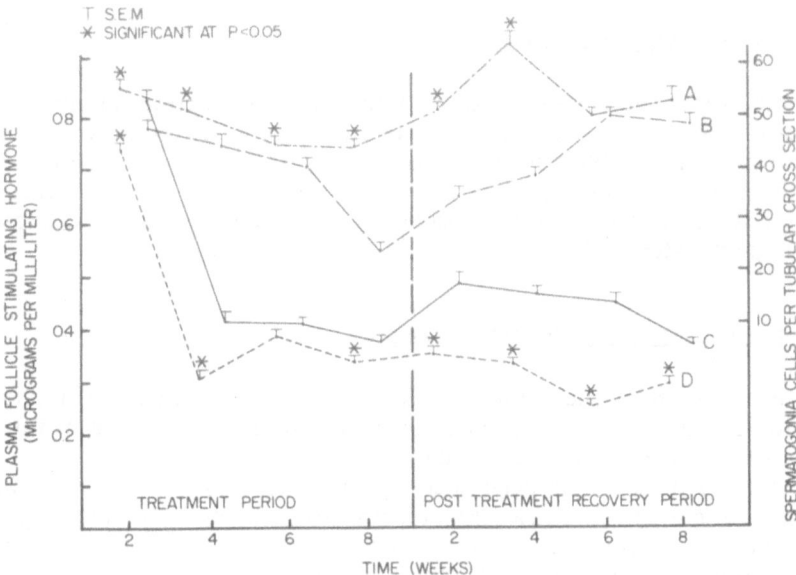

Fig. 2.4 The effect of physiological saline or adriamycin (1.0 mg/kg body weight per week) for eight weeks on circulating levels of follicle stimulating hormone (FSH) and spermatogonial cell count in prepubertal male rats. (A) Spermatogonial cell count in saline-inhected rats. (B) Spermatogonial cell count in adriamycin-treated rats. (C) Serum FSH in adriamycin-treated rats. (D) Serum FSH in saline-injected rats (Reproduced from Giffin, 1981)

the serum are not significantly altered by adriamycin treatment. Adriamycin induces decreased testis and seminal vesicle weights in prepubertal rats but does not affect ventral prostate weights (Giffin, 1981). However, short-term (3 days) treatment with large doses of adriamycin (2–11 mg/kg body weight) can inhibit testosterone-induced growth of the ventral prostate (Sloan *et al.*, 1975).

A wide range of cell types in the germinal epithelium are susceptible to the cytotoxic action of adriamycin. These include primary and secondary spermatocytes (Parvinen and Parvinen, 1978), differentiated spermatogonia and, notably, germinal stem cells (Lu and Meistrich, 1979).

Although adriamycin does disrupt reproductive physiology in the prepubertal male, recovery and progression to a normal pubertal state can occur (Giffin, 1981). Two patients receiving high doses of adriamycin as a part of a combination chemotherapy regimen were reported to be fertile. One of these two patients also fathered two children while he was undergoing chemotherapy (Da Cunha *et al.*, 1979). There was no impairment of fertilizing ability of adriamycin-treated rats after 14 weeks of recovery. However, these rats sired a smaller number of pups. Fetuses fathered by adriamycin-treated rats were also aborted spontaneously (Whitely *et al.*, 1981).

OTHER INDIVIDUAL AGENTS

Potential reproductive injury due to the cytotoxic action of many anti-cancer drugs has not been fully investigated. However, the following drugs are considered possible risks to the male reproductive system: methotrexate (Shamberger *et al.*, 1981), procarbazine (Ettlin *et al.*, 1982), vincristine, vinblastine (Cooke *et al.*, 1978), cytosine arabinoside, bleomycin and hydroxy-urea (Lu and Meistrich, 1979).

COMBINATION CHEMOTHERAPY

The use of a single chemotherapeutic agent in the treatment of malignant conditions has, for the most part, given way to administration of multiple cytotoxic agents in various combinations.

Hodgkin's disease has been successfully treated by a cyclic schedule of an alkylating agent, a vinca alkyloid, procarbazine and the steroid predni-sone. Severe reproductive damage occurs as a result of this regimen (Asbjornsen *et al.*, 1976). Adult males exhibit azoospermia or oligospermia following six cycles of treatment. Serum levels of FSH and LH as well as the FSH and LH responses to luteinizing hormone releasing hormone (LHRH) injections are elevated in these subjects. In addition, serum testo-sterone levels are below those of age-matched controls indicating damage to Leydig cells as well as to seminiferous tubule elements (Whitehead *et al.*, 1982). Severe germinal aplasia associated with increased serum FSH and LH levels and reduced serum testosterone levels is a consequence of the above therapy in adolescent boys. Gynaecomastia in the presence of normal serum prolactin and oestradiol levels in boys may be a manifestation of Leydig cell dysfunction (Sherins *et al.*, 1978).

Recovery from male reproductive damage induced by this combination therapy for Hodgkin's disease is doubtful at this time. Azoospermia or severe oligospermia and elevated serum gonadotrophin levels persist in the majority of men six to nine years after the end of the treatment regimen (Waxman *et al.*, 1982). Return of reproductive potential appears to be much greater when procarbazine is not included in the chemotherapy regimen (Roesser *et al.*, 1978).

The use of some combination therapies which do not include alkylating agents also produce seminiferous injury in adults. This appears to be re-lated to duration of therapy rather than to total dosage or particular agents used (Maguire *et al.*, 1981). Treatment of leukemia in boys with a combi-nation of methotrexate, vincristine, 6-mercaptopurine and prednisone allows normal reproductive development five years following the treatment (Blatt *et al.*, 1981). Boys treated with combination therapy regimen for acute lymphoblastic leukemia exhibit a normal testosterone response to human chorionic gonadotrophin (HCG) stimulation (Shalet *et al.*, 1981).

Azoospermia (Waxman *et al.*, 1982), interstitial fibrosis, thickening of the seminiferous tubule basement membrane and a decrease in the tubular fertility index occurs as a result of combination chemotherapy including adriamycin (Lendon *et al.*, 1978).

PHYSIOLOGICAL SIGNIFICANCE OF REPRODUCTIVE DAMAGE INDUCED BY CYTOTOXIC ANTICANCER AGENT

Injury to testicular germinal epithelium induced by chemotherapeutic agents conclusively correlates with elevated levels of serum FSH in adults. These levels are high despite adequate levels of circulating testosterone. Thus, it appears that a factor of seminiferous tubule origin which acts to inhibit FSH release is absent in males treated with anti-cancer drugs. This information supports the existence of an inhibin, a hormone of Sertoli cell (Chowdhury *et al.*, 1978) or germinal cell (Hopkinson *et al.*, 1978) origin.

The normal regulatory relationship between serum LH and testosterone is altered by chemotherapy in adults, as increased LH levels should stimulate testosterone production. In some treated adult males, especially following cyclical combination chemotherapy, serum LH levels are distinctly elevated despite normal or slightly depressed serum testosterone levels. The lack of LH stimulated testosterone production may be due to desensitization of Leydig cells by chronically elevated serum LH levels (Hseuh *et al.*, 1976). It appears that chemotherapeutic agents induce a state of compensated Leydig cell failure in these patients. Relative decreases in testosterone production by Leydig cells in this compensated state may be responsible for the gynaecomastia observed in some males undergoing chemotherapy (Friedman and Plymate, 1980).

CONCLUDING REMARKS

Anti-cancer chemotherapeutics have profound adverse effects on male reproduction. In general cytotoxic agents (1) cause severe damage to germinal elements within the seminiferous tubules which results in oligospermia or azoospermia; (2) increase serum FSH levels secondary to germinal cell destruction; (c) increase serum LH levels; (d) induce Leydig cell dysfunction and subsequent reductions in serum testosterone.

As the population of cancer survivors increases, longer recovery periods will be available for observation. Reversibility of chemotherapy-induced infertility in man is doubtful at this time. The proper reproductive management of male chemotherapy recipients should probably include collection of sperm prior to initiation of chemical treatment regimens. Thus, a normal family life is possible via artificial insemination should the patient become azoospermic. A new approach to consider for protection of reproductive potential could be the reversion of the testis to a prepubertal state prior to initiation of anti-cancer drug therapy (Glode *et al.*, 1981). More study is needed to provide important clinical information as well as clues to the regulation of reproduction in the male.

Acknowledgments

We thank the Department of Biology and Research Council of the University of Dayton, Dayton, Ohio, USA, Dr. R. Amster for interpreting photomicrographs of tissue sections, B.F. Giffin, J.C. Lee, G.A. Bonanni and Margaret McGuire for technical assistance and Ann Feldmann for typing the manuscript.

References

Adams, P.M., Fabricant, J.D. and Legator, M.S. (1980). Cyclophosphamide-induced spermatogenic effect detected in F_1 generation by behavior testing. *Science*, **211**, 80-2

Anderson, K.J. (1981). The effect of adriamycin on the repoductive system of the male rat. *MSc Thesis*, University of Dayton, Dayton, Ohio, USA. pp. 38-45

Arneil, G.C. (1972). Cyclophosphamide and the prepubertal testis. *Lancet*, **2**, 1259-60

Asbjornsen, G., Molne, K., Klepp, O. and Aakvag, A. (1976). Testicular function after combination chemotherapy for Hodgkin's disease. *Scand. J. Haematol.*, **16**, 66-9

Barber, H.R.K. (1981). The effect of cancer and its therapy upon fertility. *Int. J. Fertil.*, **26**, 250-9.

Blake, D.A., Heller, R.H., Hsu, S.H. and Schacter, B.Z. (1976). Return of fertility in a patient with cyclophosphamide-induced azoospermia. *Johns Hopkins Med. J.*, **139**, 20-2

Blatt, J., Poplack, D.G. and Sherins, R.J. (1981). Testicular function in boys after chemotherapy for acute lymphoblastic leukemia. *N. Engl. J. Med.*, **304**, 1121-4

Bonanni, G.A., Lee, J.C. and Bajpai, P.K. (1983). Effect of adriamycin on the morphology of the testis of adult rats. *Ohio J. Sci.*, **83**, 101

Buchanan, J.D., Fairley, K.F. and Barrie, J.U. (1975). Return of spermatogenesis after stopping cyclophosphamide therapy. Lancet, **2**, 156-7

Carter, S.K. (1975). Adriamycin—A Review. *J. Natl. Cancer Inst.*, **55**, 1265-74

Chowdhury, M., Steinberger, A. and Steinberger, E. (1978). Inhibition of *de novo* synthesis of FSH by the Sertoli cell factor. *Endocrinol.*, **103**, 644-7

Cooke, R.A., Nikles, A. and Roeser, H.P. (1978). A comparison of the anti-fertility effects of alkylating agents and vinca alkaloids in male rats. *Br. J. Pharmacol.*, **63**, 677-81

Da Cunha, M.F., Meistrich, M.L., Reid, H.L. and Powell, M.L. (1979). Effect of chemotherapy on human sperm production. *Am. Assoc. Cancer Res.*, **20**, 100

Debujlek, L., Arimura, A. and Schally, A.V. (1973). Pituitary and serum FSH and LH levels after massive and selective depletion of the germinal epithelium in the rat restis. *Endocrinology*, **92**, 48-54

Etteldorf, J.N., West, C.D., Pitcock, J.A. and Williams, D.L. (1976). Gonadal function, testicular histology, and meiosis following cyclophosphamide therapy in patients with nephrotic syndrome. *J. Pediatr.*, **88**, 206-12

Ettlin, R.A., Bechter, R. and Dixon, R.L. (1982). Assessment of testicular toxicity associated with anticancer agents I. Histopathology. *Proc. West. Pharmacol. Soc.*, **25**, 381-4

Forrest, J.B., Turner, T.T. and Howard, S.S. (1981). Cyclophosphamide vincristine and the blood-testis barrier. *Invest. Urol.*, **18**, 443-4

Friedman, N.M. and Plymate, S.R. (1980). Leydig cell dysfunction and gynecomastia in adult males treated with alkylating agents. *Clin. Endocrinol.*, **12**, 553-6

Fukutani, K., Ishida, H., Shinohara, M., Niijima, K., Hijikata, Y., Izawa, Y. and Minowada, S. (1981). Suppression of spermatogenesis in patients with Bechet's disease treated with cyclophosphamide and colchicine. *Fertil. Ster.*, **36**, 76-80

Giffin, B.F. (1981). Effect of adriamycin on the reproductive system of the male prepubertal rat. *MSc Thesis*, University of Dayton, Dayton, Ohio, USA. pp. 30-43

Ginsberg, L.C., Johnson, S.C., Salama, N. and Ficsor, G. (1981). Acrosomal proteolytic assay for detection of mutagens in mammals. *Mutation Res.*, **91**, 413-18

Glode, L.M., Robinson, J. and Gould, S.F. (1981). Protection from cyclophosphamide-induced testicular damage with an analog of GnRH. *Lancet*, **1**, 1132-4

Hopkinson, C.R.W., Dulisch, B., Gauss, G., Hilscher, W. and Hirschhaueser, C. (1978). The effect of local testicular irradiation on testicular histology and plasma hormone levels in the male rat. *Acta Endocrinol.*, **87**, 413–23

Hseuh, A.J.W., Dufau, M.L. and Katt, K.J. (1976). Regulation of luteinizing hormone receptors in testicular interstitial cells by gonadotropin. *Biochem. Biophys. Res. Commun.* **72**, 1145–52

Hsu, A.C., Folami, A.O., Bain, J. and Rance, C.P. (1979). Gonadal function in males treated with cyclophosphamide for nephrotic syndrome. *Fertil. Ster.*, **31**, 173–7

Lendon, M., Palmer, M.K., Hann, I.M., Shalet, S.M. and Morris-Jones, P.H. (1978). Testicular histology after combination chemotherapy in childhood for acute lymphoblastic leukemia. *Lancet*, **2**, 439–41

Lentz, R.D., Bergstein, J., Steffes, M.W., Brown, D.R., Pem, K., Michael, A.F. and Vernier, R.L. (1977). Postpubertal evaluation of gonadal function following cyclophosphamide therapy before and after puberty. *J. Pediatr.*, **91**, 385–94

Lu, C.C. and Meistrich, M.L. (1979). Cytotoxic effects of chemotherapeutic drugs on mouse testis cells. *Cancer Res.*, **39**, 3575–82

Maquire, L.C., Dick, F.R. and Sherman, B.M. (1981). The effects of anti-leukemia therapy on gonadal histology in adult males. *Cancer*, **48**, 1967–71

Parra, A., Santos, D., Cervantes, C., Sojo, I., Carranco, A. and Cortes-Gallegos, V. (1978). Plasma gonadotropins and gonadal steroids in children treated with cyclophosphamide. *J. Pediatr.*, **92**, 117–24

Parvinen, L.M. and Parvinen, M. (1978). Biochemical studies of the rat seminiferous epithelial wave: DNA and RNA synthesis and effects of adriamycin. *Ann. Biol. Anim. Biochem. Biophys.*, **18**, 585–94

Penso, J., Lippe, B., Erlich, R. and Smith F. (1974). Testicular function in prepubertal and pubertal male patients treated with cyclophosphamide for nephrotic syndrome. *J. Pediatr.*, **84**, 831–6

Rapola, J., Koskimies, O., Huttuman, N.P., Floman, P., Vilska, J. and Hallman, N. (1973). Cyclophosphamide and the pubertal testis. *Lancet*, **1**, 98–9

Richter, P., Calamera, J.C., Morganfeld, M.C., Kierszenbaum, A.L., Lavieri, J.C. and Mancini, R.E. (1970). Effect of chlorambucil on spermatogenesis in humans with malignant lymphoma. *Cancer*, **25**, 1026–30

Roesser, H.P., Stolks, A.E. and Smith, A.J. (1978). Testicular damage due to cytotoxic drugs and recovery after cessation of therapy. *Aust. N.Z. J. Med.*, **8**, 250–4

Schilsky, R.L., Lewis, B.J., Sherins, R.J. and Young, R.C. (1980). Gonadal dysfunction in patients receiving chemotherapy for cancer. *Ann. Intern. Med.*, **93**, 109–14

Schmid, B. and Zbinden, G. (1979). Unscheduled DNA synthesis in male rabbit germ cells induced by methyl methane sulfonate, cyclophosphamide and adriamycin. *Arch. Toxicol.* (Suppl.), **2**, 503–7

Schoerer, A.E., Ohen, M.M. and Johnson, C.J. (1978). Gynecomastia with nitrosourea therapy. *Cancer Treat. Rep.*, **62**, 574–6

Schwartz, H.S. and Kanter, P.M. (1975). Cell interactions: Determinants of selective toxicity of adriamycin (NSC-123127) and daunorubicin (NSC-82151). *Cancer Chemother. Rep.*, **6**, 107–14

Shalet, S.M., Lendon, M. and Morris-Jones, P.H. (1981). Testicular function after chemotherapy for ALL. *N. Eng. J. Med.*, **305**, 520

Shamberger, R.C., Rosenberg, S.A., Seipp, C.A. and Sherins, R.J. (1981). Effects of high-dose methotrexate and vincristine on ovarian and testicular functions in patients undergoing postoperative adjuvant treatment of osteosarcoma. *Cancer Treat. Rep.*, **65**, 739–46

Sherins, R.J., Olweny, C.L.M. and Ziegler, J.L. (1978). Gynecomastia and gonadal dysfunction in adolescent boys treated with combination chemotherapy for Hodgkin's disease. *N. Engl. J. Med.*, **229**, 12–16

Sloan, W.R., Heston, W.D. and Coffey, D.S. (1975). New model for studying the effects of cancer chemotherapeutic agents in the growth of the prostate gland. *Cancer Chemother. Rep.*, **59**, 185–94

Smalley, R.V. and Wall, R.L. (1966). Two cases of busulphan toxicity. *Ann. Intern. Med.*, **64**, 154–64

Tritton, T.R., Yee, G. and Wingard, Jr., L.B. (1983). Immobilized adriamycin: A tool for separating cell surface from intracellular mechanisms. *Fed. Proc.*, **42**, 284–7

Trompter, R.S., Evans, P.R. and Barret, T.M. (1981). Gonadal function in boys with steroid responsive nephrotic syndrome with cyclophosphamide for short periods. *Lancet*, **1,** 1177-9

Waxman, J.H.X., Terry, Y.A., Wrigley, P.F.M., Malpas, J.S., Rees, L.H. and Besser, G.M. (1982). Gonadal function in Hodgkin's disease: long-term follow-up of chemotherapy. *Br. Med. J.*, **285,** 1612-13

Whitehead, E., Shalet, S.M., Blackledge, G., Todd, I., Crowther, D. and Beardwell, C.G. (1982). The effects of Hodgkin's disease and combination chemotherapy on gonadal function in the adult male. *Cancer*, **49,** 418-22

Whitely, W.P., Giffin, B.F., Bonanni, G.A. and Bajpai, P.K. (1981). The effect of adriamycin on the fertility of male rats. *Ohio J. Sci.*, **81,** 90

Wierzba, K., Danysz, A. and Pierkarczyk, A. (1982). Cytostatic and immunosuppressive drugs. In Dukes, M.N.G. and Elis, J. (eds.) *Side Effects of Drugs. Annual*, 6, pp. 490-495. (Amsterdam: *Excerpta Medica*)

3
Effects of 5-thio-D-glucose on male fertility

J.R. DANIEL and R.L. WHISTLER

Glucose provides more than 50% of human caloric requirements and is the principal carbohydrate metabolite of most organisms. 5-Thio-D-glucose (Fig. 3.1) is the nearest chemical analogue of natural D-glucose with only a sulphur atom replacing the oxygen atom in the pyranose ring structure. This sulphur sugar is conformationally and chemically similar to D-glucose but is quite different from D-glucose in its biochemical reactions and physiological effects. Because of its unique biochemical properties, 5-thio-D-glucose provides a valuable probe in studying aspects of carbohydrate metabolism and may have useful medicinal properties.

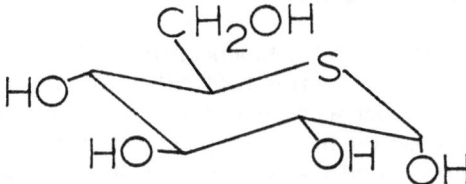

Fig. 3.1   Structure of 5-thio-D-glucose

PREPARATION AND PROPERTIES OF 5-THIO-D-GLUCOSE

The first synthesis of 5-thio-D-glucose was reported in 1962 (Feather and Whistler, 1962) and was later the subject of a patent (Whistler, 1966). This synthesis is laborious and yields are variable. The preparation has since been improved and shortened (Nayak and Whistler, 1969; Chiu and Whistler, 1973; El-Rahman and Whistler, 1973) and 5-thio-D-glucose can now be produced in better than 30% overall yield from D-glucose and is commercially available.

The thioacetal structure is unusually stable as 5-thio-D-glucose exhibits no tendency to form a disulphide open-chain dimer nor does it exhibit much mutarotation (Grimshaw *et al.*, 1979). Its stability is a consequence of the thioacetal stability as compared to the normal oxygen hemiacetal of

25

D-glucose. Thus, 5-thio-D-glucose, in solution, exists largely in a stable ring form. Interestingly, 5-thio-D-glucose crystallizes as the α-D-anomer. This raises a question as to whether or not the anomeric effect can be induced or enhanced by replacing the oxygen atom at C-5 by other heteroatoms. Nuclear magnetic resonance spectra of 5-thio-D-glucose (Suzuki and Whistler, 1972) have chemical shifts and coupling constants which are consistant with a $^4C_1$ conformation of the pyranose ring, as shown in Fig. 3.1.

5-Thio-D-glucose pentacetate may be partially oxidized to the sulphoxide with sodium metaperiodate and then to the sulphone with hydrogen peroxide in glacial acetic acid (Rowell and Whistler, 1966). Even under these strongly oxidizing conditions there is no evidence of disulphide formation, a further indication of the extreme stability of the thiopyranose ring.

Early work (Whistler and Van Es, 1963) showed that sugar glycosides containing a sulphur ring atom are more susceptible to acid-catalysed hydrolysis than their oxygen analogues. Presumably this is because of the greater stability of the carbosulphonium ion compared to the carboxonium ion intermediate.

5-Thio-D-glucose is nearly as sweet as its ring oxygen counterpart (Lindley et al., 1976). This observation, along with its low metabolic conversion, to be discussed later, makes it potentially useful as a synthetic non-caloric sweetener.

EFFECT OF 5-THIO-D-GLUCOSE ON MEMBRANE TRANSPORT PHENOMENA

Early work (Feather, 1963) on the biochemistry of 5-thio-D-glucose showed that it would not support the growth of either *Lactobacillus casei* or *Saccharomyces cerevisiae*. Other workers (Shankland et al., 1968) examined the effect of 5-thio-D-glucose on the development of larvae of the vinegar fly, *Drosophila melanogaster*, and absorption of 5-thio-D-glucose by the American cockroach, *Periplaneta americana*. The sugar analogue was found to interfere with the utilization of D-glucose in the vinegar fly larvae. This nutritional interference was evidenced even at ratios of D-glucose:5-thio-D-glucose as high as 30. The thiosugar was found to be absorbed from the gut of the American cockroach and distributed throughout the body in essentially the same way as D-glucose. Differences in distribution exist, however, but are due to differences between the metabolism of the natural sugar and the sulphur analogue. Examination of distribution of 5-thio-D-glucose in the haemolymph and midgut suggest possible metabolic utilization of the sulphur analogue since these sites contain a number of intermediates and enzymes for the Krebs cycle and glycolysis (Chefurka, 1965; Kilby, 1963).

The effect of 5-thio-D-glucose in rats was examined (Hoffman and Whistler, 1968) and it was found to be essentially non-toxic with an LD_{50} of 14 g/kg. Intraperitonal injections of large single doses of 5-thio-D-glucose in the range of 50–100 mg/kg led to a sharp increase in blood sugar concentration. A hyperglycaemic maximum occurred about 2.5 h after oral administration with the sugar level returning to normal in about 6 h. With high doses glycosuria occurred from renal spill-over of blood D-glucose. Insulin administration completely prevented the hyperglycaemia. Clearance studies of 5-thio-D-glucose showed that 97.3% of a single dose was excreted *via* the urine in 24 h, with the bulk being lost in the first 6 h. A rapid increase in fatty acid blood levels following 5-thio-D-glucose injection suggests that the thiosugar inhibits cellular uptake of D-glucose and leads to increased lipid catabolism. Other investigations (Lobl and Porteus, 1978) showed that rats may become resistant to the hyperglycaemic (diabetogenic) action of 5-thio-D-glucose. Male rats receiving oral doses of 50 mg/kg of 5-thio-D-glucose for 30 days have blood D-glucose levels within the normal range. The blood D-glucose levels were unaffected by insulin administration.

Early work indicating that 5-thio-D-glucose interferes with carbohydrate utilization by blocking transport of D-glucose was later verified (Whistler and Lake, 1972). These workers examined the effect of 5-thio-D-glucose on D-glucose transport in rat kidney, diaphragm and liver. Tissue uptake of D-glucose transport in the kidney and diaphram was decreased by 35% and 76%, respectively. However, in liver a net output of D-glucose occurred, probably due to glycolysis. Others (Critchley *et al.*, 1970; Barnett *et al.*, 1970) found inhibition of active transport of D-galactose in hamster small intestine when 5-thio-D-glucose was administered. Methyl α-D-glucopyranoside transport in *Escherichia coli* was inhibited by the thiosugar (Kaback, 1968). The suggestion was made that non-competitive inhibition of the phosphoenolpyruvate–phosphotransferase system occurred. It was also observed that 5-thio-D-glucose inhibits methyl α-D-glucopyranoside transport in kidney cortex (Critchley *et al.*, 1970). Additionally, it was found (Hellman *et al.*, 1973) that 5-thio-D-glucose at 10 mmol/l will completely inhibit insulin release by the pancreatic beta cells.

The extent of sugar transport inhibition by 5-thio-D-glucose has been quantitated (Whistler and Lake, 1972). These workers found an inhibition constant, K_i, of 4.85 mmol/l for D-galactose transport in kidney cortex slices. The thiosugar also interfered with the facilitated diffusion of D-xylose in rat diaphragm but was ineffective in inhibiting passive diffusion of D-arabinose. These observations indicate that the stereochemistry of the transported sugar and the inhibiting analogue are closely related. Further, the hydroxymethyl group at C-5 is apparently of little importance since the thiosugar can inhibit the transport of both pentoses and hexoses.

5-Thio-D-glucose inhibits active transport of neutral amino acids in rat kidney cortex (Whistler and Lake, 1972) and has a lower binding affinity for human erythrocytes than D-glucose (Kahlenberg and Dolansky, 1972). The clear inference is that sulphur in the pyranose ring lowers the sugar affinity for the D-glucose receptor site. Very likely this altered affinity at various receptor sites for 5-thio-D-glucose is the basis for its physiological/biochemical effects. However, it is puzzling that the thiosugar produces such profound effects when present at a concentration many times lower than that of the natural substrate and it is interesting that 5-thio-D-glucose does not interfere with D-glucose transport in rat erythrocytes (Hoffman, 1969).

5-Thio-D-glucose is actively transported by the D-glucose transport system (Whistler and Lake, 1972) in kidney cortex tissue and also in hamster intestine (Critchley *et al.*, 1970). A Lineweaver–Burk plot of 5-thio-D-glucose uptake in kidney cells provides a K_m of 2.4 mmol/l and a V_{max} of 70 μmol h^{-1} g^{-1} cell water. Other workers have demonstrated active uptake of 5-thio-D-glucose in renal clearance tests in the winter flounder (Pritchard and Kleinzeller, 1976).

ANTISPERMATOGENIC ACTION OF 5-THIO-D-GLUCOSE AND ITS POSSIBLE APPLICATION AS A CONTRACEPTIVE

The observation that 5-thio-D-glucose interferes with D-glucose transport led to examination of possible biomedical or pharmaceutical applications of this effect. Tissues or organs most dependent on D-glucose transport and metabolism are prime targets for biological effects. One such organ is testis.

A large body of knowledge indicates that testis' prime function (spermatogenesis) is quite sensitive to D-glucose concentration (Davis, 1969). Addition of D-glucose to incubated rat testis increases the rate of amino acid incorporation into protein. Diabetic men with lower total D-glucose have an increased incidence of impotence (Schoffling *et al.*, 1963), a lowered sperm count, atrophic changes in the germinal epithelium of the testes (Babbott *et al.*, 1958), and poor sperm motility (Klebanow and MacCleod, 1960). It is well known that an adequate supply of D-glucose is necessary for maintenance of normal testis function and morphology.

The effect of 5-thio-D-glucose on sperm production in mice has been investigated (Zysk *et al.*, 1975). The sugar analogue mixed with the mouse ration at a level of 30 mg kg^{-1} day^{-1} induced complete inhibition of spermatogenesis within two weeks. Inhibition could be maintained as long as the sugar derivative was administered and had no effect on animal libido or blood sugar level. Histological studies on the testes showed changes within one week for animals receiving 100 mg kg^{-1} day^{-1} and within two weeks for animals receiving 20 mg kg^{-1} day^{-1}. Initially, a few enlarged spermatogenic cells were observed in the lumen of the seminiferous tubules or in the spermatid zone of the germinal epithelium. Later the number of hypertrophied cells increased, with the largest number in the lumina of tubules that contained fewest spermatids. However, spermatogenesis was still observed in most tubules and spermatozoa were present in the epididymal tubules. On continued treatment with 5-thio-D-glucose there is a drastic reduction in spermatogenic cells and a complete absence of spermatozoa in the epididymal tubules.

During this treatment giant cells appeared in some of the seminiferous tubules and some of these cells had undergone necrosis. As more of the giant cells became necrotic, the tubules filled with these cells, atrophied, and developed calcified debris.

After the 30 mg kg^{-1} day^{-1} dosage was discontinued normal sperm development was observed in about 5–6 weeks. The time required for regeneration of testis function and appearance was directly related to the dose level. Sperm regeneration was noted after 8 weeks for all dose levels. Both F_1 and F_2 progeny of the males tested were normal in size and general health.

Rats fed 5-thio-D-glucose ($50\,\text{mg}\,\text{kg}^{-1}\,\text{day}^{-1}$) for two weeks show a 50% inhibition of incorporation of uridine into testicular RNA (Bushway, 1975). Similarly, incorporation of radioactive lysine was reduced by 40%.

It has been observed that 5-thio-D-glucose does not affect incorporation of L-[U-^{14}C]-phenylalanine into protein in whole rat testis but does inhibit incorporation of the amino acid by immature spermatids (Nakamura and Hall, 1976, 1977). Inhibition is independent of added D-glucose and is concentration dependent in the range 1–50 mmol/l. A similar type of inhibition is observed with L-leucine, L-lysine and L-glutamate. Mature spermatids also show inhibition of phenylalanine incorporation by 5-thio-D-glucose but the effect is not so pronounced as in immature spermatids. *In vivo* inhibition of protein synthesis is observed at a dosage of $33\,\text{mg}\,\text{kg}^{-1}$ body weight day^{-1} and this, coincidentally, is the minimum dose necessary to produce an antispermatogenic effect and consequent infertility in rats. These workers observed no significant changes in 14-day-old testicular suspensions, Sertoli cells, or Leydig cells and postulated that if the spermatids are most sensitive to 5-thio-D-glucose this might be a result of interference in cellular differentiation. In this case spermatogenesis would be disrupted for a whole generation of spermatids and the likely result would be the observed infertility.

The effect of 5-thio-D-glucose on spermatogenesis in rats has been examined (Homm *et al.*, 1977). Loss of germinal epithelium and permanent sterility was induced in rats given the thiosugar at 25 mg/kg or 50 mg/kg for 8 weeks. Similar dosages in mice produced temporary, reversible sterility. At a dosage of 12.5 mg/kg, 14 weeks were required to produce infertility but permanent sterility occurred in more than half the test group. Histology showed loss of all germ cells except spermatogonia and, rarely, primary spermatocytes. Leydig cells, Sertoli cells, and other body tissues appeared normal. Weight gain and libido were unaffected at all dose levels and of the organs examined, only testis weight was below normal. Thus, in rats, as opposed to mice, 5-thio-D-glucose is not a reversible antispermatogenic agent.

The effect of 5-thio-D-glucose on *myo*-inositol metabolism in male mice has been investigated (Burton and Wells, 1977). On administration of thiosugar by intraperitoneal injection (50 mg/kg or 250 mg/kg over 7 days) significantly reduced sperm counts were observed. 5-Thio-D-glucose caused hyperglycaemia and, at the higher dosage, produced increased testicular D-glucose 6-phosphate and free, but not lipid-bound, *myo*-inositol concentrations. 5-Thio-D-glucose 6-phosphate is a competitive inhibitor of rat testis *myo*-inositol 1-phosphate synthetase ($K_i = 3.3 \times 10^{-4}$ mol/l).

Re-examination of the effect of 5-thio-D-glucose in mice (Lobl and Porteus, 1978) showed that inhibition of spermatogenesis and infertility could be induced by orally administered thiosugar at a dosage of $50\,\text{mg}\,\text{kg}^{-1}\,\text{day}^{-1}$. However, these workers concluded on the basis of testicular morphology and mating experiments that the infertility was only partially reversible.

They also examined whether the effect of 5-thio-D-glucose would be manifested under conditions where thiosugar hyperglycaemia was suppressed. The antispermatogenic effect was seen in rats given both 5-thio-D-glucose ($50\,mg\,kg^{-1}\,day^{-1}$) and insulin ($0.5\,U/day$) and it was concluded that the sulphur sugar has intrinsic activity independent of its effect on D-glucose blood concentrations.

Whereas 5-thio-D-glucose is an effective antispermatogen in mice and rats, other species are not so sensitive to the thiosugar. 5-Thio-D-glucose, administered to male hamsters in silastic capsules, had very little effect on spermatogenesis even after 5 weeks of treatment (Das and Yanagimachi, 1978). In the test group only one out of six animals became sterile. More recently the effect of 5-thio-D-glucose in the musk shrew has been examined (Singh and Dominic, 1981). The sugar was orally administered at dosages of $50\,mg\,kg^{-1}\,day^{-1}$, $100\,mg\,kg^{-1}\,day^{-1}$, or $150\,mg\,kg^{-1}\,day^{-1}$ for 30 days. Regardless of the dose level, 5-thio-D-glucose did not induce changes in the epididymis and testis. Likewise, test and control groups showed no difference in testis weight or protein, RNA, and DNA testis concentrations. Thus, as compared to mice and rats, the hamster and musk shrew testes are relatively insensitive to 5-thio-D-glucose.

Inhibition of spermatogenesis by 5-thio-D-glucose in mice has been confirmed (Basu et al., 1979). It was noted that orally administered thiosugar was an effective dosage route whereas dosage by injection had little or no effect on the testis. They suggested, as have others, that the effect of 5-thio-D-glucose is due to decreased D-glucose testis metabolism by competition of the sulphur sugar for D-glucose metabolizing enzymes. These workers also noted that treated males were able to fertilize females 8–10 weeks after withdrawal of treatment and that the litter size of the subsequent generation was 1–3 in all cases.

Several investigations have been made into the mutagenic and teratogenic effects of 5-thio-D-glucose (Majumdar et al., 1979a, 1979b, 1982). In one investigation (Majumdar et al., 1979a) male mice were treated with 40 or $60\,mg\,kg^{-1}\,day^{-1}$ of the thiosugar for 7 or 35 successive days. Mating with treated males did not cause significant differences in average implantations or intrauterine postimplantation losses in pregnant females in comparison with controls. As previously observed, 5-thio-D-glucose treatment did not affect the mating behaviour of male mice. These workers conclude that under the conditions employed the thiosugar is not mutagenic as regards induction of a dominant lethal mutation in mice. In other work (Majumdar et al., 1979b), male mice were treated with 40 or $60\,mg\,kg^{-1}\,day^{-1}$ for 28 to 35 days and germinal cell degeneration and total inhibition of spermatogenesis in the seminiferous tubules was observed. Attendant sterility lasted for several weeks. After discontinuing treatment, sperm development resumed in 5–6 weeks. Treatment of the males did not affect libido, Leydig cells, Sertoli cells, or spermatogonia. Pregnant females were also treated with 5-thio-D-glucose on days 6 to 12 of gestation. No embryotoxic or tetratogenic effects were noted in the offspring. More recently 5-thio-D-glucose has been tested in the Ames assay (Majumdar et al., 1982). The sulphur sugar showed no evidence of mutagenicity in any of four tester strains of *Salmonella typhimurium*, either with or without S-9 (rat liver homogenate) activation. These investigations, coupled with its high LD_{50}, suggest that 5-thio-D-glucose is likely to be safe in humans.

The fine structure of the mouse testis after 5-thio-D-glucose treatment has been examined by Majumdar and Udelsman (1979). C3H/HeJ mice received intraperitoneal injections of $40\,mg\,kg^{-1}\,day^{-1}$ for 21, 28, or 35 days. Three other groups of mice received injections for 35 days and were then allowed to recover from treatment for 21, 42, and 75 days. Electron microscopy and histology revealed significant changes in the testis as early as 21 days after the start of administration. Complete eradication of spermatogenesis was noted at 35 days. Alterations in mouse testes included degradation of germinal epithelium and germ cells, formation of giant, multinucleated cells, and the presence of cellular debris in the tubule lumina. Lysosome accumulation and an increase in lipid droplets and vacuoles resembling bodies containing membrane and cellular debris were found in the Sertoli cell cytoplasm. In the recovery groups spermatogenesis began after 21 to 42 days and testicular cells in the 75-day recovery group appeared identical to the control group of testis cells.

It has been found that 5-thio-D-glucose significantly reduces the rate of D-glucose uptake in testis tissue slices and isolated rat epididymis cells (Brooks, 1979). It was concluded that the primary effect of 5-thio-D-glucose in reducing sterility is on D-glucose uptake. Some D-glucose enters epididymal cells with difficulty and uptake is a facilitated diffusion process.

In work reminiscent of earlier investigations *in vitro*, the cell-specific effects of 5-thio-D-glucose on mouse testis *in vivo* have been investigated (Brady and Majumdar, 1981). 5-Thio-D-glucose ($40\,mg\,kg^{-1}\,day^{-1}$) was administered to male C3H mice. Direct counts of spermatogenic cells revealed that immature spermatids were first affected, followed by a significant reduction in number of spermatocytes. Neither Sertoli cells nor spermatogonia were significantly affected by the thiosugar. Following discontinuation of 5-thio-D-glucose treatment, recovery of testicular architecture began in about 3 weeks and although epididymal sperm counts returned to 91% of that of the controls, testis weights were slightly below normal.

Recently, animal experiments using 5-thio-D-glucose were reviewed by Davies and Meanock (1981) and these workers are less optimistic about its potential for human use. They pointed out that in both mice and rats, regimens of 7 to 8 weeks have been shown to cause permanent sterility and that the smallest doses causing infertility are associated with transient hyperglycaemia. In large doses in rats, the thiosugar caused an increased concentration of non-esterified fatty acids in the blood and repeated smaller doses increased catecholamine excretion.

The effect of 5-thio-D-glucose on reproduction in Coturnix quail has recently been reported (Schafer *et al.*, 1982). The method used involves gavaging groups of seven male quail once with about 50% of the estimated LD_{50} of 5-thio-D-glucose ($>316\,mg/kg$) and observing the egg fertility of their female mates over six or seven periods of 5 days duration. 5-Thio-D-glucose had no effect on fertility since fertility, as measured by the percentage of eggs laid that were fertile, was 86% that of the control group over days 1–35 and 91% of that of the control group over days 20–35. Interestingly, and in opposition to the results found in selected rodent species, quail testes weight increased in the test group (4.432 g) as compared to the control group (2.854 g). The authors did not comment on this weight increase.

The effect of orally administered 5-thio-D-glucose on testis metabolism in albino mice has been examined by Veeraragavan and Ramakrishnan (1982). Dosage was 33 mg kg^{-1} day^{-1} for 21 days. In testicular tissue there was an increase in the activity of hexokinase, D-glucose 6-phosphate dehydrogenase, and sorbitol dehydrogenase. There was also an increase in the concentrations of D-fructose, pentoses and ascorbic acid as compared to the control group. However, testes weight and total protein content were decreased in the test group. These workers conclude that aerobic glycolysis is inhibited *in vivo* in mouse testes by 5-thio-D-glucose and that D-glucose is utilized by alternative pathways such as the uronic acid pathway, the hexose monophosphate shunt, and in D-fructose formation.

Results indicate that 5-thio-D-glucose has potential as a non-hormonal reversible contraceptive. Human testing has not been conducted but the possibility of developing a non-toxic, non-hormonal male contraceptive would seem to be a useful and attainable application.

EFFECT OF 5-THIO-D-GLUCOSE ON MEMORY AND LEARNING IN RATS

It has been known for sometime (Himwich *et al.*, 1939; Olson *et al.*, 1950) that normal brain tissue function is dependent on D-glucose. Because of the inhibition of D-glucose transport by 5-thio-D-glucose it was important to ascertain the effect of the thiosugar on the blood–brain barrier and on the brain itself. Behavioural experiments on rats showed no noticeable effects on learning or memory (Bushway, 1975). Rats fed 100 mg kg^{-1} day^{-1} of the sugar analogue had normal ability to learn and remember maze problems. Hebb-Williams maze problems were employed to test intelligence. Close observation of animals receiving the analogue revealed no abnormal behaviour although it is possible that 5-thio-D-glucose may affect untested brain centres.

METABOLISM OF 5-THIO-D-GLUCOSE

Intravenous or oral administration of radioactive 5-thio-D-glucose to rats result in the rapid excretion of 95% of the compound, largely in the urine (Pitts *et al.*, 1975). A small amount is converted into carbon dioxide and excreted by respiration, as shown in Table 3.1. 5-Thio-D-glucose 1-phosphate (Whistler and Stark, 1970) was tested with rabbit skeletal muscle phosphoglucomutase and was found to be converted into the 6-phosphate at 25% the rate observed for the natural oxygen analogue (Chen and Whistler, 1975a). The thiosugar 1-phosphate was also found to be a competitive

Table 3.1 Distribution of radioactivity after administration of 5-thio-D-[U-¹⁴C] glucopyranose

	5-thio-D-[U-¹⁴C]-glucopyranose	
Radioactive component	i.v. (%)	oral (%)
CO₂ 6 h	1.0	1.0
12 h	—	0.1
24 h	—	0.05
48 h	—	0.08
72 h	—	<0.01
Total	1.0	1.0
Urine	93.0	54.0
Faeces	—	37.0
Total Excreted	95.0	93.0
Carcass	1.6	4.0
Intestine	—	0.2
Glycogen	0.5	0.08

From: Pitts *et al.* (1975)

inhibitor of the enzymatic glucose 1-phosphate → glucose 6-phosphate isomerization ($K_i = 16.2 \, \mu mol/l$).

5-Thio-D-glucose 6-phosphate can be synthesized chemically and enzymatically (Whistler and Stark, 1970; Chen and Whistler, 1975a) at pH 8. It is a strong inhibitor of yeast glucose 6-phosphate dehydrogenase (Chen and Whistler, 1975a).

Chemical preparation of uridine-(5-thio-α-D-glucopyranosyl pyrophosphate) (UDPTG) was accomplished by Graham and Whistler (1975) and involves the coupling of the salt of uridine 5-monophosphate 4-morpholine-N,N-dicyclohexylcarboxamide with 5-thio-D-glucose 1-phosphate. This nucleotide analogue has also been prepared enzymatically. These sugar phosphate and nucleotide analogues have a potential for application as very senstive probes in the study of enzymatic mechanisms.

5-THIO-D-GLUCOSE AND RELATED COMPOUNDS: EFFECT OF ENZYMATIC ACTION

5-Thio-D-glucose is a substrate for yeast hexokinase and inhibits D-glucose phosphorylation. The thiosugar 1-phosphate is a substrate for phosphoglucomutase and is a potent inhibitor of the D-glucose 1-phosphate → D-glucose-6-phosphate conversion (Chen and Whistler, 1975a). 5-Thio-D-glucose 6-phosphate is a substrate for glucose 6-phosphate dehydrogenase and, thus, the thio analogue may be metabolized *via* the pentose phosphate shunt.

5-Thio-D-glucose will not replace D-glucose-1-phosphate as a substrate in enzymatic reactions but is a competitive inhibitor of enzymes acting on D-glucose-1-phosphate. It is also a non-competitive inhibitor of phosphorylase acting on amylopectin and glycogen. 5-Thio-D-glucose competitively inhibits the action of potato phosphorylase on amylopectin and the action of glycogen phosphorylase a and b on D-glucose-1-phosphate. Thus, it is possible that the thiosugar might interfere with the supply of D-glucose from polysaccharide catabolism (Chen and Whistler, 1975b, 1975c).

UDPG is the primary sugar carrier in the enzymatic synthesis of oligo- and polysaccharides from monosaccharides. UDPTG is identical in structure to UDPG except for the sulphur atom in the pyranose ring. UDPTG also has similar physical and chemical properties to UDPG. However, its biochemical properties are quite different from UDPG. UDPTG, at a concentration of 10 mmol/l, causes an increase in glycogen synthetase a activity of over 400%, even though the thionucleotide is not a substrate for the enzyme. Normalization of the otherwise sigmoidal kinetics for the reaction of UDPG with glycogen synthetase a was noted, and the K_m decreased from 2.0 mmol/l to 0.62 mmol/l. UDPTG apparently has no effect on glycogen synthetase b activity. UDPTG is inhibitory for glycogen synthetase a at higher concentration.

The initial catalytic activation at low concentration by UDPTG followed by inhibition of catalytic activity of glycogen synthetase a suggests that the thionucleotide can bind initially to a limited number of UDPG sites, thereby stimulating binding at the unoccupied sites. As the concentration of UDPTG is increased, it saturates the UDPG binding sites but is not converted into product. This makes it quite useful as a probe of enzymatic mechanism and/or the relation of substrate interaction and allosteric effects.

References

Babbott, D., Rubin, A. and Ginsburg, S. J. (1958). The reproductive characteristics of diabetic men. *Diabetes*, **7**, 33

Barnett, J.E.G., Ralph, A. and Monday, K.A. (1970). Structural requirements for active intestinal transport, the nature of the carrier-sugar bonding at C-2 and the ring oxygen of the sugar. *Biochem. J.*, **118**, 843

Basu, S.L., Ramakrishnan, S., Prasannan, K.G., Sarma, P.R.R. and Sundaresan, R. (1979). Reversible sterility due to diminished glucose metabolism in male mice treated with 5-thio-D-glucose. *Indian J. Exp. Biol.*, **17**, 632

Brady, K.D. and Majumdar, S.K. (1981). Cell specific action of 5-thio-D-glucose in mouse testis. *J. Hered.*, **72**, 347

Brooks, D.E. (1979). Carbohydrate metabolism in the rat epididymis. Evidence that glucose is taken up by tissue slices and isolated cells by a process of facilitated transport. *Biol. Reprod.*, **21**, 19

Burton, L.E. and Wells, W.W. (1977). Studies on the effect of 5-thio-D-glucose and 2-deoxy-D-glucose on myo-inositol metabolism. *Arch. Biochem. Biophys.*, **181**, 384

Bushway, A.A. (1975). Investigation of the effect of 5-thio-D-glucose on learning and intelligence of male rats. *MS Thesis*, Purdue University, W. Lafayette, IN, USA

Chefurka, W. (1965). Some comparative aspects of the metabolism of carbohydrates in insects. *Ann. Rev. Ent.*, **10**, 345

Chen, M. and Whistler, R.L. (1975a). Action of 5-thio-D-glucose and its l-phosphate with hexokinase and phosphoglucomutase. *Arch. Biochem. Biophys.*, **169**, 392

Chen, M. and Whistler, R.L. (1975b). Action of 5-thio-D-glucose and its l-phosphate with glycolytic enzymes. Abstracts of Papers, No. 143, Division of Biol. Chemistry, 170th ACS National Meeting

Chen, M. and Whistler, R.L. (1975c). Inhibition of α-glucan phosphorylases by 5-thio-D-glucose and its phosphates. Abstracts of Papers, No. 3, Division of Cellulose, Paper, and Textile Chemistry, 170th ACS National Meeting

Chiu, C.W. and Whistler, R.L. (1973). An alternate synthesis of 5-thio-D-glucose pentaacetate. *J. Org. Chem.*, **38**, 832

Critchley, D.R., Eichholz, A. and Crane, R.K. (1970). Transport of 5-thio-D-glucose in hamster small intestine. *Biochim. Biophys. Acta*, **211**, 244

Das, R.D. and Yanagimachi, R. (1978). Effects of monothioglycerol, alpha-chlorohydrin and 5-thio-D-glucose on the fertility of male hamster. *Contraception*, **17**, 413

Davies, A.G. and Meanock, S.J. (1981). Potential of 5-thio-D-glucose as an agent for controlling male fertility. *Arch. Androl.*, **7**, 153

Davis, J.R. (1969). Metabolic aspects of spermatogenesis. *Biol. Reprod.* **1** (Suppl. 1), 93

El-Rahman, M.M.A.A. and Whistler, R.L. (1973). A shorter synthesis of 5-thio-α-D-glucose pentaacetate. *Org. Prep. Proc. Int.*, **5**, 245

Feather, M.S. (1963). Synthesis of derivatives of 5-deoxy-5-mercapto-D-glucose and 6-deoxy-6-mercapto-D-fructose. *PhD Thesis*, Purdue University, W. Lafayette, IN, USA

Feather, M.S. and Whistler, R.L. (1962). Derivatives of 5-deoxy-5-mercapto-D-glucose. *Tetrahedron Lett.*, **15**, 667

Graham, T.L. and Whistler, R.L. (1975). Enzymatic synthesis and reactions of uridine 5-(5-thio-α-D-glucopyranosyl pyrophosphate). *Arch. Biochem. Biophys.*, **171**, 721

Grimshaw, C.E., Whistler, R.L. and Cleland, W.W. (1979). Ring opening and closing rates for thiosugars. *J. Am. Chem. Soc.*, **101**, 1521

Hellman, B., Lernmark, A., Sehlin, J., Taljedal, I.-B. and Whistler, R.L. (1973). The pancreatic β-cell recognition of insulin secretagogues-III. Effects of substituting sulphur for oxygen in the D-glucose molecule. *Biochem. Pharmacol.*, **22**, 29

Himwich, H.E., Hadidian, Z., Fazekas, J.F. and Hogland, H. (1939). Cerebral metabolism and electrical activity during insulin hypoglycemia in man. *Am. J. Physiol.*, **125**, 578

Hoffman, D.J. (1969). I. Diabetogenic action of 5-thio-D-glucopyranose. II. Synthesis and properties of nucleotides containing 4-thio-D-ribofuranose. *PhD Thesis*, Purdue University, W. Lafayette, IN, USA

Hoffman, D.J. and Whistler, R.L. (1968). Diabetogenic action of 5-thio-D-glucopyranose in rats. *Biochemistry*, **7**, 4479

Homm, R.E., Rusticus, C. and Hahn, D.W. (1977). The antispermatogenic effects of 5-thio-D-glucose in male rats. *Biol. Reprod.*, **17**, 697

Kaback, H.R. (1968). The role of the phosphoenolpyruvate-phosphotransferase system in the transport of sugars by isolated membrane preparations of *Escherichia coli*. *J. Biol. Chem.*, **243**, 3711

Kahlenberg, A. and Dolanskey, D. (1972). Structural requirements of D-glucose for its binding to isolated human erythrocyte membranes. *Can. J. Biochem.*, **50**, 638

Kilby, B.A. (1963). The biochemistry of the insect fat body. *Adv. Insect Physiol*, **1**, 111

Klebanow, D. and MacLeod, J. (1960). Semen quality and certain disturbances of reproduction in diabetic men. *Fertil. Steril.*, **11**, 255

Lindley, M.G., Shallenberger, R.S. and Whistler, R.L. (1976). Comparison of the sweetness of glucose and fructose with their ring-thio analogs. *J. Food Sci.*, **41**, 575

Lobl. T.J. and Porteus, S.F. (1978). Anti-fertility activities of 5-thio-D-glucose in mice and rats. *Contraception*, **17**, 123

Majumdar, S.K., Brady, K.D., Ringer, L.D., Natoli, J., Killian, C.M., Portnoy, J.A. and Koury, P. (1979b). Reproduction and teratogenic studies of 5-thio-D-glucose in mice. *J. Hered.*, **70**, 142

Majumdar, S.K., Ringer, L.D. and McFadden, L. (1979a). Genetic effects of 5-thio-D-glucose in male mice. *J. Hered.*, **70**, 75

Majumdar, S.K., Thatcher, J.D., Dennis, E.H., Cutrone, A., Stockage, M. and Hammond, M. (1982). Mutagenic evaluation of 2 male contraceptives, 5-thio-D-glucose and gossypol acetic-acid. *J. Hered.*, **73**, 76

Majumdar, S.K. and Udelsman, R. (1979). Fine structure of mouse testes following intraperitoneal treatment with 5-thio-D-glucose. *J. Hered.*, **70**, 194

Nakamura, M. and Hall, P.F. (1976). Inhibition by 5-thio-D-glucopyranose of protein biosynthesis *in vitro* in spermatids from rat testis. *Biochim. Biophys. Acta*, **447**, 474

Nakamura, M. and Hall, P.F. (1977). Effect of 5-thio-D-glucose on protein synthesis *in vitro* by various types of cells from rat testes. *J. Reprod. Fertil.*, **49**, 395

Nayak, U.G. and Whistler, R.L. (1969). Improved synthesis of 5-thio-D-glucose. *J. Org. Chem.*, **34,** 97

Olson, R.O., Robson, J.S., Richards, M. and Hirsch, E.G. (1950). Comparative metabolism of radioactive glucose in heart, brain, kidney and liver slices. *Fed. Proc.*, **9,** 211

Pitts, M.J., Chemielewski, M., Chen, M.S., El-Rahman, M.M.A.A. and Whistler, R.L. (1975). Metabolism of 5-thio-D-glucopyranose and 6-thio-D-fructopyranose in rats. *Arch. Biochem. Biophys.* **169,** 384

Pritchard, J.B. and Kleinzeller, A. (1976). Renal sugar transport in the winter flounder. I. Renal clerance studies. *Am. J. Physiol.*, **231,** 603

Rowell, R.M. and Whistler, R.L. (1966). Derivatives of α-D-glucothiopyranose. *J. Org. Chem.*, **31,** 1514

Schafer, E.W. Jr., Brunton, R.B., Schafer, E.C. and Chavez, G. (1982). Effects of 77 chemicals on reproduction in male and female Coturnix quail. *Ecotoxicol. Environ. Saf.*, **6,** 149

Schoffling, K., Federlin, K., Ditschoneit, H. and Pfeiffer, E.F. (1963). Disorders of sexual function in male diabetics. *Diabetes*, **12,** 519

Shankland, D.L., Stark, J.H. and Whistler, R.L. (1968). The effect of 5-thio-D-glucose on insect development and its absorption by insects. *J. Insect Physiol.*, **14,** 63

Singh, S.K. and Dominic, C.J. (1981). Failure of 5-thio-D-glucose to induce antispermatogenic effects in the musk shrew, *Suncus murinus* L. *Biol. Reprod.*, **24,** 655

Suzuki, M. and Whistler, R.L. (1972). 1,2,3,4,6-Penta-*O*-acetyl-5-thio-β-D-glucopyranose. *Carbohydr. Res.*, **22,** 473

Veeraragavan, K. and Ramakrishnan, S. (1982). Effect of 5-thio-D-glucose on alternative pathways of carbohydrate metabolism in mice testes. *Indian J. Biochem. Biophys.*, **19,** 201

Whistler, R.L. (1966). Novel sulfur containing compounds. U.S. Pat. 3, 243, 425. March 29, 1966 (assignee, Purdue Research Foundation)

Whistler, R.L. and Lake, W.C. (1972). Inhibition of cellular transport processes by 5-thio-D-glucopyranose. *Biochem. J.*, **130,** 919

Whistler, R.L. and Stark, J.H. (1970). 5-Thio-D-glucopyranose l-phosphate and 6-phosphate. *Carbohydr. Res.*, **13,** 15

Whistler, R.L. and Van Es, T. (1963). Solvolysis of methyl D-xylothiapyranosides and 2,3,4-tri-*O*-acetyl-α-D-xylothiapyranosyl bromide. *J. Org. Chem.* **28,** 2303

Zysk, J.R., Bushway, A.A., Whistler, R.L. and Carlton, W.W. (1975). Temporary sterility produced in male mice by 5-thio-D-glucose. *J. Reprod. Fertil.* **45,** 69

Section II

DRUGS AND MALE FERTILITY

4
Therapeutic drug effects on male reproductive function

C.G. SMITH and J.E. HARCLERODE

Some of the most commonly used drugs in therapeutics can cause impairment of sexual function in men. The reproductive system is unusual among the bodily systems in the complexity of the mechanisms that control it and that must operate in order for it to function properly. If one carefully examines the physiological control of the male reproductive system, it is clear that virtually all of the mechanisms are possible targets of primary drug effects and side-effects of drugs.

The hypothalamic–pituitary axis serves as a complex control center for the many factors that impinge on the reproductive system. Although the exact neural pathways have yet to be thoroughly described, we now know that various neurotransmitter substances in the hypothalamus are necessary to trigger the release of the gonadotropic hormones. We also know that these hypothalamic neurotransmitters are (as in other areas of the brain) sensitive to the effects of the drugs that alter their synthesis, release, or actions. Disruption of these pathways results in changes in the levels or patterns of secretion of the pituitary gonadotropins.

A second level for the observed effects of drugs is by direct action of drugs on the gonadal functions of androgen production and spermatogenesis. The synthesis of cholesterol and steroid hormones within the body is not readily inhibited by direct effects of drugs. Several drugs, most notably alcohol, can inhibit testosterone synthesis directly, but by far the major mechanism of lowered testosterone levels by drugs is disruption of hypothalamic–pituitary function with secondary effects on testosterone synthesis and secretion. Drugs that decrease testosterone levels can be expected to produce a multitude of subsequent effects on male reproductive function, since all parts of the male reproductive system are target organs for androgens. Plasma testosterone levels also exert a direct influence on libido, such that loss of sexual desire and impotence may result from use of certain drugs. A more likely target for drug effects is the rapid cell division and specialized processes involved in spermatogenesis. Spermatogenesis in man takes approximately 76 days. Thus, a drug that has an effect on the early stages of sperm production will not produce detectable effects for many weeks. However, because spermatogenesis is a renewable process, it may be possible to restore full sperm production even after a virtually complete loss of developing sperm cells. Additionally, the later stages of spermatogenesis are relatively protected from exogenous toxins by the blood–testes barrier. Because of these factors, it is sometimes difficult to predict the extent of testicular toxicity of drugs.

Drug effects on the functioning of the sex accessory organs is a very interesting example of the particular vulnerability of the reproductive system. Endocrine disruptions can be reflected in the function of the sex accessory organs. Disruption of nervous function, either voluntary or autonomic, can produce effects on these organs. Drugs that act on protein synthesis or rapidly dividing cells such as the chemotherapeutic agents can also produce effects on these tissues.

The mechanisms for drug-induced changes in sexual function are complex and may involve actions at more than one level of the reproductive system. It is often difficult to identify the precise mechanism for the disruptive effects of a particular drug or drug class. Therefore, the outline that will be used here to summarize the effects of drugs on male reproduction is based on the pharmacological properties of the various drug classes. There are few clinical studies that have examined the reproductive consequences of the use of therapeutic agents. Most information comes from case reports and reported side-effects in the product information inserts for the prescription medications. The drug classes that are included in this review were chosen because their reproductive effects are well recognized. The generic or chemical names of the drugs have been used, but an example of the trade names for the commonly used drugs has been provided.

CENTRAL NERVOUS SYSTEM (CNS) DRUGS

It is now well established that certain of the CNS drugs exert an inhibitory action on hypothalamic–pituitary function. In laboratory animals these effects can be seen as suppression of oestrus, ovulation and fertility in females and inhibition of testosterone and suppression of spermatogenesis in male animals. The primary endocrine effects on the gonadotropins are seen as secondary effects on sex steroids and subsequent effects on the growth, development and function of the sex accessory organs.

The evidence now strongly indicates that the major pathways that are involved in the hypothalamic control of gonadotropins in primates are adrenergic and dopaminergic. There are a multitude of pharmacological agents that can modify catecholamine levels by altering synthesis, release, receptor activation, re-uptake, etc. The best-known drugs that produce actions of this type are the neuropharmacological agents that either inhibit CNS activities—the anaesthetics, analgesics, sedatives, and tranquilizers; or that stimulate CNS activities—the antidepressants, stimulants, and hallucinogens. These drugs can modify the hypothalamic–pituitary control of the gonadotropins and prolactin because of their action on CNS pathways. The changes in LH, FSH and prolactin result in adverse side-effects on the reproductive system including changes in libido, impotence, inability to ejaculate, testicular swelling and gynaecomastia. In some cases it is difficult to separate the CNS effects of these drugs from their effects on the peripheral autonomic nervous system.

Antidepressants

The tricyclic antidepressants and related drugs affect adrenergic function in the CNS and have a central anticholinergic effect. These drugs block the transport system of the axonal membranes for the re-uptake of norepinephrine. Blockade of this transport mechanism causes higher levels of neurotransmitter in the synaptic cleft and potentiates sympathetic responses. In response to this drug action, libido may be increased or decreased and impotence has been reported as a side-effect. Examples of the tricyclic antidepressants include imipramine HCl (Tofranil), desipramine HCl (Norpramin) and amitriptyline HCl (Elavil HCl).

Tranquillizers/antianxiety agents/antipsychotics— phenothiazines, benzodiazepines, butyrophenones

The phenothiazines, such as chloropromazine HCl (Thoraxine) and thioridazine HCl (Mellaril), have strong antiadrenergic and weaker anticholinergic activity. They also have some antihistaminic and antiserotonin activity. Side-effects in men include decreased libido, impotence and inhibition of ejaculation. Lactation and breast engorgement may occur in women. Endocrine disruptions, especially increased prolactin levels, are thought to produce these side-effects.

The benzodiazepines, such as diazepam (Valium) and chlordiazepoxide (Librium), are commonly used antianxiety agents. These drugs have CNS depressant activity but no demonstrable peripheral autonomic actions. While changes in libido have been reported, the incidence of this side-effect is low.

The antipsychotic butyrophenone, haloperidol (Haldol), has been reported to cause impotence. Increased levels of prolactin are observed during chronic administration, but the clinical significance of elevated serum prolactin levels is unknown. Neuroleptic drugs are thought to raise prolactin levels by blocking dopamine receptors in the hypothalamus.

Centrally-acting antihypertensive drugs

There are at present two important antihypertensive drugs, alpha-methyldopa (Aldomet) and clonidine HCl (Catapres), that lower blood pressure by acting primarily on the brain to decrease sympathetic tone. Adverse side-effects including impotence, urinary retention and gynaecomastia, are characteristic of interference with sympathetic function. The degree to which these antihypertensive drugs act through central and peripheral mechanisms to produce these effects is not well established.

In patients treated with methyldopa the incidence of impotence has been reported to be as high as 30% (Bullpitt and Dollery, 1973). In studies showing a lower incidence of impotence as a side-effect of methyldopa, a uniform finding has been a decrease in the frequency of intercourse in the methyldopa groups. The antihypertensive action of methyldopa involves disruption of norepinephrine in the CNS, but some peripheral actions have been observed as well, so that possible mechanisms for this side-effect could include sedation and depression with a decrease in libido. Increases in serum prolactin levels caused by methyldopa could also directly disrupt testicular function.

Clonidine is a newer antihypertensive agent with a mechanism similar to methyldopa. It has α-adrenergic blocking activity, can inhibit the release of norepinephrine in the CNS, and also appears to produce some peripheral vasodilation. The incidence of impotence associated with the use of clonidine (alone rarely or in combination) ranges from 10 to 20%. This side-effect appears to be related to dose and is very infrequent in patients receiving 600 μg or less (Khan et al., 1970).

Narcotics

The principal site of action of narcotics is within the central nervous system, where they mediate analgesic activities, but they also act on areas of the hypothalamus that are important in the regulation of gonadotropins. Efforts have been made to determine the actions of narcotics on various areas of the hypothalamus involved in regulating pituitary function. Recent studies with endogenous opioid peptides (EOP) indicate that they may be involved in the control of gonadotropin secretion. Experiments in male Rhesus monkeys showed that stimulation of opiate receptors by opiates or EOPs exerts a negative effect on LH and testosterone levels, and administration of an opiate receptor antagonist caused an increase in LH and testosterone levels (Scher et al., 1983).

Clinical reports indicate that heroin addicts experience both diminished sexual drive and impairment of sexual function. Sperm count and sperm motility are also decreased. The exact mechanism by which narcotics suppress sexual function and desire is not known. The endorphins may have a role in influencing sexual behaviour, but it is also likely that decreased testosterone levels may be responsible for decreased libido. It is clear, that the narcotic drugs can decrease gonadotropin secretion and stimulate the secretion of prolactin. Both of these effects are likely to be inhibitory to male sexual function.

Results of both human and animal experimentation reveal that the effects of morphine, methadone, heroin and closely related agents produce widely varying discrepancies in sex steroid levels in the plasma. The levels of circulating hormones are related to the dose and duration of the narcotic administered; thus, one would expect greater changes after chronic administration. However, serum LH levels were within normal values in human narcotic addicts (Cushman, 1972) and serum FSH levels were similarly not affected (Azizi et al., 1973). There are conflicting reports regarding the actual plasma testosterone levels in men with a history of drug addiction. For instance, serum testosterone levels were reported to be unchanged

(Cushman, 1973), depressed (Azizi *et al.*, 1973), or slightly but statistically insignificantly increased (Cicero *et al.*, 1975) in drug users. A recent study by Mendelson and Mello (1982) showed that plasma testosterone and luteinizing hormone levels did not differ between former heroin addicts and normal control subjects, but were significantly suppressed in current heroin users. They also observed that recurrent heroin use during puberty did not significantly disrupt pubertal development in males, indicating that tolerance to opiate-induced suppression of pituitary and gonadal hormones occurs in both puberty and adulthood.

AUTONOMIC NERVOUS SYSTEM DRUGS

The group of drugs that are probably most likely to affect sexual function are those that act on the sympathetic and parasympathetic nervous systems. Both erection and ejaculation are under dual autonomic nervous control. Reflexogenic stimuli initiated by tactile stimulation of the genital regions are transmitted via the pudendal nerves of the spinal cord. Efferent impulses transmitted via the parasympathetic fibres arising from S-2, 3, and 4 initiate penile erection. Emission of semen is largely controlled by sympathetic nerve fibres originating from L-2, 3 segments. This apparent alpha response induces contraction of the seminal vesicles and vas deferens and triggers contraction of the bulbar muscles which induces ejaculation.

Antihypertensive drugs

The antihypertensive drugs are the best example of drugs that are likely to alter sexual function by interfering with autonomic transmission. Reports in the literature have associated the development of impotence or failure of ejaculation with virtually every antihypertensive drug in current use. The exact incidence of impaired sexual function associated with each agent is difficult to assess. The frequent use of combinations of antihypertensive drugs increases the difficulty in making this determination. For example, Hogen *et al.* (1980) studied 861 male patients receiving antihypertensive medication and included, in the evaluation, questions regarding sexual function. The reported incidence of sexual dysfunction in 177 control (non-hypertensive) patients was 4%; 9% in patients on a thiazide diuretic alone; 13% in patients on methyldopa plus diuretic; 15% in patients on clonidine plus diuretic; and 23% in patients on propranolol and hydralazine in combination plus a diuretic. Sexual dysfunction due to diuretic therapy alone is difficult to interpret. It may be a true complication of therapy, but more likely it is a consequence of the underlying hypertension and arteriosclerosis.

Hydralazine (Apresoline) decreases blood pressure by direct relaxation of vascular smooth muscle. Its effects in combination antihypertensive therapy on sexual dysfunction have been reported (Koch-Weser, 1976; Schmidt and Lucas, 1977). Propranolol (Inderal), a beta adrenergic blocking drug, was originally thought to be free of side-effects on sexual functioning. Several reports, however, show a dose-related increase in the incidence of impotence with propranolol (Miller, 1976). It is possible that this complication may be rarer with the use of a related drug, atenolol, which does not penetrate the blood–brain barrier as well. The evolution of drugs that have combined alpha and beta receptor antagonism may cause further problems with sexual dysfunction. The alpha antagonist, phenoxybenzamine (Dibenzyline), induces sexual dysfunction frequently, Prazosin (Minipress) exerts its antihypertensive effect by selective blockage of post-synaptic alpha receptors which should theoretically be associated with an increased risk of failure of ejaculation (Pitts, 1974).

Depression of libido and impotence have been frequently associated with reserpine (alone or in combination), a drug that disrupts adrenergic function (Bullpitt and Dollery, 1973; Hollander and Wilkins, 1966). This is probably due in part to the mental depression caused by reserpine. Large dose levels of reserpine have been associated with elevated prolactin levels which could also impair testicular function. Boyden et al. (1980) examined pituitary and gonadal hormones before and after three months of antihypertensive therapy with either hydrochlorothiazide (100 mg/day) or reserpine (0.25 mg daily). They were able to show no significant differences in hormone levels as a result of drug therapy and no significant impairment of sexual function.

It has been difficult to determine if the increased incidence of impotence with antihypertensive drugs is entirely a drug side-effect or a cardiovascular complication of blood pressure changes (McNay, 1974). Studies that have attempted to correlate extent of control of hypertension with incidence of impotence have been complicated by the complexities inherent in antihypertensive therapy. In summary, it appears that impairment of sexual function is an important adverse effect of a number of antihypertensive drugs as well as hypertension itself. Possible mechanisms include disruption of autonomic function to the reproductive system, CNS sedation and depression, disturbances in reproductive hormones, and direct effects on arterial vascular smooth muscle. Attention to this adverse effect is imperative, since patient compliance is a problem in antihypertensive therapy. Further, dosage adjustments can sometimes result in an improvement in sexual functioning while the drug therapy continues.

CHEMOTHERAPEUTIC DRUGS

The third group of agents that may have effects on the reproductive system are the cancer chemotherapeutic agents. The targets of the anticancer drugs are the rapidly dividing cancer cells. These agents inhibit cell division by inhibiting the various steps in DNA, RNA and protein synthesis. Because these drugs lack selective toxicity, the major adverse side-effects are due to their toxic effects on other rapidly dividing cells including the germinal epithelium and glandular elements of the sex accessory organs (Schilsky and Erlichman, 1982; Sieber and Adamson, 1975).

The primary testicular lesion caused by anticancer drugs is depletion of the germinal epithelium lining the seminiferous tubules. In severe cases, testicular biopsy reveals complete germinal aplasia with only Sertoli cells left lining the tubule. The tubules appear atrophic and peritubular fibrosis is sometimes observed. There is a marked decrease in testicular volume with a marked increase in serum FSH levels. Subtle changes in Leydig cell function may be observed, but abnormalities in serum testosterone or changes in sex accessory gland function are not common.

The alkylating agents, particularly chlorambucil and cyclophosphamide, have been most fully investigated. Alkylating agents cause testicular damage with resultant azoospermia and absence of germinal cells on testicular biopsy. Fairley *et al.* (1972) reported that all samples of seminal fluid from 31 adult male patients who had received cyclophosphamide showed low sperm-counts. Serial counts that were done in six patients showed that 4 months or more of drug therapy was uniformly associated with azoospermia.

Sherins and De Vita (1973) evaluated reproductive function in 16 men who had been given combination cancer chemotherapy (an alkylating agent, vincristine, procarbazine or methotrexate, and steroid). When these patients were examined shortly after therapy, the combination drug therapy had produced germinal aplasia with resultant azoospermia in most patients. Biopsy specimens generally showed preservation of Sertoli and Leydig cells. Libido and potency were generally normal in these patients. In two men, in remission 4 and 7 years, spermatogenesis was normal at the time of evaluation. The data from this and other studies suggest that spermatogenesis may return after extensive chemotherapy, but it is more likely to return several years after drug treatment. Studies in children treated with cyclophosphamide for nephrotic syndrome show that young males are not spared the effects of these agents. In fact, it has been suggested that the pubertal male gonad is most sensitive to the effects of these agents (Kirkland, 1976). In summary, infertility caused by cancer chemotherapeutic agents is a common occurrence, and although it is likely to be reversible, it may last for up to 5 years after cessation of therapy. Testosterone levels, libido and secondary sex characteristics will be less affected than fertility, since the hormone producing cells apear to be more resistant to the drugs than the germinal epithelium. Nonetheless, patients on alkylating agents and combination chemotherapy should be warned of the possibility of permanent sterility but should also be informed that they may recover fertility with time.

DRUGS THAT INHIBIT THE SYNTHESIS, TRANSPORT, OR ACTIONS OF ANDROGENS

Cholesterol and steroid hormone synthesis are not easily inhibited by drugs. The synthesis of steroids is critically important to various aspects of bodily functions. There are agents (experimentally and clinically useful) that inhibit steroid synthesis. For example, metyrapone inhibits synthesis of certain adrenal steroids. *In vitro* testosterone synthesis can be inhibited by a number of other natural and synthetic steroids. In *in vivo* studies, however, most of these agents also have hypothalamic/pituitary actions as well.

It has been recently postulated that a number of drugs, particularly drugs of abuse, inhibit testosterone synthesis. Marijuana derivatives, phencyclidine (PCP) and alcohol are examples. Apparently, testicular metabolism of these drugs inhibits the enzymatic machinery for synthesis of testosterone. This direct effect has been difficult to demonstrate because some of these drugs have hypothalamic/pituitary effects as well. *In vitro* studies of isolated Leydig cells or decapsulated testis preparations have been used to demonstrate possible direct testicular effects. Interpretation of these studies is sometimes difficult because the active form of the drug may not be the parent compound that is added to the incubation medium. An interesting example of a drug that apparently works by this direct mechanism is alcohol. In 1977, Mendelson *et al.* published a study of 16 normal adult males during acute alcohol intoxication. The testosterone levels began to fall during the ascending phase of the blood alcohol curve, but LH levels were not altered. At peak blood alcohol levels (100 mg/dl), plasma testosterone levels were significantly depressed, and a significant increase in LH occurred. During the descending phase of the blood alcohol curve, testosterone levels remained depressed and LH decreased toward baseline. These results indicate that alcohol acts by a direct mechanism on testosterone synthesis and/or secretion.

Alcoholic cirrhosis is associated with hypogonadism, including testicular atrophy, abnormal testicular histology, seminal fluid defects, decreased libido and potency, and gynaecomastia (Chopra *et al.*, 1973; Gordon *et al.*, 1978). It has been assumed that defective hepatic metabolism in patients with liver disease leads to retention of oestrogens in the blood. These oestrogens suppress pituitary function and further decrease androgen secretion. These studies demonstrate the importance of normal liver function to the health of the reproductive system.

Administration of oestrogens in large doses to men is often asociated with decreased or absent libido, impotence and diminished formation of prostatic and seminal vesicle secretions. Oestrogen-induced alterations in hypothalamic function can affect both autonomic and hormonal activity.

Certain other drugs can be classified as having antiandrogenic properties because they antagonize the actions of androgens. These drugs produce their adverse side-effects at least in part by competing for androgen receptors in the androgenic target organs. Clofibrate and spironolactone probably act through this mechanism (Greenblatt and Koch-Weser, 1973). Medroxyprogesterone also antagonizes the action of androgens and can directly inhibit spermatogenesis.

MISCELLANEOUS DRUGS

There are other drugs, that have been reported to cause problems with sexual function, whose mechanisms are not at all well understood. Cimetidine, a new H_2 receptor blocker used to inhibit gastric hyperacidity, apparently causes some impairment of male sexual function, although its clinical use is too recent to make firm conclusions (Van Thiel *et al.*, 1979). Metronidazole, an antitrichamonal drug, is reported to cause a change in libido, but again the mechanism for this side-effect is not known.

Three commonly used anticholinergic drugs, clindinium bromide, dicyclomine HCl and isopropamide iodide, list impotence among the adverse side-effects of drug use. It is likely that impotence may result from inhibition of peripheral cholinergic sites. Other drugs that possess anticholinergic activity (e.g. tricyclic antidepressants) can also cause similar effects probably due in part to a peripheral mechanism.

CONCLUDING REMARKS

There are a number of types or classes of drugs that have potential for inhibiting the male reproductive system. This side-effect has received renewed attention for several important classes of drugs including CNS drugs, the chemotherapeutic agents, antihypertensive drugs, and a number of commonly abused drugs including alcohol and marijuana. Figure 4.1 summarizes the proposed sites of action for a number of these drug classes.

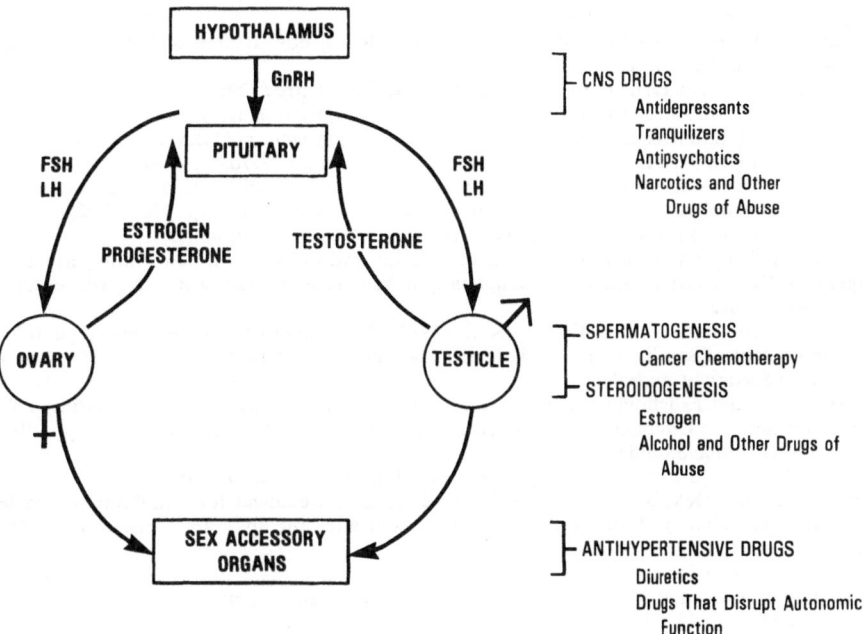

SUMMARY OF DRUG EFFECTS ON REPRODUCTIVE FUNCTION

Fig. 4.1 Summary of drug effects on reproductive function

MALE FERTILITY AND ITS REGULATION

References

Azizi, F., Vagenaki, A.G., Longcope, C., Ingbar, S.H., and Braverman, L.E. (1973). Decreased serum testosterone concentration in male heroin and methadone addicts. *Steroids*, **22**, 467-72

Boyden, T.W., Nugent, C.A., Ogihara, T, and Maeda T, (1980). Reserpine, hydrochlorothiazide and pituitary gonadal hormones in hypertensive patients. *Eur. J. Clin. Pharmacol.*, **17**, 329-32

Bullpitt. C.J., and Dollery, C.T., (1973). Side effects of hypertensive agents evaluated by a self-administered questionnaire. *Br. Med. J.*,**3**, 485-90

Chopra, I.J., Tulchinsky, D. and Greenway, F.L., (1973). Estrogen-androgen imbalance in men with hepatic cirrhosis. *Ann. Intern. Med.*, **79**, 198-203

Cicero, T., Bell, R., Weist, W., Allison, J.H., Polakoski, K. and Robins, E. (1975a). Function of the male sex organs in heroin and methadone users. *N. Engl. J. Med.*, **292**, 882-7

Cushman, P. (1972). Sexual behavior in heroin addiction and methadone maintenance. *N.Y. State J. Med.*, **72**, 1261-5

Fairley, K.F., Barrie, J.A. and Johnson, W. (1972). Sterility and testicular atrophy related to cyclophosphamine therapy. *Lancet*, **1**, 568-9

Gordon, G.G., Southern, A.L. and Lieber, C.S. (1978). The effects of alcoholic liver disease and alcohol ingestion on sex hormone levels. *Alcoholism: Clinical and Experimental Research*, **2**, 259-63

Greenblatt, D.J. and Koch-Weser, J. (1973). Gynecomastia and impotence: Complications of spironolactone therapy. *J. Am. Med. Assoc.*, **223**, 82

Hogen, M.J., Wallin, J.D. and Baer, R.M. (1980). Antihypertensive therapy and male sexual dysfunction. *Psychosomatics*, **21**, 234-7

Hollander, W. and Wilkins, R.W. (1966). The pharmacology and clinical use of rauwolfia, hydralazine, thiazides, and aldosterone antagonists in arterial hypertension. *Prog. Cardiovasc. Dis.*, **8**, 291-318

Khan, A., Camel, G. and Perry, H.M.J. (1970), Clonidine (catapres): A new antihypertensive agent. *Curr. Ther. Res.*, **12**, 10-12

Kirkland, R.T. (1976). Gonadotropin responses to LRF in boys treated with cyclophosphamide for nephrotic syndrome. *J. Pediatr.*, **89**, 941-4

Koch-Weser, J. (1976). Drug therapy: hydralazine. *N. Engl. J. Med.*, **295**, 68-9

McNay, J.L. (1974). Adrenolytic and vasodilator therapy. *Postgrad. Med.*, **56**, 76-80

Mendelson, J.H. and Mello, N.K. (1982). Hormones and psycho-sexual development in young men following chronic heroin use. *Neurobehavioral Toxicol and Teratol.*, **4**, 441-5

Mendelson, J.H., Mello, N.K. and Ellingboe, J (1977). Effects of acute alcohol intake on pituitary-gonadal hormones in normal human males. *J. Pharmacol. Exp. Ther.*, **202**, 676-82

Miller, R.A. (1976). Propranolol and impotence. *Ann. Intern. Med.*, **85**, 682-3

Pitts, N.E. (1974). The clinical evaluation of prazosin hydrochloride, a new antihypertensive agent. In Cotton (ed.), *Prazosin: Evaluation of a New Antihypertensive Agent*. (Amsterdam: Excerpta Medica)

Scher, P.M., Smith, C.G. and Almirez, R.G. (1983). The role of endogenous opioid peptides in the control of sex hormone levels in the male non-human primate. *Annual Meeting of American Society of Andrology*

Schilsky, R.L. and Erlichman, C. (1982). Late complications of chemotherapy: infertility and carcinogenesis. In Chabner, B. (ed.) *Pharmacologic Principles of Cancer Treatment*, pp. 109-131. (Philadelphia; Saunders)

Schmidt, C.W. and Lucas, M.J. (1977). Impotence. *Primary Care*, **2**, 275-80

Sherins, R.J. and DeVita, V.T. Jr. (1973). Effect of drug treatment for lymphoma on male reproductive capacity: Studies of men in remission after therapy. *Ann. Intern. Med.*, **79**, 216-20

Sieber, S.M. and Adamson, R.H. (1975). Toxicity of antineoplastic agents in man: chromosomal aberrations, antifertility effects, congenital malformations and carcinogenic potential. *Adv. Cancer Res.*, **22**, 57-144

Van Thiel, D.H., Gavaler. B.S., Smith, W.I. Jr. and Paul, G. (1979). Hypothalamic-pituitary-gonadal dysfunction in men using cimetidine. *N. Engl. J. Med.*, **300**, 1012-15

5
Reversible male infertility induced by sulphasalazine

C. O'MORAIN, P. SMETHURST, and A.J. LEVI

Sulphasalazine (Azulfidine) was first introduced over 40 years ago as treatment for rheumatoid arthritis. The idea was to use two 'wonder drugs' as one compound, sulphapyridine and 5'-aminosalicylate. It was noticed that a patient who had coexisting ulcerative colitis had a marked improvement in his bowel symptoms when taking sulphasalazine (Swartz, 1942). Since then many controlled trials have confirmed this fortuitous observation and its efficiency as treatment of both the acute form of the disease and as long-term therapy to prevent relapses (Misecwitz *et al.*, 1965). It has also been shown to be effective treatment of Crohn's disease particularly when it involves the large bowel (Summers *et al.*, 1979).

Ulcerative colitis and Crohn's disease have a peak age of onset in the late teens. The incidence of Crohn's disease is rising and is estimated to be 8 per 100 000, with more than a two fold increase in the last 20 years. The incidence of ulcerative colitis is static but is still more common than Crohn's disease. Both diseases are commonest in North Eastern Europe and the USA. The sex ratio of male to female is roughly equal. The cause of both conditions is unknown, as is the exact relationship of one to another and it is possible that they are a spectrum of one disease (Kirsner and Shorter, 1982a, b).

SULPHASALAZINE METABOLISM

Sulphasalazine is a compound drug (Fig. 5.1) consisting of sulphapyridine linked by an azo bond to 5'-aminosalicylic acid. A small amount of the parent molecule is absorbed in the small intestine and the remainder is split

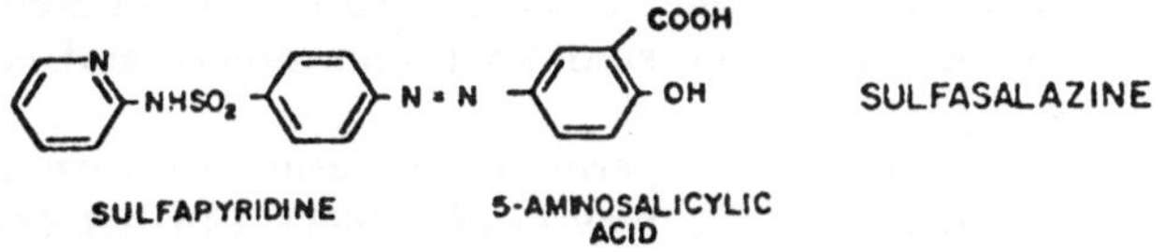

SULFAPYRIDINE   5-AMINOSALICYLIC ACID   SULFASALAZINE

Fig. 5.1 Structure of sulphasalazine

49

by caecal bacteria to its component molecules. Eighty per cent of the sul-phapyridine is absorbed and is either glucuronated or acetylated or both in the liver and excreted by the kidneys. Circulating blood levels of sulpha-pyridine can be used to monitor therapeutic levels. The rate of acetylation is genetically determined. Slow acetylators are more prone to side-effects and have high circulating levels of sulphapyridine (Das et al., 1973). The 5'-aminosalicylic acid is thought to be the therapeutically active part and to exert its effect locally. There is, however, evidence that the parent molecule is the active component. The exact way in which sulphasalazine exerts its therapeutic effect is not known. However, it has anti-prostaglandin effects, causes a decreased leukocyte chemotaxis, may alter immune function and has antibacterial properties.

SIDE-EFFECTS OF SULPHASALAZINE

The side-effects of sulphasalazine can be divided into two groups. The incidence of side-effects is estimated to occur in 30% of patients but are relatively mild. The first group is dose related, acetylator phenotype depen-dent and therefore predictable. These would include generalized side-effects such as nausea, vomiting, malaise as well as haemolytic anaemia, reticulo-cytosis and methaemoglobulinaemia. The second major group of side-effects are hypersensitivity reactions that occur in an idiosyncratic manner, skin rash, aplastic anaemia, hepatic and pulmonary dysfunction and auto-immune haemolysis. These side-effects are not dose related and usually occur soon after commencement of treatment. Some side-effects can be overcome by a desensitization programme of slowly introducing the drug (Taffet and Das, 1983). Reversible male infertility has only recently been described as a side-effect of sulphasalazine and is dose related. It has been estimated by Pharmacia that approximately 1.8–2.5 million people are tak-ing sulphasalazine in the USA, a significant proportion of whom will be males in the reproductive age.

REVERSIBLE MALE INFERTILITY INDUCED BY SULPHASALAZINE

Male infertility due to sulphasalazine was first described by our group in Great Britain (Levi et al., 1979) and simultaneously and independently by Toth (1979) in the USA. Since then there have been numerous reports confirming this observation from many different parts of the world (Birnie et al., 1981; Freeman et al., 1982; Collen, 1980.). This side-effect is dose related, appears to be due to the sulphapyridine moiety and is more pro-nounced in slow acetylator phenotypes.

The effect is reversible in that sperm counts return to normal 3 months after withdrawal of the drug (Toovey et al., 1981). Further evidence that the antifertility effect is reversible in humans is that pregnancies occurred following drug withdrawal. One resulted in early abortion but the rest were all full-term normal deliveries and there were no fetal abnormalities. The median time of conception was 2.5 months, suggesting an effect on early spermatogenesis (O'Morain et al., 1983a).

ANIMAL MODELS OF SULPHASALAZINE-INDUCED REVERSIBLE MALE INFERTILITY

In an effort to understand the mechanism by which sulphasalazine exerts its effect on sperm function, male Sprague-Dawley rats were fed sulphasalazine. Subsequently the treated animals bred and the litter size from bred females were significantly decreased compared to controls. The effect was dose related and more marked at the higher doses but the litter size was never reduced to zero (O'Morain et al., 1983a). A time course was plotted by serially introducing two virgin females to the males at 3 weeks and 5 weeks. The number of females pregnant at 5 weeks in the control and treated groups increased but the litter size was as low as at 3 weeks in the treated groups. This was evidence that sulphasalazine did not interfere with libido. When the component molecules, sulphapyridine and 5'-aminosalicylic acid were given to male rats and then mated, the litter size was only reduced in those who recovered sulphapyridine. A closer analysis of the reversibility was performed by mating the treated animals with two successive females at 6–10, 10–14 and 14–18 days after sulphasalazine withdrawal. The effect was fully reversible at 18 days (O'Morain et al., 1983a).

The effect was dose related and litter size was most reduced in animals receiving the higher dose of 617 mg/kg bodyweight. These results suggest that the drug may exert its effect on sperm function by disabling sperm stored in the epididymis or by a direct effect on the sperm. Other drugs such as α-chlorohydrin and chlorinated sugars have been shown to affect stored sperm (Ford, 1980). These drugs inhibit glyceraldehyde phosphate dehydrogenase activity resulting in insufficient energy for motility (Ford and Waites, 1980). Because sulphasalazine and the chlorinated sugars have similar recovery time courses spermatozoa were collected from the caput epididymis of rats treated with sulphasalazine (617 mg/kg weight for 8 weeks) and who had reduced litter size when mated. Controls were fed a normal diet. Sperm motility was assessed by measuring the area change frequency with an image analysing computer.

[U-^{14}C] glucose was incubated with sperm and seminiferous tubules and the energy change and $^{14}CO_2$ production was measured. The testes and accessory sex glands were weighed and examined histologically. There was no difference in sperm count, motility or production of energy and CO_2. Further there were no gross weight or histological changes in the sex glands. This suggests that sulphasalazine has a direct effect on the sperm and that its mechanism of action differs from that of α-chlorohydrin and the chlorinated sugars (O'Morain et al., 1983b).

Studies on the mouse and the hamster have confirmed these observations in the rat. Spermatozoa obtained from mice fed 617 mg/kg body weight were unable to undergo the acrosome reaction but had normal whiplash motility, Spermatozoa from hamsters fed sulphasalazine (617 mg/kg body weight) were incubated with eggs *in vitro*. A significantly decreased sperm penetration rate was observed despite their normal motility and count (O'Morain *et al.*, 1983c).

This qualitative abnormality of rat sperm has also been confirmed *in vivo*. Female rats bred to treated males were killed 24 hours after mating. The number of eggs at the two cell stage was dratically reduced compared to controls, indicating an inability of the treated sperm to penetrate the egg.

In summary the animal experiments show that sulphasalazine induces a reversible dose-dependent infertility in rat, mouse and hamster. The sperm count, motility and glucose metabolism appears normal. There was both *in vivo* and *in vitro* evidence to indicate a qualitative effect on sperm function (functional sterility). The time course suggests that the effect is on the later stages of sperm maturation. The sperm also appear unable to undergo the acrosome reaction.

HUMAN STUDIES

Further studies in humans, taking sulphasalazine have shown that a significant fall in sperm count, a decrease in motility and an increase in the number of abnormal forms occurs. Some patients apparently conceived children while on the drug. This emphasizes that the laboratory parameters are not absolute indicators of fertility. The effect was not due to inflammatory bowel disease as patients on no treatment had normal semen parameters even though these patients were more ill than treated patients. The effect is not mediated hormonally as gonadotrophin-releasing hormone test profiles while on and off the drug, were almost identical. Seminal plasma parameters including acid phosphatase, and fructose were normal in treated patients (O'Morain *et al.*, 1983a). Zinc has been reported to be low in inflammatory bowel disease (Solomons *et al.*, 1977) and low zinc levels have been implicated in male infertility (Stanwell-Smith *et al.*, 1983). However the seminal zinc levels were normal. It was also noted that the sperm of patients on sulphasalazine treatment had a characteristic 'megalo' form head. This had been confirmed by flow cytometry (O'Morain *et al.*, 1983d). Folate deficiency is associated with megaloblastic anaemia. Sulphasalazine has been shown to inhibit intestinal folate transport and the enzymes dihydrofolate reductase, methylenetetrahydrofolate reductase and serine transhydromethylene (Selhub *et al.*, 1978). The megalo form head could be induced by the anti-folate effects of sulphasalazine. However, giving patients large doses of folate failed to improve the sperm counts whereas withdrawal of sulphasalazine did. In addition seminal folate was normal in treated patients. Large doses of aspirin have been reported to induce male infertility through its antiprostaglandin effect (Didolkar *et al.*, 1980), however very little of the 5'-aminosalicylic acid (a similar compound to aspirin) is absorbed and seminal prostaglandin levels were normal.

Another hypothesis for the mechanism of action is that sulphasalazine and sulphapyridine inhibit enzymes in the acrosomal membrane. The large head may merely reflect membrane damage due to the resulting leakage. It may also represent the release of immature sperm as condensation of the sperm head occurs late in sperm maturation.

The sperm function of sulphasalazine-treated patients, even those with good sperm counts is impaired as assessed by their ability to penetrate zona free hamster eggs *in vitro* (O'Morain *et al.* 1984). Fertilization rates indicate that sperm from fertile males penetrate zona free hamster eggs at a greater rate than sperm from infertile males, this effect is independent of normal semen analysis parameters (Rogers *et al.*, 1979). *In vitro* fertilization using the zona free hamster egg model detects qualitative sperm abnormalities (Hall, 1981). Sulphasalazine therefore induces a qualitative as well as a quantitative abnormality of sperm.

CONCLUDING REMARKS

Sulphasalazine has been available for the past 40 years but an important side-effect, reversible male infertility, has only been described recently. With present screening procedures for new drugs, this side-effect would be noted earlier. It is important that doctors should be aware of the side-effects of this drug commonly prescribed for inflammatory bowel disease. This observation has given a stimulus to drug manufacturers to search for more effective and side-effect free drugs for the treatment of inflammatory bowel disease. Sulphasalazine is thought only to act as a carrier molecule. Other drugs are currently available which will deliver 5'-aminosalicylic acid to the colon and avert this side-effect.

Sulphasalazine also induces a reversible infertility in humans and in laboratory animals. Research to date indicates that it has both a qualitative and quantitative effect on human sperm, but only a qualitative effect on the sperm of other animals.

Sulphapyridine induces this effect. The relative non-toxicity of this compound makes it an attractive compound to investigate as a possible male contraceptive. The exact mechanism still remains to be elucidated. Further research with this class of chemicals may lead to an effective male contraceptive.

Acknowledgements

We are grateful to Mrs Maureen Moriarty for secretarial assistance.

References

Birnie, G.G., McLeod, T.I.F. and Watkinson, G. (1981). Incidence of sulfasalazine induced male infertility. *Gut*, **22**, 452–5

Collen, MJ. (1980). Azulfidine induced oligospermia. *Am, J. Gastrol.*, **74**, 441–2

Das, K.M., Eastwood, M.A., McManus, J.P.A. and Sircus, W. (1973). The metabolism of salicylazosulphapyridine in ulcerative colitis. I. The relationship between metabolites and response to treatment in inpatients. II. The relationship between metabolism and progress of the disease studied in outpatients. *Gut*, **14**, 631–6

Didolkar, A.K., Gurjar, A., Joshi, U.M., Sheth, A.R. and Roychowdhury, D. (1980). Effects of aspirin on blood plasma levels of testosterone, LH and FSH in maturing male rats. *Int. J. Andrology*, **3**, 312–18

Ford, W.C.L. (1980). The contraceptive effect of 6-chloro-6-deoxysugars in the male. In Cunningham, G.R., Schill, W.B. and Hafez, E.S.E. (eds.) *Regulation of Male Fertility*. Vol. 1, pp. 123–126. (London: Martinus Nighoff).

Ford, W.C.L. and Waites, G.M.H. (1980). The control of male infertility by 6-chloro-6-deoxysugars. *Reprod. Nutr. Dev.*, **20**, 101–9

Freeman, J.G., Reece, V.A.C. and Venables, C.W. (1982). Sulfasalazine and spermatogenesis. *Digestion*, **23**, 68–71

Hall, J.R. (1981). Relationship between semen quality and human sperm penetration of zona free hamster ova. *Fertil. Steril.*, **35**, 457–63

Hudson, E., Doré, C., Sowter, C., Toovey, S. and Levi, A.J. (1982). Sperm size in patients with inflammatory bowel disease on sulfasalazine therapy. *Fertil. Steril.*, **38**, 77–83

Kirsner, J.B. and Shorter, R.G. (1982a). Recent developments in non-specific inflammatory bowel disease (first of two parts). *N. Engl. J. Med.*, **306**, 775–85

Kirsner, J.B. and Shorter, R.G. (1982b). Recent developments in non-specific inflammatory bowel disease (second of two parts). *N. Engl. J. Med.*, **306**, 837–48

Levi, A.J., Fisher, A.M., Hughes, L. and Hendry, W.F. (1979). Male infertility due to sulfasalazine. *Lancet*, **2**, 276–8

Misecwitz, J.J., Lennard Jones, J.F., Connell, A.M., Baron, J.H. and Jones, F.A. (1965). Controlled trial of sulfasalazine in maintenance therapy of ulcerative colitis. *Lancet*, **1**, 185–8

O'Morain, C., Smethurst, P., Levi, A. (1983a). Reversible male infertility due to sulfasalazine. Studies in man and rat. *Gut*, in press.

O'Morain, C., Smethurst, P., Levi, A.J., Ford, W.C.L., Harrison, A., Setchell, B.P. and Dott, H.M. (1983b). The effect of sulfasalazine on motility and glucose oxidation in rat spermatozoa. Manuscript in preparation.

O'Morain, C., Smethurst, P., Levi, A.J., Fraser, L. and Moore, H.D. (1983c). Male infertility due to sulfasalazine in laboratory animals. In press.

O'Morain, C., Edwards, A., Smethurst, P. and Levi A.J. (1983d). Abnormal sperm morphology induced by sulfasalazine assessed by flow cytometry. Manuscript in preparation.

O'Morain, C., Moore, H., Smethurst, P. and Levi, A.J. (1984). Sulfasalazine inhibits sperm penetration of the zona free hamster egg. Submitted for publication.

Rogers, B.J., Van Campen, H., Ueno, M., Lamber, H., Bronson, R. and Hale, R. (1979). Analysis of human spermatozoa fertilizing ability using zona free ova. *Fertil. Steril.* **32**, 664–70

Selhub, J., Dhar, G.J. and Rosenberg, I.H. (1978). Inhibition of folate enzymes by sulfasalazine. *J. Clin. Invest.*, **61**, 221–4

Solomons, N.W., Rosenberg, I.H., Sandstead, H.H. and Vo-Khachu, K. (197). Zinc deficiency in Crohn's disease. *Digestion*, **16**, 87–95

Stanwell-Smith, R., Thompson, S.G., Haines, A.P., Ward, R.J., Cashmore, C., Hendry, W.F. and Stedronska, J. (1983). A comparative study of fertile and infertile men: I. Zinc Copper, cadmium and lead levels. *Fertil. Steril.* In press.

Summers, R.W., Switz, D.M., Sessions, J.T., Becktel, J.M., Best, W.R., Kern, F. and Singleton, J.W. (1979). National cooperative Crohn's disease study. Results of drug treatment. *Gastroenterology*, **77**, 847–9

Swartz, N. (1942). Salazopyrin, a new sulfanilamide preparation. *Acta Med. Scand.*, **110**, 185–8

Taffet, S.L. and Das, K.M. (1983). Sulfasalazine adverse effects and desensitization. *Am. J. Dig. Dis.*, **28**, 833–42

Toovey, S., Hudson, E., Hendry, W. and Levi, A.J. (1981). Sulfasalazine and male infertility. Reversibility and possible mechanism. *Gut*, **22**, 443–51

Toth, A. (1979). Reversible toxic effects of salicylazosulphapyridine on semen quality. *Fertil. Steril.*, **31**, 538–40

6
Effects of illicit drugs on male reproduction

J. HARCLERODE and C.G. SMITH

Maturation, maintenance, and regulation of normal reproductive capacity in the male is a complex and highly integrated phenomenon. It requires proper nutritional and hormonal support, not only by the hormones directly involved in reproduction, but also the synergistic action of hormones produced by other endocrine organs throughout the body. The regulation of many endocrine organs in the body is through the hypothalamus, an area of the central nervous system (CNS) which is sensitive to chemical, hormonal, and sensory input from all parts of the body. Therefore, one can understand why drugs which alter neural function in various parts of the CNS so powerfully affect the output of hormones from the hypothalamus and trophic hormones from the pituitary. This review will attempt to summarize the effects that illicit drugs of abuse have on the male reproductive system.

The hypothalamus contains neurosecretory neurons which are responsible for the synthesis and secretion of factors that regulate the release of the hormones elaborated by the anterior lobe of the pituitary gland. A single hypothalamic factor seems to be responsible for the release of both luteinizing hormone (LH) and follicle stimulating hormone (FSH) and this factor is gonadotropin releasing hormone (GnRH). The secretion of GnRH is affected by a variety of factors which include neural, chemical, hormonal, and drugs. Release of GnRH is regulated by the neural transmitters of the hypothalamus. Thus, factors which alter dopamine and norepinephrine also alter GnRH release. Generally, substances which enhance the release of norepinephrine stimulate the release of GnRH. Those substances, such as drugs which stimulate dopaminergic release, inhibit the hypothalamic release of GnRH with subsequent reduction in LH secretion (Yen *et al.*, 1978).

The regulation of the hormonal events involved in the regulation of reproductive function in the male is summarized in Fig. 6.1. The gonadotropins, FSH and LH, are released in response to GnRH and transported to the testis via the general circulation. LH stimulates the Leydig cells between the seminiferous tubules to produce testosterone. FSH stimulates the seminiferous tubules to induce sperm production. Testosterone, necessary

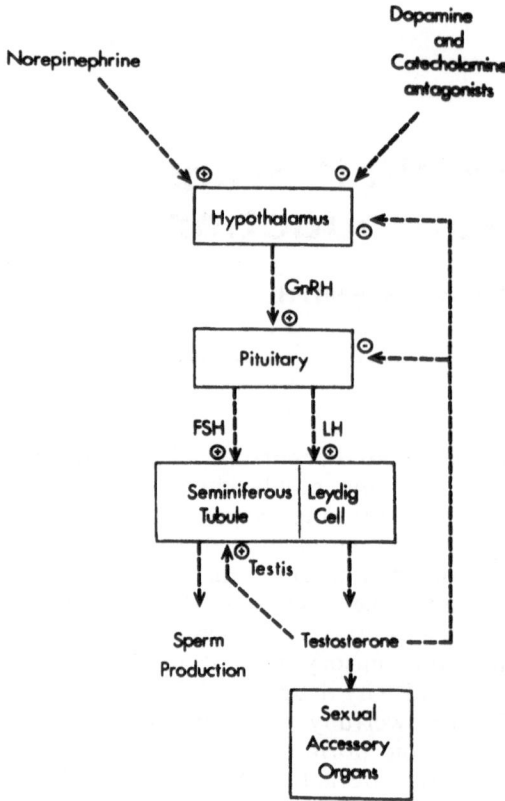

Fig. 6.1 Hormonal regulation of male reproductive function

for proper sperm production, is also needed for growth and normal secretory activity of the sexual accessory organs such as the prostate and seminal vesicles. Testosterone acts at the hypothalamus to inhibit GnRH release and at the pituitary to inhibit LH release, thus decreasing the Leydig cell stimulation of its own production. Testosterone acts at other levels of the central nervous system to elicit sexual behaviour.

Drugs of abuse may affect male reproduction by acting at several different levels. Some drugs such as the CNS stimulants and CNS depressants alter norepinephrine and dopaminergic pathways. The exact mechanism for this is not known but it may involve interference with synthesis, reuptake, or release of the neural transmitters in the area of the hypothalamus that controls the GnRH release. The drug-induced alteration of GnRH levels produce a corresponding alteration of LH and FSH release from the pituitary with a subsequent effect on the seminiferous tubules and Leydig cells of the testis. Thus, in an indirect manner, the drugs may alter sperm production or testosterone synthesis due to action on the CNS. Drugs that act in this fashion usually produce changes in the reproductive system that are reversible upon cessation of drug treatment. Such changes might include production of abnormal sperm, impotency, reduced seminal volume, and ejaculatory problems.

Drugs of abuse may have a direct action on the various organs of the male reproductive system. Drugs that act directly on the testis may produce irreversible damage and cause infertility. Such damage may be exhibited by genetic damage as a result of alteration of spermatogenesis in the tubules. There may also be direct action of drugs on various enzyme systems involved in the biosynthesis of testosterone by the Leydig cells or inhibition of certain enzyme systems needed for proper functioning of accessory organs so that the quality and quantity of semen may be altered.

MARIJUANA

The marijuana plant (*Cannabis sativa*) grows ubiquitously throughout the temperate regions of the world. Although it contains many compounds, only one of these, delta-9-tetrahydrocannabinol (THC) is responsible for the major psychotrophic effects. It is possible that the non-psychoactive compounds in marijuana may have a direct effect on the organs associated with reproduction in the male. However, it appears that the psychoactive ingredient, THC, is responsible for most of the hormonal changes that are seen after marijuana use. Figure 6.2 summarizes most of these changes. There are reports in the literature that marijuana use causes disruption of normal reproductive function in male laboratory animals, Rhesus monkeys, and man.

Considerable research effort was expended over the past 10 years to examine the effects of marijuana on male reproductive function. In 1973, Marks reported that luteinizing hormone levels in ovariectomized rats were inhibited by THC. He concluded that the action of THC may be due to its ability to increase the uptake and retention of catecholamines by the brain tissues which would, in effect, produce an inhibition of GnRH release from the hypothalamus. Symons *et al.* (1976) showed that either acute or chronic treatment of rats with THC produced a decrease in both plasma luteinizing hormone and testosterone. Although Collu *et al.* (1975) reported a reduction of plasma LH levels in prepubertal male rats treated with THC they were unable to find any change in FSH. Dalterio *et al.* (1978) showed that oral administration of THC to male mice resulted in reduced plasma testosterone, LH, and FSH levels. However, cannabinol (CBN), a non-psychoactive ingredient, had no effect on these three hormones.

Male Rhesus monkeys responded to THC treatment with a 65% reduction in serum testosterone levels which returned to normal over a three-day period. The depression in LH levels was comparable in magnitude and duration to the depression in testosterone (Smith *et al.*, 1976) indicating that the THC-induced inhibition of male sex hormones was due to its action on the hypothalamus or pituitary. THC treatment of female ovariectomized monkeys produced a 68% reduction in LH levels and a 56% reduction in FSH levels. The maximum decrease occurred at the same time for both gonadotropins. Moreover, the decrease in both LH and FSH were equiva-

MARIJUANA

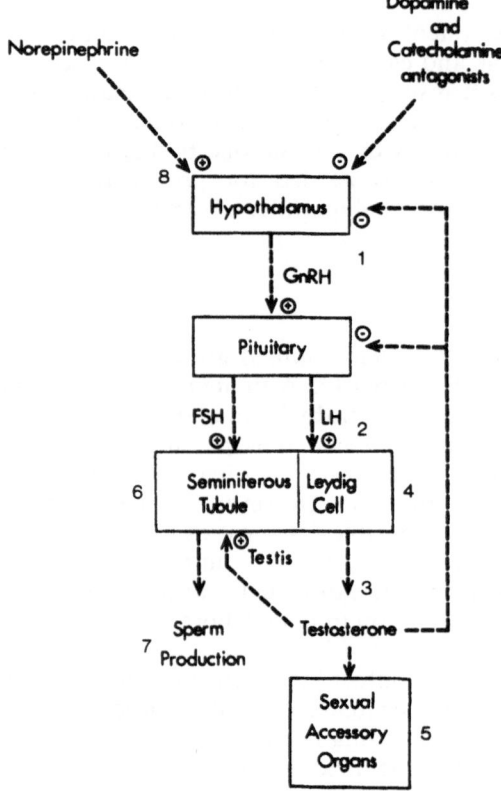

Fig. 6.2 Sites of action of marijuana (THC) on the male reproductive system. The psychoactive THC in marijuana causes decreased release of GnRH (1). The THC-induced decrease in GnRH yields reduced FSH and LH (2) secretion from the anterior pituitary with subsequent reduction in testosterone production by the testis (3). There may be direct effects of THC, and perhaps some of the non-psychoactive cannabinoids found in marijuana, on the sexual accessory organs (5) and on the seminiferous tubules (6) to affect sperm production (7), although some of the effects on sperm are due to lowered testosterone production (3) and perhaps due to reduced FSH (2). THC affects other hypothalamic releasing hormones to cause hormonal changes which might indirectly have an effect on male reproductive function (8). These include decreased prolactin, increased ACTH with subsequent adrenal cortical hormone elevations, and depressed thyroid hormone levels

lent in response to equal doses of THC. This response was found whether the THC was administered as a pure substance or as the same percentage in crude marijuana extract (CME) (Smith *et al.*, 1979a). These data indicate that the inhibitory action of marijuana on gonadotropin levels is produced by THC. Other cannabis derivatives contained in marijuana do not contribute to the effect since neither cannabidiol (CBD) nor CBN had any significant effect on gonadotropin levels at reasonable dosages. Thus, it appears that the inhibitory effect of cannabis derivatives on gonatrophins is related to their psychoactivity.

It is also possible that certain non-psychoactive cannabinoids found in marijuana smoke, which may not be involved in altering hormonal changes in the hypothalamus, pituitary, or the testis, may contribute to a direct effect on other reproductive structures. Such effects may be on sperm production, interference with hormonal effects on growth and secretory activity of accessory sex organs, interaction with hormones at the target tissue level, and altering the receptors for hormones at target tissues.

The pharmacological site of action of THC on gonadotropin levels is probably mediated through some action to reduce GnRH secretion. Administration of GnRH to Rhesus monkeys that had previously received a blocking dosage of THC reversed the THC-induced reduction in LH and FSH (Smith *et al.*, 1979a). Similar data have been reported for the ovariectomized rat (Tyrey, 1978). Thus, it appears that THC blocks GnRH release from the hypothalamus since the pituitary is capable of responding to exogenous GnRH in the presence of THC.

It seems likely that the observed THC-induced suppression of gonadotropin output arises indirectly from an action of THC upon the hypothalamus and not through a direct effect on the pituitary. In view of the psychoactive nature of THC, it is possible that it alters neural transmitter substances throughout the brain, and, especially in that region of the hypothalamus that regulates GnRH release. Some studies have shown that THC affects neural transmitter substances in certain areas of the brain. Kramer and Ben-David (1974) have shown that alteration of serotonin and dopamine may be responsible for the inhibitory effect of THC on prolactin. THC also prevented reuptake of dopamine, norepinephrine, and serotonin into respective nerve endings throughout the brain (Hershkowitz *et al.*, 1977).

Testis and accessory reproductive organs

Prolonged exposure to THC significantly reduced the weight of ventral prostate, seminal vesicles, and epididymis in rats which was correlated with decreased plasma testosterone levels and accompanied by a reduced number of sperm in the fluids of the epididymis (Fujimoto *et al.*, 1978). These effects were reversible for the organ weights returned to control levels by 30 days after cessation of drug treatment. Similar findings were reported by Dixit and Lohiya (1975) for the castrated male mouse and by Vyas and Singh (1976) for pigeons.

THC may have a direct affect on the tissue of the testis. Administration of THC to hypophysectomized rats blocked the stimulatory effect of human chorionic gonadotropin on ventral prostate and seminal vesicle weights (Purohit *et al.*, 1979). Also, THC prevented the testosterone-induced changes in DNA, RNA, protein content, acid phosphatase, and an isoenzyme variant of acid phosphatase in the ventral prostate tissues of adult castrated rats (Ghosh *et al.*, 1981).

Both marijuana smoking and exposure to THC affect the quality and quantity of sperm produced by the testis. Among the testicular changes that have been reported are seminal tubule degeneration, interference with sperm maturation (Rosenkrantz and Hayden, 1979), increased numbers of abnormal sperm (including ring and chain translocation), heads without hooks, banana shaped heads, amorphous heads, and folded heads (Zimmerman *et al.*, 1979a). Rats exposed to marijuana smoke for 75 days had a decreased number of epididymal sperm and an increased number of sperm with head to tail dissociations. The testes were reduced in weight as were the seminal vesicles.

THC may interfere with meiotic processes involved in sperm production. Mice treated with THC had a higher frequency of unpaired sex chromosomes at metaphase than did controls. Other chromosomal aberrations reported to be produced by cannabinoids included ring and chain translocation, and an increased incidence of aneuploidy. Also, the F_1 male offspring of cannabinoid-exposed males that successfully impregnated females produced litters with a higher incidence of developmental anomalies or litters that exhibited chromosomal rearrangements (Dalterio *et al.*, 1982).

Several studies may help to explain the reduced sperm production as well as the abnormal sperm that were reported in the semen after treatment of animals with various cannabinoids. *In vitro* studies by Jacubovic and McGeer (1977), where various cannabinoids were incubated with testicular slices or testicular cell suspensions, showed suppression of incorporation of radioactive amino acids into nucleic acids, lipids, and proteins. It appears that the consequence of cannabinoid treatment may be direct inhibition of the kinases and/or polymerases involved in nucleic acid synthesis. The inhibition of protein synthesis may be a result of decreased nucleic acids which could ultimately lead to alterations in spermatogenesis.

Cannabinoids may affect various enzymes in the testis. Cannabidiol and THC produced a decrease in both microsomal cytochrome P-450 from Leydig cells (an enzyme which is involved in the biosynthesis of testosterone) and γ-glutamyl transpeptidase (GTP) (a marker protein for Sertoli cells in the seminiferous tubules of the testis). Normal levels of cytochrome P-450 and GTP were restored when exogenous LH and FSH were supplied to the THC-treated animals. Therefore, some of the enzymatic defects caused by cannabinoid exposure may be prevented if normal levels of gonadotropins are maintained. These data also indicate that cannabinoid effects on the testis might be due to defects of pituitary hormones rather than by direct action of the drug on the testis.

In vitro studies have also indicated that THC may affect the enzymes that are involved in the biosynthesis of testosterone by Leydig cells. Among the enzymatic steps that appear to be affected are the conversion of pregnenolone into progesterone, the conversion of cholesterol into pregnenolone, and the alteration of enzymes which affect the availability of precursor cholesterol thereby inhibiting cholesterol esterase (Burstein *et al.*, 1978a, b, 1979; Shoupe *et al.*, 1980).

Human males

Controversy exists about the effects of marijuana smoking on reproductive functions of the human male. For instance, acute marijuana smoking decreased both LH and testosterone levels in the blood, an effect that lasted for up to 3 hours; however, no change was detected in FSH levels (Cohen, 1976; Kolodny et al., 1976; Jones, 1977). Also, Kolodny et al. (1974) reported that marijuana smoking decreased the blood levels of testosterone but had no effect on LH, FSH, or prolactin. Other workers (Coggins et al., 1976; Mendelson et al., 1974b, 1976; Nahas, 1976) were unable to find any changes in plasma testosterone.

Marijuana smoking by human males appears to affect the quality of the semen. Among the seminal alterations reported were decreased sperm count, reduced concentration of sperm, decreased sperm motility, and an increase in the number of sperm exhibiting abnormal morphology including aberrations of the nucleus. The sperm aberrations may be due to an effect of marijuana on spermatogenesis, due to changes in the sperm as they pass through the epididymis, or due to failure to complete sperm maturation. As in the studies with laboratory animals, once marijuana treatment ended there was a gradual return to apparently normal gonadal activity (Hembree et al., 1979). Several other studies (Issidorides, 1979; Stefanis and Issidorides, 1976) reported sperm aberrations in ejaculated semen. Among the abnormalities reported were spongy, fuzzy, and disorganized layers of acrosomal substance, sperm with incomplete condensation of chromatin, sperm with no acrosomes, and sperm which had arrested maturation.

Prolactin

There are conflicting reports on the effect of THC to increase or decrease prolactin levels in the pituitary and in the serum. Some of the apparent conflicts can be explained by method of administration and dosage of THC. Intraventricular injection of THC in prepubertal and adult rats caused an increased level of prolactin in the pituitary which was not accompanied by changes in brain levels of norepinephrine, dopamine, or serotonin (Collu, 1976). Kramer and Ben-David (1974) however, reported suppression of prolactin release by acute THC treatment, an effect that was abolished by administration of the serotonin antagonist, cyprohepatidine, or with the dopamine antagonists, perphenazine and chemozine. High doses of THC administered to male rats produced a marked suppression of prolactin as short as 15 minutes after injection, and the release of prolactin in ether-stressed rats was blocked by THC (Bromley et al., 1977). Similarly, mice had reduced plasma prolactin levels in stressed and non-stressed males after a single dose of THC (Dalterio et al., 1981). Smith et al. (1979b) and Asch et al. (1979) have shown that administration of THC produced a short-lived inhibition of prolactin levels in the serum of male Rhesus monkeys. Administration of thyrotropin releasing hormone (TRH) reversed the suppression indicating that the hypothalamus was the site of action of the THC-induced depression of prolactin release.

From these data and other experiments it appears that THC produces a prompt depression of prolactin secretion from the pituitary gland of the male. The exact mechanism of this inhibition is not known, but it probably acts on the hypothalamus to alter secretion of the several neural trasmitters which are involved in regulating prolactin release from the pituitary gland. The effect of THC to inhibit release of prolactin, LH, and FSH from the pituitary appears to be unique and in apparent contrast to many other psychoactive drugs which stimulate prolactin release while inhibiting secretion of both LH and FSH.

Adrenal cortical hormones

Marijuana has been shown to affect plasma levels of other hormones which are not directly involved in reproduction but whose secretion is needed for proper support and function of the reproductive organs. Adrenal cortical hormones may alter reproductive function of the male, especially in those instances when the animal is stressed. Exposure to cannabinoids prompted a rise in corticosterone levels in the plasma of both rats and mice over a wide range of dosages. Other indications of adrenal cortical activation by THC treatment are a decrease in adrenal ascorbic acid (Dewey et al., 1970), a decrease in adrenal cortical cholesterol, and an increase in unesterified fatty acids (Maier and Maitre, 1975).

There is conflicting evidence regarding the acquisition of tolerance to the plasma corticosterone elevation of THC. Birmingham and Bartova (1976) reported a disappearance of the response of THC to elevate plasma corticosterone after 8 days of treatment and Pertwee (1974) showed a developing tolerance to the effects of THC on corticosterone levels in mouse plasma. However, Mitra et al. (1977) found no evidence of tolerance after 21 days of THC treatment using fairly high dosages of THC.

The question of whether THC acts as a general systemic stressor to elicit the elevation of plasma corticosterone was examined by Bromley and Zimmerman (1976). Their results indicated that, unlike most stressful stimuli, acute administration of THC caused a depression of prolactin but stimulated corticosterone release. Generally, stress causes an increase in both prolactin and corticosterone levels in male rats.

Several studies have examined whether THC acts directly on the adrenal cortex or whether it acts by way of the central nervous system to stimulate release of ACTH, thereby increasing the stimulation of adrenal cortical hormones. Hypophysectomized rats treated with THC were unable to respond with an increase in plasma corticosterone levels which eliminated the possibility that THC acts directly on adrenal cortex (Barry et al., 1973). Puder et al. (1982) showed that when adult male rats with a completely deafferentiated hypothalamus were injected with THC, there was no significantly altered serum concentration of either ACTH or corticosteroids.

These results demonstrated that extrahypothalamic sites and/or neural pathways mediate the affect of THC to increase corticosterone secretion. Further evidence for central action of THC comes from a study that employed the dopamine receptor antagonists, perphenazine and pimazide (Malor et al., 1978). Dopamine is involved in eliciting the response of ACTH release. The two dopamine receptor antagonists blocked the THC-induced rise in plasma corticosterone which increased plasma non-esterified fatty acids. Agents which block ACTH secretion from the pituitary (pentobarbitol and dexamethasone) prevented the adrenal cortical response to THC which indicated that the response was centrally mediated and required the presence of functional dopaminergic receptors for it to be elicited (Malor *et al.*, 1978; Mitra *et al.*, 1977).

Not all the effects of cannabinoids on adrenal cortical function are due to the effect they have to stimulate ACTH release. Several investigators have shown that addition of various cannabinoids to incubation medium in which cultured adrenal cortical cells were grown prevented the cells from responding to added ACTH (Carchman *et al.*, 1976; Warner *et al.*, 1977). There is evidence of a direct effect of THC on enzymatic processes involved in steroidogenesis presumably at a biochemical step between cyclic AMP production and pregnenolone production (Warner *et al.*, 1977) and perhaps inhibition of cholesterol esterase activity similar to that found in Leydig cells (Burstein *et al.*, 1978b).

Thyroid hormones

Thyroid function is apparently altered by marijuana. Among the alterations reported were depressed accumulation of radioactive iodine in the thyroid gland (Miras, 1965) and decreased release of radioactive iodine from the thyroid glands which was reversed by injection of thyroid stimulating hormone (TSH) (Lomax, 1970). A depression of serum thyroxine levels in the rat has also been reported (Nazar *et al.*, 1977). Administration of TSH, however, elevated serum thyroxine indicating that the THC action was at the level of the hypothalamus and not on the thyroid gland directly. Tolerance was reported to develop after 14 days of twice daily treatment.

ALCOHOL

A very high proportion of alcoholics complain of sexual dysfunction. Among the complaints most frequently reported for alcoholic men are: feminization (including gynaecomastia and changes in bodily hair), impotence, decreased libido, testicular atrophy, and sterility. Research workers have examined the effect of alcohol in altering hormone biosynthesis and metabolism, hormone transport by binding proteins in the plasma, conversion of androgen precursors into oestrogenic substances, and metabolism of sex steroids in the cirrhotic liver (Fig. 6.3).

Van Thiel *et al.* (1975a) showed that the alcohol-reduced plasma testosterone levels in rats was accompanied by marked testicular, prostatic, and seminal vesicle atrophy. Nutritional factors could not account for the sexual defects, since the rats received a diet that was nutritionally balanced but had a high proportion of its caloric content (36%) as alcohol. Bard and Bartke (1974) found similar decrements in testosterone levels in mice. Mendelson and Mello (1974) had also reported reduced plasma testosterone levels in alcoholic men, and Gordon *et al.* (1976) showed that normal adult men maintained on chronic ethanol administration had episodic bursts of

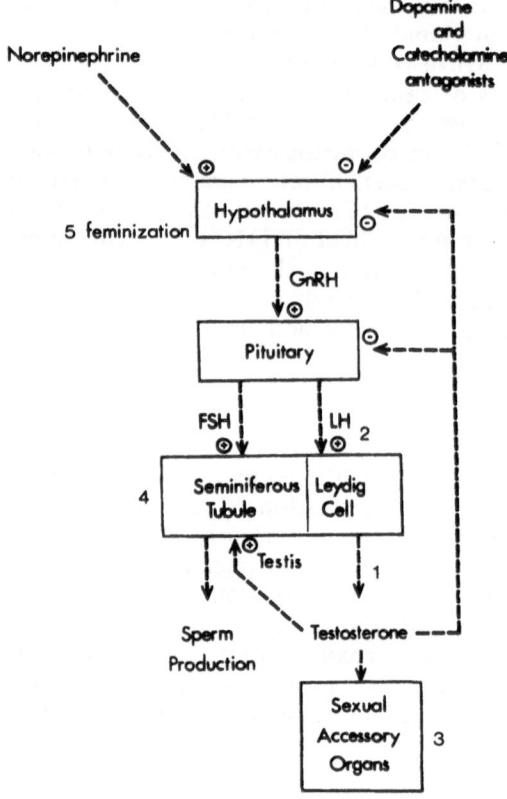

Fig. 6.3 Effects of alcohol on male reproductive function. Alcohol affects the Leydig cells directly to inhibit testosterone biosynthesis (1). The lower blood levels of testosterone cause an increase in LH release and LH levels in the blood become elevated (2). Reduced testosterone levels result in alteration of the sexual accessory organs (3) and, perhaps, sperm production (4); however, alcohol inhibition of vitamin A activation may also affect sperm production. The feminization (5) observed in many chronic alcoholic men is probably due to a multitude of factors including reduced testosterone (1), increased production of oestrogenic substances, hyperprolactinaemia, increased hepatic clearance of testosterone, and an increased plasma binding of testosterone

testosterone secretion which were reduced in magnitude and decreased plasma level of testosterone. They also showed an increased metabolic clearance rate of testosterone as well as a decreased rate of testosterone production following chronic alcohol intake. The fall in plasma testosterone concentration appeared to cause an increase in secretion of LH in some subjects, but in others a decreased plasma level of the steroid was associated with the fall in the secretion of LH. They postulated that the gonadal effect of alcohol was due both to an action on the hypothalamo-pituitary axis and to a direct gonadal effect.

The conflicting results reported by a number of investigators (Toro *et al.*, 1973; Dotson *et al.*, 1975) on the effect of alcohol on testosterone production by the testis have been explained by Mendelson *et al.* (1977) as being due to procedural problems of analysing plasma hormones, differences in time of blood collection, and circadian variation in plasma levels of the gonadal and gonadotropic hormones. To minimize the effect of these variables, Mendelson *et al.* (1977) collected blood specimens at consecutive 20-minute intervals over a 6-hour period, both before and during alcohol consumption. The changes in gonadotropic and gonadal hormones in the serum were correlated with actual blood alcohol levels. When blood alcohol was at its peak level, plasma testosterone was significantly depressed and plasma luteinizing hormone was significantly increased. As blood alcohol levels decreased, plasma LH decreased toward baseline values while plasma testosterone remained depressed. They concluded that alcohol ingestion suppressed plasma testosterone by interfering with biosynthesis or biotransformation of testosterone, and the surge of LH during intoxication was due to lack of suppression by testosterone on GnRH release.

The effect of alcohol to produce feminization of men was examined by several investigators. The level of oestradiol circulating in the plasma of 50 hard-core alcoholics was within the normal range and could not be used to explain the symptoms of hyperoestrogenization such as changes in bodily hair distribution, decreased beard growth, and female escutcheon that were present in half of them. Plasma testosterone binding globulins were approximately eight times those of normal subjects (Van Thiel *et al.*, 1975b) and plasma concentrations of oestrogen-responsive neurophysin were also increased to approximately three times the level found in normal men, while that portion of neurophysin which was not oestrogen-responsive was normal. They also showed that plasma oestrone concentrations, a relatively weak oestrogenic material, were increased two and a half times and plasma prolactin concentrations were doubled in alcoholic subjects. The elevated oestrone production, which may have been due to conversion of androstenedione into oestrone by peripheral metabolism in liver and fat, probably could not account for the severe hyperoestrogenization observed in their subjects.

In addition to the direct gonadal effects of alcohol, Van Thiel *et al.* (1974a) presented evidence of an inadequate hypothalamo-pituitary response in alcoholic patients. Although FSH and LH concentrations were high in a majority of their patients, an adequate response to clomiphene stimulation of FSH and LH release was lacking in two-thirds of their patients. Therefore, they postulated a double effect of alcohol: gross hypothalamo-pituitary dysfunction and a gross defect of gonadal function.

Among the other reproductive defects noted in alcohol-fed rats and alcoholic men were reduction in the mass of testes, ventral prostate, and seminal vesicles relative to body mass. There was also a reduction in the mean seminiferous tubular diameter and the amount of germinal epithelium contained within the tubules (Lieber, 1968). Sperm from these animals had an increased number of abnormal cell types and a decrease in the number of cells. The mechanism by which alcohol produced these effects on the gonads is unclear, but one possibility is that alcohol somehow affects the metabolism of vitamin A, which is necessary for spermatogenesis. Alcohol concentrations as low as 6×10^{-8}M inhibit oxidation of retinol to retinal by testicular alcohol dehydrogenase, levels which are much lower than the plasma concentration found in alcoholics. Thus, if vitamin A activation is inhibited by alcohol-depressed retinal formation, one would also expect spermatogenesis to be inhibited (Van Thiel et al., 1975b).

Cicero et al. (1979) observed that alcohol inhibited testosterone production in vivo in laboratory animals. The conversion of pregnenolone into progesterone in the biosynthesis of testosterone requires NAD. Alteration of the NAD/NADH ratio by the oxidation of ethanol by the testicular alcohol dehydrogenases with excessive conversion of NAD into NADH may produce adverse effects at this stage of steroidogenesis (Van Thiel et al., 1974b). Hepatic steroid A ring reductase activity was increased in both humans (measured from liver biopsy specimens) and in rats following chronic alcohol administration. This enzyme is responsible for metabolism of testosterone by the liver and is responsible for its clearance from the blood. Increased activity of this enzyme could account for lower levels of circulating testosterone. These data indicate that the decreased level of testosterone found in the circulation after excessive alcohol consumption was due, at least in part, to two actions of alcohol: to decreased synthesis of testosterone by interference with the biosynthetic enzymes in the testes, and production of an increased metabolism of testosterone by the liver.

COCAINE

Cocaine is an alkaloid of the *Erythroxylum coca* plant. It is most generally seen as the salt cocaine hydrochloride. At low plasma concentration, cocaine is a central nervous system stimulant, acting mainly on the catecholamine neurotransmitters. Many of the common names of cocaine imply that it is an aphrodisiac. Some reports indicate that cocaine may actually heighten sexual powers and sexual arousal temporarily. A recent report demonstrated that cocaine improved sexual performance in male rats as measured by the number of ejaculations per half hour (Grinspoon and Bakalar, 1976). Cocaine has been applied topically to male and female genitalia to increase sexual performance in human males, probably due to its effect as a local anaesthetic, thereby prolonging erection and delaying ejaculation. In addition, many claims that cocaine is an aphrodisiac may be attributed to the facts that, like most other drugs, it removes or suppresses inhibitions; thus the aphrodisiac effect of cocaine may be psychological rather than physiological. High doses, however, tend to inhibit sexual activity.

In adult male rats, cocaine biphasically altered the level of serum testosterone (Gordon et al., 1980), apparently by disrupting the hypothalamo-pituitary axis with a minor effect on testosterone synthesis and secretion (Fig. 6.4). The effect of acute use of cocaine seems to be dosage-dependent, for low to moderate dosages produce an increase in luteinizing hormone,

COCAINE

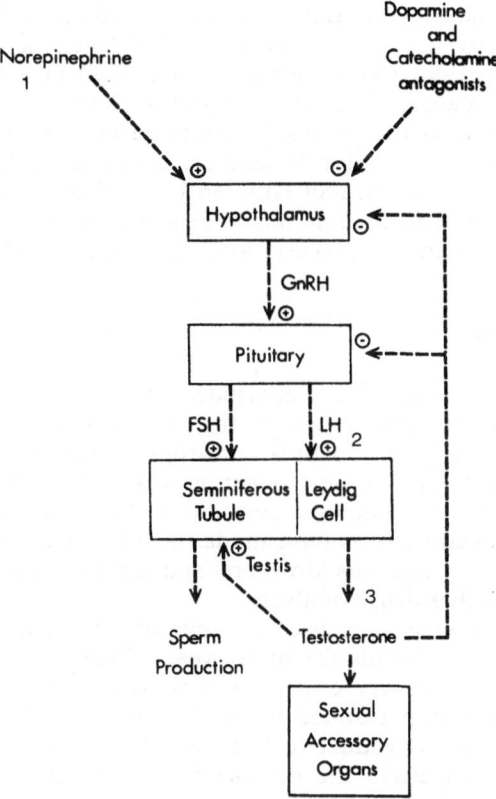

Fig. 6.4 Effects of cocaine on male reproductive function. The primary effect of cocaine appears to be in the CNS where it prevents reuptake of norepinephrine (which increases LH release from the pituitary) and dopamine (which inhibits prolactin release from the pituitary) (1). Cocaine has a biphasic effect on LH secretion at the hypothalamo-pituitary axis (2). Low dosages increase LH with a subsequent increase in testosterone production (3), while high dosages of cocaine inhibit LH with a subsequent decrease in testosterone production

whereas at higher doses cocaine seems to inhibit luteinizing hormone release. Interestingly, cocaine does not appear to affect the level of FSH at any dosage. Therefore, at low to moderate dosage, so-called recreational levels, an increase in testosterone should be expected, and at higher dosages testosterone levels should be inhibited. The data using female ovariectomized rats show that moderate doses (10–20 mg/kg of cocaine) produced an increase in serum LH whereas high dosages (40 mg/kg cocaine) caused a decrease in serum LH. FSH was unaffected at any dosage, and serum prolactin levels were decreased by cocaine at either dosage level (Steger *et al.*, 1981).

The effects of cocaine on LH and prolactin appear to be due, in part, to their effect on the neurotransmitters, norepinephrine and dopamine.

Muscholl (1961) showed that cocaine prevented reuptake of released nore-pinephrine at peripheral nerve endings which led to increased levels of catecholamine in the nerve terminals and enhanced effect. Thus changes in norepinephrine closely parallel changes in LH levels so that when nor-epinephrine is increased, LH is increased, and when norepinephrine is de-creased, LH is decreased. Cocaine has also been shown to block the reup-take of dopamine; thus the previously reported inhibition of prolactin by cocaine may be due to its action to increase dopamine. Although Steger *et al.* (1981) did not find a parallel between dopamine levels and decreased levels of serum prolactin, cocaine has been shown to decrease prolactin in rats by increasing dopamine release (Ravitz and Moore, 1977).

BARBITURATES

The barbiturates are classified pharmacologically as sedative–hypnotic agents. The major therapeutic uses of the drugs are as sedatives and anti-convulsants. They are general depressant drugs, and the CNS is particularly sensitive. Although the exact mechanism of action of the barbiturates is not known, they are known to depress neural activity in various brain regions. Their potent depressant effects have made them popular as drugs of abuse, both for their primary effect as 'downers' and for the effect they produce in combination with other drugs of abuse.

The barbiturates have been used as anaesthetic agents in reproductive studies in laboratory animals for many years. These studies provided the description of the inhibitory effects of these drugs on reproductive hor-mones, observations that resulted in the use of these drugs as important tools in the study of reproductive function (Fig. 6.5). Most of these in-vestigations have concerned the neuroendocrine control of female repro-ductive cycles, but some information is available on the effects of barbitur-ates in male animals. The results of these studies have important implications in the therapeutic use of barbiturates and in studying the abuse of these drugs by young men.

The general effect of the barbiturates is an inhibition of both LH and FSH with subsequent depression of steroid hormone secretion. Barbiturate anaesthesia blocked both spontaneous and steroid-induced LH release in rats (Everett and Sawyer, 1950) and hamsters (Siegel *et al.*, 1976). In these animals, the spontaneous release of LH is controlled by the light–dark cycle and occurs at a specific hour and day of the oestrous cycle. Prolonged barbiturate anaesthesia did not block the steroid-induced LH surge in Rhe-sus monkeys (Knobil, 1974). This suggests that barbiturates act on neural elements in the medial preoptic area that generate the circadian stimulus mediating LH release and not at the medial basal hypothalamus where steroid hormones have their action.

The effect of barbiturate anaesthesia in male animals is similar to the effect in females. Phenobarbital inhibits gonadotropin secretion, and blocks the rise in serum gonadotropin levels that normally follows castration (Nan-sel *et al.*, 1979). Both of these effects can be reversed by the administration

BARBITURATES

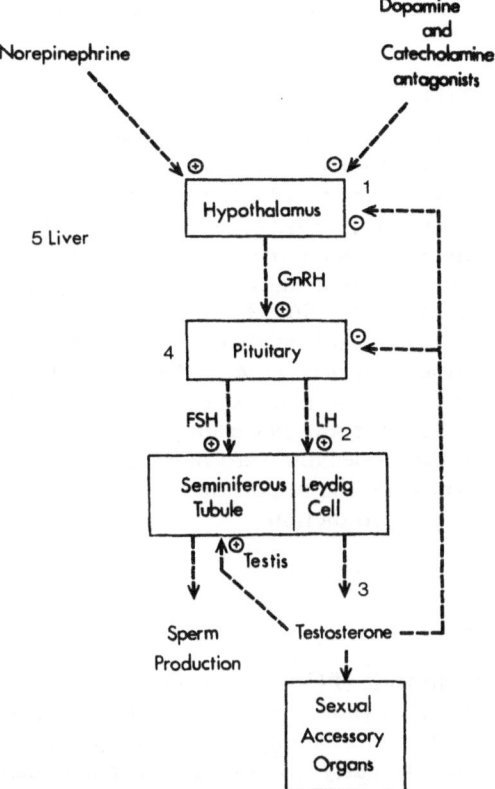

Fig. 6.5 Effect of barbiturates on male reproductive function. Barbiturates act primarily on the hypothalamus to suppress GnRH release (1) with subsequent reduction in pituitary LH secretion (2) and reduced Leydig cell production of testosterone (3). Small doses of barbiturates cause prolactin release from the pituitary (4) while large doses block prolactin release. Barbiturates increase liver enzymes which increase testosterone metabolism and reduce the amount of testosterone available

of GnRH. LH secretion and ovulation can be restored in barbiturate-treated animals by infusion of GnRH (Arimura *et al.*, 1967), indicating a hypothalamic site of action for the barbiturates. Studies in both male and female animals showed that barbiturate pretreatment can even potentiate the effect of GnRH on LH release (Nansel *et al.*, 1979; Wedig and Gay, 1973).

The effect of barbiturates on prolactin levels is less well established. The factors controlling prolactin release are complex and incompletely understood. Non-specific stress increases prolactin release. For example, anaesthesia and blood drawing can cause the release of prolactin and thus the results of studies which employ these techniques are complicated by these methods. Acute administration of barbiturates in relatively small doses appears to cause the release of prolactin (Ajika *et al.*, 1972a; Wuttke and Meites, 1970). However, barbiturate anaesthesia blocks the release of prolactin caused by ether or oestrogen administration (Ajika *et al.*, 1972b).

Barbiturates and liver metabolism

Certain of the barbiturates are among a group of drugs and chemicals that increase the activity of the liver enzymes (hydroxylases) resulting in an increased rate of biotransformation of steroid hormones. This metabolism of testosterone may cause a substantial decrease in its biological action. Pretreatment of rats with phenobarbital inhibits the growth-promoting effects of testosterone by decreasing the concentration and biological action of the androgen (Levin *et al.*, 1969; Fahim *et al.*, 1970). The alteration in testosterone biotransformation is evidenced by increased excretion of polar metabolites in the urine (Southren *et al.*, 1969). Testosterone stimulation of erythropoiesis can also be antagonized by phenobarbital pretreatment in rats. These findings illustrate another example of how drugs can indirectly modify reproductive hormones and thus have effects on reproductive function. They also demonstrate the importance of normal liver function to the maintenance of normal reproduction.

PHENCYCLIDINE

Phencyclidine hydrochloride (PCP) first made its appearance on the streets under the trade name 'Sernylan', an animal tranquillizer, in 1967. Frequent bad experiences made the drug unpopular and it all but vanished from common use by 1968. The early seventies saw a sharp renewal of interest in the drug, more commonly referred to as 'angel dust' at the street level, which resulted in its being classified as a major drug of abuse. Legal manufacture and sale of the drug were stopped in 1978 (Dipalma, 1979).

Many areas of the brain are affected by phencyclidine. The drug has been shown to act upon the cerebral cortex of rabbits (Van Meter *et al.*, 1960), and to have a thalamocortical action (Miyasaia and Domino, 1968).

PCP has also been shown to alter the catabolism, steady-state levels, and turnover rates of most of the reported neurotransmitters in the central nervous system. It has dopaminergic (DA) properties and acts by bringing about an increase in DA activity in the brain (Garey, 1979). Tyrosine, a precursor for both dopamine and norepinephrine (NE) synthesis, was found in elevated levels by Wurtman *et al.* (1974). Leonard and Tong (1969) reported a substantial decrease in whole brain NE concentrations and a slight increase in DA levels. PCP appeared to antagonize acetylcholine (ACh) receptors and the overall activity of the drug was seen to be anticholinergic (Leonard and Tong, 1970; Domino and Wilson 1972); therefore, the effects of phencyclidine are most likely caused by an alteration in function of several neurotransmitters and are not limited to any one system.

Little research effort has been reported on the effect of phencyclidine on the reproductive system. Several authors have indicated that PCP at anaesthetic dosages affects the endocrine system of monkeys and cows. Himsworth *et al.* (1972) showed that monkeys sedated with PCP had significantly lower plasma growth hormone concentrations. Setchell *et al.* (1975a, b) have found that prolonged sedation of Rhesus monkeys with PCP was associated with a gradual increase in plasma cortisol concentration and the hypothalamic–pituitary–adrenal system responded rapidly to alterations in the level of steroids in the circulation. Belchetz *et al.* (1978) reported that protracted sedation of normal monkeys with PCP resulted in a decline of tri-iodothyronine in the plasma within a few hours with no alteration in thyroxine. However, both thyroxine and thyroid stimulating hormone were increased in the plasma 24 hours later. Anaesthetization of young heifers with phencyclidine caused a release of prolactin (Tucker *et al.*, 1973). Ferin *et al.* (1976) showed that release of LH, GH, and prolactin persisted even under prolonged sedation with phencyclidine and that the secretion of prolactin in response to the administration of TRH was increased in animals under sedation. Zaidi *et al.* (1982) reported that serum testosterone levels and production rates were not significantly different in conscious or ketamine (a closely related compound to PCP) anaesthetized male Rhesus monkeys.

Several studies have been reported which have examined the effect of smaller dosages of PCP on reproductive hormone levels in male rats. Acute administration of PCP at recreational dosage levels produced only a slight depression of serum testosterone and LH levels. However, both hormones were strongly reduced after 9 daily treatments (Harclerode *et al.*, 1982). Upon cessation of drug treatment, both hormones were significantly elevated above control hormone levels, but returned to normal by 60 days postinjection. A similar period of elevated serum testosterone and LH was found in adult male rats that received 9 daily injections of PCP during sexual maturation (Mooney and Harclerode, 1982). The magnitude of the increased hormone levels of the PCP-injected juvenile rats was several times that of the rats that received the drug as adults, and the period of elevation persisted for 80 days.

References

Ajika, K., Kalra, S.P., Krulich, L., Fawcett, C.P. and McCann, S.M. (1972b). The effect of stress and Nembutal on plasma levels of gonadotropins and prolactin in ovariectomized rats. *Endocrinology*, **90**, 707–15

Ajika, D., Krulich, L. and McCann, S.M. (1972a). The effect of pentobarbital (Nembutal) on prolactin release in the rat. *Proc. Soc. Exp. Biol. Med.*, **141**, 203–5

Arimura, A., Schally, A.V., Saito, T., Miller, E. and Bowers, C.Y. (1967). Induction of ovulation in rats by highly purified pig LH-releasing factor (LRF). *Endocrinology*, **80**, 515–20

Asch, R.H., Smith, C.G., Siler-Khodr, T.M. and Pauerstein, C.J. (1979). Acute decreases in serum prolactin concentrations caused by $\triangle^9$-tetrahydrocannabinol in nonhuman primates. *Fertil. Steril.*, **32**, 571–5

Bard, F. and Bartke, A. (1974). Effect of ethyl alcohol on plasma testosterone level in mice. *Steroids*, **23**, 921–8

Barry, J. 3rd, Kubena, R.K. and Perhach, J.L. Jr. (1973). Pituitary-adrenal activation and related responses to delta-9-tetrahydrocannabinol. *Prog. Brain Res.*, **39**, 323–30

MALE FERTILITY AND ITS REGULATION

Belchetz, P.E., Gredley, G. and Himsworth, R.L., (1978). Pituitary-thyroid function in the Rhesus monkey (*Macaca mulatta*). *J. Endocrinol.*, **76**, 427–38

Birmingham, M.K. and Bartova, A. (1976). Effects of cannabinol derivatives on blood pressure, body weight, pituitary-adrenal function, and mitochondrial respiration in the rat. In Nahas, G.G. *et al.* (eds) *Marihuana; Chemistry, Biochemistry and Cellular Effects*. 556 pp. (New York: Springer)

Bromley, B., Gordon, J. and Zimmerman, E. (1977). Delta-9-tetrahydrocannabinol inhibition of ether and perphenazine induced release of prolactin in male rats. *Fed. Proc.*, **36**, 1026

Bromley, B. and Zimmerman, E. (1976). Divergent release of prolactin and corticosterone following $\triangle^9$-tetrahydrocannabinol injection in male rats. *Fed. Proc. Am. Soc. Exp. Biol.*, **35**, 220

Burstein, S., Hunter, S.A. and Shoupe, T.S. (1978b). Inhibition of cholesterol esterases by $\triangle^1$-tetrahydrocannabinol. *Life Sci.*, **23**, 979–82

Burstein, S., Hunter, S.A., and Shoupe, T.S. (1979). Site of inhibition of Leydig cell testosterone synthesis by $\triangle^1$-tetrahydrocannabinol. *Mol. Pharmacol.*, **15**, 633–40

Burstein, S., Hunter, S.A., Shoupe, T.S. and Taylor, P. (1978a). Cannabinoid inhibition of testosterone synthesis by mouse Leydig cells. *Res. Commun. Chem. Pathol. Pharmacol.*, **19**, 557–60

Carchman, R.A., Warner, W., White, A.C. and Harris, L.S., (1976). Cannabinoids and neoplastic growth. In Nahas, G.G. (ed.) *Marihuana: Chemistry, Biochemistry and Cellular Effects*. pp. 329–345. (New York: Springer-Verlag.)

Cicero, T.J., Schainker, B.A. and Meyer, E.R. (1979). Endogenous opioids participate in regulation of the hypothalamic–pituitary–luteinizing hormone axis and testosterone's negative feedback control of luteinizing hormone. *Endocrinology*, **104**, 1286–91

Coggins, W.J., Swenson, E.W., Dawson, W.W., Fernandez-Salas, A., Hernandez-Bolanos, J., Jiminez-Antillon, C.F., Solano, J.R., Vinocour, R. and Faerron-Valdez, F. (1976). Health status of chronic heavy cannabis users. *Ann. N.Y. Acad. Sci.*, **282**, 148–61

Cohen, S. (1976). The 94-day cannabis study. *Ann. N.Y. Acad. Sci.*, **282**, 211–20

Collu, R. (1976). Endocrine effects of chronic intraventricular administration of $\triangle^9$-tetrahydrocannabinol to prepubertal and adult male rats. *Life Sci.*, **18**, 223–30

Collu, R., Letarte, J., Leboeuf, G. and Ducharme, J.R. (1975). Endocrine effects of chronic administration of psychoactive drugs to prepuberal male rats. I: $\triangle^9$-tetrahydrocannabinol. *Life Sci.*, **16**, 533–42

Dalterio, S., Badr, F., Bartke, A. and Mayfield, D. (1982). Cannabinoids in male mice: effects of fertility and spermatogenesis. *Science*, **216**, 315–6

Dalterio, S., Bartke, A., Roberson, C., Watson, D. and Burstein, S. (1978). Direct and pituitary-mediated effects of $\triangle^9$-THC and cannabinol on the testis. *Pharmacol. Biochem. Behav.*, **8**, 673–8

Dalterio, S.L., Michael, S.D., MacMillan, B.T. and Bartke, A. (1981). Differential plasma prolactin growth hormone and corticosterone levels in male mice. *Life Sci.*, **28**, 761–6

Dewey, W.L., Peng, T.C. and Harris, L.S. (1970). The effect of 1-trans-delta-9-tetrahydrocannabinol on the hypothalamo-hypophyseal-adrenal axis of rats. *Eur. J. Pharmacol.*, **12**, 382–4

Dipalma, J.R. (1979). Phencyclidine: angel dust. *Am. Fam. Physician*, **20**, 120–2

Dixit, V.P. and Lohiya, N.K. (1975). Effects of cannabis extract on the response of accessory sex organs of adult male mice to testosterone. *Indian J. Physiol. Pharmacol.*, **19**, 98–100

Domino, E.F. and Wilson, A.E., (1972). Psychotropic drug influences on brain acetocholine utilization. *Psychopharmacologia*, **25**, 291–8

Dotson, L.E., Robertson, L.S. and Tuchfeld, B. (1975). Plasma alcohol, smoking, hormone concentrations and self-reported aggression. A study of social-drinking situations. *J. Stud. Alcohol*, **36**, 578–86

Everett, J.W. and Sawyer, C.H. (1950). A 24-hour periodicity in the 'LH-release apparatus' of female rats, disclosed by barbiturate sedation. *Endocrinology*, **47**, 198–218

Fahim, M.S., Fahim, Z., Dement, G. and Hall, D.G., (1970). Induced alteration in the hepatic metabolism of androgens in the rat. *Am. J. Obstet. Gynecol.*, **107**, 1085–91

Ferin, M., Carmel, P.W., Warren, M.P., Himsworth, R.L. and Frantz, A.G. (1976). Phencyclidine sedation as a technique for handling Rhesus monkeys: effects on LH, GH, and prolactin secretion. *Proc. Soc. Exp. Biol. Med.*, **151**, 428–33

72

Fujimoto, G.I., Rosenbaum, R.M., Ziegler, D., Retture, G. and Morrill, G.A. (1978). Effects of marihuana extract given orally on male rat reproduction and gonads. *Proc. 60th Ann. Meet. Endocrinol. Soc.*

Garey, R.E. (1979). PCP (phencyclidine): an update. *J. Psychedelic Drugs*, 11, 265–75

Ghosh, S.P., Chatterjee, T.K. and Ghosh, J.J. (1981). Antiandrogenic effect of delta-9-tetrahydrocannabinol in adult castrated rats. *J. Reprod. Fertil.*, 62, 513–17

Gordon, G.G., Altman, K., Southren, A.L., Rubin, E. and Lieber, C.S. (1976). Effect of alcohol (ethanol) administration on sex-hormone metabolism in normal men. *N. Engl. J. Med.*, 295, 793–7

Gordon, L.A., Mostofsky, D.I. and Gordon, G.G. (1980). Changes in testosterone levels in the rat following intraperitoneal cocaine HCl. *Int. J. Neurosci.*, 11, 139–41

Grinspoon, L. and Bakalar, J.B. (1976). *Cocaine*. (New York: Basic Books)

Harclerode, J., Bird, L., Sawyer, H., Berger, V., Mooney, R. and Smith, R. (1982). Sex hormone levels in adult rats injected with $\triangle^9$-tetrahydrocannabinol and phencyclidine hydrochloride. Presented at *Cannabinoid '82 Meetings*, Louisville, KY

Hembree, W.C., Nahas, G.G. and Huang, H.F.S. (1979). Changes in human spermatozoa associated with high dose marihuana smoking. In Nahas, G.G. and Paton, W.D.M. (eds.) *Marihuana: Biological Effects*, pp. 429–439. (New York: Pergamon)

Hershkowitz, M., Goldman, R. and Raz, A. (1977). Effect of cannabinoids on neuotransmitter uptake, ATPase activity and morphology of mouse brain synaptosomes. *Biochem. Pharmacol.*, 26, 1327–31

Himsworth, R.L., Carmel, P.W. and Frantz, A.G. (1972). The location of the chemoreceptor controlling growth hormone secretion during hypoglycemia in primates. *Endocrinology*, 91, 217–26

Issidorides, M.R. (1979). Observations in chronic hashish users: nuclear aberrations in blood and sperm and abnormal acrosomes in spermatozoa. In Nahas, G.G. and Paton, W.D.M. (eds.) *Marihuana: Biological Effects*, pp. 377–388. (New York: Pergamon)

Jakubovic, A. and McGeer, P.L. (1977). Biochemical changes in rat testicular cells in vitro produced by cannabinoids and alcohol: metabolism and incorporation of labeled glucose, amino acids, and nucleic acid precursors. *Toxicol. Appl. Pharmacol.*, 41, 473–86

Jones, R. (1977). Human effects. In Petersen, R.C. (ed.) *Marihuana Research Findings*, pp. 128–178. National Institute on Drug Abuse Research Monograph 14. DHEW Pub. No. (ADM) 78–501. Washington, D.C.: Superintendent of Documents, U.S. Government Printing Office

Knobil, E. (1974). On the control of gonadotropin secretion in the Rhesus monkey. *Recent Prog. Horm. Res.*, 30, 1–46

Kolodny, R.C., Lessin, R.C., Toro, G., Masters, W.H. and Cohen, S. (1976). Depression of plasma testosterone with acute marihuana administration. In Braude, M.C. and Szara, S. (eds.) *The Pharmacology of Marihuana*, pp. 217–225. (New York: Raven Press)

Kolodny, R.G., Masters, W.H., Kolodner, R.M. and Toro, G. (1974). Depression of plasma testosterone levels after chronic intensive marihuana use. *N. Engl. J. Med.*, 290, 872–4

Kolodny, R.C., Toro, G. and Masters, W.H. (1975). Letter to the editor in response to Schaefer, Gunn and Dubowski. *N. Engl. J. Med.*, 292, 868

Kramer, J. and Ben-David, M. (1974). Suppression of prolactin secretion by acute administration of delta-9-THC in rats. *Proc. Soc. Exp. Biol. Med.*, 147, 482–4

Leonard, B.E. and Tong, S.R. (1969). The effects of some hallucinogenic drugs upon the metabolism of noradrenaline. *Life Sci.* 8, 815–25

Leonard, B.E. and Tong, S.R. (1970). Some effects of an hallucinogenic drug (phencyclidine) on neurohumoral substances. *Life Sci.* 9, 1141–52

Levin, W., Welch, R.M. and Conney, A.H. (1969). Inhibitory effect of phenobarbital or chlordane pretreatment on the androgen-induced increase in seminal vesicle weight in the rat. *Steroids*, 13, 155–61

Lieber, C.S. (1968). Metabolic effects produced by alcohol in the liver and other tissues. In Snapper, I. and Stollerman, G.H. (eds.) *Advances in Internal Medicine*, Vol. 14, pp. 151–199. (Chicago: Year Book Medical Publishers)

Lomax, P. (1970). The effect of marijuana on pituitary-thyroid activity in the rat. *Agents and Actions*, 1, 252–7

Maier, R. and Maitre, L. (1975). Steroidogenic and lipolytic effects of cannabinoids in the rat and the rabbit. *Biochem. Pharmacol.*, 24, 1695–9

73

Malor, R., Jackson, D.M. and Chesher, G.B. (1978). Possible central dopaminergic modulation of the rise in plasma concentration of nonesterified fatty-acids produced in the mouse by levo-trans-delta-9-tetrahydrocannabinol. *Biochem. Pharmacol.*, **27**, 407-14

Marks, B.H. (1973). Δ^1-tetrahydrocannabinol and luteinizing hormone secretion. *Prog. Brain Res.*, **39**, 331-8

Mendelson, J.H., Babor, T.F., Kuehnle, J.C., Rossi, A.M., Bernstein, J.G., Mello, N.K. and Greenberg, I. (1976). Behavioral and biological aspects of marihuana use. *Ann. N.Y. Acad. Sci.*, **282**, 186-210

Mendelson, J.H., Kuehnle, J.C., Ellingboe, J. and Babor, T.F. (1974). Plasma testosterone levels before, during and after chronic marihuana smoking. *N. Eng. J. Med.*, **291**, 1051-5

Mendelson, J.H. and Mello, N.K. (1974). Alcohol, aggression and androgens. In Frazier, S.H. (ed.) *Aggression*. pp. 225-247. (Baltimore: Williams and Wilkins)

Mendelson, J.H., Mello, N.K. and Ellingboe, J. (1977). Effects of acute alcohol intake on pituitary-gonadal hormones in normal human males. *J. Pharmacol. Exp. Ther.*, **202**, 676-82

Miras, C.J. (1965). Some aspects of cannabis action. In Wolstenholme, G.E.W. and Knight, J. (eds.) *Hashish: its Chemistry and Pharmacology*, CIBA Foundation. Study group 21. pp. 37-52. (Boston: Little, Brown)

Mitra, G., Poddar, M.K. and Ghosh, J.J. (1977). Interaction of delta-9-tetrahydrocannabinol with reserpine, phenobarbital, and LSD-25 on plasma and adrenal corticosterone. *Toxicol. Appl. Pharmacol.*, **42**, 505-12

Miyasaia, M. and Domino, E.F. (1968). Neuronal mechanisms of ketamine-induced anesthesia. *Int. J. Neuropharmacol.*, **7**, 557-73

Mooney, R.P. Jr. and Harclerode, J. (1982). Sex hormone levels in adult male rats injected during sexual maturation with Δ^9-tetrahydrocannabinol and phencyclidine hydrochloride. *Fed. Proc.*, **41**

Muscholl, E. (1961). Effect of cocaine and related drugs on the uptake of noradrenaline by heart and spleen. *Br. J. Pharmacol.*, **16**, 352-9

Nahas, G.G. (1976). *Marijuana: Chemistry, Biochemistry and Cellular Effects.* 556 pp. (New York: Springer-Verlag)

Nansel, D.D., Aiyer, M.S., Meinzer, W.H. II and Bogdanove, E.M. (1979). Rapid direct effects of castration and androgen treatment on luteinizing hormone-releasing hormone-induced luteinizing hormone release in the phenobarbital-treated male rat: examination of the roles direct and indirect androgen feedback mechanisms might play in the physiological control of luteinizing hormone release. *Endocrinology*, **104**, 524-31

Nazar, B., Kairys, D.J., Fowler, R. and Harclerode, J. (1977). Effects of delta-9-tetrahydrocannabinol on serum thyroxine concentrations in the rat. *J. Pharm. Pharmacol.*, **29**, 778-9

Pertwee, R.G. (1974). Tolerance to the effect of delta-1-tetrahydrocannabinol on corticosterone levels in mouse plasma produced by repeated administration of cannabis extract or delta-1-tetrahydrocannabinol. *Br. J. Pharmacol.*, **51**, 391-7

Puder, M., Weidenfeld, J., Chowers, I., Nir, I., Conforti, N. and Siegel, R.A. (1982). Corticotrophin and corticosterone secretion following delta-1-cannabinol, in intact and in hypothalamic deafferentated male rats. *Exp. Brain Res.* (West Germany), **46**, 85-8

Purohit, V., Singh, H.H. and Ahluwalia, B.S. (1979). Evidence that the effects of methadone and marihuana on male reproductive organs are mediated at different sites in rats. *Biol. Reprod.*, **20**, 1039-44

Ravitz, A.J. and Moore, K.E. (1977). Effects of amphetamine, methylphenidate and cocaine on serum prolactin concentrations in the male rat. *Life Sci.*, **21**, 267-72

Rosenkrantz, H. and Hayden, D.W. (1979). Acute and subacute inhalation toxicity of Turkish marihuana, cannabichromene, and cannabidiol in rats. *Toxicol. Appl. Pharmacol.*, **48**, 357-86

Setchell, K.D.R., Shackleton, C.H.L. and Himsworth, R.L. (1975a). Effect of acute inhibition of adrenocorticotrophin secretion on plasma corticosteroids in the Rhesus monkey (*Macaca mulatta*). *J. Endocrinol.* **76**, 251-7

Setchell, K.D.R., Shackleton, C.H.L. and Himsworth, R.L. (1975b). Studies on plasma corticosteroids in the Rhesus monkey (*Macaca mulatta*). *J. Endocrinol.*, **67**, 241-50

Shoupe, T.S., Hunter, S.A., Burstein, S.H. and Hubbard, C.D. (1980). The nature of the inhibition of cholesterol esterase by delta-1-tetrahydrocannabinol. *Enzyme*, **25**, 87-91

Siegel, H.I., Bast, J.D. and Greenwald, G.S. (1976). The effects of phenobarbital and gonadal steroids on periovulatory serum levels of luteinizing hormone and follicle stimulating hormone in the hamster. *Endocrinology*, **98**, 48–55

Smith, C.G., Moore, C.E., Besch, N.F. and Besch, P.K. (1976). The effect of marihuana delta-9-tetrahydrocannabinol on the secretion of sex hormones in the mature male Rhesus monkey. *Clin. Chem.*, **22**, 1184

Smith, C.G., Ruppert, M.J., Asch, R.H. and Siler-Khodr, T. (1979b). The effects of tetrahydrocannabinol on prolactin in the Rhesus monkey. Presented at the *NIDA Conference on Genetic, Perinatal, and Developmental Effects of Abused Substances*, Airlie, Virginia

Smith, C.G., Smith, M.T., Besch, N.F., Smith, R.G. and Asch, R.H. (1979a). Effect of $\triangle^9$-tetrahydrocannabinol (THC) on female reproductive function. In Nahas, G.G. and Paton, W.D.M. (eds.) *Marihuana: Biological Effects. pp.* 449–67. (New York: Pergamon)

Southren, A.L., Gordon, G.G., Tochimoto, S., Kuntzman, R., Krikun, E., Krieger, D. and Jacobson, H. (1969). Effect of N-phenylbarbital (phetharbital) on the metabolism of testosterone and cortisol in man. *J. Clin. Endocrinol.*, **29**, 251–6

Stefanis, C.N. and Issidorides, M.R. (1976). Cellular effects of chronic cannabis use in man. In Nahas, G.G. (ed.) *Marihuana: Chemistry, Biochemistry, and Cellular Effects*, pp. 533–550 (New York: Springer-Verlag)

Steger, R., Silverman, A., Johns, A. and Asch, R.H. (1981). Interactions of cocaine and delta-9-tetrahydrocannabinol with the hypothalamic-hypophyseal axis of the female rat. *Fertil. Steril.*, **35**, 567–72

Symons, A.M., Teale, J.D. and Marks, V. (1976). Proceedings: Effect of delta-9-tetrahydrocannabinol on the hypothalamic-pituitary-gonadal system in the maturing male rat. *J. Endocrinol.*, **68**, 43–4

Toro, G., Kolodny, R.C., Jacobs, L.S., Masters, W.H. and Daughaday, W.H. (1973). Failure of alcohol to alter pituitary and target organ hormone levels. *Clin. Res.*, **21**, 505

Tucker, H.A., Koprowski, J.A. and Oxender, W.D. (1973). Relationships among mammary nucleic acids, milk yield, serum prolactin, and growth hormone in heifers from 3 months to age of lactation. *Dairy Sci.*, **56**, 184–8

Tyrey, L. (1978). $\triangle$-9-tetrahydrocannabinol suppression of episodic luteinizing hormone secretion in the ovariectomized rat. *Endocrinology*, **102**, 1808–14

Van Meter, W.G., Owens, H.F. and Himwich, H.E. (1960). The effects on rabbit brain of a new drug with psychomimetic properties. *J. Neurol. Neurosurg. Psychiatry*, **1**, 129–34

Van Thiel, D.H., Gavaler, J.S. and Lester, R. (1974b). Ethanol inhibition of vitamin A metabolism in the testes: possible mechanism for sterility in alcoholics. *Science*, **186**, 941–2

Van Thiel, D.H., Gavaler, J.S., Lester, R. and Goodman, M.D. (1975a). Alcohol-induced testicular atrophy: An experimental model for hypogonadism occurring in chronic alcoholic men. *Gastroenterology*, **69**, 326–32

Van Thiel, D.H., Gavaler, J.S., Lester, R. Loriaux, D.L. and Braunstein, G.D. (1975b). Plasma estrone, prolactin, neurophysin, and sex steroid binding globulin in chronic alcoholic men. *Metabolism*, **24**, 1015–19

Van Thiel, D.H., Lester, R. and Sherins, R.J. (1974a). Hypogonadism in alcoholic liver disease: evidence for a double defect. *Gastroenterology*, **67**, 1188–99

Vyas, D.K. and Singh, R. (1976). Effect of cannabis and opium on the testis of the pigeon *Columbia livia* Gmelin. *Indian J. Exp. Biol.*, **14**, 22–5

Warner, W., Harris, L.S. and Carchman, R.A. (1977). Inhibition of corticosteroidogenesis by delta-9-tetrahydrocannabinol. *Endocrinology*, **101**, 1815–20

Wedig, J.H. and Gay, V.L. (1973). Potentiation of luteinizing hormone-releasing factor activities following pentobarbital anesthesia in the steroid-blocked castrated rat. *Proc. Soc. Exp. Biol. Med.*, **144**, 993–8

Wurtman, R.J., Larin, F. and Mastafapour, S. (1974). Brain catechol synthesis: control by brain tyrosine concentration. *Science*, **185**, 183–4

Wuttke, W. and Meites, J. (1970). Effects of ether and pentobarbital on serum prolactin on LH levels in proestrous rats. *Proc. Soc. Exp. Biol. Med.*, **135**, 648–52

Yen, S.S.C. and Jaffe, R.B. (1978). In *Reproductive Endocrinology*, Clinics *in Endocrinology and Metabolism*, Vol. 7. (Philadelphia: Saunders)

Zaidi, P., Wickings, E.J. and Nieschlag, E. (1982). Effects of ketamine hydrochloride and barbiturate anesthesia on the metabolic clearance and production rates of testosterone in the male Rhesus monkey *Macaca mulatta. J. Steroid Biochem.*, **16,** 436–66

Zimmerman, A.M., Bruce, W.R. and Zimmerman, S. (1979a). Effects of cannabinoids on sperm morphology. *Pharmacology,* **18,** 143–8

Zimmerman, A.M., Zimmerman, S. and Raj, A.Y. (1979b). Effects of cannabinoids on spermatogenesis in mice. In Nahas, G.G. and Paton, W.D.M. (eds.) *Marihuana: Biological Effects.* pp. 407–18. (New York: Pergamon)

7
Effects of abused substances on male reproductive development

S. DALTERIO and A. BARTKE

A wide variety of pharmacological agents, both medically prescribed and recreationally abused, can affect endocrine and reproductive functions in the male. Alcohol, opiates, barbiturates and marijuana have been reported to suppress gonadal function, impair spermatogenesis and decrease sexual activity in men (Bloch et al., 1978).

Androgen production by the fetal testis plays a critical organizational role in the development of male reproductive structures and in the establishment of male patterns of neuroendocrine function and sexual behaviour (Barraclough, 1967). It is well established that fetal or neonatal castration, suppression of the steroidogenic function of the testis by stress or treatment with antibodies to gonadotropins, as well as interference with the action of testicular androgens by administration of anti-androgens or antibodies to steroid hormones can produce long-term consequences on the development of the reproductive system and its function (see Table 7.1 for literature review).

Table 7.1 Effects of perinatal treatments on male reproductive functions

Treatment	Period	Species	Effect
castration	neonatal	rat	two-fold ↑ in LH-cells in pituitary (Matsumura and Daikoku, 1978)
castration	neonatal	mouse	↓ penis size, testes weights and sexual behaviour (Quadagno et al., 1975)
anti-LRF	neonatal	rat	infertility, ↓ testis size (Bercu et al., 1977)
anti-LH	neonatal	mouse	↓ in penis size, seminal vesicle weights, sexual behaviour, fertility (Goldman, 1972; Quadagno, et al., 1975)
anti-PRL	neonatal	rat	↑ plasma LH at 49 days of age, ↓ prostate and seminal vesicle weights (Hostetter and Piaczek, 1977)

Table 7.1 cont.   Effects of perinatal treatments on male reproductive functions

Treatment	Period	Species	Effect
anti-testosterone	prenatal	rabbit	feminization of internal and external reproductive structures; prostate absent (Bidlingmaier *et al.*, 1977)
anti-testosterone	prenatal	rat	↑ T production by neonatal testes *in vitro* (Goldman, A.S. *et al.*, 1972)
anti-oestrogens	neonatal	rat	↑ lordosis response, ↓ body and testes weights, delayed testicular descent (Clark and McCormack, 1977)
anti-androgens	prenatal	rat	↓ penis size, ejaculations, fetal growth, ano-genital distance; ↑ uptake of oestradiol by adult hypothalamus (Neumann *et al.*, 1977)
protein malnutrition	prenatal	rat	↓ testosterone production *in vitro*, ↓ seminal vesicles and testes weights, ABP absent, ↑ FSH post-castration (Glass *et al.*, 1979)
monosodium glutamate (MSG)	neonatal / neonatal	rat / mouse	↑ body weight, ↓ pituitary, thyroid, adrenal, testes, and prostate weights; ↓ serum TSH, GH, and LH; impaired fertility (Nemeroff *et al.*, 1978; Bakke *et al.*, 1978)
stress	prenatal	rat	↓ ano-genital distance, body and adrenal weights (Dahloff, 1978); ↓ male sex behaviour and fetal T (Ward, 1972, 1980).
dihydrotestosterone	neonatal	rat	↓ testes weight and testosterone content; ↓ gonadotropins after neonatal castration (Van der Schoot *et al.*, 1976)
oestrogens	neonatal	rat	↓ in hypothalamic uptake of testosterone (Tuohima and Niemi, 1972); ↓ binding of LH to testes and receptor synthesis (Kolena *et al.*, 1978)
testosterone	neonatal	rat	↓ in 17-oxo reduction and ↑ 17-β-hydroxylase in testis (Kincl and Henderson, 1978), ↓ ejaculation (Zadina *et al.*, 1979)
testosterone	neonatal	mouse	↑ plasma testosterone and sexual behaviour (Campbell and McGill, 1970)
progesterone	perinatal	rat	↓ sexual behaviour (Hull *et al.*, 1980)
phenobarbital	prenatal	mouse	dose-dependent ↓ in male sex behaviour; ↑ female behaviour at lower doses (Clemens, 1974)
chlorpromazine	neonatal	mouse	↑ testis wt., ↑ spermatogenesis (Hogarth and Chalmers, 1973)
methadone	prenatal	rat	↑ plasma androgens (Soyka *et al.*, 1978).

Table 7.1 cont. Effects of perinatal treatments on male reproductive functions

Treatment	Period	Species	Effect
morphine	neonatal	rat	↑ pituitary size and testes weights (Bakke *et al.*, 1973)
alcohol	perinatal	mouse	↓ testes wt., plasma T and *in vitro* T production (Dalterio *et al.*, 1981)
alcohol	prenatal	rat	↓ ano-genital distance, prolonged gestation and ↑ penile reflex (Chen and Smith, 1979).
Antabuse (disulphiram)	prenatal	rat	↓ fertility (Holck *et al.*, 1970)
cannabinoids	perinatal	mouse	alterations in body weight regulation, pituitary-gonadal function and ↓ sexual behaviour (Dalterio and Bartke, 1979)
cannabinoids	prenatal	mouse	↓ in fetal T (Dalterio *et al.*, 1981)
nicotine	prenatal	rat	↑ number of ♂/litter and ↑ fetal resorptions (Abel *et al.*, 1979)

Thus, it seems reasonable to expect that exposure to substances of abuse during the 'critical' (fetal or neonatal) periods of differentiation could compromise the hormonal function of the developing testes and/or interfere with 'organizational' effects of androgenic steroids and, thus, lead to alterations in reproductive and sexual functions. In this chapter we will review evidence that several of the commonly abused substances can, indeed, interfere with male sexual development in experimental animals, and that some of them appear to be able to exert similar effects also in the human.

BARBITURATES

In the rat, exposure to phenobarbital during late fetal development reduced ano-genital distance, delayed testicular descent, decreased fertility and reduced adult plasma levels of testosterone (T) and luteinizing hormone (LH) (Gupta *et al.*, 1980). In addition, a decrease in the weights of the seminal vesicles, with a concomitant increase in the concentration of androgen receptors was observed in these animals. Another study reported a decrease in adult mating behaviour subsequent to neonatal exposure of rats to phenobarbital (Clemens, 1974). Results obtained in mice following prenatal phenobarbital exposure suggested that the behavioural teratogenicity of this drug could be related to neuronal deficits induced in cerebellar and hippocampal tissues, (*Bergman et al.*, 1980) rather than to effects on pituitary or testicular function.

OPIATES

Early exposure to opiates has also been observed to influence subsequent development of reproductive and endocrine functions. In male rats, morphine exposure during the second half of gestation decreased T and $\triangle^4$-androstenedione levels in male fetuses (Singh *et al.*, 1980). However, effects of perinatal morphine exposure included an increase in relative testicular weights later in life, possibly due to enhanced gonadotropin secretion (Bakke *et al.*, 1973). It has also been reported that untreated offspring of male rats addicted neonatally to morphine exhibit a delay in postnatal growth and a reduction in body weights (Friedler and Cochin, 1968; Sonderegger *et al.*, 1979), although tolerance to such effects in both sire and offspring has been observed after repeated methadone administration (Soyka *et al.*, 1978). Maternal methadone exposure during the last part of gestation has been linked to disruption of endocrine function in fetal rats. Male, but not female, fetuses showed reductions in plasma T and $\triangle^4$-androstenedione levels and these changes could be prevented by naloxone adminstration (Singh *et al.*, 1980).

ALCOHOL

Maternal alcohol abuse, both severe and moderate, has now been associated with a number of congenital anomalies, including growth impairment and mental retardation. Animal models of the 'fetal alcohol syndrome' allowed control of such factors as maternal undernutrition or life-style variables, and substantiated the conclusion that exposure to alcohol, even at fairly low levels, may compromise fetal development (Weathersbee and Lodge 1978).

In adulthood, after prenatal alcohol exposure, males exhibited normal levels of sexual behaviour and plasma T, as well as normal weights of accessory reproductive glands (Chen and Smith, 1979). In mice, alcohol exposure early in gestation delayed sexual maturation in females, and resulted in kidney abnormalities in both sexes (Boggan *et al.*, 1979).

In adult male mice perinatally exposed to alcohol, we observed significant reduction in the weights of the kidneys and testes, in the concentration of T in plasma, as well as in testicular responsiveness to gonadotropic stimulation in vitro (Dalterio *et al.*, 1981). The possible mechanisms of these effects of pre- or perinatal exposure to alcohol on the subsequent development of male reproductive functions are not well understood. However, a toxic metabolite of ethyl alcohol, acetaldehyde, appears to be particularly deleterious to testicular function (Badr *et al.*, 1977); Cicero *et al*, 1980).

CANNABINOIDS

Reports from our laboratory have demonstrated long-term alterations in reproductive function in male mice whose mothers received cannabinoids during late pregnancy and early lactation (Dalterio 1980). In these studies, exposure to the main psychoactive constituent of marijuana, $\triangle^9$-tetra-hydrocannabinol (THC), or to a relatively non-psychoactive constituent, cannabinol (CBN), during the last part of gestation and for six days postpartum, resulted in alterations in body weight regulation, pituitary-gonadal function, responsivity to stimuli originating from conspecifics, and adult sexual activity. It is of particular interest that perinatal exposure of male mice to either the psychoactive, or a relatively non-psychoactive cannabinoid, resulted in significant suppression of adult copulatory behaviour (Dalterio et al., 1980).

Reports from several laboratories indicate that prenatal exposure to cannabis or its purified constituents can affect the content of proteins and nucleic acids (Luthra, 1980), as well as lipid and water concentrations (Greizerstein and Abel, 1980) in neonatal rats. In addition, several investigators have noted maturational delays and learning deficits in rats exposed to cannabinoids during early development (Fried, 1976; Gianutsos and Abbatiello, 1972). The possible relevance of these findings to human users of cannabis is suggested by a report that marijuana use by pregnant women is associated with a significant increase in symptoms associated with nervous system anomalies in their newborn infants (Fried, 1980). However, the mechanisms responsible for these cannabinoid-induced alterations in male reproductive function and sexual behaviour, and in learning and development remain to be elucidated.

STRESS

Stress may accompany any experimental treatments directed toward a pregnant or lactating female. Thus, the interpretation of results may be complicated by the possible direct or indirect effects of stress on any of the parameters measured. Studies have indicated that maternal stress alters the developmental pattern and maximal volumes of T levels in fetal rats (Ward and Weisz, 1980), and the development of the fetal genital system, as indicated by a decrease in testes weights (Dahlof, 1978). In addition, stress during pregnancy has been shown to decrease steroid aromatase activity in the brains of fetal male and female rats (Weisz et al., 1982), and reduce adult male copulatory behaviour (Ward, 1972).

MECHANISMS RESPONSIBLE FOR THE EFFECTS OF CANNABINOIDS AND ALCOHOL ON THE REPRODUCTIVE DEVELOPMENT OF MALE MICE

Introduction

As mentioned above alterations in the hormonal milieu during critical periods of sexual development may result in dramatic long-term consequences for the development of male reproductive functions, with effects quite similar to those reported after perinatal exposure to barbiturates, opiates or alcohol. The present experiments were designed to determine whether perinatal exposure to the major psychoactive constituent of marijuana, Δ^9-tetrahydrocannabinol (THC), or to its non-psychoactive constituents cannabinol (CBN) or cannabidiol (CBD), could influence the function of the hypothalamo-pituitary-gonadal (HPG) axis in adulthood. Specifically, we determined the reproductive organ weights, plasma levels of T, LH and FSH, androgen production by the testes *in vitro*, and the release of pituitary gonadotropins in response to castration in adult male mice exposed to THC, CBN or CBD early in development. In addition, we attempted to identify possible critical periods for the effects of cannabinoids on the development of the male reproductive system.

The *in vitro* responsiveness to gonadotropins of the testes obtained from adult mice perinatally exposed to alcohol or disulphiram was also examined. Disulphiram blocks the activity of aldehyde dehydrogenase, an enzyme involved not only in the metabolism of alcohol, but also that of the catecholamines (Holck *et al.*, 1970). Therefore, disulphiram results in acetaldehyde accumulation even in the absence of alcohol. This treatment permits evaluation of the effects of acetaldehyde without alcohol-related effects on maternal weight gain, fluid or caloric intake and this may indicate whether alcohol or its metabolites are responsible for observed disruptions in testicular function.

Methods

Animals

Animals were obtained from our colony of random-bred mice, housed on a 14 h light:10 h dark, lighting schedule and provided with a commercial feed and tap water *ad libitum*.

Procedures

Female mice received 50 mg/kg body weight THC, CBN or CBD orally in a 20 μl volume of sesame oil. Ethanol (40% w/v; 0.33 g/kg body weight) was administered orally in a 50 μl volume. The disulphiram was also administered by oral feeding in 20 μl of sesame oil at a dose of 250 μg/kg body weight.

Adult female mice were housed with an adult male and checked daily for the presence of a vaginal plug (considered day 1 of pregnancy). Treatments were administered either 1-3 days before parturition (prenatally), one day before parturition and for six days postpartum (perinatally), or on the first day postpartum (postnatally). The young were weaned at 21 days of age and housed in groups of three per cage until adulthood, i.e. aged 60-80 days.

Testes were removed from animals killed by cervical dislocation, weighed, decapsulated, and incubated in Krebs–Ringer bicarbonate buffer in the presence of 12.5 mIU/ml human chorionic gonadotropin (hCG; Follutein, Squibb), unless indicated otherwise. The accumulation of T in the medium after a 4 h incubation was measured by radioimmunoassay without extraction, as described in previous reports (Dalterio 1980).

Some males from the prenatal and postnatal treatment groups were castrated under ether anaesthesia using a mid-ventral incision. Animals were killed two weeks later by cervical dislocation and trunk blood was collected for radioimmunoassay determination of LH and FSH in plasma.

Results

Organ weights and plasma T, LH and FSH in intact males

Perinatal exposure to THC resulted in a significant reduction in testicular weights in adulthood. While the weights of the seminal vesicles appeared lower, this effect was not statistically significant. Plasma LH levels were significantly higher in THC-exposed mice, compared to those of oil-exposed males, although plasma T concentrations were in the normal range. Perinatal exposure to CBN did not appear to influence any of these parameters, although the levels of FSH in the plasma appeared reduced.

Prenatal exposure to CBN did not affect the weights of the testes, but the weights of the seminal vesicles were significantly lower than those in the controls. Plasma levels of FSH were also reduced by prenatal CBN treatment. In contrast, prenatal exposure to CBD increased weights of the seminal vesicles, although plasma hormone levels were not affected. Prenatal THC exposure did not influence these parameters.

In contrast to the results of prenatal exposure, adult male mice postnatally exposed to CBD had a significant reduction in testicular weights, while similar postnatal exposure to THC or CBN did not affect the weights of the testes. Plasma concentrations of gonadotropins were reduced in animals exposed to cannabinoids postnatally.

Testicular T production in vitro

Perinatal exposure to disulphiram significantly reduced the responsiveness of the testes to gonadotropin stimulation *in vitro* by 36% ($p < 0.05$) (Fig. 7.1A), although the weights of the testes were not different from control [$265 \pm 9(n = 16)$ vs 270 ± 14 ($n = 16$) mg]. Perinatal exposure to ethanol resulted in a marked decrease in the production of T by decapsulated testes (Fig. 7.1A, left), and testicular weights were also significantly reduced [255 ± 18 ($n = 12$) vs 324 ± 12 ($n = 16$) mg; $p < 0.05$]. In contrast, perinatal exposure to THC did not affect the ability of the testis to respond to gonadotropin *in vitro* and, in fact, concomitant perinatal THC treatment prevented the effects of ethanol on this parameter (Fig. 7.1A).

Prenatal exposure to CBN significantly enhanced testicular responsiveness to hCG *in vitro*, while prenatal exposure to THC tended to increase hCG-stimulated T production, although this effect was not significant (Fig. 7.1A middle).

Postnatal exposure to CBD significantly enhanced *in vitro* T production by decapsulated testes in the presence of hCG, while postnatal treatment with THC or CBN had little, if any, effect on testicular responsiveness to hCG *in vitro*. Basal T production was not affected by postnatal cannabinoid exposure.

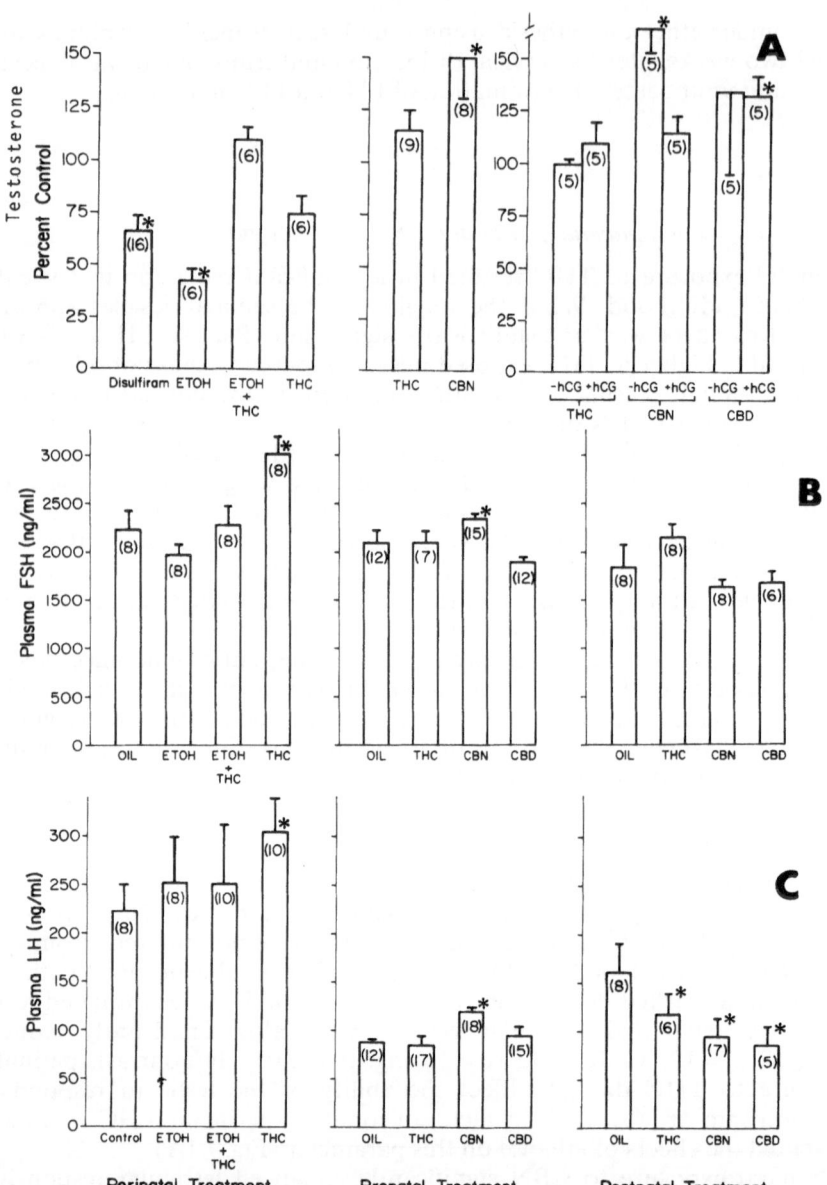

Fig. 7.1 A. Testicular testosterone (T) production, expressed as a percentage of the control, by decapsulated testes obtained from adult male mice after perinatal, prenatal, or postnatal exposure to disulphiram, ethanol (ETOH), and/or $\triangle^9$-tetrahydrocannabinol (THC), cannabinol (CBN) or cannabidiol (CBD), after a 4 h incubation in the presence of 12.5 mlU/ml human chorionic gonadotropin (hCG). B. Plasma levels of LH in castrated adult male mice exposed to ethanol (ETOH), and/or $\triangle^9$-tetrahydrocannabinol (THC), cannabinol (CBN), or cannabidiol (CBD) during either perinatal, prenatal or postnatal periods. C. Plasma levels of FSH in the animals described in B [mean $\pm$ SE (N)]. *significantly different from control ($p < 0.05$)

Pituitary gonadotrophins post-castration

Perinatal exposure to THC resulted in significantly higher levels of LH in the peripheral plasma of adult castrated males, compared to that in castrated controls, while ethanol or THC plus ethanol were without effect on post-castration LH levels.

Prenatal exposure to CBN resulted in significantly higher ($p<0.05$) plasma LH and FSH levels in castrated adult male mice compared to those of castrated controls (Fig. 7.1B, middle), while CBD and THC did not affect these measures.

Postnatal cannabinoid exposure resulted in decreased concentrations of LH post-castration, compared to those in castrated controls (Fig. 7.1C right). Plasma levels of FSH tended to be higher in the THC-exposed, but lower in CBN- and CBD-exposed animals compared to control castrates, although these changes were not statistically significant.

DISCUSSION

The ability of cannabinoids to suppress gonadotropin release is well documented (Bloch *et al.*, 1978). Previously, we have suggested that cannabinoids can inhibit the biosynthesis of T also by a direct action on the testis. In support of this possibility, cannabinoids added *in vitro* are capable of interfering with the steroidogenic activity of incubated testes (Dalterio *et al.*, 1977), ovaries (Burstein *et al.*, 1979) and adrenals (Warner *et al.*, 1977). Regardless of the mechanism of action, cannabinoids can interfere with androgen production in adult, immature, and fetal male mice (Dalterio *et al.*, 1980, 1981).

Cannabinoids cross the placental barrier and are transferred through the milk in lactating females (Bloch *et al.*, 1978). It is, therefore, not surprising that exposure to these compounds during pre- and postnatal periods of sexual differentiation is capable of interfering with the endocrine milieu of the developing fetus or neonate, thus producing long-term consequences for the establishment of the physical and behavioural characteristics normally associated with the male genotype.

One of the most consistent findings in these, and previous studies, is the alteration in testicular responsivity to gonadotropins in cannabinoid-exposed animals. In the case of perinatal exposure to THC, plasma levels of LH were observed to be considerably elevated, both before and after sexual maturation. Yet, the levels of plasma T were either normal or slightly decreased, and testes weights were significantly reduced. Although plasma LH and T levels were normal in males prenatally exposed to THC, we observed increased testicular responsiveness *in vitro* to exogeneous gonadotropins. Concomitant perinatal treatment with THC can block the decrease in gonadotropin-stimulated T production by decapsulated testes from animals perinatally exposed to alcohol. It seems likely that exposure to THC during critical periods of sexual differentiation can directly alter the steroidogenic function of the testis.

The similarity in the effects of perinatal ethanol and disulphiram exposure on testicular T production *in vitro* may indicate that ethanol-induced alterations in subsequent testicular responsiveness to gonadotropins may be due, at least in part, to the acetaldehyde derived from the metabolism of ethanol. This suggestion is consistent with our earlier finding that T production by decapsulated mouse testes was considerably more sensitive to the inhibitory effects of acetaldehyde added to the medium than to the action of ethanol (Badr *et al.*, 1977). Other investigators have also specifically implicated the accumulation of acetaldehyde as being particularly deleterious to male reproductive functions (Cicero *et al.*, 1980).

In the laboratory rodent, the 'critical period' of development and differentiation of the male reproductive system spans both the prenatal and early postnatal periods. It is quite evident from the literature that a number of manipulations, including exposure to drugs used therapeutically, steroid hormones, or environmental factors, such as protein malnutrition or stress, can interfere with the normal development of the fetus or the neonate. It is also evident that whereas some agents evoke gross alterations in phenotypic characteristics, such as the genital feminization induced by antiandrogens (Neumann *et al.*, 1977), other treatments produce more subtle effects, such as the deficits in sexual behaviour observed after prenatal barbiturate exposure (Clemens *et al.*, 1974). Indeed, behavioural teratogenesis may be but one expression of underlying alterations in the biochemical processes within the central nervous system. It is also apparent from the observed effects of maternal stress on sexual differentiation that, while stress may indeed represent a confounding variable that may interact with any treatment in complex ways, by itself, it cannot account for the multitude of effects reported after the described perinatal manipulations.

The possible contribution of stress to the effects of cannabinoids discussed in this chapter should also be considered from another point of view. Namely, cannabinoid-induced alterations in stress responsivity could reverse or prevent stress reactions to handling or injection in a pregnant or lactating animal. Thus, while some effects of cannabinoids reported herein may be critically dependent on the time of exposure, such as the reduction in testes weights after postnatal CBD exposure, compared to the increase in testicular weights after prenatal CBD, it is also possible that cannabinoid treatment differentially affected stress responses to oral drug feeding to the pregnant or lactating female. In addition, we have provided evidence that the long-term consequences of perinatal exposure to the psychoactive THC differ considerably from those of the chemically related, but non-psychoactive, CBN and CBD. This strongly argues against important contributions of non-specific stress effects to these findings.

The effects of castration on the release of pituitary gonadotropins appear to be altered by exposure to cannabinoids during early development. A postnatal period of exposure appears to be required for THC and CBD to be effective in this regard, while CBN also seems to be effective after exposure *in utero*. However, the possible importance of the differential behavioural effects of these two compounds on the female must be considered. Although cannabinoids affect post-castration gonadotropin release, this is not a typical consequence of any interference in the perinatal hormonal milieu. Indeed, we have failed to observe any results of perinatal treatment with either morphine or naloxone on this parameter (Dalterio, unpublished observations), although, in the adult, both compounds readily affect adult pituitary function (Teiri *et al.*, 1979).

Thus, it is apparent that maternal exposure to either psychoactive or non-psychoactive cannabinoids, whether during late pregnancy, early lactation, or both, can result in long-term alterations in the function of the HPG axis in their male offspring. In addition, perinatal exposure to ethanol or disulphiram also appear capable of influencing the development of testicular functions. All of these agents influence the development of the reproductive system in males, and it appears that many of the sequelae of early exposure to any one of them reflects their specific ability to alter the hormonal milieu in the developing individual.

Acknowledgements

We thank Denise Mayfield for her excellent technical assistance in these experiments. This work was supported by a grant from NIH (DA16329, S.D.).

References

Abel, E.L., Dintcheff, B.A. and Day, N. (1979). Effects of *in utero* exposure to alcohol, nicotine and alcohol plus nicotine, on growth and development in rats. *Neurobehavioural Toxicol.*, **1**, 153–9

Badr, F.M., Bartke, A., Dalterio, S. and Bulger, W. (1977). Suppression of testosterone production by ethyl alcohol. Possible mode of action. *Steroids*, **30**, 647–53

Bakke, J.L., Lawrence, N.L. and Bennett, J. (1973). Late effects of perinatal morphine administration on the pituitary-thyroidal and gonadal function. *Biol. Neon.*, **23**, 59–77

Bakke, J.L., Lawrence, N. and Bennett, J. (1978). Late endocrine effects of administering monosodium glutamate to neonatal rats. *Neuroendocrinology*, **26**, 220–8

Barraclough, C.A. (1967). Modifications in reproductive functions after exposure to hormones during the prenatal and early postnatal period. *Neuroendocrinology*, **11**, 61–100

Bercu, B.B., Jackson, I.M.D., Sawin, C.T., Safail, H. and Reichlin, S. (1977). Permanent impairment of testicular development after transient immunological blockade of endogeneous luteinizing hormone in the neonatal rat. *Endocrinology*, **101**, 1871–9

Bergman, A., Rosselli-Austin, L., Yedwab, G. and Yanai, J. (1980). Neuronal deficits in mice following phenobarbital exposure during various periods in fetal development. *Acta Anat.*, **108**, 370–3

Bidlingmaier, F., Knorr, D. and Neumann, F. (1977). Inhibition of masculine differentiation in male offspring of rabbits actively immunized against testosterone before pregnancy. *Nature*, **266**, 647–8

Bloch, E., Thysen, B., Morrill, G.A., Gardner, E. and Fujimoto, G. (1978). Effects of cannabinoids on reproduction and development. *Vit. Horm.*, **36**, 203–58

Boggan, W.O., Randall, C.L. and Dodds, H.M. (1979). Delayed sexual maturation in female C57 Bl/6J mice prenatally exposed to alcohol. *Res. Commun. Chem. Pathol. Pharmacol.*, **23**, 117–25

Burstein, S., Hunter, S.A. and Shoupe, T.S. (1979). Cannabinoid inhibition of rat luteal cell progesterone synthesis. *Res. Commun. Chem. Path. Pharmacol.*, **24**, 413–16

Campbell, A.B. and McGill, T.E. (1970). Neonatal hormone treatment and sexual behaviour in male mice. *Horm. Behav.*, **1**, 145–50

Chen, J.J. and Smith, E.R. (1979). Effects of perinatal alcohol on sexual differentiation and open-field behaviour in rats. *Horm. Behav.*, **13**, 219–31

Cicero, T.J., Bell, R.D., Meyer, E.R. and Badger, T.M. (1980). Ethanol and acetaldehyde directly inhibit testicular steroidogenesis. *J. Pharmacol. Exp. Ther.*, **213**, 228-33

Clark, J.H. and McCormack, S. (1977). Clomid or nafoxidine administratered to neonatal rats causes reproductive tract abnormalities. *Science*, **197**, 164-5

Clemens, L.G. (1974). Neurohormonal control of male sexual behaviour. In *Advances in Behavioral Biology*, pp. 23-53. (New York: Plenum)

Dahlof, L.C. (1978). Influence of maternal stress on the development of the fetal genital system. *Physiol. Behav.*, **20**, 193-5

Dalterio, S. (1980). Perinatal or adult exposure to cannabinoids alters functions in mice. *Pharmacol. Biochem. Behav.*, **12**, 143-53

Dalterio, S., Bartke, A. and Burstein, S. (1980). Cannabinoids inhibit testosterone secretion by mouse testes *in vitro*. *Science.*, **196**, 1472-3

Dalterio, S. and Bartke, A. (1981). Fetal testosterone in mice: Effect of gestational age and cannabinoid exposure. *J. Endocrinol.*, **91**, 509-14

Dalterio, S., Bartke, A. and Sweeney, C. (1981). Interactive effects of ethanol and Δ^9-tetrahydrocannabinol on endocrine functions in male mice. *J. Andrology*, **2**, 87-93

Fried, P.A. (1976). Short- and long-term effects of pre-natal cannabis inhalation upon rat offspring. *Psychopharmacology*, **50**. 285-91

Fried, P.A., (1980). Marihuana use by pregant women: Neurobehavioral effects in neonates. *Drug Alcohol Dependence*, **6**, 415-24

Friedler, G. and Cochin, J. (1968). The effect of cross-fostering on growth patterns in offspring of morphinized and withdrawn female rats. *Fed. Proc.*, **27**, 754

Gianutsos, G. and Abbatiello, R.R. (1972). The effect of pre-natal *Cannabis sativa* on maze learning ability in the rat. *Psychopharmacologia (Berl.)*, **27**, 117-22

Glass, A.R., Mellitt, R., Vigersky, R.A. and Swerdloff, R.S. (1979). Hypoandrogenism and abnormal regulation of gonadotropin secretion in rats fed a low protein diet. *Endocrinology*, **104**, 438-42

Goldman, A.S., Baker, M.K., Chen, J.C. and Wieland, R.G. (1972). Blockade of masculine differentiation in male rat fetuses by maternal injection of antibodies to testosterone-3-Bovine serum albumin. *Endocrinology*, **90**, 716-21

Goldman, B.D., Quadagno, D.M., Shyrne, J. and Gorski, R.A. (1972). Modifications of phallus development and sexual behavior in rats treated with gonadotropin antiserum neonatally. *Endocrinology*, **90**, 1025-31

Griezerstein, H.B. and Abel, E.L. (1980). *In utero* exposure to marihuana extract: Changes in neonate rat body composition. *Neurobehav. Toxicol.*, **3**, 53-6

Gupta, C., Shapiro, S.J., and Yaffe, S.J. (1980). Reproductive dysfunction in male rats following prenatal exposure to phenobarbital. *Pediatr. Pharmacol.*, **1**, 55-62

Gupta, C., Yaffe, S.J. and Shapiro, B.H. (1982). Prenatal exposure to phenobarbital permanently decreases testosterone and causes reproductive dysfunction. *Science*, **216**, 640-2

Hogarth, P.J. and Chalmers, P. (1973). Effect of the neonatal administration of a single dose of chlorpromazine on the subsequent sexual development of male mice. *J. Reprod. Fertil.*, **34**, 539-41

Holck, H.G.O., Lish, P.M., Sjorgen, D.W., Westerfeld, W.W. and Malone, M.H. (1970). Effects of disulfiram on growth, longevity and reproduction of the albino rat. *J. Pharm. Sci.*, **59**, 1267-8

Hostetter, M.W. and Placzek, B.E. (1977). The effect of prolactin deficiency during sexual maturation in the male rat. *Biol. Reprod.*, **17**, 574-7

Hull, E.M., Franz, J.R., Snyder, A. and Nishita, J.K. (1980). Perinatal progesterone treatment and learning, social and reproductive behavior in rats. *Physiol. Behav.*, **24**, 251-6

Ieiri, T., Chen, H.T. and Meites, J. (1979). Effects of morphine and naloxone on serum levels of luteinizing hormone and prolactin in prepubertal male and female rats. *Neuroendocrinology*, **29**, 288-92

Kincl, F.A. and Henderson, S.B. (1978). The influence of neonatal steroid exposure on testosterone metabolism in adult male rats. In Dorner, G. and Kawakami, M. (eds.) *Hormones and Brain Development*, pp. 147-152. (Amsterdam: Elsevier/North Holland)

Kolena, J., Sebokova, E. and Jezova-Repcekova,. D. (1978). Gonadotropin receptors, cAMP and testosterone in estrogenized male rats. *Experientia*, **34**, 266-7

Luthra, Y.K. (1979). Brain biochemical alterations in neonate of dams treated orally with

Δ^9-tetrahydrocannabinol during gestation and lactation. In Nahas, G.G. and Paton, W.D.M. (eds.) *Marihuana: Biochemical Effects*, pp. 531–537. (New York: Pergamon)

Matsumura, H. and Daikoku, S. (1978). Quantitative observation of the effects of sex-steroids on the postnatal development of LH-cells. An immuno-histochemical study. *Cell Tissue Res.*, **188**, 491–6

Nemeroff, C.B., Lipton, M.A. and Kizer, J.S. (1978). Models of neuroendocrine regulations: Use of monosodium glutamate as an investigational tool. *Dev. Neurosci.*, **1**, 102–9

Neumann, F., Graf, K.J., Hasan, S.H., Schenck, B. and Steinbeck, H. (1977). Central actions of anti-androgens. In Martini, L. and Motta, M. (eds.) *Androgens and Antiandrogens*, pp. 163–177. (New York: Raven)

Quadagno, D.M., Wolfe, H.G., Kan Wha Ho, G. and Goldman, B. (1975). Influence of neonatal castration or neonatal anti-gonadotropin treatment on fertility, phallus development and male sexual behavior in the mouse. *Fertil. Steril.*, **26**, 939–44

Singh, H.H., Purohit, V. and Ahluwalia, B.S. (1980). Effect of methadone treatment during pregnancy on the fetal testes and hypothalamus in rats. *Biol. Reprod.*, **22**, 480–5

Sonderegger, T., O'Shea, S. and Zimmerman, E. (1979). Progeny of male rats addicted neonatally to morphine. *Proc. West. Pharmacol. Soc.*, **22**, 137–9

Soyka, L.F., Jaffee, J.M., Peterson, J.M. and Smith, S.M. (1978). Chronic methadone administration to male rats: Tolerance to adverse effects on sires and their progeny. *Pharmacol. Biochem. Behav.*, **9**, 405–9

Tuohima, P. and Niemi, M. (1972). Uptake of sex steroids by the hypothalamus and anterior pituitary of pre- and neonatal rats. *Acta Endocrinol. (Scand.)* **71**, 45–54

Van der Schoot, P., Van der Voort, P.D.M. and Vreeburg, J.T.M. (1976). Masculinization in male rats is inhibited by neonatal injections of dihydrotestosterone. *J. Reprod. Fertil.*, **48**, 385–7

Ward, I.L. (1972). Prenatal stress feminizes and demasculines the behavior of males. *Science*, **175**, 82–4

Ward, I.L. and Weisz, J. (1980). Maternal stress alters plasma testosterone in fetal males. *Science*, **207**, 328–9

Warner, W., Harris, L.S. and Carchman, R.A. (1977). Inhibition of adrenal steroidogenesis by delta-9-tetrahydrocannabinol. *Endocrinology*, **101**, 1815–20

Weathersbee, P.S. and Lodge, J.R. (1978). A review of ethanol's effects on the reproductive process. *J. Reprod. Med.*, **21**, 63–78

Wehmer, F., Porter, R.H. and Scales, B. (1970). Pre-mating and pregnancy stress in rats affects behavior of grandpups. *Nature*, **227**, 622

Weisz, J., Brown, B.L. and Ward, I.L. (1982). Maternal stress decreases steroid aromatase activity in brains of male and female rat fetuses. *Neuroendocrinology* **35**, 374–9

Zadina, J.E., Dunlap, J.L. and Gerall, A.A. (1978). Modifications induced by neonatal steroids in reproductive organs and behaviors of male rats. *J. Comp. Physiol. Psych.*, **93**, 314–22

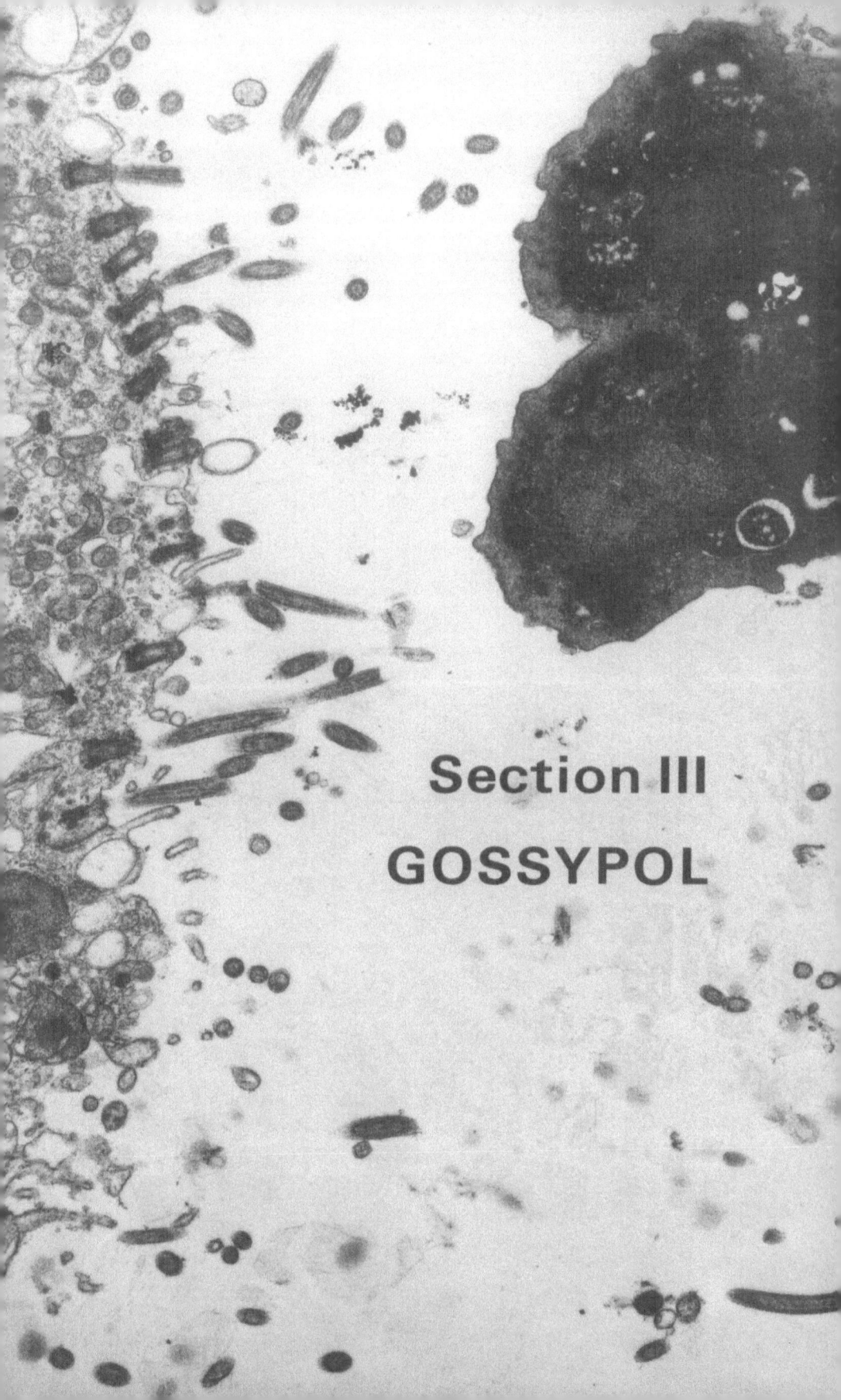

Section III

GOSSYPOL

8
Gossypol chemistry and plant distribution

L.A. JONES

The cotton plant is indigenous to many locations throughout the world. There is a major production of cotton in Brazil, Egypt, India, Mexico, Pakistan, the U.S., and China, as well as in the Soviet Union. Due to variations in density there is appreciably more seed derived from the seed cotton which is plucked directly from the cotton boll than there is lint produced. Of a given weight of seed cotton which is processed through a cotton gin, 62% results as cotton seeds and 38% of the weight is accounted for by the actual cotton fibre. Cotton is frequently measured in units of 480 lb bales and from that bale there is 1.6 times as much cottonseed produced at the gin. While the recent world production of cotton has ranged in the area of 67 million bales per year, the amount of cottonseed produced has been in the area of 28 million metric tonnes per year. United States production of cottonseed has averaged approximately 4.8 million metric tonnes per year over the past five years. When cottonseed is processed, approximately 9% of the weight of the original ginned seed becomes cotton linters which are short cellulose fibres used in paper manufacture and other cellulose applications; 25% are hulls which are used as an animal feed and for other specialized industrial applications; 16% is crude cottonseed oil which is predominately used for salad oil and other lipid applications for human consumption; the bulk of the seed at 45% is cottonseed meal which is a high protein supplement primarily used in animal feeds; the remaining 5% is attributed to waste.

Native gossypol is not a rare commodity. A yearly cottonseed crop in the United States of 4.54 million metric tonnes would contain approximately 27.3 million kilograms of gossypol. In some years the amount may reach 45 million kilograms. Worldwide, the production of gossypol reaches approximately 0.15 million metric tonnes per year. Koltun *et al.* (1959) considered the cost of producing gossypol in either the crude state, as gossypol acetic acid, or as pure gossypol and estimated a cost of $12.21/kg of pure gossypol in 1959 dollars. The process they considered was the gossypol recovery process described by Pons *et al.* (1959) which is capable of isolating approximately 99% pure gossypol from the gums obtained by water washings of crude hexane-extracted cottonseed oil. These gums are a product of the direct solvent process of cottonseed oil extraction, and are regularly added back into various points of the process stream in cottonseed meal production.

OCCURRENCE OF GOSSYPOL

Gossypol distribution

The distribution of gossypol in the cotton plant is a subject of interest to the entomologist as well as the agronomist and has been found to be of economic importance because gossypol can act as a natural insect deterrent (Lukefahr and Houghtaling, 1969). Integrated pest management programmes work well with cotton containing naturally high gossypol levels in plant parts subject to insect feeding. Genetic manipulation of the cotton plant to increase tissue gossypol levels which also produce higher levels of gossypol in the seed result in a potential reduction in the value of the seed. The higher the level of gossypol in the seed, the more appears in the meal derived from that seed, which in turn reduces its value for animal feeding (Phelps, 1966).

Gossypol, as well as a number of other similar pigments, is contained in discrete subepidermal glands dispersed in the above ground plant parts and in the cotyledons of the seed. Gossypol is also present in the root bark of the plant (Royce et al., 1941; Stipanovic et al., 1975). Several workers have shown that gossypol levels in the cotton seed and plant vary with the cultivar being tested (Pons et al., 1953) as well as with the location (Cherry et al., 1978). In common varieties of cotton, gossypol occurs in the kernel at levels from 0.4 to 1.7%.

Since the early 1950s, considerable effort has gone into the development of a genetic variety of cotton without the gossypol containing glands in the seed (McMichael, 1954). Present cultivars of this glandless cotton have been developed to the extent of being able to produce similar lint quantities as glanded varieties in many cases. Glandless cottonseed contains little or no gossypol and produces a high quality clear oil and leaves a meal or protein fraction much better suited as an animal feed and with potential as a human food.

Gossypol is not peculiar to cotton, but is present in many members of the order Malvaceae. Okra belongs to this order, and reportedly contains 3.2 mg of gossypol per 100 g of dried seed, a level believed to be too low to be toxic. A vegetable curd made from okra seed was reported to contain from 0.011% to 0.039% gossypol, depending on the method of preparation (Martin et al., 1979), a level well within the food levels of 0.045% free-gossypol required by the US Food and Drug Administration, or the 0.06% free-gossypol or 1.2% total gossypol recommended by the Food and Agricultural Organization of the United Nations.

Twenty-one different characteristics of cottonseed grown at eight locations in Texas during the 1974 growing season have been examined (Cherry et al., 1978) relative to the effect of both genetic and growing location effects. The results are representative of other studies. Variation in total

Table 8.1   Mean total gossypol in kernels
from eight locations in Texas, 1974 (From
Cherry *et al.*, 1978)

Location	Percent*
A	1.00 c
B	0.88 a
C	0.96 bc
D	0.92 ab
E	1.00 cb
F	0.92 ab
G	0.89 a
H	0.99 c

*Means with the same letter are not sig-
nificantly different according to the Newman–Keuls multiple range test.

gossypol was seen to be highly significant between both locations and cultivars as was their interaction. Table 8.1 gives the total gossypol as determined on moisture-free cottonseed kernels (seeds with the hull removed).

Effects of commercial processing on gossypol

The method of commercial processing of cottonseed determines the form
and amount of gossypol found in the resulting products. In processing, the
rupture of the pigment glands containing gossypol and other complex
polyphenols allows binding of these highly reactive compounds with components of the meal. Thus, that portion of gossypol which has combined is
known as 'bound' gossypol. The remaining, uncombined gossypol is called
'free' gossypol. In raw, unprocessed cottonseed the gossypol is considered
to be all in the 'free' form since it is protected by its pigment gland
membrane from degradation. Therefore, the 'total' gossypol in raw seed
will be all in the 'free' form whereas the 'total' gossypol in products will be
a combination of both 'free' and 'bound' forms.

The analytical method for determining the amounts of free and bound
gossypol in a sample is based on extraction by an acetone:water solvent.
By current definition, free gossypol is that which is readily extracted by
70% aqueous acetone. The sample is then hydrolysed with oxalic acid which
renders all the gossypol and some gossypol-like pigments soluble in the
aqueous acetone. The additional gossypol extracted after hydrolysis is considered to be the 'total' gossypol present in the sample. The calculated
difference between 'total' and 'free' yields the amount of 'bound' gossypol
(Berardi and Goldblatt, 1980).

Since rupture of pigment glands and the exposure of gossypol is necessary
for binding of gossypol, the method of processing will determine the free
and bound levels of end products. There are four methods used for extraction of oil from cottonseed. 'Hydraulic pressing', which was the original
method using flat presses, has been replaced with more efficient technology
so that today less than 1% of cottonseed is processed that way. Mechanical

extraction by 'screw pressing' now accounts for about 20% of the total crush. Solvent extraction, either 'direct' or prepress', is the technique used on most of the seed processed—approximately 80%.

In preparation for extraction, seed follows a similar path regardless of the process. Seed kernels (meats) are separated from the seed coat (hull) and then flaked to a thickness of about 0.01 inches. Under controlled moisture conditions the flakes are cooked for 60-90 minutes at temperatures ranging from 93 to 135°C. Flaking and cooking are essential for effective removal of oil and binding of free gossypol (Berardi and Goldblatt, 1980).

From this point on processing conditions vary widely. Total gossypol in meal after extraction varies according to preparation conditions and the native amount of gossypol in the particular lot of crushed seed. It usually ranges from 0.5 to 1.2%. Free gossypol can range from 0.02 to 0.5% in the meal and depends on the extraction method (Table 8.2).

Table 8.2 Free gossypol and oil contents of meals from four cottonseed processing methods (From Berardi and Goldblatt, 1980)

Method	Residual oil %	Free gossypol %
Hydraulic Pressing (2000 psi)	4.5–7.5	0.04–0.10
Screw Pressing (20 000 psi)	2.5–5	0.02–0.05
Prepress solvent	0.4–1	0.02–0.07
Direct solvent	1	0.1 –0.5

Gossypol not finding its way to the meal fraction is extracted in the oil and removed from the oil in the refining process. Almost all the gossypol in crude cottonseed oil is in the free form. As in the meal, the amount of gossypol in crude oil varies with processing (Table 8.3).

Refining of crude cottonseed oil yields soapstock (foots) as the principal by-product. Gossypol is concentrated in the soap stock but the amount can be quite variable ranging from less than 1 to over 10%. Most of this gossypol is in the free form. Approximately 100 million pounds (45 500 metric tonnes) of cottonseed oil soapstock are produced annually in the United States (Berardi and Goldblatt, 1980).

Table 8.3 Gossypol in crude cottonseed oil

Oil extraction method	Gossypol content %
Hydraulic pressed	0.02 –0.11
Screw pressed	0.25 –0.47
Hexane extracted	0.05 –0.42
Cold pressed	0.005–0.009

Isolation of gossypol

Crude gossypol was first extracted from the soapstock of cottonseed oil resulting from the hydraulic pressing of seeds (Longmore, 1886). Marchlewski (1899) used the same process in purifying the pigment and after demonstrating that it was a polyphenol, called the product gossypol as a contraction of the genus (*Gossypium*), and its chemical form, as a phenol. As reviewed by Berardi and Goldblatt (1980), many procedures for the preparation of gossypol are derived from three steps originally published by Carruth (1918) and reviewed by Boatner (1948). These three procedures include (1) formation of an ether-insoluble gossypol–acetic acid complex, (2) formation of a water-soluble sodium salt followed by purification by way of the acetic acid complex, and (3) reaction with aniline to form ether-insoluble dianilinogossypol, which is followed by hydrolysis and purification as the acetic acid complex.

Preparation of pure gossypol from flaked cottonseed meats, an intermediary product of most modern cottonseed processing mills, via dianilinogossypol has been described (Smith, 1960). Gossypol removal is accomplished by means of extraction with peroxide-free ether. Dianilinogossypol is formed by the addition of aniline which is followed by acid hydrolysis to produce gossypol–acetic acid. Crystallization from a mixture of ether, ethanol, and water from the dianilinogossypol yields about 75% gossypol with a high degree of purity.

A further procedure for the isolation of gossypol from cottonseed gums by water washing of crude, direct solvent extracted cottonseed oil was described by Pons *et al.* (1959). A gossypol–acetic acid complex of better than 98% purity results from the process which involves the refluxing of methyl ethyl ketone containing oxalic or phosphoric acid; 25 g of gossypol–acetic acid can be extracted from a kilogram of gums. Pure gossypol can then be prepared from the acetic acid complex (Boatner, 1948).

The starting material for the isolation of gossypol can determine the preferred method of removal. When the older hydraulic press soapstocks were still available, they were adequate starting materials, but present cottonseed oils are extracted by means of a mechanical screw press or by hexane extraction, or by a combination of both methods, and the resulting soapstock is reputed not to be a suitable starting source for gossypol isolation. Other methods have been described for the removal of gossypol from glandular pigments or from cotton root bark (Royce *et al.*, 1941). A thorough review of isolation techniques is presented by Markman and Rzhekhin (1965).

GOSSYPOL AND GOSSYPOL-LIKE PIGMENTS

Chemical form of gossypol

The structure of gossypol was verified and shown to have the following structure: 1,1',6,6',7,7'-hexahydroxy-5,5'-diisopropyl-3,3'-dimethyl (2,2'-binaphthalene)-8,8'-dicarboxaldehyde (Adams *et al.*, 1960). Whereas the structure of gossypol was first proposed by Adams *et al.*, (1938), it was corroborated in other work and confirmed through the full synthesis of gossypol (Edwards, 1958).

Gossypol is soluble in most organic solvents. It is most soluble in the more polar solvents and insoluble in the non-polar solvents. It is very soluble in methyl, ethyl, isopropyl, and butyl alcohols. It is also soluble in the following solvents: ethylene glycol, dioxane, diethyl ether, acetone, ethyl acetate, chloroform, carbon tetrachloride, ethylene dichloride, phenol, pyridine, and heated napthalene and vegetable oils. It is much less soluble in glycerine, cyclohexane, benzene, and gasoline, and it is insoluble in low-boiling point petroleum ether (b.p. 30–60°C) and in water (Markham and Rhekhin, 1965; Berardi and Goldblatt, 1980.)

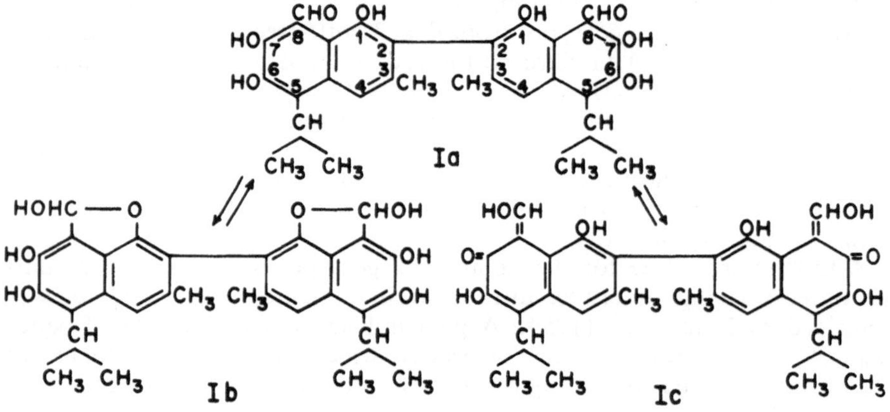

Fig. 8.1 Structures of the various tautomeric forms of gossypol where (a) represents the hydroxy aldehyde tautomer; (b) the lactol tautomer; and (c) the cyclic carbonyl tautomer

The terpenoid compound, gossypol, historically has been the compound of greatest concern in cottonseed. The chemical characteristics have been outlined (Berardi and Goldblatt, 1980; Markman and Rzhekhin, 1965). Gossypol is markedly reactive and shows strongly acidic properties. It can act as a phenolic and as an aldehydic compound. The phenolic groups react readily to form esters and ethers. The aldehyde groups react with amines to form Schiff bases and with organic acids to form heat-labile compounds (Adams *et al.*, 1960). The reaction with aromatic amines such as aniline is important in analysis. Gossypol has a molecular weight of 518.5. Gossypol of m.p. 184°C is obtained upon crystallization from ether, of m.p. 199°C from chloroform, and of m.p. 214°C from ligroin. Such a wide range of melting temperatures is attributed to the polymorphism of gossypol.

The postulation of three tautomeric forms of gossypol (Adams *et al.*, 1938) was necessary to explain many of the reactions of the compound. As shown in Fig. 8.1, (a) represents the hydroxy aldehyde tautomer, (b) the lactol tautomer, and (c) the cyclic carbonyl tautomer.

Absorption spectra of gossypol

A number of factors influence the characteristics of the spectral curves of gossypol. Among them are the conditions under which the gossypol was prepared, or crystallized, the duration of the storage period, the temperature used to dissolve the crystals, and also the solvent used for any particular determination. A review of spectral characteristics is given by Markman and Rzhekhin (1965) and Boatner (1948). Most of the differences in spectra may be due to the different tautomeric forms and to the reactivity of the molecule. A comparison of the spectra of gossypol in cyclohexane, chloroform, and ethanol shows that the absorption maxima are shifted toward longer wave lengths in the polar solvents and their intensity is lower in the cyclohexane solution. Table 8.4 lists the ultraviolet and visible absorption maxima of chloroform or ethanol solutions of gossypol pigments (Berardi and Goldblatt, 1980).

Table 8.4 Ultraviolet and visible absorption maxima of gossypol pigments (From Berardi and Goldblatt, 1980)

Pigment	Solvent	Maxima (nm)
Gossypol	$CHCl_3$	276–279, 288–289, 362–365
Gossycaerulin	$CHCl_3$	605
Diaminogossypol	$CHCl_3$	250, 378
Gossypurpurin	$CHCl_3$	326–327, 370, 530–532, 565–568
Gossyfulvin	$CHCl_3$	250–251, 312–313, 439–440
Gossyverdurin	$CHCl_3$	250, 370, 560
6-Methoxygossypol	EtOH	235, 288, 369
6, 6′-Dimethoxygossypol	EtOH	231, 253, 287, 360, 390

Analysis of gossypol

A thorough review of gossypol analytical techniques up to the mid 1970s has been presented (Pons, 1977). At the present time the procedure for the analysis of free-gossypol (Ba7-58 of the American Oil Chemists Society (AOCS) employs an extraction method suggested by Pons and Guthrie (1949) which uses an acetone-water (70:30 v/v) mix for extraction of free-gossypol in 1 h on a shaker with minimal extraction of lipids and minimal hydrolysis of bound gossypol. At about the same time that this method was developed another method using ethanol-water–ether (57:27:17, by vol.) was developed by Smith (1946) and required five minutes extraction in a high speed blender. Both of these procedures were culminations of several decades of work employing single or multiple solvents with extraction periods of up to three days time.

The initial attempts at the quantitative estimation of extracted free-gossypol were based on gravimetric precipitation of gossypol as the dianilino derivative but gave way to spectrophotometric methods employing p-anisidine (Pons and Guthrie, 1949). Antimony trichloride and phloroglucinol were also tried with varying degrees of sensitivity. The present AOCS method employs an adaptation of the technique of Smith (1946).

The National Cottonseed Products Association (NCPA) speciifies an analytical technique for the analysis of free-gossypol, but not for total gossypol. The specified procedure for free-gossypol is that of the AOCS. The NCPA also has a three part standard for glandless cottonseed which requires the total gossypol of undelinted seed to be less than 400, 100 and 10 parts/10^6 respectively, with the analytical method being specified.

The AOCS official method for analysis of total gossypol is Ba8-78. It is based on a spectrophotometric method in which bound gossypol is hydrolysed and allowed to react with analine. For purposes of trade the total gossypol technique using aminopropanol hydrolysis seems to be accurate, reproducible and fully suitable for the purpose (Pons, 1977). Table 8.5 presents detection limits for several quantitative methods for gossypol.

In considering the progress made in gossypol analysis (Pons, 1977) it was mentioned that high performance liquid chromatography (HPLC) offered great potential for gossypol determination. In response to both academic and industry calls for the development of an HPLC method for gossypol, work has recently been completed on such a technique (Nomeir and Abou-Donia, 1982). It was indicated that the minimum detectable limits of the HPLC technique were 10 ng whereas the minimum detection limits for traditional spectrophotometric methods are in the range of 10 to 25 μg. In addition to having advantages in detection limits, HPLC also offers the advantage of fewer steps, and can also distinguish between gossypol and some closely related metabolites or cottonseed pigments. It is also non-destructive and the eluted gossypol can be used for further identification techniques. It should be noted that there have also been methods published for the gas–liquid chromatographic (Raju and Cater, 1967), infrared spectrophotometric (Abou-Donia and Dieckert, 1975) and mass spectrophotometric (Abou-Donia and Dieckert, 1975) and mass spectrophotometric (Abou-Donia et al., 1970) analysis of gossypol.

Table 8.5 Sensitivity and detection limits of gossypol quantitative methods (Adapted from Pons, 1977)

Type of measurement	Reference	Sensitivity (μg)	Detection limit (parts/10^6)
Spectrophotometry	AOCS (Ba7–58)	10	50–100
Paper chromato-graphy	Schramm and Benedict (1958)	0.5	10
Gas–liquid chromato-graphy	Raju and Cater (1967)	0.2–1.0	1–2
HPLC	Nomeir and Abou-Donia (1982)	–	0.01

Gossypol as a terpenoid of cotton

Gossypol and other terpenoids of cottonseed, as well as flavonoids and phenols, have been the subject of periodic review (Bell and Stipanovic, 1977; Jones, 1979).

Gossypol is concentrated in discrete glands within the leaves, stems, roots, and seeds of the cotton plant. The pigment glands in the foliage parts of the plant are located below the epidermis and hypodermis. In the seed embryo, or kernel, these pigment-containing glands are 100 to 400 μm in diameter. Gossypol makes up approximately 20–40% of the weight of these glands and results in levels of gossypol in the whole kernels of 0.4 to 1.7% (Bell and Stipanovic, 1977).

Concern about the toxicity and contraceptive activity of gossypol has resulted in a series of events in the past two or three decades that have recently led to a great expansion of knowledge about cotton plant pigments. These events have altered the historical emphasis of gossypol research away from its effect in cottonseed protein for feed and food uses.

In the early 1960s, commercial development of genetically glandless varieties of cotton was undertaken on the basis that the value of cottonseed oil and meal could be improved and its usefulness extended if gossypol were not present. That assumption is still valid and is the basis for continued productive work on glandless varieties. With the advent of glandless varieties, it was found that many of the insects which did not attack glanded cotton inflicted damage on glandless strains in areas where the insect infestation was heavy (Bell and Stipanovic, 1977; Stipanovic *et al.*, 1977). Such observations stimulated studies on the importance of pigment glands in host plant resistance. Concern with regard to agricultural chemicals also emphasized the need for natural control measures.

Toxicity of glanded flower buds to some insects has been correlated with gossypol content. The traditional method of analysis commonly used employed aniline which is a non-specific reagent for aromatic aldehydes. It is not known exactly how many aromatic aldehydes exist in glands, and this left the above correlation in doubt. In addition to this, other workers (Bell and Stipanovic, 1977) suspected that some wild types of cotton had more insecticidal activity than could be accounted for by the gossypol concentration alone. This set the stage for the extensive work on terpenoids in cotton glands. Initially, the toxic activity was attributed to 'X-factors'. These X-factors have recently been identified as two sesquiterpenoids and a series of eight derived sesterterpenoids called heliocides. The sesquiterpenoids are illustrated in Fig. 8.2 as HGQ and mHGQ while the sesterterpenoids are heliocides H1, H2, H3, and H4, and also B1, B2, B3, and B4.

Although commonly cultivated varieties of cotton are presently almost all glanded, they are by no means insect free. The common cotton cultivars contain gossypol, hemigossypolone, and the heliocides H1, H2, H3, and H4 (Fig. 8.2). Insect-resistant wild types of cotton are observed to contain these same compounds, but the concentrations are as much as three times as great. This is especially true of heliocides H1 and H4. True glandless cotton cultivars do not contain the terpenoid aldehydes (Bell and Stipanovic, 1977).

The above research is directed toward insect control and not toward gossypol in seed products. Since the seed is not the site of the heaviest

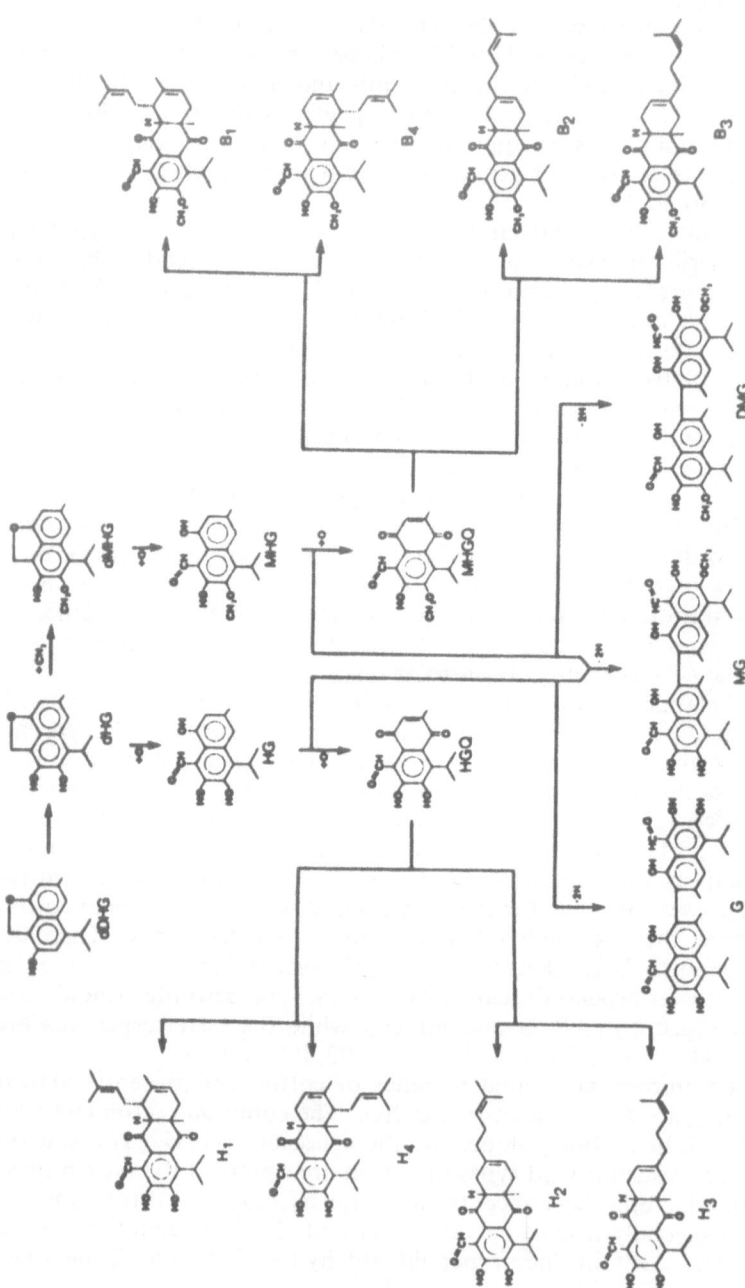

Fig. 8.2 Proposed pathway for biosynthesis of terpenoid aldehydes in cotton. dDHG = desoxy-6-deoxyhemigossypol; dHG = desoxyhemigossypol; dMHG = desoxy-6-methoxyhemigossypol; HG = hemigossypol; MHG = 6-methoxyhemigossypol; HGQ = hemigossypolone; MHGQ = 6-methoxyhemigossypolone; G = gossypol; MG = 6-methoxygossypol; DMG = 6,6'-dimethoxygossypol; H_1-H_4 = heliocides H_1-H_4; B_1-B_4 = heliocides B_1-B_4. Adapted from Stipanovic, Bell and Lukefahr (1977)

insect attack, it has been somewhat neglected in the most recent gossypol research. One of the long-range goals of host plant resistance researchers is to develop cotton lines with optimum terpenoid biosynthesis for pest control while preserving the value of the seed products. The beneficial terpenoids thus might be concentrated in the vegetable plant parts, while the seed, which is not the first point of insect attack, could be kept terpenoid-free, and thus be more valuable for food and feed.

Not all pigment glands in all locations of the cotton plant have a similar terpenoid make up. The predominant terpenoid aldehyde of the seed is gossypol, but Bell and his coworkers have shown that it is not the only one (Stipanovic *et al.*, 1975) although gossypol is by far the most predominant terpenoid aldehyde. The triterpenoids 6-methoxygossypol and 6,6'-dimethoxygossypol are present in much lower relative amounts, while the sesquiterpenoids hemigossypol and 6-methoxyhemigossypol appear in only trace amounts. There is no indication that there may be any heliocides in the seed itself (Stipanovic *et al.*, 1977). Figure 8.2 illustrates the structures of gossypol as well as 6-methoxygossypol and 6,6'-dimethyoxygossypol which are present in slight but quantifiable amounts.

Hemigossypol may possibly be a branch point to either the heliocides or gossypol and its related compounds. If chlorophyll is present in plant tissue, then the path may lead to heliocides, whereas if it is not present, as in the seed, then the path may go to gossypol (Stipanovic *et al.*, 1977).

Several gossypol-related compounds that have not been included in these biochemical schemes should be noted. These gossypol-like pigments of the seed have been mentioned in the older literature and in review articles on gossypol. Recent analytical techniques, however, raise some questions as to the actual presence of them in the intact seed. Two of these gossypol-like pigments that have long been thought to occur in seed are gossypurpurin and gossyfulvin (Berardi and Goldblatt, 1980). Gossypurpurin has been measured at about 1% of the gland contents, while gossyfulvin has been measured at about 2% of the gland contents. The structure of gossyfulvin has not been elucidated, but a structure for gossypurpurin has been proposed (Berardi and Goldblatt, 1980). Several others had been historically identified as occurring in various steps of cottonseed processing, either in the meal or the oil or the soapstock. These other products have been called gossyverdurin, gossycaerulin, and diaminogossypol. The possibility exists that these other pigments, long thought to exist in cottonseed, might actually be oxidation or condensation products of gossypol. HPLC techniques for the analysis of gossypol (Nomeir and Abou-Donia, 1982) should aid in this determination.

REACTIVITY OF GOSSYPOL

Specific chemical reactions of gossypol in the formation of ethers, esters, anils, and in oxidation reactions have been competently reviewed by Berardi and Goldblatt (1980) and others (Abou-Donia, 1976; Markman and Rzhekhin, 1965; Boatner, 1948) and will not be duplicated here. Some biological actions however, will be considered.

The effect of gossypol on monogastric animals has been the subject of intensive research over the past century. Recently this investigation has included ruminants. Practical limitations on the use of cottonseed meal because of reactions of gossypol in the animal body have been established through extensive research and practical work. The pathological effects of gossypol in animals have been examined by Smith and Clawson (1970).

The activity of gossypol in specific biological enzyme systems has not been as fully examined as the gross effect of gossypol, but has been the subject of some work over the years. The effect of gossypol on the enzymatic activity of crystalline trypsin, pepsin, muscle aldolase, and in the activation of pepsinogen was studied in vitro (Tanksley et al., 1970). It was found that trypsin activity was completely inhibited, while pepsin activity was not inhibited after prolonged incubation. The activation of pepsinogen was completely prevented. Muscle aldolase activity was likewise inhibited.

When the activities of certain respiratory enzyme systems were examined in pigs, rabbits and rats (Meksongsee et al., 1970), it was found that cyto-chrome oxidase and succinoxidase activities in the liver of the three species were not markedly affected by gossypol in vivo, even when the gossypol dosage levels were toxic to the animals. Similarly, no effect was shown in succinic dehydrogenase activity in pig liver. Reports by other workers showed variation in the effects of gossypol on these enzymes, especially in vitro. Other work on rat liver microsomal oxidases (Abou-Donia and Dieckert, 1971) found that gossypol appeared to stimulate these enzymes through an increase in enzyme synthesis. It was not shown if the response was an adaptive detoxification reaction, or a pathological response.

In other work examining the effect of gossypol in liver activity (Skutches and Smith, 1974), it was found that gossypol inhibits liver microsomal peroxidation by chelating with iron. Liver lipid peroxidation activity was found to be inversely related to liver gossypol concentrations.

In work to investigate the effect of gossypol as a male contraceptive, there is a preliminary indication that gossypol may act by inhibiting several key enzymes, including lactate dehydrogenase-X, which is the form of the enzyme found only in the testes and sperm. Gossypol may also have a species specific effect on malate dehydrogenase, and may also affect the glutathione S-transferase system.

An area of gossypol activity which has received little attention has been the interaction of the compound with the transport systems of the gut. Studies with rats (Jones and Smith, 1975) indicate that bound gossypol in the diet can cause an increase in the faecal nitrogen level compared to controls and can decrease amino acid absorption. Increased rate of passage of digesta, the reported inhibition of gossypol on proteolytic enzymes of digestion (Lyman et al., 1959; Tanksley et al., 1970), and an action of gossypol on amino acid absorption are all possible factors involved in such an observation. It has also been observed (Tone and Jensen, 1969) that rats fed on a diet with 0.18% total gossypol exhibited a greater rate of cell extrusion and a larger mitotic index in the duodenum compared to rats fed on the same diet without gossypol. Such pathology may affect absorption.

The possibility that the reduced nutritional value of gossypol containing cottonseed meal may be due to actions of gossypol other than the pathological effects mentioned (Tone and Jensen, 1969) on the amino acid absorptive systems of the small intestine has not been thoroughly investigated.

Carrier-mediated intestinal transport systems have been adequately demonstrated for neutral, basic, and acidic amino acids. Some hint of how gossypol may affect these enzyme systems may be found in studies on the effect of gossypol on the rat intestinal amino acid transfer mechanism (Jones and Smith, 1975). In these studies, *in vitro* determiniations of the effects of two forms of gossypol on the kinetic values K_t and V_{max} for intestinal transport of labelled L-lysine, L-methionine, and L-valine were determined. While gossypol alone was not actively transported, it did have the ability to alter the kinetic transport parameters for the three amino acids. Ability to alter these enzyme mediated transport functions may indicate a potential ability to alter other enzyme activities as well.

Reactions of gossypol with nutrients

Since researchers first suggested that cottonseed meal caused injury to livestock, a voluminous amount of literature has been published on the nature and control of gossypol effects. The influence of diet is chronicled by many reviews (Adams *et al.*, 1960; Phelps, 1966; Abou-Donia, 1976; Berardi and Goldblatt, 1980).

Shortly after early workers had demonstrated the toxicity of gossypol, Withers and Brewster (1913) observed that iron salts alleviated cottonseed toxicity. It was also noted that steaming raw cottonseed reduced toxicity and that heat and moisture applied during processing of seed tended to render gossypol less toxic. It was proposed that gossypol reacted with the free amino groups of proteins to form an insoluble complex. Reactions with various nutrients that are based on these hypotheses will be briefly discussed.

Proteins

It is quite evident that both dietary protein quantity and quality affect response to ingested gossypol. Many studies did not adequately distinguish between the quantity and quality. Indeed, both may be related to the availability of reactive amino groups, especially the epsilon-amino group of lysine (Berardi and Goldblatt, 1980).

After preliminary work showed that including casein in rat diets containing cottonseed meal accelerated gain, Gallup and Reder (1935) reported that a short-term sublethal but growth-retarding level of gossypol in rat diets permitted marked increases in gain when protein was increased from 13 to 35% by adding casein. Later, Woronick and Grau (1955) reported that gossypol aldehyde groups condense with free amino groups of egg cephalin to form a Shiff's base in egg yolk. Narain *et al.* (1958) observed that the amount of gossypol–cephalin transferred to eggs was halved by increasing protein from 17.5 to 30% in the diet. They surprisingly failed to find the same response when soybean meal was used in a separate trial. These observations assumed added importance since the egg is an important pathway of the hen's elimination of absorbed gossypol.

Both quality and quantity of protein can affect gains of protein-depleted rats. Hale and Lyman (1957) eliminated swine mortality and gross pathological abnormality by increasing protein from 15% to 30% in diets containing 200 to 300 parts/10^6 of gossypol. Swine mortality at a constant gossypol and protein level is lower with soybean meal than with peanut or cottonseed meals, probably because there is more lysine in soy. This contrasted with evidence that heat-damaged soybean and cottonseed meals, which were probably made about equally poor in available essential amino acids, were not different in their effects upon gain, feed efficiency, pathology, and mortality of pigs fed gossypol. Increasing dietary protein as much as threefold did not prevent damage by intraperitoneally injected gossypol.

The review by Phelps (1966) presents support for the hypothesis that L-lysine supplementation may improve chicken performance but it lacks the gossypol detoxifying effects of protein. The work of Lyman et al. (1959) and others indicates the same response with swine and rats. Cater and Lyman (1969) found good evidence that gossypol reacts progressively with free amino groups as they are exposed by enzymatic digestion of protein in the gut eventually to form cross-linked insoluble complexes.

The accumulated research indicates that the physiological effects of ingested gossypol may be reduced or eliminated, within limits, by increasing the dietary level or quality of protein and that a major function is reduced gossypol absorption.

Minerals

Most investigative studies with minerals have involved iron salts. The ferrous form has been more thoroughly explored than ferric iron. Ferrous sulphate appears to be the most generally suitable salt.

Withers and Brewster (1913) successfully fed citrate of iron and ammonia to rabbits and also alleviated gossypol toxicity in pigs with ferrous sulphate and ferric chloride. Ferric citrate and ferrous ammonium sulphate, but not ferric oxide, were found to be effective in rats. Eagle (1949) protected rats from a high level of ingested gossypol with ferrous sulphate. Lyman (1966) defined the observations of his group on the separate and additive effects of protein quantity and quality and iron supplementation of cottonseed meals of high gossypol content in practical swine feeding. In the 1930s, researchers noted that ferrous sulphate tended to prevent gossypol discoloration of eggs, findings which have proven to be important in the commercial poultry industry.

Clawson et al. (1962) clarified the role of iron in preventing gossypol toxicity. They provided support for the hypothesis that iron forms an insoluble complex with gossypol in the pig gut since liver iron was inversely related to dietary gossypol and dietary iron did not prevent injected gossypol toxicity. Abou-Donia *et al*. (1970) noted that the biological half-life of radiolabelled gossypol in the rat was 23 h with ferrous sulphate supplementation and 48 hours without. Iron appeared to increase expiration of labelled carbon dioxide in the rat, but this is apparently not a major pathway of gossypol detoxification in the pig (Abou Donia and Dieckert, 1975) and the chicken. It has been shown, however, that iron has a poor therapeutic value for gossypol-poisoned rats. Adding iron to a diet to deplete gossypol already present in pig tissue is also ineffective. Work by several authors (Skutches *et al*., 1973; Tone and Jensen, 1976) indicates gossypol can cause anaemia by binding to iron.

Gallup and Reder (1935) concluded that alkaline diets high in calcium stimulated growth of rats fed gossypol, and also reported that calcium carbonate and sodium bicarbonate detoxify gossypol. Sodium, potassium, ammonium, and calcium ions contribute to gossypol detoxifications probably through creation of alkaline conditions in which gossypol is less stable. Supplementing with both iron and calcium resulted in full protection against gossypol but calcium alone resulted in lowered haematological values. Possibly the biologically synergistic effect of calcium with iron is explained by the formation of an insoluble complex. Smith and Clawson (1970) studied copper, zinc, manganese, and iron, alone and in combination, in rat diets. Only iron increased gains and it reduced liver bound and free gossypol most effectively. Zinc and manganese individually lowered bound gossypol but were less effective in combination. Copper interacted with zinc and with manganese to increase liver bound gossypol.

Other nutrients

Rojas and Scott (1969) noted that ferrous sulphate improved metabolizable energy of high-gossypol meal for chicks but not of essentially gossypol-free glandless meal and that there was a synergistic effect with hydrolysis of phytin. Phytase treatment also appeared to exert a gossypol detoxifying effect. It is unclear as to whether this effect is by release of protein from protein–phytate complex and/or release of minerals which might participate in gossypol binding.

Berardi and Goldblatt (1980) interpret the reports of several workers to indicate that carbohydrates, phospholipids, and flavones have an effect on gossypol activity. The evidence appears to be very good for phospholipids and fairly good for flavones but the effect noted for carbohydrates might be more related to reduction of protein quality during processing of cottonseed protein. Gallup and Reder (1935) found that lactose had only a slight effect on gossypol fed rats but diet acidity may have been a confounding factor. Addition of refined, edible oil increased gain slightly, perhaps by energy intake. A higher level of toxicity has also been noted in vitamin A-deficient rats but no relationship was found between deficiencies of the vitamin B complex or vitamin D and toxicity. The flavonal glycosides rutin and isoquercetin seem to have an adverse effect upon rat response to gossypol. Rincon *et al*. (1978) reported that propionic acid, added as a mould inhibitor, appeared to reduce iron–gossypol binding during wet treatment of whole cottonseed with ferrous sulphate but did not appear to increase liver deposits of gossypol nor reduce performance of rats. Their data do not support any conclusion on how the preservative may have caused results contrary to those expected. Phelps *et al.* (1965) cited studies which show that dietary cyclopropenoid fatty acids enhance the yolk discoloration of gossypol-containing eggs but there is no evidence that gossypol toxicity is related to the presence of cyclopropenes.

It appears quite conclusive that ingested gossypol may be materially influenced by diet. In studies with laboratory and farm species iron and protein quantity and quality have been the major factors employed to modify toxicity. If the human species reacts to gossypol comparably to these test animals, uncontrolled diet could affect either the efficacy or the safety of its administration as an anti-fertility drug. Eagle's caution in 1949 to proceed slowly before prescribing gossypol to depress appetite for prevention of obesity appears to be an excellent precedent. Techniques for avoidance of gossypol hazards in feeding farm animals are generally known. It is hoped that careful design of experiments on the reproduction effects of gossypol and a thorough analysis of the composition of all experimental diets plus reporting the diets and results precisely in publications, will help to avoid much of the confusion and misinterpretation encountered for so many years when gossypol was tested with farm animals.

References

Abou-Donia, M.B. (1976). Physiological effects and metabolism of gossypol. In Gunther, F.A. (ed.) *Residue Reviews*, Vol. 61, pp. 125-160 (New York: Springer-Verlag).

Abou-Donia, M.B. and Dieckert, J.W. (1971). Gossypol; subcellular localization and stimulation of rat liver microsomal oxidases. *Toxicol. Appl. Pharmacol.*, **18**, 507-16

Abou-Donia, M.B. and Dieckert, J.W. (1975). Metabolic fate of gossypol: The metabolism of 14C-gossypol in swine. *Toxicol. Appl. Pharmacol.*, **31**, 32

Abou-Donia, M.B., Dieckert, J.W. and Lyman, C.M. (1970). Mass spectrometry of some gossypol ethers. *J. Agr. Food Chem.*, **18**, 534-5

Adams, R., Geissman, T.A. and Edwards, J.D., (1960). Gossypol, a pigment of cottonseed. *Chem. Rev.*, **60**, 555-74

Adams, R., Morris, R.C., Geissman T.A., Butterbaugh, D.J. and Kirkpatrick, E.C. (1938). Structure of gossypol. XV. An interpretation of its reactions. *J. Am. Chem. Soc.*, **60**, 2193-204

Bell, A.A., and Stipanovic, R.D. (1977). The chemical composition, biological activity, and genetics of pigment glands in cotton. *Beltwide Cotton Production Research Conferences Proceedings*, Jan 10-12, Atlanta, pp. 244-258. (Memphis: National Cotton Council)

Berardi, L.C. and Goldblatt, L.A. (1980). Gossypol. In Liener, D.E. (ed.) *Toxic Constituents of Plant Foodstuffs*, Chap. 7, (New York: Academic Press)

Boatner, C.H. (1948). Pigments of cottonseed. In Bailey, A.E. (ed.) pp. 213-363. (New York: Interscience Publishers)

Carruth, F.E. (1918). Contribution to the chemistry of gossypol, the toxic principle of cottonseed. *J. Am. Chem. Soc.*, **40**, 647-63

Cater, C.M. and Lyman, C.M. (1969). Reactions of gossypol with amino acids and other compounds. *J. Am. Oil Chem. Soc.*, **46**, 649-53

Cherry, J.P., Simmons, J.G. and Kohel, R.J. (1978). Cottonseed composition of National Variety Test cultivars grown at different Texas locations. *Beltwide Cotton Production Research Conference Proceedings*, Jan. 9-11, Dallas, pp. 47-50. (Memphis: National Cotton Council).

Clawson, A.J., Smith, F.H. and Barrick, E.R. (1962). Accumulation of gossypol in the liver and factors influencing the toxicity of injected gossypol. *J. Anim. Sci.*, **21**, 911–15

Eagle, E. (1949). Detoxification of cottonseed pigment glands with ferrous sulfate. *Proc. Soc. Exp. Biol. Med.*, **72**, 444–6

Edwards, J.D. Jr. (1958). Total synthesis of gossypol. *J. Am. Chem. Soc.*, **80**, 3798–9

Gallup, W.D. and Reder, R. (1935). The influence of certain dietary constituents on the response of rats to gossypol ingestion. *J. Agr. Res.*, **51**, 259–66

Hale, F. and Lyman, C.M. (1957). Effect of protein level in the ration on gossypol tolerance in growing fattening pigs. *J. Anim. Sci.*, **16**, 364–9

Jones, L.A. (1979). Gossypol and some other terpenoids, flavonoids, and phenols that affect quality of cottonseed protein. *J. Am. Oil Chem. Soc.*, **56**, 727–30

Jones, L.A. and Smith, F.H. (1975). Effect of free and bound gossypol on the absorption of L-(^{14}C)Lysine, L-(^{14}C)Methionine, and L-(^{14}C)Valine from the rat intestine. *J. Agr. Food Chem.*, **23**, 647–53

Koltun, S.P., Decossas, K.M., Pominski, J., Pons, W.A. Jr and Patton, E.L. (1959). Production of gossypol from cottonseed gums. Preliminary cost study. *J. Am. Oil Chem. Soc.*, **36**, 349–52

Longmore, J. (1886). Cottonseed oil: Its coloring matter mucilage, and description of a new method of recovering the loss occurring in the refining process. *J. Soc. Chem. Ind.*, **5**, 200–5

Lukefahr, M.J. and Houghtaling, J.E. (1969). Resistance of cotton strains with gossypol content to *Heliothis* spp. *J. Econ. Entomol.*, **62**, 588–91

Lyman, C.M. (1966). The effect of gossypol and gossypol-like compounds upon swine in the presence and absence of iron salts and/or protein of high biological value. *Proceedings Conference on Inactivation of Gossypol with Mineral Salts*, pp. 104–106. (Memphis: National Cottonseed Products Association)

Lyman, C.M., Baliga, B.P. and Slay, W. (1959). Reaction of protein with gossypol. *Arch. Biochem. Biophys.*, **84**, 486

Marchlewski, L. (1899). Gossypol, ein bestandtheil der bauwollsamen. *J. Prakt. Chem.*, **60**, 84

Markman, A.L. and Rzhekhin, V.P., (1965). *Gossypol and its Derivatives*. English translation. Published for the USDA & NSF, Available from U.S. Dept. Commerce, Clearinghouse for Federal Scientific & Technical Information, Springfield, VA, 22151

Martin, F.W., Telek, L., Ruberte', R. and Santiago, A.G. (1979). Protein, oil and gossypol contents of a vegetable curd made from okra seeds. *J. Food Sci.*, **44**, 1517–19

McMichael, S.C. (1954). Glandless boll in upland cotton and its use in the study of natural crossing. *Agron. J.*, **46**, 527–8

Meksongsee, L.A., Clawson, A.J. and Smith, F.H. (1970). The *in vivo* effect of gossypol on cytochrome oxidase, succinoxidase, and succinic dehydrogenase in animal tissues. *J. Agr. Food Chem.*, **18**, 917–20

Narain, R.C., Lyman, C.M. and Couch, J.R. (1958). Effect of increased protein level in the hen diet on the transfer of gossypol cephelen to the egg. *Poultry Sci.*, **37**, 893–6

Nomeir, A.A. and Abou-Donia, M.B. (1982). Gossypol: high-performance liquid chromatographic analysis and stability in various solvents. *J. Am. Oil. Chem. Soc.*, **59**, 546–9

Phelps, R.A. (1966). Cottonseed meal for poultry: from research to practical application. *World's Poult. Sci. J.*, **22**

Phelps, R.A., Shenstone, F.S., Kemmerer, A.R. and Evans, R.J. (1965). A review of cyclopropenoid compounds: biological effects of some derivatives. *Poultry Sci.*, **44**, 359–94

Pons, W.A. Jr. (1977). Gossypol analysis: past and present. *J. Assoc. Off. Anal. Chem.*, **60**, 252–9

Pons, W.A. and Guthrie, J.D. (1949). Determination of free gossypol in cottonseed materials. *J. Am. Oil Chem. Soc.*, **26**, 671–6

Pons, W.A. Jr., Hoffpauir, C.L. and O'Connor, R.T. (1950). Determination of total gossypol pigments in cottonseed materials. *J. Am. Oil Chem. Soc.*, **27**, 390–3

Pons, W.A. Jr., Hoffpauir, C.L. and Hooper, T.H. (1953). Gossypol in cottonseed: influence of variety of cottonseed and environment. *J. Agr. Food Chem.*, **1**, 1115–18

Pons, W.A. Jr., Pominski, J. King, W.H., Harris, J.A. and Hopper, T.H. (1959). Recovery of gossypol from cottonseed gums. *J. Am. Oil. Chem. Soc.*, **36**, 328–32

Raju, P.U. and Cater, C.M. (1967). Gas-liquid chromomatographic determination of gossypol as the trimethylsilyl ether derivative. *J. Am. Oil Chem. Soc.*, **44,** 465-6

Rincon, R., Smith, F.H. and Clawson, A.J. (1978). Detoxification of gossypol in raw cottonseed and the use of raw cottonseed meats as a replacement for soybean meal in diets for growing-finishing pigs. *J. Anim. Sci.*, **47,** 865-73

Rojas, S.W. and Scott, M.L. (1969). Factors affecting the nutritive value of cottonseed meal as a protein source in chick diets. *Poultry Sci.* **48,** 819-35

Royce, H.D., Harrison, J.R. and Hahan, E.R. (1941). Cotton root bark as a source of gossypol. *Oil & Soap*, **18,** 27-9

Schramm, G. and Benedict, J.H. (1958). Quantitative determination of traces of free gossypol in fats, oils, and fatty acids by paper chromatography. *J. Am. Oil Chem. Soc.*, **35,** 371-3

Skutches, C.L., Herman, D.L. and Smith, F.H. (1973). The effect of intravenous gossypol injection on iron utilization in swine. *J. Nutr.*, **103,** 851-5

Skutches, C.L. and Smith, F.H. (1974). Metabolism of gossypol synthesized from methyl-[14]C- and carboxyl-^{14}C-labeled sodium acetate in the rat. *J. Am. Oil Chem. Soc.*, **51,** 413-15

Smith, F.H. (1946). Estimation of gossypol in cottonseed meal and cottonseed meats. *Ind. Eng. Chem.*, **18,** 43-5

Smith, F.H. (1960). Preparation of pure gossypol from dianilinogossypol. *J. Am. Oil Chem. Soc.*, **37,** 286-8

Smith, F.H. and Clawson, A.J. (1970). The effects of dietary gossypol on animals. *J. Am. Oil Chem. Soc.*, **47,** 443-7

Stipanovic, R.D., Bell, A.A. and Lukefahr, M.J. (1977). Am. Chem. Soc. Symposium Series No. 62, Host Plant Resistance to Pests. Hedin, P.A. (ed.) p. 197.

Stipanovic, R.D., Bell, A.A., Mace, M.E. and Howell, C.R. (1975). Antimicrobial terpenoids of gossypium: 6-methoxygossypol and 6,6'-dimethoxygossypol. *Phytochem.*, **14,** 1077-81

Tanksley, T.D. Jr., Neumann, H., Lyman, C.M., Pace, C.N. and Prescott, J.M. (1970). Inhibition of pepsinogen activation by gossypol. *J. Biol. Chem.*, **245,** 6456-61

Tone, J.N. and Jensen, D.R. (1969). Effects of ingested gossypol on the duodenum of rats. *Trans. Ill. State Acad. Sci.*, **62,** 388-90

Tone, J.N. and Jensen, D.R. (1976). The accumulation pattern of ingested gossypol in selected organs of the rat. *Experientia*, **32,** 369-71

Withers, W.A. and Brewster, J.F. (1913). Studies on cottonseed meal toxicity. II. Iron as an antidote. *J. Biol. Chem.*, **15,** 161-6

Woronick, C.L. and Grau, C.R. (1955). Gossypol-cephalin compound from fresh eggs of hens fed cottonseed meal. *J. Agr. Food Chem.*, **3,** 706-7

9
Toxicological effects of gossypol

A.A. NOMEIR and M.B. ABOU-DONIA

Gossypol [1,1′,6,6′,7,7′-hexahydroxy-5,5′-diisopropyl-3,3′-dimethyl (2,2′-binaphthalene)-8,8′-dicarboxyaldehyde] is a yellow phenolic substance present in various parts of cotton plants (Abou-Donia, 1976). Kuhlman first isolated gossypol in 1861 when he obtained a crude form that he called 'cottonseed blue' (Adams *et al.*, 1960). Twenty five years later Longmore isolated a brown, pungent, alkali-soluble solid from the cottonseed 'foots'; this was impure gossypol (Adams *et al.*, 1960). In 1899 Marchlewski isolated the compound in a pure form and named it gossypol, which recalls its plant origin (genus *Gossypium* sub-tribe Hibisceae order Malvaceae) as well as its phenolic nature (Marchlewski, 1899). Gossypol synthesis in cotton plants is believed to be induced in response to such irritants as pathogens, metabolic inhibitors and cupric and mercuric ions (Abou-Donia, 1976).

Gossypol is located in the glands (ovoid spherical bodies, 100–400 μm in length) of the seeds, leaf, stem, taproot bark, and root of the cotton plant (Abou-Donia, 1976). The compound constitutes 20 to 40% of the weight of the pigment glands in cotton seed. The amount of gossypol in raw cottonseed kernels varies considerably and depends on the species, the environment, and specific varieties. Within several varieties of *G. hirsutum* the gossypol content varies from 0.4 to 1.7% (Adams *et al.*, 1960).

The total world production of cotton seed is about 25 million tonnes/year (containing approximately 78 000 tonnes of gossypol) and approximately 3–6 million tonnes are produced in the USA (Singleton and Kratzer, 1973). An average tonne of cottonseed gives approximately 335 pounds of oil and 945 pounds of meal (Altschul *et al.*, 1958). It is estimated that one quarter of the cottonseed flour potentially available could alleviate the present worldwide shortage of protein (Singleton and Kratzer, 1973). However, the presence of gossypol in the seeds has limited its use for human consumption.

Recently, gossypol has been proposed as a male contraceptive agent, which renews concern about it toxicological effects. This chapter stresses primarily these toxicological effects of gossypol. Some aspects of gossypol chemistry, its stability, and analysis are also briefly discussed. In addition, the physiological and biochemical aspects of gossypol in relation to its toxicological actions are presented.

CHEMISTRY

Chemical structure

Gossypol has a molecular formula of $C_{30}H_{30}O_8$ which corresponds to a molecular weight of 518.54. Its structure was proposed and subsequently confirmed to be a symmetrically substituted 2,2'-di-(1-napththol) derivative (Adams *et al.*, 1938; Edwards, 1958). The UV, IR, and mass spectra of gossypol fit the structure as described (Abou-Donia, 1976).

Gossypol was found to be a polymorphic compound (Adams *et al.*, 1960). When crystallized from diethyl ether, it melts at 184°C; from chloroform, at 199°C, and from petroleum ether (b.p. 60-110°C), at 214°C. All of these forms of gossypol have the same chemical structure. Gossypol is soluble in organic solvents of intermediate polarity such as methanol, acetone, ether,

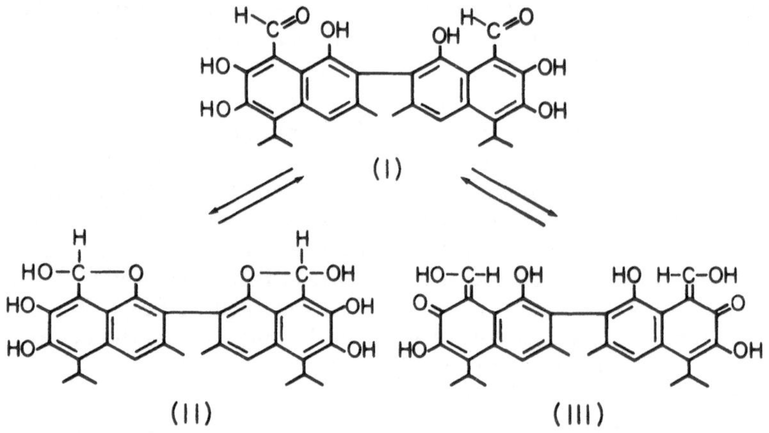

Fig. 9.1 Tautomeric forms of gossypol

chloroform, but it is not readily soluble in water or hexane (Singleton and Kratzer, 1973). The addition of acetic acid to its solution in many solvents causes the separation of gossypol-acetic acid, which is a loosely bound complex of one molecule of gossypol and one molecule of acetic acid. Gossypol is present in three tautomeric forms: the aldehyde, the hemiacetal, and the enolic quinoid tautomer (Fig. 9.1).

Gossypol isolated from the tropical tree *Thespesia populnea* (Corr.) (order Malvaceae) is optically active ($[\alpha]_D^{19} + 445$ in chloroform), whereas the cottonseed pigment is produced as a racemate (Abou-Donia, 1976). The optical activity of *Thespesia* gossypol results from the restricted rotation around the bond that joins the naphthalene nuclei. The restricted rotation results in a non-planar molecule which lacks the presence of a plane of symmetry giving the strong optical activity.

Chemical reactions

Gossypol is a highly reactive molecule. The presence of the phenolic hydroxyl as well as the aldehydic groups allows the molecule to react with a wide variety of reagents. It is strongly acidic for a phenol, with pK_a value of 7.2 (Abou-Donia, 1976), is readily oxidizable and acts as an antioxidant. Gossypol, through its aldehyde groups, reacts with two molecules of aniline and similarly with a number of other primary aromatic and aliphatic amines to yield condensation products with the loss of two molecules of water (an imine or Schiff's base). Many arylimino derivatives of gossypol have been synthesized and characterized (Adams *et al.*, 1938; Abou-Donia, 1976). Liquid ammonia reacts similarly to give diaminogossypol (Adams *et al.*, 1960). The aldehyde groups of gossypol are oxidizable to carboxylic acid and the resulting carboxylic groups may react with the hydroxyl groups in the 1,1′ positions to form lactone. These aldehyde groups also may be removed by the action of alkali to form the unstable product apogossypol (Adams *et al.*, 1960). The phenolic groups of gossypol are oxidized by the action of ferric chloride to form the 1:4-binaphthoquinone, gossypolone (Hass and Shirley, 1965); acylated; and methylated and ethylated to form methyl and ethyl ethers, respectively. Reactions involving the degradation of the naphthalene nuclei into many decomposition products of gossypol have also been reported (see review by Adams *et al.*, 1960).

Stability

The stability of gossypol solutions in methanol, ethanol, chloroform, acetonitrile, and acetone as solvents was studied during storage in the dark at 37, 22, 5, −10, −25, and −80°C (Nomeir and Abou-Donia, 1982). The study showed that both the type of solvent and the storage temperature affect the rate of decomposition of gossypol. Gossypol is highly unstable at 37°C in all solvents studied with a half-life ranging from 0.7 to 33 days. At room temperature, 22°C, gossypol has a half-life ranging from 2.5 to 90 days, a stability that increased as the storage temperature was decreased. At all temperatures, depending on the solvent used, the rate of decomposition of gossypol increased in the following order: acetone < acetonitrile < chloroform < ethanol < methanol. The results indicate that gossypol solutions in any of the solvents studied should not be stored at 5°C, or even at −10°C, for long periods of time. However, under very low temperatures (−25°C and −80°C) gossypol in solution showed greater stability, with only 2-5% decomposition observed after three months of storage. The stability of gossypol under the UV light was also studied (Nomeir and Abou-Donia, unpublished data) and the results showed that gossypol was unstable when exposed to the UV light.

Isolation

Gossypol is isolated from ground cottonseed kernels first by extraction with low boiling petroleum ether to remove the oil, followed by extraction with diethyl ether (peroxide free) to remove gossypol (Adams *et al.*, 1960). The pigment can be separated as gossypol–acetic acid complex by the addition of acetic acid to the concentrated ether solution. This procedure was first developed by Withers and Carruth (1915) and refined by several other groups (Adams *et al.*, 1960). Crystalline free gossypol is also separated by allowing an ether solution of gossypol–acetic acid to evaporate in contact with an aqueous layer. Chloroform, ethanol–water (60:40,v/v) and acetone–water (70:30,v/v) were also used to extract gossypol (Pons, 1977). Gossypol can be extracted from the leaves and flower buds of cotton plants (Smith, 1967), cottonseed meal and cottonseed meats (Smith, 1968) and roots, stems, and seeds of cotton plants (Abou-Donia *et al.*, 1981; Nomeir and Abou-Donia, 1982) by a solvent system developed earlier (Smith, 1968) and consisting of ethanol–water–glacial acetic acid–ether (715:285:0.2:200, by vol.). Gossypol was also extracted with methylene chloride from hexane-defatted meal which resulted in the reduction of the content of gossypol from 2.6% to 0.013% (Cherry and Gray, 1981).

Analysis

Analyses of gossypol in cottonseeds, cottonseed meal, cottonseed oil, mixed feeds, various animal tissues, and other parts of the cotton plant have been reviewed (Pons, 1977). A gravimetric procedure based on the conversion of gossypol into its dianilino derivative was developed (Carruth, 1918) and refined later (Adams *et al.*, 1960). A titrimetric procedure for gossypol analysis based on the reduction of cupric ion has been used (Pons, 1977). Many of the current analytical procedures for the determination of gossypol utilize the reaction of gossypol with aniline or *p*-anisidine to form a Schiff's base derivative, which is determined by spectrophotometric measurement at 440 or 447 nm (Smith, 1967, 1968). This reagent also reacts with bound gossypol to form the same product. Total gossypol (free and bound) is that extracted after hydrolysis with oxalic acid in methyl ethyl ketone or after heating with 3-amino-1-propanol in *N,N*-dimethylformamide (Singleton and Kratzer, 1973). Antimony trichloride forms a stable red complex with gossypol, which is used as the basis of another procedure for its determination (Pons, 1977). Recently, an equilibrium spectrophotometric method based on a fixed-time kinetic measurement was reported (Crouch and Bryant, 1982). The method involves the reaction of gossypol with 1,3,5-trihydroxybenzene (phloroglucinol) in concentrated hydrochloric acid for a fixed time and measurement of the absorbance at 550 nm. Trace amounts of gossypol in fats, oil, and fatty acids have been determined by paper chromatography (Pons, 1977). Other analytical methods include: nuclear magnetic resonance (NMR), polarography, optical microscopy (Crouch and Bryant, 1982), thin-layer chromatography (Abou-Donia and Dieckert, 1975), and quenching of fluorescin luminescence (Pons, 1977). A gas chromatographic method was used to analyse gossypol as the trimethylsilyl ether derivative utilizing a 3% JXR on 80/100 mesh Gaschrom-G column (Abou-Donia, 1976).

Recently high performance liquid chromatography (HPLC) has been used successfully, with a high sensitivity, for the qualitative and quantitative anlysis of gossypol (Hanny, 1980; Abou-Donia *et al.*, 1981; Nomeir and Abou-Donia, 1982). Gossypol was extracted from cotton seeds, roots, and stems of cotton plants and analysed on a reversed-phase C_{18} cartridge, which was eluted isocratically by 0.1% phosphoric acid in methanol–water (9:1, v/v). This method, which can detect amounts as small as 5 ng, was used successfully to study the stability of gossypol in various solutions. When the HPLC and spectrophotometric methods are compared, spectrophotometry is not specific, especially in the presence of some of gossypol degradation product(s) (Nomeir and Abou-Donia, 1982). Furthermore, the HPLC method was approximately 5000 times as sensitive as the spectrophotometric method.

Biosynthesis

Gossypol is synthesized in various parts of cotton plants. The biosynthesis of gossypol was studied using [1-^{14}C]acetate [2-^{14}C]acetate and [2-^{14}C]mevalonate and an enzyme system that is located in the 105 000 g supernatant of cotton root homogenate (Heinstein *et al.*, 1970). Six molecules of [2-^{14}C]mevalonate are stereospecifically incorporated into one molecule of gossypol. The pattern of labelling indicates that gossypol is biosynthesized via the isoprenoid pathway by a specific cyclization of *cis-cis*-farnesyl pyrophosphate. A method for biosynthesis, isolation, and purification of gossypol from [^{14}C]acetate is available (Smith, 1974).

Detoxification

Moist heat treatment or cooking during processing of cottonseed largely detoxifies gossypol (Abou-Donia, 1976). Inactivation of gossypol seems to involve the reaction of free amino groups (largely lysine) of protein molecules with the aldehyde groups of gossypol to form (Schiff's base) bound gossypol (Clark, 1928). Although bound gossypol can be chemically liberated from its Schiff's base combination, this does not happen in digestion (Singleton and Kratzer, 1969). Gossypol reacts with many metals to form complex compounds. This reaction has been utilized in the detoxification of gossypol in cottonseed meal. It has been postulated that ferrous ions detoxify gossypol by catalysing its decarbonylation (Abou-Donia *et al.*, 1970). Sodium, potassium, ammonium, and calcium were also shown to be capable of detoxifying gossypol in cottonseed (Abou-Donia, 1976). Other detoxification methods suggested include treatment with a mixture of steam and alkali, steam and sulphur dioxide, steam and ammonia, steam and methanol, and phloroglucinol (Adams *et al.*, 1960). Gossypol was detoxified when cottonseed meal was fermented with a strain of fungus *Diplodia*. Both fermentation with *Diplodia* and the addition of ferrous sulphate are effective in detoxifying gossypol (Abou-Donia, 1976). All present commercial processes for cottonseed meal production involve the use of heat and other processes to remove, destroy, or bind as much as 80–99% of the gossypol (Singleton and Kratzer, 1973).

TOXICOLOGY

The presence of gossypol in cottonseeds presents two separate problems. The first of these is the presence of high levels of gossypol which may cause unfavourable toxic effects. The second factor is the chemical reactions between gossypol and protein and other nutrients resulting in the reduction in nutritional quality of the diet.

Toxicity to ruminant animals

Earlier studies concluded that ruminant animals appear to be resistant to gossypol toxicity (Adams *et al.*, 1960; Singleton and Kratzer, 1973; Abou-Donia, 1976). This lack of toxicity after consuming small amounts of cottonseed, even with intact gland, to these animals is attributed to prolonged mastication, water contents, and increased time in the rumen, which result in binding of gossypol to protein (Abou-Donia, 1976). For this reason, cottonseed meal is used widely as a protein supplement in the diets of cattle and sheep but not of young calves whose rumen are not yet fully functioning (Adams *et al.*, 1960). A recent study, however, has reported that feeding of large amounts of cottonseed meal to dairy cows in early lactation can be toxic (Lindsey *et al.*, 1980). In this study cows were given cottonseed meal rations containing 6.6 and 42.7 mg of free gossypol kg^{-1} body weight day^{-1} for 14 weeks. Haemoglobin was depressed and total plasma protein was elevated by the ninth week in cows fed a diet high in free gossypol (42.7 mg/ kg body weight for 14 weeks). Erythrocyte fragility was detected in these cows by the seventh week. Cows fed rations containing lower levels of free gossypol (6.6 mg kg^{-1} body weight day^{-1}) developed this abnormality later in the experimental period. The study concluded that intoxication is possible in mature ruminants consuming cottonseed meal containing high levels of free gossypol.

Toxicity to non-ruminant animals

It has been known for many years that non-ruminant animals are more sensitive to gossypol toxicity than are ruminants (Adams *et al.*, 1960; Singleton and Kratzer, 1973). However, the acute toxicity of gossypol is not high for most animals following a single administration. The ranges of the oral LD_{50} values for rats, mice, rabbits, and guinea pigs fed gossypol in water were 2400–3340, 500–950, 350–600, and 280–300 mg/kg, respectively (Abou-Donia, 1976). The toxicity to rats increases by about 10% when administered in oil, probably due to possible enhancement of absorption by oil. Intact cotton glands were two to four times as toxic as gossypol; which suggests the presence of some other chemicals in the glands which may be more toxic or may potentiate the toxicity of gossypol.

Tolerance to gossypol varies with the species. Dogs appear to be quite sensitive. Repeated oral doses of 10–200 mg/kg were reported to be fatal (Eagle, 1960). Chickens are about as sensitive as rats, but pigs are more sensitive. The oral LD_{50} for gossypol in pigs was 550 mg/kg (Lyman *et al.*,

1963). Pigs may appear normal for a few weeks to a year when fed toxic levels of gossypol, then abruptly they begin to gasp for breath (thump) and die in a few days with severe anaemia and other complications (Singleton and Kratzer, 1969, 1973). The safe level of gossypol for pigs has been set at 0.01% or less, or a diet containing not over 9% cottonseed meal. Cats fed gossypol develop spastic paralysis in the hind legs, oedema of the lungs, rapid pulse, and dyspnoea (Schwartz and Alsberg, 1924). Dutch-belted male rabbits fed daily does of 80, 40 and 20 mg gossypol kg^{-1} day^{-1} died within 8–17, 23–35, and 35–84 days after the initiation of treatment. The animals lost their appetite and body weight, developed hind limb paralysis, breathing difficulties and collapsed (Saksena et al., 1981). Water-soluble condensation products of gossypol with carbohydrates, amino acids, and proteins were reported to be harmful to aquarium fish and mice, but none of these condensation products has been isolated or characterized, leading to some doubt as to whether they actually exist (Adams et al., 1960).

Toxicity to humans

Prior to 1976, low levels of gossypol were believed to produce no toxic effects in humans. Reports indicated that heated cottonseed cakes with 0.11–0.2% free gossypol content, consumed in moderate amounts (60 g daily), for 4.5 months has no adverse effects. However, it is not known how much gossypol, if any, remains after heating and cooking the cottonseed meal. The United States has set maximum free gossypol levels in cottonseed preparations for human use at 0.045% (450 mg/kg) while international groups allow higher concentrations: 0.06% (600 mg/kg) for free gossypol and 1.2% total gossypol (Abou-Donia, 1976). Incaprina, a food containing 38% cottonseed flour for human consumption developed by Panama, produces no noticable toxicity in small children fed the supplement while under close clinical supervision for over 2 years. The product is already a commercial nutrient in some countries and some families have used it for more than 4 years without any obvious indication of difficulty (Singleton and Kratzer, 1973).

Recent reports from China indicate that gossypol causes antifertility in human males. This antifertility property, discovered by accident, was later proved by epidemilogical studies. In the late 1950s, a doctor working in Jiangsu Province, East China, found a high incidence of childless marriages among people consuming large quantities of crudely processed cottonseed oil (Wen, 1980). Later, doctors in Central China's Hubei Province found that girls brought up on a cottonseed oil diet who wed men outside the region were having children at a normal rate, whereas many girls who wed men from the same area remained childless (Wen, 1980). Clinical and experimental studies indicate that gossypol is indeed a male antifertility agent in humans as well as other animals. This property is discussed later in this chapter.

Toxicity to insects

It has been reported that gossypol is ineffective as either contact or stomach poison for aphids and Mexican bean beetles (Abou-Donia, 1976). However, cotton plants devoid of the pigment gland were more susceptible than their glanded counterparts to attack by several insect species (Bottger *et al.*, 1964). Gossypol incorporated into an artificial diet was toxic to the bollworm, *Heliothis zea* (Boddie), and the tobacco budworm, *Heliothis virescens* (*f.*) (Abou-Donia, 1976). Gossypol was found to be toxic to pink bollworms, *Pectinophora gossypiella* (Saunders) and to *Heliothis* spp. (Shaver and Lukefahr, 1969). Cotton plants containing 1.7% gossypol were not damaged as much by the bollworm *Heliothis zea* (Boddie) as cotton containing 0.5% gossypol (Abou-Donia, 1976). Gossypol was found to antagonize the toxicity of some insecticides to the Egyptian cotton leafworm *Spodoptera littoralis* (Boisduval) (Abou-Donia, 1976). It was suggested that gossypol may either reduce the penetration of these insecticides into the body or it may enhance detoxification of the absorbed insecticide. The latter assumption is in agreement with the finding that gossypol increased the activity of rat liver microsomal oxidases (Abou-Donia and Dieckert, 1971).

Toxicity to microorganisms

Gossypol was reported to induce complete immobilization of *Trypanosoma cruzi*, the parasite that causes Chagas disease (Montamat *et al.*, 1982). This effect of gossypol was attributed to its powerful inhibition of NAD-linked enzymes (α-hydroxy acid dehydrogenase and malate dehydrogenase). The study suggested the possible value of gossypol as a therapeutic agent for Chagas disease and other trypanosomiases (Montamat *et al.*, 1982).

Gossypol inactivates influenza virus infectivity *in vitro*. Mice treated with gossypol showed a 96-100% protection rate against the virus (Dorsett *et al.*, 1975). Apogossypol, the decarbonylation derivative of gossypol, and gossypol were found to inactivate the enveloped parainfluenza-3 and herpes simplex viruses *in vitro* using HEp-2 cells in cultures (Dorsett *et al.*, 1975). The study also showed that when infected cells were incubated with gossypol or apogossypol no alteration in the subsequent plaque formation was observed, indicating that the antiviral effect does not occur within the cell. Gossypol–acetic acid showed a clear-cut effect on herpes simplex virus type-2 infecting culture of human amniotic epithelial cells (Wichmann *et al.*, 1982). Gossypol inhibited the development of virus-induced cytopathic products and also inhibited the viral multiplication in these cells which were chosen to mimic the natural target cells of herpes genitalis infection *in vivo* (Wichmann *et al.*, 1982).

Gossypol may also act as a general antifungal antibotic, with differential toxicity to fungal species (Abou-Donia, 1976). Gossypol has been shown to have antibacterial and antitumour activities as well (Abou-Donia, 1976).

Signs of toxicity

The signs of gossypol toxicity have been reported in many reviews (Adams *et al.*, 1960; Eagle, 1960; Abou-Donia, 1976). Dogs treated orally with gossypol manifested lassitude, diarrhoea, anorexia, and weight loss. Vomiting occurred at high doses. Autopsy showed haemorrhagic intestines, hydrothorax, oedema of the lungs, excessive fluid in the peritoneal cavity, hydropericardium, and congestion of the splanchnic organs (Eagle, 1960). Haemolytic anaemia developed in chicks fed gossypol and ceroid-like pigment appears in the duodenal villi and sinusoids of liver and spleen (Adams *et al.*, 1960). Eggs from hens fed cottonseed meal are generally normal in appearance but after several months of storage, a discoloration may be found in the yolks and albumin which makes them unsalable. Gossypol also reduces egg weight and hatchability (Adams *et al.*, 1960).

Rats poisoned by pigment glands showed haemorrhage, gastritis, enteritis in the lower parts of the duodenum, and in some cases, congestion throughout the intestine. The liver had prominent lobules and the kidneys were badly congested (Abou-Donia, 1976). Gossypol might inhibit haematopoiesis in rats, with a resultant decrease in erythrocytes (Abou-Donia, 1976). Administration of gossypol to rats caused depression of appetite and growth performance (Tone and Jensen, 1970). Gossypol resulted in increased erythrocyte packed-cell volumes and haemoglobin concentration during the first seven days after its injection into rats. These parameters fell to below normal values by day 14. Iron injection showed a normal erythrocyte population in rats treated with gossypol (Tone and Jensen, 1974). When hamsters inhaled gossypol in aerosol form (in sterile deionized water at concentrations of $0.1–1.0\,mg/100\,ml$) it caused damage to the epithelial cells of the airway all the way to the respiratory bronchioles. Ciliated cells showed occasional extrusion with some vacuolization of mitrochondria; the secretory cells (Clara cells) showed vacuolization beneath the nuclei, nuclear extrusion, mitochondrial swelling, marked vacuolization of the endoplasmic reticulum, Golgi vesicles, and Golgi appratus as well as cell extrusion (Abou-Donia, 1976).

Intravenous and intraperitoneal injection of gossypol in rabbits caused loss of appetite, collapse, haemoglobinaemia, suffocation, and death (Menaul, 1923). Parenterally injected gossypol in rabbits caused an immediate drop in blood pressure, lung oedema, alveolar congestion and ascites (Schwartz and Alsberg, 1924). Rabbits fed gossypol also develop loss of appetite, diarrhoea, spastic paralysis, and hypoprothrombinaemia (Schwartz and Alsberg, 1924; Adams *et al.*, 1960).

Pigs are known to be one of the most sensitive animals to gossypol toxicity. Gossypol fed to pigs caused hypoprothrombinaemia and haemorrhages of liver, small intestine, and stomach. When cottonseed ration containing 0.03% gossypol was fed to pigs, dyspnoea, anorexia, weight loss, diarrhoea, and hair discoloration were observed (Smith, 1957). Post-mortem examination showed oedematous fluid in the pleural, pericardial, and peritoneal cavities; oedema of the lungs, heart, and lymph nodes; degeneration of liver, spleen, and cardiac muscle, intralobular hepatic necrosis; hypertrophy and dilation of the heart; and deficiency of lymphoid cells. Pigs fed gossypol showed dyspnoea, characterized by thumping, progressive weakness, and emaciation. Widespread congestion and oedema were the dominant post-mortem lesions (Hale *et al.*, 1958). Feeding pigs on rations contain 240 parts/10^6 of gossypol for 15 weeks lowered haemoglobin and haematocrit levels (Abou-Donia, 1976). Gossypol also altered the electrocardiogram in swine (Abou-Donia, 1976).

Common signs for gossypol toxicity can be summarized as: loss of appetite; weight loss; hypoprothrombinaemia; diarrhoea; hair discoloration; lowering of haemoglobin, red cell count, and serum protein; oedematous fluid in body cavities, lungs and heart; degenerative changes in the liver and spleen; haemorrhages of liver, small intestine, and stomach; yolk discoloration and decreased hatchability of eggs.

Gossypol interaction with protein, iron and other components in the body

Some of the toxic effects of gossypol may result from its interaction with some components of the diet and/or in the body of the animal. Intravenous injection of gossypol in swine increased the concentration of iron in the liver and bile (Skutches *et al.*, 1973), suggesting that initially gossypol chelates liver iron, thereby interfering with the normal utilization of iron in the synthesis of haemoglobin and respiratory enzymes (Skutches *et al.*, 1973). This is supported by the fact that iron deficiency is frequently associated with gossypol toxicity. Iron was partially effective in preventing the accumulation of gossypol in porcine liver (Buitrago *et al.*, 1970). Iron dextran injected into the peritoneal cavity of the rat simultaneously with corn oil containing gossypol was partially effective in preventing the growth depression resulting from the injected gossypol (Clawson *et al.*, 1962). When iron was injected with gossypol in rats, the animals showed a normal erythrocyte population whereas gossypol alone showed an increase in erythrocytes (Tone and Jensen, 1974). Gossypol reduces the uptake of iron by everted segments of rat duodenum when it is present with the iron simultaneously in the mucosal medium (Herman and Smith, 1975). Absorption of the iron is decreased when bound gossypol is fed to rats (Herman and Smith, 1973). When rats were fed varying amounts of free gossypol in their diet, iron absorption decreased as the levels of gossypol in the ration increased (Braham and Bressani, 1975). The discoloration of the yolk during storage of eggs from chickens treated with gossypol was attributed to the reaction between gossypol and ferric ions released from yolk protein. This discoloration was prevented by the addition of ferrous sulphate to the diet of laying hens (Abou-Donia, 1976). It appears that gossypol produces anaemia by its binding of iron. It is noteworthy, however, that iron catalyses the loss of formyl groups of gossypol thus reducing its ability to bind to proteins.

The carbonyl groups of gossypol react with the amino groups of the amino acids and proteins to form a Schiff's base type of derivative. This reaction is a major factor in the toxicity of gossypol since it can take place with dietary protein as well as tissue protein. This can result in rendering amino acids unavailable, particularly lysine via its terminal amino group, thus lowering the nutritional value of the diet. Other chemical bonds are also thought to be involved in the interaction between gossypol and proteins

(Abou-Donia, 1976). The phenolic groups may combine with protein reversibly by hydrogen bonding and also irreversibly by oxidation to quinones, which may react with proteins. Van Der Waals and charge transfer forces play a minor role in the binding of gossypol to protein since they are weak, short lived and effective only in short distance. Considerable attraction can result, however, when non-polar groups come closer in the aqueous solution to form hydrophobic bonds, which may take place via the hydrocarbon structure of gossypol (Abou-Donia, 1976). It has been reported that gossypol complexes are formed with several free amino acids including L-lysine, L-glutamine, L-ornithine, L-arginine, DL-asparagine, glycine and γ-aminobutyric acid (Abou-Donia, 1976). Since both carbonyl groups of gossypol can link with amino groups, cross linking between protein chains could have a profound effect on enzymatic hydrolysis (Abou-Donia, 1976).

All analysed amino acids were present in the partially digested chyme of the proximal gut of rats fed a diet containing gossypol in a significantly greater degree than the amount present in the non-gossypol treated rat chyme (Jones and Smith, 1977a). Addition of L-lysine, L-isoleucine, L-valine, and L-threonine to a diet containing gossypol significantly improved weight gain of rats when compared to diet enriched by gossypol alone (Jones and Smith, 1977b). Rat growth was markedly depressed with levels of bound gossypol above 0.75%. It was shown that increasing the level of bound gossypol from 0.45 to 1.3% required an increase in the level of dietary protein of approximately 4% to produce approximately the same rate of gain in weanling rats (Smith, 1972). Accumulations of gossypol in the livers of rats injected with gossypol were found and attributed to its binding with protein (Tone and Jensen, 1974). Gossypol reduced the serum iron-binding capacity and total serum protein by approximately 20% when pigs were fed a diet containing 0.06% free gossypol for 43 days (Skutches *et al.*, 1974). These effects were attributed to the interference of gossypol with protein synthesis. Injection of free gossypol in swine (15 mg/kg of body weight) resulted in binding of approximately 90% of the compound 15 min after injection indicating that gossypol binds to serum protein, serum iron, and perhaps other substances (Albrecht *et al.*, 1972).

Gossypol significantly decreased the levels of total plasma cholesterol, low density lipoprotein, very low density lipoprotein, and very low density lipoprotein–cholesterol concentration in adult male cynomolgus monkeys consuming a diet containing 0.19 mg of cholesterol/kcal (Shandilya and Clarkson, 1982). These results suggest that gossypol may be a useful drug in lowering plasma cholesterol concentrations.

Gossypol showed a transient decrease in plasma K^+ levels after 2 weeks of administration of gossypol–acetic acid to rat at a dose level of 5 mg rat^{-1} day^{-1}. The potassium level returned to normal after 4 weeks of gossypol treatment (Kalla *et al.*, 1981). Gossypol was found to cause hypokalaemia or depletion of potassium in a small portion of human volunteers (less than 1%) who were given a daily dose of gossypol (National Coordinating Group on Male Antifertility Agents, 1978).

Effect on specific enzymes

Gossypol, in addition to its non-specific reactions with proteins in the body, also affects many enzymatic reactions, resulting in the interference with many vital biological processes. Such effects may take place by reacting with the substrate thereby blocking the action of the enzyme and/or by combining with the enzyme itself. Several studies indicate that gossypol can reduce the action of proteolytic enzymes by forming complexes with their substrates. The *in vitro* digestion of casein and cottonseed globulin by pepsin and trypsin, acting successively, was reduced when gossypol was added prior to enzymatic digestion (Abou-Donia, 1976). Gossypol inhibited trypsin and competitively inhibited pepsin (Abou-Donia, 1976). Gossypol reacts with pepsinogen, in the presence of 10% ethanol, to form gossypolpepsinogen, a zymogen which cannot be autocatalytically activated to pepsin (Tanksley *et al.*, 1970). The study suggests that lysyl residues in pepsinogen are involved in the reaction which apparently resulted in a change in protein conformation. After the reaction has occurred, the conformation of native pepsinogen cannot be re-established (Tanksley *et al.*, 1970). The modified zymogen–gossypol complex was digested and a gossypol–containing portion was isolated and purified (Wong *et al.*, 1972). The purified material was found to be a decapeptide which originated from the amino terminal portion of the protein and a heptapeptide obtained from the carboxyl terminus. The two peptides were cross-linked by gossypol through the epsilon-NH_2 groups of lysine 18 and 358. It is apparent from this study that intra- as well as intermolecular cross-linkage may occur as a result of gossypol reaction with pepsinogen (Wong *et al.*, 1972).

Gossypol in the diet reduced succinic dehydrogenase and cytochrome oxidase activities in chick but not in hen liver homogenates (Abou-Donia, 1976). *In vitro* studies using liver homogenates of the normal hen showed gossypol capable of markedly reducing succinic dehydrogenase, cytochrome oxidase and xanthine oxidase activities (Abou-Donia, 1976). Gossypol uncoupled succinate oxidation with active mitochondria isolated from soybeans (Abou-Donia, 1976). Gossypol uncouples the respiratory chain phosphorylation, *in vitro*, of rat liver mitochondria (Abou-Donia and Dieckert, 1974a). Dietary gossypol stimulated the oxidative N-demethylation of p-chloro-N-methyl aniline and some other carbamate pesticides of rat liver microsomes (Abou-Donia and Diekert, 1971). Glutathione S-transferase isoenzymes were reversibly inhibited by gossypol in a competitive kinetics model with respect to the substrate 1-chloro-2,4-dinitrobenzene (Lee *et al.*, 1982).

The effect of gossypol on rat liver catechol-o-methyltransferase, a key enzyme in the metabolism of catecholamines, was studied *in vitro* (Tang *et al.*, 1982). Gossypol non-competitively inhibited catechol-o-methyltransferase with an I_{50} of 0.01 mol/l. Blood serum albumin significantly reduced the inhibitory effect of gossypol. The effect of gossypol on liver microsomal p-nitroanisole demethylase and lipid peroxidation was studied in both sodium phenobarbital-treated and non-treated rats (Skutches and Smith, 1974a). Liver lipid peroxidation activity was found to be inversely related to gossypol concentration in the liver. In a liver postmitochondrial supernatant fraction prepared from rats that were given oral doses of 25, 50, or 100 mg of gossypol/kg body weight, lipid peroxidation activity was inhibited whereas O-demethylation of p-nitroanisole was not affected. Intraperitoneal injection of sodium phenobarbital increased p-nitroanisole demethylase activity but did not overcome the gossypol-inhibited lipid peroxidation (Skutches and Smith, 1974a). The activities of glutamic–oxaloacetic and glutamic–pyruvic transaminases increased in blood serum and decreased in liver when gossypol was fed to rats (Braham and Bressani, 1975). Similar results were reported in pigs fed rations containing gossypol (Abou-Donia, 1976). These results are in agreement with the fact that gossypol causes liver necrosis since the activity of these enzymes in plasma is indicative of such toxic condition.

Antifertility action of gossypol

As stated above, Chinese scientists have recently reported that gossypol is capable of inhibiting the fertility of male rats (National Coordinating Group on Male Antifertility Agents, 1978). The compound was also tested in humans as a male contraceptive drug in which over 4000 healthy men were given gossypol at a dose level of 20 mg daily for approximately 2 months. The antifertility efficacy, evaluated by semen examination, was 99.89%. After achievement of infertility, the subjects were moved to the maintenance dose of 150-200 mg/month given in divided doses (National Coordinating Group on Male Antifertility Agents, 1978). Since then, massive experimental testing has been carried out to determine the possible use of gossypol as a male contraceptive in humans. Since these studies are discussed in detail elsewhere in this book, we will only briefly summarize them in this chapter.

Gossypol is found to be a non-mutagen in the Ames-*Salmonella* mammalian microsomal test system with or without metabolic activation, a finding which increases its chances for human use (Peyster and Wang, 1979). Gossypol causes reversible male infertility when given orally on a daily basis to some animal species such as rats, cynomolgus monkeys, hamsters, and humans but not in mice and rabbits. The dose and duration of treatment required to induce infertility varies and depends on the species. This infertility effect of gossypol is not observed in females (Chang *et al.*, 1980; Hahn *et al.*, 1981; Saksena *et al.*, 1981; Waller *et al.*, 1981; Kalla *et al.*, 1982; Shandilya *et al.*, 1982; Saksena and Salmonsen, 1982; Weinbauer *et al.*, 1982; Wu *et al.*, 1981). Infertility in male rats is also produced by cottonseed flour which contains low levels of gossypol. This infertility is reversible at least as early as 6 weeks after cessation of the gossypol-containing diet (Sotelo *et al.*, 1982).

Several studies have been done to determine the mechanism of gossypol action. The earliest signs of gossypol's effect were seen in the spermatids, which displayed nuclear vacuolation and swelling (National Coordinating Group on Male Antifertility Agents, 1978). Obvious changes such as pyknosis, karyorrhexis, or cytolysis were present in spermatocytes and spermatids. Exfoliation of the cells of the germinal epithelium with resultant desquamation and formation of multinucleated giant cells of spermatid and spermatocytic derivation were readily discernible. Many spermatozoa had their heads and tails separated. Electron-microscopic examination revealed swelling, dissociation, and fragmentation of the acrosome and head caps of the spermatids. The mitochondrial spiral sheath of the midpeice was deranged and swollen and the cristae decreased in number (National Coordinating Group on Male Antifertility Agents, 1978). Missing members of both outer fibres and inner microtubules of the principal piece and broken cell membrane of the sperm head were observed (Nadakavukaren *et al.*, 1979).

Gossypol was found to immobilize human sperm rapidly *in vitro*, an effect which is attributed to its inhibition of energy metabolism by blocking the degradation of glucose or fructose to CO_2 (Poso *et al.*, 1980). Human spermatozoa incubated with gossypol showed a significant decrease in the activities of Ca^{2+} and Mg^{2+}-activated ATPase; this may be responsible for the inhibition of sperm motility (Kalla and Vasudev, 1981). Spermatozoa from humans treated with gossypol showed a decrease in succinic dehydrogenase and lactic dehydrogenase activities in the midpiece (National Coordinating Group on Male Antifertility Agents, 1978). Gossypol was found to inhibit rat testes cytosolic lactic dehydrogenase-X activity in a dose-dependent manner. Such inhibition of the enzyme was competitive with respect to NADH.and non-competitive with respect to α-ketoglutarate (Giridharan *et al.*, 1982). A preliminary study also indicated that gossypol inhibits other dehydrogenases such as glutamic dehydrogenase, glutathione reductase, and malic dehydrogenase as well (Giridharan *et al.*, 1982).

Disposition, excretion and metabolism

The disposition and excretion of gossypol have been studied in many animal species; however, its biotransformation received little attention. When gossypol was fed to rainbow trout at a concentration of 1000 parts/10^6 in the diet for 18 months, large amounts of gossypol accumulated in the tissues, with the highest concentration being observed in the liver and the lowest in the muscle (Abou-Donia, 1976). Gossypol administered to dogs was excreted in the faeces in almost the same quantity (Abou-Donia, 1976). Gossypol was isolated and crystallized as dianilinogossypol from the livers of pigs fed cottonseed meal (Smith, 1963). Of the gossypol injected into swine 40% was eliminated in the faeces over a 93 h period (Albrecht *et al.*, 1972). Gossypol disposition in the pig liver was found to be directly related to the total gossypol contents in the diet (Buitrago *et al.*, 1970). The study concluded that gossypol was apparently eliminated via the bile (Buitrago *et al.*, 1970).

Dietary ferrous sulphate decreased the amount of both free and bound gossypol in the faeces and in certain organs of swine (Smith and Clawson, 1965). Buitrago *et al.* (1970) reported that free and bound gossypol levels in pig liver were markedly reduced by the presence of high levels (2400 and

3200 mg/kg) of ferrous sulphate in the diet. The ratio of free to bound gossypol deposited in the liver was dependent on the iron concentration in the pig liver (Skutches et al., 1974). It was postulated that iron may react with gossypol upon ingestion, thereby reducing its absorption; also iron may have detoxified the gossypol molecule to a compound that no longer responds to the reagents of the analytical procedure (Smith and Clawson, 1965). This observation is in agreement with the suggestion that iron cata-lyses the decarbonylation of gossypol to CO and presumably the unstable apogossypol (Abou-Donia et al., 1970).

A study of the metabolic fate of [^{14}C]gossypol in the pig indicated that decarbonylation of gossypol is not the major route of metabolism (Abou-Donia and Deickert, 1975). Twenty days after a single oral dose of 6.7 mg/kg, the total radioactivity recovered in the faeces was 94.6% of the admin-istered dose; another 2.1% was recovered in the expired CO_2. The urine contained only 0.7% of the administered dose. Approximately 33% of the dose was recovered from tissues one day after administration; this fell to 1.2% by day 20. The highest concentration of radioactivity was found in the liver, bile, and gall bladder, especially at the early time points. The gastrointestinal tract, spleen, kidneys, and lungs also contained high con-centrations of radioactivity. The half-life for the disappearance of radio-activity from the animal body was 78 h (Abou-Donia and Dieckert, 1975).

The metabolism of a single oral 10 mg/kg dose of [^{14}C]gossypol in the laying hen results in high excretion via the combined urine/faeces contents (78.6% of the administered dose in 8 days) (Abou-Donia and Lyman, 1970). A total of 3.2% of the administered dose was recovered in the expired CO_2 over a period of 20 days. At the end of the eighth day the total radioactivity accumulated in egg albumin and egg yolk was 4.6 and 9.1%, respectively. The high ^{14}C in the egg was attributed to high protein content in eggs. A small portion of the orally administered gossypol was deposited in the tissues. One day after administration the tissues had 8.1% of the admin-istered dose; this fell to 0.9% at day eight. The highest concentration of radioactivity was observed in the bile, liver, gastrointestinal tract parts and contents, followed by residue in spleen, blood, and kidneys. The biological half-life of ^{14}C in laying hens was 30 h (Abou-Donia and Lyman, 1970).

In rats the major portion of labelled gossypol is also excreted in the faeces. The results of a study in which radioactive gossypol was admin-istered by stomach tube to two rats, showed that the binaphthalene nucleus of gossypol molecule was not degraded to CO_2 (Skutches and Smith, 1974b). The major portion of the radioactivity was excreted in the faeces while a low level of radioactivity was found in the urine. The highest concentration of radioactivity was associated with the gastrointestinal tract, liver, kidneys, and spleen (Skutches and Smith, 1974b). In another study, rats given a single oral dose of [^{14}C]gossypol (25 mg/kg) excreted most of the compound in the faeces (74.4% of the dose) (Abou-Donia et al., 1970). Appreciable amounts of radioactivity (12.1% of the dose) were recovered in the expired CO_2 while little (2.3% of the dose) was excreted in the urine. Liver, gastrointestinal tract parts and its contents contained the highest concentrations while brain, testes, and adipose tissues contained the lowest concentrations of radioactivity. Addition of iron to the diet reduced ^{14}C in the animal body and increased the amount of radioactivity in the exhaled air. The biological half-life of ^{14}C-containing materials in the rat body was 48 h without and 23 h with added iron (Abou-Donia et al., 1970). When male rats were treated orally with gossypol at a dose level of 40mg kg^{-1} body weight day^{-1} for 2, 4, or 8 weeks, free and bound gossypol was found in all tissues analysed (Jensen et al., 1982). Based on μg of total gossypol (free and bound)/g wet tissue, the spleen showed the highest tissue concentration, followed by heart, kidneys, liver, lungs, and testes. Gossypol also showed an accumulative trend in all of these tissues (Jensen et al., 1982).

The absorption, distribution, and excretion of gossypol were studied in mice, rats, dogs, and rhesus monkeys (National Coordinating Group on Male Antifertility Agents, 1978). The biological half-life of gossypol in rat gastrointestinal tract was 9.6 h, indicating a relatively slow rate of absorption. The biological half-life of the radioactivity was 60 h and it took 19 days to eliminate 97.24% of the dose from the male rat body.

Gossypol was retained longer in the body of dogs and mice relative to monkeys and rats. There was a close similarity between the patterns of gossypol distribution in the bodies of mice, rats, rabbits, dogs, and monkeys. In all animals studied, the liver contained the highest concentrations of radioactovity at 5 or 48 h after oral administration. The spleen, lungs, kidneys, heart, blood, and fat also contained some of the labelled compounds at 5 or 6 h after administration. Gossypol was found to be subjected to enterohepatic recirculation and this, in turn, probably played a part both in the delay of elimination from the body and in the presence of high concentrations in the intestine. Radioactivity was low in the testes within 48 h after a single oral dose; this gradually increased and reached its peak by day 9 after gossypol administration. In the rat, most of the ingested radioactivity was eliminated in the faeces (83% in 19 days) while a smaller fraction was in the exhaled CO_2 (11.73%) and in the urine (2.5%) (National Coordinating Group on Male Antifertility Agents, 1978). These results are in complete agreement with the data reported earlier (Abou-Donia et al., 1970). In rhesus monkeys, the pattern of gossypol elimination was very similar to that of the rat, i.e. mainly eliminated in the faeces. After oral administration of gossypol to rhesus monkeys, about 50% of the administered dose was eliminated in the faeces within 48 h (National Coordinating Group on Male Antifertility Agents, 1978).

In all animals studied a very small portion (less than 3% of the dose) of the ingested [^{14}C]gossypol was excreted via urine. Reabsorption of gossypol-derived radioactivity from the renal tubules by non-ionic absorption may account for this despite the high radioactivity present in the kidney (Abou-Donia, 1976). It has been reported that the mechanism of non-ionic diffusion in the renal tubules has a profound effect on the excretory rate of any drug that is reasonably lipid soluble and has an appropriate pK_a (Abou-Donia, 1976). Gossypol is a weak acid and may be filtered and secreted by the tubular mechanism for organic acids (Abou-Donia, 1976). Such compounds are reabsorbed from the tubules by non-ionic diffusion.

The tubular epithelium of the distal convoluted tubule is selectively permeable or more permeable to the un-ionized lipid-soluble molecule than the poorly lipid-soluble corresponding anion or cation (Abou-Donia, 1976). In the case of gossypol, which has a pK_a value of 7.2, reabsorption is favoured by the low urinary pH (around 6 for rats, and 5.5 for pigs) (Abou-Donia and Dieckert, 1975). This increases the proportion of non-ionized molecules. Also, the high solubility of gossypol in organic solvents results in a high rate of absorption.

Unlike the urine, excretion into the intestine via the bile is a major pathway by which absorbed gossypol is removed from the body of all animals studied. The concentration of radioactivity in the bile was much greater than in any other tissue. These results suggest that gossypol and metabolites are concentratively transferred from the blood to the bile. The bile/plasma concentration ratio ranged between 10.3 and 29.5 in hens and in pigs, respectively (Abou-Donia and Lyman, 1970; Abou-Donia and Dieckert, 1975). This puts gossypol in class B of Brauer's classification which divided the substances that are excreted into bile into three classes according to their bile/plasma concentration ratios usually ranging from 10 to 1000. The high concentration of gossypol in the bile suggests that it is actively secreted into bile. This is in agreement with the concept that the transport of compounds in class B across the biliary epithelium into bile appears to require some kind of active secretory process. The assumed high rate of bile secretion of gossypol observed is in harmony with the conclusion that compounds of high molecular weight (more than 300) and with two or more aromatic rings tends to be excreted into bile (Williams et al., 1965). It is also in agreement with the suggestion that for appreciable biliary excretion, a compound should have polar anionic groups and a molecular weight about 350 (Millburn et al., 1967). Gossypol possesses these properties with six polar hydroxyl groups and two carbonyl groups with a molecular weight of 518. The bulk of radioactivity in the bile from pigs fed [14C]gossypol was in the form of glucuronides, with most of the remaining appearing as sulphate conjugates and water-soluble metabolites (Abou-Donia and Dieckert, 1974b).

Some of the gossypol metabolites formed in pigs after administration of [14C]gossypol were identified (Abou-Donia and Dieckert, 1975). The identification was carried out by UV, IR, and mass spectrometry along with thin-layer chromatography and autoradiography. The formation of $^{14}CO_2$ from the carbonyl-labelled gossypol suggests the formation of the decarbonylation product, apogossypol, which was not identified, probably because of its instability (Abou-Donia, 1976). It was suggested that gossypol was oxidized to gossypolone [6,6',7,7'-tetrahydroxy-5,5'-diisopropyl-3,3'-dimethyl-(2,2'-binaphthalene)-1,1',4,4'-tetraone-8,8'dicarboxaldehyde] which was subsequently oxidized to gossypolonic acid [6,6',7,7'-tetrahydroxy-5,5'-diisopropyl-3,3'-dimethyl-(2,2'-binaphthalene)-1,1',4,4'-tetraone-8,8'-dicarboxylic acid]. Gossypol as well as its metabolites may be conjugated to form the more water–soluble glucuronides, sulphate, and glucuronide sulphate hybrids (Abou-Donia and Dieckert, 1974b). These metabolic pathways could be considered detoxifications since they should enhance the excretion of gossypol from the animal body and render it less toxic.

Selective toxicity and metabolism of gossypol

Gossypol is known to be more toxic to pigs than to rats with oral LD_{50} values of 550 and 2630 mg/kg, respectively (Lyman *et al.*, 1963; Eagle, 1960). It is interesting to know that only 2.1% of radioactive gossypol administered to pigs was recovered in the expired air during 20 days, whereas it was approximately 12% from rats (Abou-Donia *et al.*, 1970; Abou-Donia and Dieckert, 1975; National Coordinating Group on Male Antifertility Agents, 1978). These results indicate that the decarbonylation of gossypol is not a major route for gossypol biodegradation in pigs, yet it seems to be a major pathway for its metabolism in rats. The selective toxicity of gossypol in various species may be related, in part, to the differential degree of decarbonylation of gossypol.

Although different animals may have different detoxification mechanisms, it is possible that the differences in tolerance to gossypol are due to the amount of gossypol absorbed by the animal through the intestinal tract and deposited in the tissues. In pigs, which are sensitive to gossypol toxicity, and in rats, which are insensitive, the maximum amounts of gossypol-derived radioactivity in the tissues were 32.9 and 16.8% of the orally administered dose, respectively. This indicates that in susceptible animals gossypol has readier access to the target, which itself may be more sensitive to gossypol toxicity.

CONCLUDING REMARKS

Gossypol, a yellow phenolic substance present in cotton plants, is a 2,2'-binaphthalene compound with a symmetrical substitution of six hydroxyl, two aldehyde, two methyl, and two isopropyl groups. An optically active type of gossypol was isolated from the tropical tree *Thespesia populnea* Corr., while the material isolated from cotton plants is a non-optically active racemate. The compound is polymorphic, readily soluble in ordinary organic solvents with intermediate polarity, and not readily soluble in water and hexane. The addition of acetic acid to its solution in many solvents causes the separation of gossypol–acetic acid, a loosely bound complex of one molecule of gossypol and one molecule of acetic acid.

Gossypol is isolated from cotton plants by extraction using a variety of solvents and solvent mixtures. The presence of the phenolic and aldehydic groups in the molecule makes it highly reactive. It is strongly acidic for a phenol, readily oxidizable and acts as an antioxidant. Gossypol is highly unstable in solutions when stored at room temperature or even upon refrigeration at 4°C. Gossypol combines with the free amino groups of proteins to form non-extractable (bound) gossypol, a process that is utilized to detoxify gossypol in cottonseed meal. Gossypol reacts with primary amines such as aniline to form dianilinogossypol, a reaction which has been used for its gravimetric and spectrophotometric determination. Many other analytical methods with higher sensitivity and accuracy, such as gas–liquid and high performance liquid chromatography, have been developed. Gossypol, which is believed to be synthesized in the plant in response to irritant, is biosynthesized via the isoprenoid pathway by specific cyclization of *cis*-*cis*-farnesyl pyrophosphate. Gossypol has a wide range of toxicological, pharmacological, physiological, and biochemical effects.

The absorption, metabolism, and toxicity of gossypol varies depending on the species. The compound is more toxic to non-ruminants than ruminants, a characteristic which limits the use of cottonseed meal as a dietary source of protein for animals and humans. The acute toxicity of gossypol is not very high on single dose basis; its medium lethal dose (LD_{50}) ranges from approximately 300 to 3500 mg/kg, depending on the species. Pigs and dogs are among the sensitive species whereas rats are not. The compound is not effective as an insecticide; however, it showed some protective effect for cotton plants against some insects when present in higher concentrations. Gossypol is effective against *Trypanosoma cruzi*, the parasite that causes Chagas disease, and against influenza, parainfluenza-3, and herpes simplex viruses. It acts as a general antifungal antibiotic, antibacterial and also antitumour agent. Signs of gossypol toxicity in higher animals include loss of appetite, weight loss, hypoprothrombinaemia, diarrhoea, hair discoloration, lowering of haemoglobin, red blood cell count and serum protein, oedematous fluid in body cavities, lungs, and heart, degenerative changes in the liver and spleen, haemorrhages of liver, small intestine and stomach, and yolk discoloration and decreased hatchability of eggs. Gossypol exerts its toxic effect by either non-specific interaction with some dietary and body components such as iron and protein and/or specific inhibition of certain enzymes. It combines with pepsinogen to form gossypol–pepsinogen which cannot be autocatalytically activated to pepsin. Gossypol inhibits succinic dehydrogenase, cytochrome oxidase, xanthene oxidase, pepsin, trypsin, glutathione-*S*-transferase isoenzymes, catechol-*o*-methyltransferase and lipid peroxidation activities. Gossypol uncouples the respiratory chain phosphorylation of rat liver mitochondria, and succinate oxidation in the mitochondria isolated from soybeans. Gossypol reduces the oxygen-carrying capacity of the blood and causes a haemolytic effect on the erythrocytes. Gossypol induces rat liver microsomal N-demethylation activity of p-chloro-N-methyl aniline. It is a non-mutagen in the Ames—*Salmonella*-mammalian microsomal test system. Gossypol decreases the total plasma cholesterol level, a characteristic which may have therapeutic application.

Gossypol causes a reversible male antifertility to rats, hamsters, cynomolgus monkeys, and humans but not to rabbits and mice. The compound inhibits sperm motility, and spermatozoal energy metabolism *in vitro*. *In vivo* treatment of gossypol showed many morphological changes in the sperm such as separation of the head and tail, swelling, dissociation, and fragmentation of the acrosome and head caps of the spermatids. Gossypol inhibits Ca^{2+} and Mg^{2+}-ATPase and also lactic dehydrogenase-X in the sperm and testes.

In all animals studied, gossypol was eliminated primarily via faeces with very little being excreted in the urine. The excretion of gossypol into the intestine via the bile seems to be the major elimination pathway. Gossypol fed to animals was deposited in various tissues with the highest concentrations being observed in the liver, gall bladder, bile, and kidneys. The biological half-life of gossypol ranges from 23 to 78 h depending on the species and the presence or absence of iron in the diet. Gossypol metabolism studies showed that the binaphthalene nucleus is not degraded and only the aldehyde carbon is metabolized to CO_2 in different proportions depending on the species. Gossypol and its metabolites may be conjugated to form glucuronides, sulphates, or hydrides. Gossypol is also deposited in the eggs of chickens fed on gossypol, with higher concentrations being observed in the yolk.

Acknowledgements

The secretarial assistance of Mrs Erna S. Daniel is acknowledged. This study was supported in part by The Rockefeller foundation Grant No. GAPS 8421.

References

Abou-Donia, M.B. (1976). Physiological effects and metabolism of gossypol. *Residue Rev.* **61**, 125-60

Abou-Donia, M.B. and Dieckert, J.W. (1971). Gossypol: Subcellular localization and stimulation of rat liver microsomal oxidases. *Toxical. Appl. Pharmacol.*, **18**, 507-16

Abou-Donia, M.B. and Dieckert, J.W. (1974a). Gossypol: Uncoupling of respiratory chain and oxidative phosphorylation. *Life Sci.*, **14**, 1955-63

Abou-Donia, M.B. and Dieckert, J.W. (1974b). Urinary and biliary excretion of ^{14}C-gossypol in swine. *J. Nutr.*, **104**, 754-60

Abou-Donia, M.B. and Dieckert, J.W. (1975). Metabolic fate of gossypol: the metabolism of [^{14}C]gossypol in swine. *Toxicol. Appl. Pharmacol.*, **31**, 32-46

Abou-Donia, S.A., Lasker, J.M. and Abou-Donia, M.B. (1981). High-performance liquid chromatographic analysis of gossypol. *J. Chromatogr.*, **206**, 606-10

Abou-Donia, M.B. and Lyman, C.M. (1970). The metabolism of ^{14}C-gossypol in laying hens. *Toxicol. Appl. Pharmacol.*, **17**, 4473-86

Abou-Donia, M.B., Lyman, C.M. and Dieckert, J.W. (1970). Metabolic fate of gossypol: the metabolism of ^{14}C-gossypol in rats. *Lipids*, **5**, 938-46

Adams, R., Geissman, T.A. and Edwards, S.D. (1960). Gossypol, a pigment of cottonseed. *Chem. Rev.*, **60**, 555-74

Adams, R., Morris, R.C., Geissman, T.A., Butterbaugh, D.J. and Kirkpatrick, E.C. (1938). Structure of gossypol. XV. An interpretation of its reactions. *J. Am. Chem. Soc.*, **60**, 2193-204

Albrecht, J.E., Clawson, A.J. and Smith, F.H. (1972). Rate of depletion and route of elimination of intravenously injected gossypol in swine. *J. Animal Sci.*, **35**, 941-6

Altschul, A.M., Lyman, C.M. and Thurber, F.H. (1958). Cottonseed meal. In Altschul, A.M. (ed.). *Processed Plant Protein Foodstuffs*, p. 469. (New York; Academic Press)

Bottger, G.T., Sheehan, E.T. and Lukefahr, M.J. (1964). Relation of gossypol content of cotton plants to insect resistance. *J. Econ. Entomol.*, **57**, 283-5

Braham, J.E. and Bressani, R. (1975). Effect of different levels of gossypol on transaminase activities on nonessential and essential amino acid ratio and on iron and nitrogen retention in rats. *J. Nutr,,* **105**, 348-55

Buitrago, J.A., Clawson, A.J. and Smith, F.H. (1970). Effects of dietary iron on gossypol accumulation in and elimination from porcine liver. *J. Animal Sci.*, **31**, 544-58

Carruth, F.E. (1918). Contribution to the chemistry of gossypol, the toxic principle of cottonseed. *J. Am. Chem. Soc.*, **40**, 647–63

Chang, M.C., Gu, Z. and Saksena, S.K. (1980). Effects of gossypol on the fertility of male rats, hamsters, and rabbits. *Contraception*, **21**, 461–9

Cherry, J.P. and Gray, M.S. (1981). Methylene chloride extraction of gossypol from cottonseed products. *J. Food Sci.*, **46**, 1726–33

Clark, E.P. (1928). Studies on gossypol II. Concerning the nature of Carruth's D Gossyol. *J. Biol. Chem.*, **76**, 229–35

Clawson, A.J., Smith, F.H. and Barrick, E.R. (1962). Accumulation of gossypol in the liver and factors influencing the toxicity of injected gossypol. *J. Animal Sci.*, **21**, 911–15

Crouch, F.W. Jr. and Bryant, M.F. (1982). Reaction-rate spectrophotometric method for analysis of gossypol in cottonseed extracts. *Anal. Chem.*, **54**, 242–6

De Peyster, A.D. and Wans, Y.Y. (1979). Gossypol-proposed contraceptive for men passes the Ames Test (letter). *N. Engl. J. Med.*, **301**, 275–6

Dorsett, P.H., Kerstine, E.E. and Powers, L.J. (1975). Letter: Antiviral activity of gossypol and apogossypol. *J. Pharm. Sci.*, **64**, 1073–5

Eagle, E. (1960). A review of some physiological effects of gossypol and cottonseed pigment glands. *J. Am. Oil. Chem. Soc.*, **37**, 40–3

Edwards, J.D. Jr. (1958). Total synthesis of gossypol. *J. Am. Chem. Soc.*, **80**, 3798–9

Giridharan, N., Bamji, M.S. and Sankaram, A.V.B. (1982). Inhibition of rat testis LDH-X activity by gossypol. *Contraception*, **26**, 607–15

Hahn, D.W., Rustious, C., Probst, A., Homm, R. and Johnson, A.N. (1981). Antifertility and endocrine activities of gossypol in rodents. *Contraception*, **24**, 97–105

Hale, F., Lyman, C.M. and Smith, H.A. (1958). Use of cottonseed meal in swine rations. *Texas Agr. Expt. Sta. Bull.*, **898**, 1–14

Hanny, B.W. (1980). Gossypol, flavonoid, and condensed tannin content of cream and yellow anthers of five cotton (*Gossypium hirsutum* L.) cultivars. *J. Agric. Food Chem.*, **28**, 504–6

Hass, R.H. and Shirley, D.A. (1965). The oxidation of gossypol. II. Formation of gossypolone with ferric chloride. *J. Am. Chem. Soc.*, 4111–13

Heinstein, P.F., Herman, D.L., Tove, S.B. and Smith, F.H. (1970). Biosynthesis of Gossypol. Incorporation of mevalonate-2-^{14}C and isoprenyl pyrophosphates. *J. Biol. Chem.*, **245**, 4658–65

Herman, D.L. and Smith, F.H. (1973). Effect of bound gossypol on the absorption of iron by rats. *J. Nutr.*, **103**, 882–9

Herman, D.L. and Smith, F.H. (1975). Effect of free gossypol on tissue uptake of iron by everted segments of rat duodenum. *J. Agric. Food Chem.*, **23**, 548–51

Jensen, D.R., Tone, J.R., Sorensen, R.H. and Bozek, S.A. (1982). Deposition pattern of the antifertility agent, gossypol, in selected organs of male rats. *Toxicology*, **24**, 65–72

Jones, L.A. and Smith, F.H. (1977a). Effect of gossypol on the removal of nitrogen and amino acids from feed in digestion by the rat. *J. Animal Sci.*, **44**, 410–16

Jones, L.A. and Smith, F.H. (1977b). Effect of bound gossypol and amino acid supplementation of glandless cottonseed meal on the growth of weanling rats. *J. Animal Sci.*, **44**, 401–9

Kalla, N.R., Foo, T.W. and Sheth, A.R. (1982). Studies on the male antifertility agent gossypol acetic acid. V. Effect of gossypol acetic acid on the fertility of male rats. *Andrologia*, **14**, 492–500

Kalla, N.R. and Vasudev, M. (1981). Studies on the male antifertility agent gossypol acetic acid. II. Effects of gossypol acetic acid on the motility and ATPase activity of human spermatozoa. *Andrologia*, **13**, 95–8

Kalla, N.R., Vasudev, M. and Arora, G. (1981). Studies on the male antifertility agent gossypol acetic acid. III. Effect of gossypol acetic acid on rat testis. *Andrologia*, **13**, 242–9

Lee, C.Y.G., Moon, Y.S., Yuan, J.H. and Chen, A.F. (1982). Enzyme inactivation and inhibition by gossypol. *Mol. Cell Biochem.*, **47**, 65–70

Lindsey, T.O., Hawkins, G.E. and Guthrie, L.D. (1980). Physiological responses of lactating cows to gossypol from cottonseed meal rations. *J. Dairy Sci.*, **63**, 562–73

Lyman, C.M., El-Nockrashy, A.S. and Dollahite, J.W. (1963). Gossyverdurin: A newly isolated pigment from cottonseed pigment glands. *J. Am. Oil Chem. Soc.*, **40**, 571–5

Marchlewski, L. (1899). Gossypol, ein Bestandtheil der Baumwollsamen. *J. Prakt. Chem.*, **60**, 84–90

Menaul, P. (1923). The physiological effect of gossypol. *J. Agr. Res.*, **26**, 233-7.

Millburn, R., Smith, R.L. and Williams, R.T. (1967). Biliary excretion of foreign compounds, biphenyl, stilbestrol, and phenolphthalein in the rat; molecular weight, polarity, and metabolism as factors in biliary excretion. *Biochem. J.*, **104**, 1275-81

Montamat, E.E., Burgos, C., Gerez de Burgos, N.M., Rovai, L.E., Blanco, A. and Segura, E.L. (1982). Inhibitory action of gossypol on enzymes and growth of *Trypanosoma Cruzi*. *Science*, **218**, 288-9

Nadakavukaren, M.J., Sorensen, R.H. and Tone, J.N. (1979). Effect of gossypol on the ultrastructure of rat spermatozoa. *Cell Tissue Res.*, **204**, 293-6

National Coordinating Group on Male Antifertility Agents (1978). Gossypol-A new antifertility agent for males. *Chinese Med. J.*, **4**, 417-28

Nomeir, A.A. and Abou-Donia, M.B. (1982). Gossypol: High-performance liquid chromatographic analysis and stability in various solvents. *J. Am. Oil Chem. Soc.*, **59**, 546-9

Peyster, A.D. and Wans, Y.Y. (1979). Gossypol-proposed contraceptive for men passes the Ames test (letter). *N. Engl. J. Med.*, **301**, 275-6

Pons, W.A. Jr. (1977). Gossypol analysis: Past and Present. *J. Am. Oil Chem. Soc.*, **60**, 252-9

Poso, H., Wichmann, K., Janne, J. and Luukkainen, T. (1980). Gossypol, a powerful inhibitor of human spermatozoal metabolism. *Lancet*, **1**, 885-6

Saksena, S.K. and Salmonsen, R.A. (1982). Antifertility effects of gossypol in male hamsters. *Fertil. Steril.*, **37**, 686-90

Sakesena, S.K., Salmonsen, R., Lau, I.F. and Chang, M.C. (1981). Gossypol: Its toxicological and endocrinological effects in male rabbits. *Contraception*, **24**, 203-14

Schwartz, E.W. and Alsberg, C.L. (1924). Pharmacology of gossypol. *J. Agr. Res.*, **28**, 191

Shandilya, L.N. and Clarkson, T.B. (1982). Hypolipidemic effects of gossypol in cynomolgus monkeys (*Macaca fascicularis*). *Lipids*, **17**, 285-90

Shandilya, L., Clarkson, T.B., Adams, M.R. and Lewis, J.C. (1982). Effect of gossypol on reproductive and endocrine functions of male cynomolgus monkeys (*Macaca fascicularis*). *Biol. Reprod.*, **27**, 241-52

Shaver, T.N. and Lukefahr, M.J. (1969). Effect of flavonoid pigments and gossypol on growth and development of the bollworm, tobacco budworm, and pink bollworm. *J. Econ. Entomol.*, **62**, 642-6

Singleton, V.L. and Kratzer, F.H. (1969). Toxicity and related physiological activity of phenolic substances of plant origin. *J. Agric. Food Chem.*, **17**, 497-512

Singleton, V.L. and Kratzer, F.H. (1973). Plant Phenolics. In Toxicants Occurring Naturally in Foods, pp. 318-23. Washington, DC: National Academy of Sciences

Skutches, C.L., Herman, D.L. and Smith, F.H. (1973). Effect of intravenous gossypol injection on iron utilization in swine. *J. Nutr.*, **103**, 851-5

Skutches, C.L., Herman, D.L. and Smith, F.H. (1974). The effect of dietary free gossypol on blood components and tissue iron in swine and rats. *J. Nutr.* **104**, 415-23

Skutches, C.L. and Smith, F.H. (1974a). Effect of phenobarbital on the level of gossypol in the liver and the effect of gossypol and phenobarbital on liver microsomal O-demethylation and lipid peroxidation activities in the rats. *J. Nutr.*, **104**, 1567-75

Skutches, C.L. and Smith, F.H. (1974b). Metabolism of gossypol, biosynthesized from methyl-^{14}C- and carboxyl-^{14}C-labeled sodium acetate in rats. *J. Am. Oil Chem. Soc.*, **51**, 413-5

Smith, F.H. (1963). Isolation of gossypol from tissue of porcine livers. *J. Am. Oil Chem. Soc.*, **40**, 60-1

Smith, F.H. (1967). Determination of gossypol in leaves and flower. *J. Am. Oil Chem. Soc.*, **44**, 267-9

Smith, F.H. (1968). Estimation of free gossypol in cottonseed meal and cottonseed meats. Modified Method. *J. Am. Oil Chem. Soc.*, **45**, 903

Smith, F.H. (1972). Effect of gossypol bond to cottonseed protein on growth of weanling rats. *J. Agric. Food Chem.*, **20**, 803-4

Smith, F.H. (1974). Preparation of ^{14}C-gossypol by incorporation of acetate-1-^{14}C and acetate 2-^{14}C by biosynthesis. *J. Am. Oil Chem. Soc.*, **51**, 410-12

Smith, F.H. and Clawson, J.A. (1965). Effect of diet on accumulation of gossypol in the organs of swine. *J. Nutr.*, **87**, 317-21

Smith, H.A. (1957). The pathology of gossypol poisoning. *Am. J. Pathol.*, **33**, 353-65

Sotelo, A., Montalvo, I., de la Luz Crail, M. and Gonzalez-Garza, M.T. (1982). Infertility in male rats induced by diets containing whole cottonseed flour. *J. Nutr.*, **112**, 2052-7

Tang, F., Tsang, A.Y., Lee, C.P. and Wong, P.Y. (1982). Inhibition of catechol-*O*-methyl-transferase by gossypol: the effect of plasma proteins. *Contraception*, **26**, 515-19

Tanksley, T.D., Neumann, H., Lyman, C.M., Pace, C.N. and Prescott, J.M. (1970). Inhibition of pepsinogen activation by gossypol. *J. Biol. Chem.*, **245**, 6456-61

Tone, J.N. and Jensen, D.R. (1970). Effect of ingested gossypol on the growth performances of rats. *Experientia*, **26**, 970-1

Tone, J.N. and Jensen, D.R. (1974). Hematological effects of injected gossypol and iron in rats. *J. Agric. Food Chem.*, **22**, 140-3

Waller, D.P., Fong, H.H., Cordell, G.A. and Soejarto, D.D. (1981). Antifertility effects of gossypol and its impurities on male hamsters. *Contraception*, **23**, 653-60

Weinbauer, G.F., Rovan, E. and Frick. J. (1982). Antifertility efficacy of gossypol acetic acid in male rats. *Andrologia*, **14**, 270-5

Wen, W. (1980). China invents male birth control pill. *Am. J. Chin. Med.*, **8**, 195-7

Wichmann, K., Vaheri, A. and Luukkainen, T. (1982). Inhibiting herpes simplex virus type 2 infection in human epithelial cells by gossypol, a potent spermicidal and contraceptive agent. *Am. J. Obstet. Gynecol.*, **1**, 593-4

Williams, R.T., Millburn, P. and Smith, R.L.(1965). The influence of enterohepatic circulation on toxicity of drugs. *Ann. NY Acad. Sci.*, **123**, 110-24

Withers, W.A. and Carruth, F.E. (1915). Gossypol—A toxic substance in cottonseed meal. A preliminary note. *Science*, **41**, 324

Wong, R.C., Nakagawa, Y. and Perlman, G.E. (1972). Studies on the nature of the inhibition by gossypol of the transformation of pepsinogen to pepsin. *J. Biol. Chem.*, **247**, 1625-31

Wu, Y.M., Chappel, S.C. and Flickinger, G.L. (1981). Effects of gossypol on pituitary-ovarian endocrine function, ovulation and fertilty in female hamsters. *Contraception*, **24**, 259-68

10
Biochemical and nutritional considerations of gossypol intake

J. E. BRAHAM and R. BRESSANI

Gossypol (1,1′,6,6′,7,7′-hexahydroxy-5,5′-diisopropyl-3,3′-dimethyl-2,2′-bi-naphthalene-8,8′-dicarboxaldehyde) is a yellow pigment present in the roots, leaves and seeds of the cotton plant. Free gossypol is contained in pigment glands together with more than 20 other pigments; gossypol, how-ever, is present in the highest amounts constituting about 40% of the gland. The ultrastructural morphology of the latter has been studied by Yatsu *et al.* (1974). The glands appear to the naked eye as black dots embedded in the tissue of the seed, and can be easily separated by floatation in hexane or as the underflow of the liquid cyclone process from which gossypol can by crystallized as the acetic acid derivative. Gossypol melts at 184°C when crystallized from ether, 199°C when crystallized from chloroform and 214°C when petroleum ether is used; it is soluble in most organic solvents, and it imparts a bright yellow colour to cottonseed products. Most of the bio-logical activity of cottonseed flours and meals has been ascribed to free gossypol which is that fraction of the pigment not bound to protein; the sum of the free and the bound fraction constitutes total gossypol. Since it has been reported (Jones, 1979) that there are present in the cotton plant more than 525 compounds with biological activity one has to wonder to what extent are the toxicity symptoms ascribed to gossypol really due to this pigment alone. Certainly some of the other pigments, such as gossy-verdurin may be more toxic than gossypol itself (Lyman *et al.*, 1963), and some of the infertility effects observed in man have been ascribed to a powerful contaminant of the gossypol molecule rather than to gossypol itself (Zatuchni and Osborn, 1981).

PROCESSING OF COTTONSEED FLOURS

Regardless of variety, the amount of gossypol in cottonseed meal depends on the process used to extract the oil. The process selected will in turn affect not only the amount of gossypol present but the quantity and quality of the protein in the flour. These two factors, gossypol and protein quantity and quality, are very important in determining the nutritional value of cottonseed flours since, as it will be discussed later, there is an interrelationship between them.

Bressani and Elías, (1968) have shown that meals extracted by the solvent extraction procedure contain more free gossypol than those extracted by press or pre-press solvent extraction procedures, while total gossypol is about the same for the three procedures (Table 10.1). Likewise, protein

Table 10.1 Proximate chemical composition of cottonseed flours according to the industrial process used (%) (Bressani *et al.*, 1968)

	Industrial process		
Component	Press	Pre-pressed solvent	Solvent
Moisture	7.5	8.6	11.0
Dry matter	92.5	91.4	89.0
Ether extract	6.9	2.9	2.5
Crude fibre	10.3	6.3	10.9
Protein (N × 6.25)	42.1	47.6	35.8
Ash	6.5	7.3	6.6
Nitrogen-free extract	26.7	27.3	33.2
Free gossypol	0.051	0.056	0.126
Total gossypol	0.991	0.853	0.996
Soluble N in NaOH	51.4	67.7	83.2

content is higher for pre-pressed solvent extraction than for the other two procedures.

The most important changes occurred during the pressing of the seed where a significant decrease in the ether extract, free gossypol and available lysine was observed. Toxicity of the meal decreased as it passed from raw to cooked and decreased still further when it was pressed. No mortality was observed in animals when the pressed meal was fed, and protein quality improved slightly. Tables 10.2 and 10.3 show the results of Bressani *et al.* (1966) on the changes that occurred in cottonseed composition when it was

Table 10.2 Changes in fat, nitrogen, free-amino groups of lysine and free and total gossypol during cottonseed processing by screw press (Bressani *et al.*, 1966)

				Gossypol[b]	
Position in process[a]	Ether extract (g/100 g)	Nitrogen (g/100 g)	Lysine (g/16 g N)	Free (mg/100 g)	Total (g/100 g)
Seed	34.4	5.01	3.13	203	1.94
Cooker	28.0	4.34	3.22	193	1.48
Dryer	29.6	4.00	3.52	200	1.46
Conditioner	30.4	4.38	3.12	200	1.49
Expeller	5.2	6.22	2.83	43	1.16
Flour[c]	4.7	5.33	2.48	46	1.14

[a] Samples taken after operation.
[b] On a fat-free basis.
[c] Ground to pass 80 mesh screen.

Table 10.3 Changes in fat, nitrogen, gossypol and nutritive value of cottonseed processed by pre-press solvent extraction (Bressani et al., 1966)

Position in process[a]	Ether extract (g/100 g)	Nitrogen (g/100 g)	Free gossypol (mg/100 g)	Mortality start/finish	Weight gain (g)
Seed	33.3	5.60	930	8/1	—
Cooker	32.8	5.29	951	8/1	—
Dryer	33.0	5.71	933	8/1	—
Conditioner	33.0	5.00	872	8/5	13
Expeller	10.0	7.09	98	8/8	76
Solvent ext.	2.8	7.85	64	8/8	58
Flour	3.4	8.28	69	8/8	62

[a] Samples taken after operation

processed by the screw press and by the prepress solvent extraction technologies. With the former, ether extract, lysine, and free gossypol levels decreased, nitrogen content increased and bound gossypol decreased slightly as the seed moved from one operation to the other. For the prepress solvent extraction method the same pattern was observed for ether extract, free gossypol and nitrogen. Biological trials with rats showed that the seed was very toxic up to the conditioner stage, after which no mortality was observed, and the animals gained a substantial amount of weight when fed the cottonseed flour at a 10% protein level in the ration. Similar results were obtained by Elías et al. (1969) when comparing the three methods of oil extraction. In this case, the PER obtained for the press, the pre-press-solvent and the solvent methods were 1.47, 1.96 and 2.86, respectively. Part of the free gossypol is dissolved in the oil especially in processes using heat and pressure, and crude cottonseed oil needs to be refined before it is used for human consumption.

Robison (1934) reported that cottonseed meal toxicity was markedly reduced by autoclaving the meal for one hour under 14 pounds of pressure. Clark (1969) reported that continuous extrusion cooking was effective in decreasing free gossypol levels in the meal. The binding of gossypol occurred during the preconditioning stage and the flours obtained conformed to the United Nations Tentative Quality and Processing Guide for Cottonseed Flour for Human Consumption. The extrusion process was effective also in binding gossypol from ground, screened meal but not from ground, unscreened meal.

Ridlehuber and Gardner (1954) used the liquid cyclone process to produce cottonseed flour for human consumption. The material obtained was light cream in colour, and contained almost 70% protein with a PER of 2.51–2.57. Since in this process the pigment glands are recovered intact in the underflow fraction, there is no gossypol present in the flour. It has been used successfully in bakery products, beef patties and sausages, and has served as a raw material for obtaining a protein isolate for human consumption.

The processes used for extracting the oil involve either heat and pressure or solvent extraction. Meals obtained by the former are usually lower in

Table. 10.4 Changes in chemical composition of cottonseed during extraction of the oil by screw press (Bressani and Elias, 1968)

Sample	Ether extract (g/100 g)	Nitrogen (g/100 g)	Gossypol (g/100 g)		ε-amino lysine groups (g/16 g N)	Temperature (°F)
			Free	Total		
Whole seed	29.8	4.84	0.91	1.02	—	—
Laminated seed	36.4	5.13	1.01	1.01	3.58	—
After:						
cooker	31.3	4.23	0.89	1.07	3.61	190
dryer	32.3	4.63	0.87	1.02	3.07	165–250
Conditioner:						
No. 1	34.6	4.32	0.91	1.09	3.27	240
No. 2	34.7	4.59	0.68	0.96	3.16	240
Press No. 1	7.8	5.81	0.053	0.78	2.82	—
Press No. 2	6.5	6.08	0.040	0.79	2.90	—
Flour	8.0	6.08	0.056	0.82	3.06	—

free gossypol than those obtained by the latter process, due to the catalytic effect of heat on the reaction between free gossypol and lysine which results in bound gossypol with no biological activity. Heat, however, will also catalyse the reaction between lysine and carbohydrates resulting therefore, in meals of lower protein quality due to a deficiency in the amino acid which is already limiting in raw cottonseed meal. Some of these results are shown in Table 10.4 where it can be seen that as ether extract decreased, protein content increased, while free gossypol decreased after passing through the conditioner and presses. There was little change in total gossypol, and available lysine started to decrease as heat was used, reaching the lowest levels during the pressing operation where considerable heat is generated (Bressani and Elías, 1968).

GOSSYPOL TOXICITY AND PATHOLOGY

The symptoms of gossypol toxicity vary with the different species studied and sometimes with the strain of animal used. They also depend on the form in which gossypol is administered (whether pure or as cottonseed meal), on the way of administration (orally or injected), and on the composition of the diet. Common symptoms obtained, however, are growth rate depression, anorexia, anaemia, hair loss or depigmentation, diarrhoea and respiratory and circulatory irregularities. The respiratory effects are prevalent in swine, where laboured breathing and dyspnoea are one of the main symptoms observed, followed by sudden death. Swine are probably the most susceptible animals to the toxic effect of gossypol, whereas chicks and rats are more resistant and can withstand higher levels of gossypol in the ration than hogs. In cats and rabbits spastic paralysis often develops (Zatuchni and Osborn, 1981). Gossypol has not shown a mutagenic effect in studies *in vitro* (de Peyster and Wang, 1979).

Pathology of gossypol ingestion

Since hogs and dogs are more susceptible to gossypol toxicity than other species, most of the studies on the pathology of gossypol have been carried out in these animals. Smith (1957) reported that the main lesions of gossypol toxicity observed in swine were congestion and oedema resulting from myocardial injury. The congestion observed in the liver was massive and most of the organ was destroyed and filled with blood. The heart was hypertrophied and appeared flabby and dilated. Some intestinal enteritis and congestion of the spleen lymph nodes and kidneys was observed, but by far the most dramatic lesions observed were congestion of the liver and congestion and oedema of the lungs. In contrast, Eagle (1949) working with dogs found lesions of focal necrosis in the caecum, ileocaecal valve and adjacent portions of the large intestine. In further studies Eagle (1950) found marked gastroenteritis in dogs with excessive fluid in the abdomen and pericardium, hydrothorax and oedema of the lungs. In most animals gossypol ingestion results in either gastrointestinal alterations, congestion of the lungs and congestion of the liver.

Findings in the blood, blood serum and other tissues

The main changes observed in the blood constituents of animals ingesting gossypol are low levels of haematocrit, haemoglobin and serum iron. This is the result of the binding of dietary iron by gossypol in the diet and in the intestine which eventually results in the anaemia observed in most species. The studies by Clawson *et al* (1962) showed that there was an inverse relationship between cottonseed meal in the ration and the levels of blood serum and liver iron. The levels of certain enzymes in the blood serum of animals ingesting gossypol have been also studied (Braham *et al.*, 1967). Of the enzymes studied only glutamic–oxalacetic transaminase (GOT) was increased, indicating some degree of hepatic damage. Since some of the symptoms of gossypol toxicity observed involve the respiratory system, the levels of some respiratory enzymes in liver homogenates of animals fed gossypol were also studied (Meksongsee *et al.*, 1970). The results showed that neither cytochrome oxidase nor succinic oxidase in liver homogenates or in mitochondria were different from the values obtained in control animals. On the other hand, gossypol has been reported to inhibit lactic dehydrogenase X (Maugh, 1981) found only in spermatozoa and testicular cells, resulting in decreased sperm production, which may explain, in part, the infertility observed in humans and animals ingesting high levels of free gossypol. The pigment can also cause inactivation of malate dehydrogenase in rodents but not in humans, and in both rodents and humans gossypol inhibits glutathione-*S*-transferase which has an active role in the detoxification process of certain organic compounds.

Effect of cottonseed products on colour and composition of eggs

Another effect associated with the ingestion of cottonseed products is the discoloration of egg yolk to an olive to brown colour (Schaible *et al.*, 1934), (Maugh, 1981) and the albumin to a salmon or pink colour of hens consuming cottonseed meal or crude cottonseed oil. The discoloration of the yolk takes place after storing the egg for some time, or when they are exposed to an atmosphere of ammonia, and it is due to gossypol since cottonseed meal, pigment glands or pure gossypol produce this effect. The occurrence of pink or salmon albumin is associated with the feeding of cottonseed meal or oil either crude or refined; the substances responsible are present in the pigment glands of cottonseed and have been identified as sterculic and malvalic acids, that is, cyclopropenoid fatty acids that give a positive Halphen reaction. These fatty acids are dissolved into the oil during the press or pre-press solvent extraction methods. The solvent extraction method results in flours and oils with a lower content of cyclopropenoid fatty acids, since no pressing is involved and therefore no rupture of glands, and since the flour will contain less residual oil it will also be lower in Halphen positive compounds than those obtained by the other processes.

The mechanism of action of cyclopropenoid acids has been reviewed by Phelps *et al.* (1965). The pH of the yolk is 6.2–6.5 and of the white 8.6–9.2;

under the influence of cyclopropenoid acids these values approach each other and may become the same. The change in pH results in the diffusion of yolk components into the white. One of the compounds diffused is iron which combines with conalbumin in the white producing a pink or salmon chelate. At the same time gossypol combines with iron in the yolk to produce the olive or black yolk characteristic of hens consuming gossypol. This reaction is favoured by the increased pH in the yolk. These changes may occur in normal eggs from hens not receiving either gossypol or cyclopropenoid fatty acids if they are stored for long periods of time; the effect of the cottonseed components appears to be in accelerating these changes so that they become evident even after only 7 days of storage. Other changes observed are a thinner vitelline membrane and a different fatty acid composition of the yolk. Frampton *et al.* (1966) postulated that in eggs from hens fed on cottonseed meal or oil the *in vivo* reaction of stearic to oleic and linoleic acids is driven to the left and this results in the accumulation of saturated fatty acids in the fat of the egg yolk. The latter shows a spherical shape and is more pasty than the yolk of eggs from hens not fed cottonseed products. This effect is due to malvalic acid.

The feeding of cottonseed meal or gossypol has a detrimental effect not only on the colour and consistency of the egg components but also on egg production, weight and hatchability (Heywang *et al.*, 1950). The studies by Fletcher *et al.* (1953), Kemmerer *et al.* (1965), Schaible *et al.* (1934) and others, have shown that the discoloration of the egg yolk caused by gossypol could be counteracted by feeding ferrous salts.

The effect of gossypol on hatchability is probably due to interference of gossypol with the utilization of some of the egg nutrients. Gossypol also interferes with semen production and viability in roosters (Akaubi *et al.*, 1981), and therefore, the gossypol fertility effect in birds is two-fold; on the one hand, spermatozoa are affected in males and on the other, the pigment is deposited by hens in the eggs and interferes with nutrient utilization and hatchability. One can conclude that in a flock where males and females were fed rations containing high enough levels of cottonseed meal or pure gossypol, hatchability of the eggs produced would be almost nil.

FACTORS THAT AFFECT GOSSYPOL TOXICITY

Protein quality and quantity

The gossypol effect observed in animals is modified or counteracted by different nutrients or additives in the diet. Hale and Lyman (1957) showed that protein level in the ration of pigs receiving gossypol was important since animals receiving 30% protein did not show symptoms of toxicity as compared with animals receiving 15% protein with the same level of gossypol in the rations, in spite of the fact that the former consumed more gossypol than the latter. Similar results were obtained by Narain *et al.* (1960) with chicks.

Most of the studies on protein quality and quantity and gossypol have been done with cottonseed meal as the protein source. Protein quality of cottonseed meal is, however, somewhat low when compared with soybean flour. Jarquín et al. (1968) used three cottonseed flours produced by three different methods in Central America, to which iron and calcium were added and then fed to growing swine. The two minerals are known to decrease gossypol toxicity and therefore, the protein effect was isolated from the gossypol effect on growth. Results showed that the meal obtained by the expeller process resulted in better growth and feed conversion, followed by solvent and pre-pressed solvent extracted meals. None of these meals, however, resulted in as good growth as that obtained with soybean meal. Similar results were obtained by Noland et al. (1968) using glandless cottonseed meal and soybean meal. Although growth improved when 0.4% lysine was added to cottonseed flour, it never reached the value obtained with soybean meal. It is therefore, important to keep in mind the protein quality of the diet especially its lysine content, when studying the toxic effects of gossypol since it has been shown that gossypol intake results in decreasing levels of free lysine in both serum and liver (Bressani, 1975).

Iron and calcium

Other diet constituents also affect the toxicity of gossypol. Iron was known to be an antidote to gossypol as early as 1913 (Withers and Brewster, 1913), and numerous studies (Jarquin et al., 1966; Clawson and Smith, 1966; Bressani et al., 1964) have ascertained the validity of this finding. Clawson and Smith (1966) found that the addition of iron to the ration in a 1:1 gossypol:iron ratio protected growing swine from gossypol toxicity; it also decreased the accumulation of the pigment in the liver. Bressani et al. (1964) showed in studies in vitro that ferrous sulphate decreased the level of gossypol in the diet and that the addition of calcium hydroxide had a synergistic effect on the reaction. Studies in swine (Braham et al., 1967) showed that although iron alone improved the weight gain in swine, it was more effective when calcium hydroxide was present in the diet. Calcium alone

Table 10.5 Effect of calcium hydroxide and ferrous sulphate in pigs fed on cottonseed flour (Braham et al., 1967)

	Treatments			
	None	$Ca(OH)_2$ (1%)	$FeSO_4$ (0.1%)	$Ca(OH)_2$ (1%) + $FeSO_4$ (0.1%)
Weight gain (kg/day)	0.27	0.25	0.33	0.43
Blood serum protein (g/100 ml)	6.87	6.70	6.74	6.98
Albumin (g/100 ml)	2.73	2.57	2.51	2.81
Haemoglobin (g/100 ml)	10.9	8.1	12.1	13.2
Haematocrit (%)	37	34	36	43
GOT (units)	175	65	74	74
Leucine amino peptidase (units)	183	165	226	139
Aldolase	21	20	57	19

was more effective than iron in protecting swine against hair depigmentation. Biochemical data indicated that the combination of both elements was more effective in maintaining adequate levels of haemoglobin and haematocrit than either one alone (Table 10.5). Serum iron and iron binding capacity also improved with the addition of both elements. The mechanism by which iron decreases gossypol toxicity seems to be through a binding reaction that takes place in the intestine, the resulting complex being unavailable for absorption. Clawson *et al.* (1961) demonstrated that the effect of iron is not evident when gossypol is injected, which indicates that the binding reaction takes place in the intestine of animals. Protein reacts in much the same way with gossypol, especially through highly reactive groups such as the ε-amino groups of lysine.

Amino acids

Other additives that have been studied are the amino acids. Table 10.3 summarizes the results obtained with the addition of lysine and methionine to swine rations containing cottonseed meal. The results showed that lysine addition improved growth in all instances while the addition of methionine, which has been reported to be also limited in cottonseed meal, showed a deleterious effect on growth. This kind of effect has been demonstrated in other species.

The symptoms of lysine deficiency and those of gossypol toxicity are very similar, and sometimes it is difficult to differentiate between the two. Table 10.6 shows some of these symptoms for both compounds. It has been suggested (Bressani, 1975) that the symptoms observed on gossypol ingestion are really those of lysine deficiency induced by the pigment, but whether this is so or not, the fact remains that there is a striking similarity between the symptoms of lysine deficiency and those of gossypol toxicity. This is not surprising since on the one hand, cottonseed protein is low in lysine and on the other, part of this amino acid may be bound, and therefore rendered unavailable, by gossypol during the extraction of the oil (Phelps, 1966), as has been shown in supplementation studies (Baliga and Lyman, 1957).

In this respect, the studies by Conkerton and Frampton (1959) demonstrated that the number of ε-amino groups of lysine in proteins which can react with 2,4-dinitrofluorobenzene is reduced when the proteins are made to react with gossypol. The reaction increased when the pH of the mixture was increased.

Athens *et al.* (1958) showed that lysine added to swine rations containing cottonseed meal increased the number of reticulocytes by 12% over those of control animals not receiving lysine in their ration. The same effect was obtained when lysine was supplied as casein in the ration.

Hale and Lyman (1961) used two cottonseed meals of different quality and incorporated them in swine rations according to the level of gossypol and available lysine in the meals. Pigs fed the lower quality cottonseed meal supplemented with 0.31% lysine gained 1.66 lbs (754 g) as compared with 0.34 lbs (154 g) for the unsupplemented meal, while for the higher quality

Table 10.6 Effects common to both gossypol toxicity and lysine deficiency

Condition	Reference–gossypol toxicity	Reference–lysine deficiency
Oedema and fluid in the body cavity	Smith (1957)	Lowrey, R.S. et al., J. Animal Sci., **20**, 941 (1961)
Albumin/globulin ratio in serum	Braham et al. (1967)	Brock, C.C. et al., J. Animal Sci., **20**, 926 (1961)
Low haemoglobin level	Braham et al. (1967)	Brock, C.C. et al., J. Animal Sci., **20**, 926 (1961)
Low liver enzymatic activity	Ferguson et al., Proc. Conf. on Chemistry of Gossypol	Bothwell, J.M. and Williams, J.N., Proc. Soc. Exp. Biol. Med., **85**, 544 (1954)
Low serum glutamic–oxalacetic transaminase	Numerous references	Wissler, R.W. et al., J. Nutr., **36**, 345 (1948)
Low weight gain	Numerous references	Numerous references
Hair depigmentation	Braham et al. (1967) and others	Kratzer, P., Science, **124**, 1145 (1956)
High liver fat	Jarquin et al. (1966)	

From Bressani et al. (1979)

Table 10.7 Effect of amino acid supplementation to cottonseed flour

Diet	Amino acid	Weight gain (lbs/day)	Feed consumed / Weight gain (lbs)	Reference
Corn + cottonseed flour	− Lysine	0.38	5.22	Clawson et al. (1961)
	+ 0.2% L-lys–HCl	1.09	3.53	
Corn + cottonseed flour	− Lysine	0.52	2.85	Noland et al. (1968)
	+ 0.4% L-lys	0.70	2.23	
	+ 0.8% L-lys	0.74	2.24	
Corn + cottonseed flour	− Lysine	0.87	4.13	Wallace et al. (1955)
	+ 0.4% DL-lys	0.80	4.28	
	+ 0.8% DL-lys	1.03	3.59	
	+ 0.4% DL-lys + 0.075% DL-Met	0.76	4.23	
Sorghum + cottonseed flour (1.99 available lysine)	− Lysine	0.34	5.88	Hale and Lyman (1961)
	+ 0.31% lys	1.66	3.44	
	+ 0.64% lys	1.74	3.40	
Sorghum + cottonseed flour (2.99 available lysine)	− Lysine	1.07	3.70	Hale and Lyman (1961)
	+ 0.31% lys	1.61	3.49	
	+ 0.62% lys	1.71	3.43	

meal the daily weight gains were 1.61 and 1.07 lbs (731 and 486 g), respectively. In both cases feed consumption and conversion increased with lysine supplementation. When 0.62% lysine was added there was a further increase in the variables studied. These data can be seen in Tables 10.7 and 10.8. Gossypol intake increased from 61.4 to 176.8 mg/day when the ration with 22.6% cottonseed flour was supplemented with 0.31% lysine, but no toxic symptoms were observed. Furthermore, the addition of lysine (Aguirre et al., 1960) or protein (Robison, 1934; Baliga and Lyman, 1957) to swine rations containing cottonseed meals has been shown to protect against the mortality observed in swine fed on cottonseed meal. This effect was very much dependent on feed consumption: in the cases where lysine supplementation resulted in an increased feed intake, there was a definite beneficial

Table 10.8 Effect of lysine supplementation to rations based on cottonseed flour used for feeding pigs (Hale and Lyman, 1961)

Cottonseed flour						
Gossypol		Available lysine (g/16 g N)	Lysine (% of ration)	Weight gain (lbs/day)	Feed consumed (lbs/day)	Feed conversion
Total (%)	Free (%)					
1.15	0.03	1.99	0	0.34[a]	2.00	5.88
			0.31	1.66[a]	5.71	3.44
			0.62	1.74[a]	5.92	3.40
0.84	0.02	2.99	0	1.07[b]	3.96	3.70
			0.31	1.61[b]	5.63	3.49
			0.62	1.71[b]	5.87	3.43

[a] Cottonseed flour in ration, 22.6%
[b] Cottonseed flour in ration, 19.6%

effect of lysine supplementation on gossypol toxicity. Numerous studies (Lyman *et al.*, 1959; Baliga and Lyman, 1957; Chang *et al.* 1955; Couch *et al.*, 1955) have shown that ingested free gossypol forms a complex with dietary lysine which is not absorbed. In some of these studies all of the lysine and gossypol ingested were recovered in the faeces of the experimental animals. It seems, therefore, that the combination of a high quality protein, good source of lysine, and iron and calcium in the diet may protect animals against the toxicity of ingested gossypol.

GOSSYPOL AND HUMAN NUTRITION

Cottonseed flour has been used in human nutrition, especially for the manufacture of vegetable high protein mixtures in underdeveloped countries where the flour is produced, and sometimes is the only high source of protein available for industrial purposes. The best known of these mixtures is Incaparina developed by a group of scientists at the Institute of Nutrition of Central America and Panama (INCAP) (Bressani *et al.*, 1961) which contained 38% cottonseed flour whose free and total gossypol content was 0.055% and 0.95%, respectively, with an ε-amino lysine content of 3.6 g/16 g N. The mixture contained 27.5% protein and it was designed for feeding children and other people suffering from protein-calorie malnutrition. After numerous studies in laboratory animals and later on in children the mixture was found to be non-toxic and placed on the market where it has enjoyed steadily increasing sales.

If the recommended amount of 75 g per day of Incaparina were ingested, the free gossypol intake would be about 15 mg/day. These levels are decreased about 50% by cooking, and since the protein digestibility of the mixture is about 72%, some gossypol would be excreted in the faeces, and the rest (about 5.4 mg) absorbed. These small amounts of gossypol can be efficiently metabolized by the organism. Bressani *et al.* (1969) ran long-term studies with rats fed Vegetable Protein Mixture 9 for 14 months (Table 10.9). Breeding performance, fertility, lactation, number of rats born and weight per rat at birth were not affected by the low levels of gossypol fed.

Ridlehuber and Gardner (1954) obtained a 70% protein flour by the liquid cyclone process which could be used as an extender in several manufactured products for human consumption. The protein isolate obtained

Table 10.9 Breeding performance of rats fed for 14 months on diets containing various levels of free gossypol

Free gossypol in diet fed (%)	Number bred (total)	Number pregnant	(%)	Total number born	Average wt. per rat at birth (g)
0 (control)	36	28	77.8	289	6.5
0.011 (K)	36	35	97.2	393	6.2
0.014 (P)	31	29	93.5	324	6.3
0.022 (B)	36	33	91.7	372	6.0
0.028 (C)	36	34	94.4	416	6.1

Source: Bressani *et al.* (1969)

from this flour had excellent whipping characteristics comparing favourably with egg white solids and sodium caseinate. Spadaro and Gardner (1979) used cottonseed flour for human consumption mixed with wheat flour in cereal-like products such as snacks, cookies, doughnuts, cakes and breads. The protein isolate obtained from the flour was white and almost completely soluble at pH 3.5 and it showed excellent whipping characteristics. A cottonseed butter was also produced by grinding roasted cottonseed kernels in equipment used for making peanut butter. Graham *et al.* (1969, 1970) studied several cottonseed flours in infants and children; the results of their metabolic studies indicated that glandless cottonseed flour was the best, and that properly processed cottonseed flour fed at adequate levels could serve as the main or only source of protein for rapidly growing infants and children.

INFERTILITY EFFECTS OF GOSSYPOL IN HUMANS AND ANIMALS

In humans

Recent studies conducted in China have shown that men who ingest relatively high levels of gossypol may become infertile. The studies were conducted after it was found that people who ingested cottonseed oil obtained from cottonseed pressed without heating developed, after a year or so, fever and dyspnoea. The women developed amenorrhoea and the men infertility, but both conditions were reversible after discontinuing the ingestion of the oil. The factor responsible was found to be gossypol. Since then numerous studies have been conducted on the effect of gossypol on fertility, both in animals and humans, and which have been reviewed by Zatuchni and Osborn (1981). The general conclusion is that gossypol in appropriate doses can cause oligospermia and azoospermia in certain species including man. All the studies with men have been conducted in China. Some of these studies showed a potential hypokalaemic effect of gossypol. Potassium in the body tissues of gossypol users was lower than controls and remained low even when blood plasma and intercellular fluid potassium levels returned to normal. Results of rat studies indicated that potassium metabolism was affected when gossypol was given with a low potassium intake. These results indicate the importance of potassium intake in gossypol users. Before using gossypol as an oral male contraceptive, further studies are necessary to try to separate the toxic from the fertility effect. This is very important for populations whose diet is deficient in some nutrients and especially when the protein is of low quality, as happens in many underdeveloped countries, which are precisely those more in need of an effective oral male contraceptive.

In animals

Results in rats, hamsters and rabbits showed that high levels of gossypol resulted in low fertility in rats and hamsters, but rabbits showed no effect on sperm production (Zatuchni and Osborn, 1981). Akaubi *et al.* (1981) using dwarf single-comb White Leghorn roosters found that when gossypol was fed at levels of 0, 20, 40 and 80 mg/kg body weight, there was a significant reduction in feed consumption, body weight, fertility, semen grade and turbidity and spermatocrit. Histopathological studies showed enlargement of the acrosomes of the spermatozoa caused by gossypol feeding. With the 40 mg level or higher, 75–100% mortality was observed.

Since in the human studies it has been observed that as gossypol is purified its effect on fertility decreases, it has been postulated that the infertility effect may be due to some contaminant of the gossypol molecule rather than the gossypol *per se*. Likewise, some of the toxic effects observed in animals consuming cottonseed meal may be due to the presence of other compounds such as gossyverdurin, which has been reported to be the most toxic of all pigments present in cottonseed (Lyman *et al.*, 1963). That this may be the case is supported by the results of El-Nockrashy *et al.* (1963) who found that pigment glands were more toxic than gossypol and those of Eagle *et al.* (1948) who found no correlation between the toxicity of pigment glands and their gossypol or gossypurpurin content, suggesting that some other pigment was responsible for the toxicity observed.

ABSORPTION AND METABOLISM OF GOSSYPOL

The absorption of gossypol has been studied in rats, dogs, swine and children (Bressani *et al.*, 1979), and the results have been very similar in all species. Figure 10.1 shows the results obtained in 10–12 week-old Duroc Jersey pigs fed 300 g of a ration containing 46% of cottonseed flour. Two animals were killed after 1, 2, 3, 4, 5, 6, 7 and 9 h after ingestion of the feed, and stomach and intestinal contents were collected and analysed for free and total gossypol. As the feed moved from the stomach to the intestine free gossypol decreased in the former. In the small intestine, however, analytical values for free gossypol were two to three times higher than ingested amounts. Total gossypol in the small intestine increased with time of death, and the sum of stomach and intestine total gossypol content was similar to the ingested amount (Fig. 10.2).

Table 10.10 shows the actual amounts of free and total gossypol found

Table 10.10 Free and total gossypol content in the digestive tract of pigs (Braham *et al.*, 1971)

Time (h)	Free gossypol (mg)		Total gossypol (mg)	
	Ingested	Total in digestive tract	Ingested	Total in digestive tract
1	128	116	1817	1522
2	128	241	1818	1731
3	128	298	1811	1811
4	127	308	1802	1783
5	125	265	1773	1691
7	120	268	1704	1447
9	97	268	1386	1461

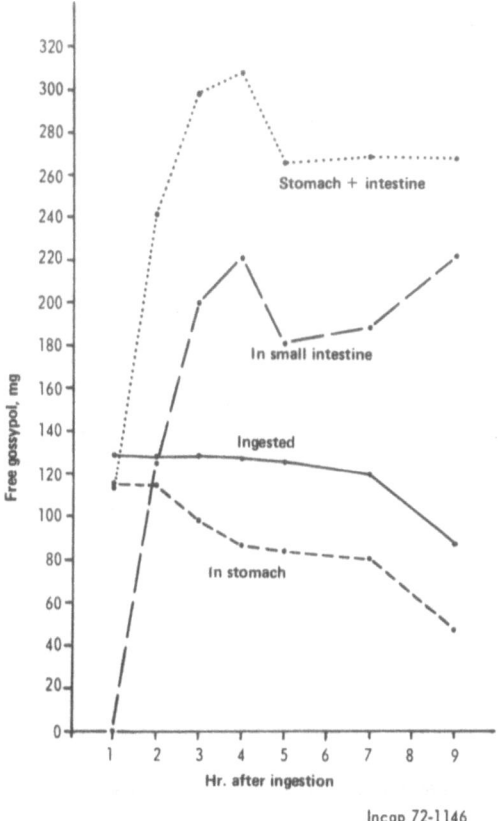

Incap 72-1146

Fig. 10.1   Free gossypol content in the digestive tract of pigs (Bressani *et al.*, 1972)

in the digestive tract, and the intake of these compounds throughout the nine hours of the experiment. As can be seen, after two hours the free gossypol content of the digestive tract was 1–2.5 times higher than ingested amounts, while total gossypol was somewhat lower than the ingested amount. The increase in free gossypol can be explained on the basis of an enterohepatic mechanisms suggested by Bressani *et al.* (1979) whereby free gossypol is absorbed by the intestinal wall, transferred to the liver and excreted via the bile to the intestine. Figures 10.3 and 10.4 show diagrammatically what may be the mechanism of gossypol absorption and toxicity. Free gossypol is absorbed by the intestinal wall and passes to the liver where it can be partially stored, passed to the blood and circulated to other organs, or excreted through the bile to the small intestine where it can be either excreted in the faeces as free gossypol, bound and excreted as bound gossypol or reabsorbed by the intestine and returned to the liver where it follows the same circle. Bound gossypol may be hydrolysed to free gossypol and follow the same pattern. This would explain the higher levels of free gossypol in faeces than ingested that have been reported in some studies.

149

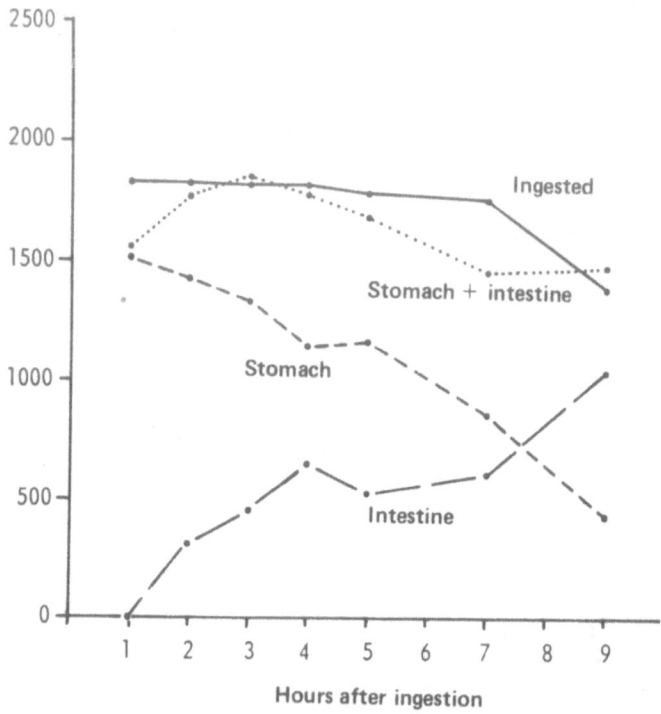

Incap 72-1145

Fig. 10.2   Free gossypol content in the digestive tract of pigs (Bressani *et al.*, 1972)

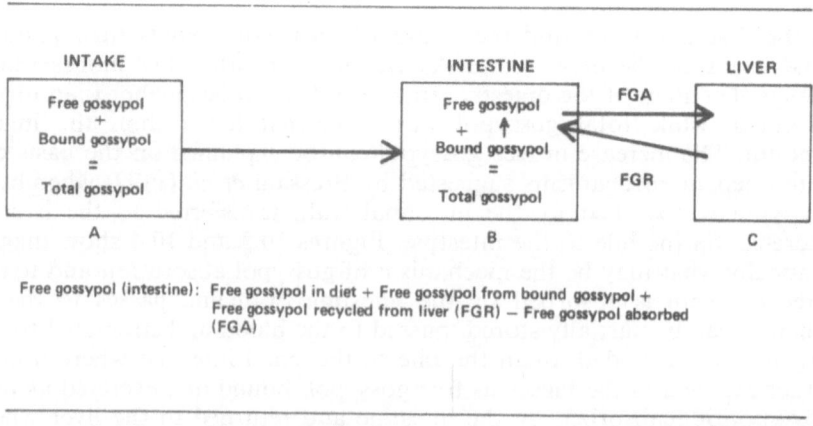

Free gossypol (intestine): Free gossypol in diet + Free gossypol from bound gossypol +
Free gossypol recycled from liver (FGR) – Free gossypol absorbed
(FGA)

Incap 80–128

Fig. 10.3   Possible balance of free and total gossypol in the small intestine (Bressani *et al.*, 1972)

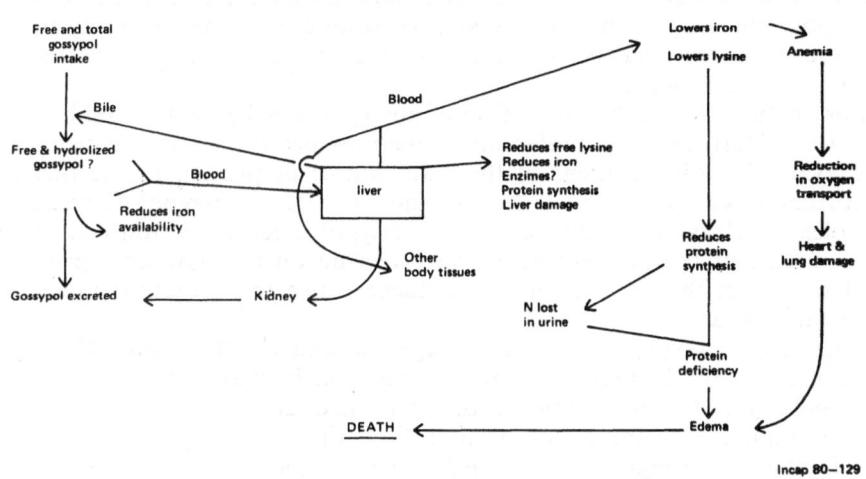

Fig. 10.4 Sequence of events that may explain gossypol toxicity (Bressani *et al.*, 1972)

That this mechanism may be the one taking place is corroborated by the results of Sharma *et al.* (1966) who found high levels of free gossypol in the bile of pigs fed rations of different gossypol and protein content, suggesting that this compound was excreted to the small intestine where it is either reabsorbed or excreted in the faeces as free or bound gossypol. The highest level of protein used in the study (28%) resulted in lower gossypol content in all organs studied. Smith and Clawson (1965) found also that free gossypol concentration was high in the bile of pigs fed free gossypol. In both these studies liver was found to be the organ storing the highest level of gossypol, whereas pancreas, lymph nodes, blood serum, diaphragm muscle, brain and other tissues and organs stored very little amounts. Gossypol levels were lower in all tissues when either high levels of protein or ferrous iron were fed. Injected iron did not have the same effect as dietary iron. The studies by Abou-Donia and Dieckert (1974) using [^{14}C-]gossypol in swine showed also that high levels of the pigment were found in bile. On the basis of these and other results it can be concluded that free gossypol is absorbed in the intestine and then passes to the liver where part is stored in the liver tissue and part excreted to the small intestine via the bile. Very little gossypol is excreted in the urine and in the expired air.

In conclusion, cottonseed flour use in human and animal nutrition is conditioned by the gossypol content of the flour, and by the composition of the diet and the presence or absence of additives. The PAG of the UN System considered that cottonseed flour could be used in human nutrition provided that its free gossypol content does not exceed 0.06%, its total gossypol content is no more than 0.95%, with an ε-amino lysine content of no less than 3.6 g/16 g N. Flours that conform to these specifications have been used successfully as components of vegetable mixtures (Incaparina) for human consumption. The numerous studies in humans and animals that

151

preceded the marketing of this mixture showed that the low levels of free gossypol remaining in the mixture after cooking did not result in any toxicity and the mixture has been on the market for more than 18 years without any report of untoward effects.

For animal feeding the toxic effect of gossypol may be neutralized by the addition of ferrous salts, preferably in the presence of calcium hydroxide. The available lysine content of the main source of protein in the diet is important since the amino acid combines with free gossypol forming a complex which is not absorbed. When gossypol is fed as cottonseed meal the amounts of the pigment in the meal depend on the industrial process used to extract the oil; this process influences also the protein content of the meal or flour.

When free gossypol is ingested in large amounts ($\geqslant 20\,mg/day$) the pigment may result in infertility both in men and in male animals, due to azoospermia and abnormalities in the sperm produced. The effects in man are reversible two to three months after discontinuation of gossypol intake. The intake of the pigment at this high level results also in hypokalaemia, therefore, both protein quality of the diet and the potassium content of the latter are of the greatest importance in gossypol users. Whether gossypol will in time become a successful 'pill' for men depends on further research to separate the toxic from the infertility effect.

References

Abou-Donia, M.B. and Dieckert, J.W. (1974). Urinary and biliary excretion of ^{14}C-gossypol in swine. *J*, Nutr., **104**, 754–60.

Aguirre, A., Wallace, H.D. and Combs, G.E. (1960). Effect of lysine added to high-gossypol cottonseed oilmeal rations for baby pigs. *J. Animal Sci.*, **19**, 1246.

Akaubi, O., Nakane, H.S. and Arscott, G.H. (1981). Effect of gossypol acetic acid on reproductive capability of dwarf single comb White Leghorn roosters. *Poultry Sci.*, **60**, 1613.

Athens, J.W., Cartwright, G.E. and Wintrobe, M.M. (1958). Hematological manifestations of lysine deficiency in swine. *Proc. Soc. Exp. Biol. Med.*, **97**, 909–12.

Baliga, B.P. and Lyman, C.M. (1957). Preliminary report on the nutritional significance of bound gossypol in cottonseed meal. *J. Am. Oil Chem. Soc.*, **34**, 21–4.

Braham, J.E., Cañas, A.G. and Bressani, R. (1971). Absorción de gosipol en ratas y cerdos. *Arch. Latinoamer. Nutr.*, **21**, 450–71

Braham, J.E., Jarquín, R., Bressani, R., González, J.M. and Elías, L.G. (1967). Effect of gossypol on the iron-binding capacity of serum in swine. *J. Nutr.*, **93**, 241–8

Braham, J.E., Jarquín, R., Elías, L.G., González, M. and Bressani, R. (1967). Effect of calcium and gossypol on the performance of swine and on certain enzymes and other blood constituents. *J. Nutr.*, **91**, 47–54

Bressani, R. (1975). Función de las especies de animales menores en la nutrición y en la producción de alimentos. Trabajo presentado en la *VIII Reunión Intermericana a Nivel Ministerial sobre el Control de la Fiebre Aftosa y Otras Zoonosis. Guatemala, del 16 al 19 de abril de 1975, bajo el patrocinio de la Organización Panamericana de la Salud*

Bressani, R., Braham, J.E. and Elías, L.G. (1979). Human nutrition and gossypol. *Food and Nutrition Bulletin (UNU)*, **2**, 24–32

Bressani, R., Braham, J.E. and Jarquín, R. (1972). Harina de torta de semilla de algodón en la alimentación de cerdos. Trabajo presentado en el Seminario sobre Sistemas de Producción Porcina en América Latina que se llevó a cabo en Cali, Colombia del 18 al 21 de septiembre, 1972 bajo los asupicios del Centro Internacional de Agricultura Tropical (CIAT)

Bressani, R. and Elías, L.G., (1968). Cambios en la composición química y en el valor nutritivo

BIOCHEMICAL CONSIDERATIONS OF GOSSYPOL INTAKE

de la proteína de la harina de algodón durante su elaboración. *Arch. Latinoamer. Nutr.*, **18**, 319-39

Bressani, R., Elías, L.G., Aguirre, A. and Scrimshaw, N.S. (1961). All-vegetable protein mixtures for human feeding. III. The development of INCAP Vegetable Mixture Nine. *J. Nutr.*, **74**, 201-8

Bressani, R., Elías, L.G. and Braham, J.E. (1966). Cottonseed protein in human foods. In Altschul, Aaron M. (ed.). *World Protein Resources*, pp. 75-100. Advances in Chemistry Series 57, American Chemical Society

Bressani, R., Elías, L.G., Braham, J.E. and Erales, M. (1969). Long-term feeding studies with vegetable mixtures containing cottonseed flour produced by different methods. *J. Agr. Food Chem.*, **17**, 1135-8

Bressani, R., Elías, L.G., Braham, J.E. and Jarquín, R. (1968). Uso de recursos alimenticios centroamericanos para el fomento de la industria animal. I. Composición química y contenido de gosipol de harinas de torta de semilla de algodón elaboradas en el área. *Turrialba*, **18**, 391-6

Bressani, R., Elías, L.G., Jarquín, R. and Braham, J.E. (1964). All-vegetable protein mixtures for human feeding. XIII. Effect of cooking mixtures containing cottonseed flour on free gossypol content. *Food Technol.*, **18**, 95-9

Chang, W.Y., Couch, J.R., Lyman, C.M., Hunter, W.L., Entwistle, V.P., Green, W.C., Watts, A.B., Pope, C.W., Cabell, C.A. and Earle, I.P. (1955). The nutrition value of prepressed-solvent cottonseed meals. *J. Am. Oil Chem. Soc.*, **32**, 103-9

Clark, S.P. (1969). Continuous extrusion cooking of cottonseed kernels and of partially defatted meal. *J. Am. Oil Chem. Soc.*, **46**, 673-7

Clawson, A.J. and Smith, F.H. (1966). Effect of dietary iron on gossypol toxicity and on residues of gossypol in porcine liver. *J. Nutr.*, **89**, 307-10

Clawson, A.J., Smith, F.H. and Barrick, E.R. (1966). Accumulation of gossypol in the liver and factors influencing the toxicity of injected gossypol. *J. Animal Sci.*, **21**, 911-15

Clawson, A.J., Smith, F.H., Osborne, J.C. and Barrick, E.R. (1961). Effect of protein source, autoclaving and lysine supplementation on gossypol toxicity. *J. Animal Sci.*, **20**, 547-52

Conkerton, E.J. and Frampton, V.L. (1959). Reaction of gossypol with free ε-amino groups of lysine in proteins. *Arch. Biochem. Biophys.*, **81**, 130-4

Couch, J.R., Chang, W.Y. and Lyman, C.M. (1955). The effect of free gossypol on chick growth. *Poultry Sci.*, **34**, 178-83

de Peyster, A. and Wang, Y.Y. (1979). Gossypol-proposed contraceptive for men passes the Ames test. *N. Engl. J. Med.*, **301**, 275-6

Eagle, E. (1949). Chronic toxicity of gossypol. *Science*, **109**, 361

Eagle, E. (1950). Effect of repeated doses of gossypol on the dog. *Arch. Biochem. Biophys.*, **26**, 68-71.

Eagle, E., Castillon, L.E., Hall, C.M. and Boatner, C.H. (1948). Acute oral toxicity of gossypol and cottonseed pigment glands for rats, mice, rabbits and guinea pigs. *Arch. Biochem.*, **18**, 271-7

Elías, L.G., Sánchez, S. and Bressani, R. (1969). Estudio comparativo de diferentes métodos para evaluación del valor proteico de harinas de semilla de algodón. *Arch. Latinoamer. Nutr.*, **19**, 279-97

El-Nockrashy, A.S., Lyman, C.M. and Dollahite, J.W. (1963). The acute oral toxicity of cottonseed pigment glands and intraglandular pigments. *J. Am. Oil Chem. Soc.*, **40**, 14-17

Fletcher, J.L., Barrentine, B.F., Dreesen, L.J., Hill, J.E. and Shawver, C.B. (1953). The use of ferrous sulfate to inactivate gossypol in diets of laying hens. *Poultry Sci.*, **32**, 340-2

Frampton, V.L., Kuck, J.C., Pepperman, A.B. Jr., Pons, W.A. Jr., Watts, A.B. and Johnston, C. (1966). Some properties of Halphen-positive cottonseed oils. *Poultry Sci.*, **45**, 527-35

Graham, G.G., Morales, E., Acevedo, G., Baertl, J.M. and Cordano, A. (1969). Dietary protein quality in infants and children. II. Metabolic studies with cottonseed flour. *J. Am. Clin. Nutr.*, **22**, 577-87

Graham, G.G., Morales, E., Acevedo, G., Baertl, J.M. and Cordano, A. (1970). Dietary protein quality in infants and children. III. Prolonged feeding of cottonseed flour. *Am. J. Clin. Nutr.*, **23**, 165-9

Hale, F. and Lyman, C.M. (1957). Effect of protein level in the ration on gossypol tolerance in growing-fattening pigs. *J. Animal Sci.*, **16**, 364-9

Hale, F. and Lyman, C.M. (1961). Lysine supplementation of sorghum grain-cottonseed meal rations for growing-fattening pigs. *J. Animal Sci.*, **20**, 734-6

Heywang, B.W., Bird, H.R. and Altschul, A.M. (1950). The effect of pure gossypol on egg hatchability and weight. *Poultry Sci.*, **29**, 916-20

Heywang, B.W., Bird, H.R. and Thurber, F.H. (1954). Observations on two components of cottonseed that cause discoloration in eggs. *Poultry Sci.*, **33**, 763-7

Jarquín, R., Bressani, R., Elías, L.G., Tejada, C. and Braham, J.E. (1966). Effect of cooking and calcium and iron supplementation on gossypol toxicity in swine. *J. Agr. Food Chem.* **14**, 275-9

Jarquín, R., González, M., Oliva, R., Lamm, L.A., Elías, L.G. and Bressani, R. (1968). Estudio del uso de harina de semilla de algodón en el crecimiento y engorde de cerdos. *Arch. Latinoamer. Nutr.*, **18**, 39-63

Jones, L.A. (1979). Gossypol and some other flavonoids and phenols that affect quality of cottonseed protein. *J. Am. Oil Chem. Soc.*, **56**, 727-30

Kemmerer, A.R., Heywang, B.W., Vavich, M.G. and Sheehan, E.T. (1965). Effect of iron sulphate on egg discoloration caused by gossypol. *Poultry Sci.*, **44**, 1389

Lyman, C.M., Baliga, B.P. and Slay, M.W. (1959). Reactions of proteins with gossypol. *Arch. Biochem.*, **84**, 486-97

Lyman, C.M., El-Nockrashy, A.S. and Dollahite, J.W. (1963). Gossyverdurin: A newly isolated pigment from cottonseed pigment glands. *J. Am. Oil Chem. Soc.*, **40**, 571-5

Maugh, T.H. (1981). Male 'pill' blocks sperm enzyme. *Science*, **212**, 317

Meksongsee, L.A., Clawson, A.J. and Smith, F.H. (1970). The *in vivo* effect of gossypol on cytochrome oxidase, succinoxidase and succinic dehydrogenase in animal tissues. *J. Agr. Food Chem.*, **18**, 917-20

Narain, R., Lyman, C.M., Deyoe, C.W. and Couch, J.R. (1960). Effect of protein level of the diet on free gossypol tolerance in chicks. *Poultry Sci.*, **39**, 1556-9

Noland, P.R., Funderburg, M., Atterberry, J. and Scott, K.W. (1968). Use of glandless cottonseed meal in diets for young pigs. *J. Animal Sci.*, **27**, 1319-21

Phelps, R.A. (1966). Cottonseed meal for poultry: from research to practical application. *World's Poultry Sci. J.*, **22**, 86-112

Phelps, R.A., Shenstone, F.S., Kemmerer, A.R. and Evans, R.J. (1965). A review of cyclopropenoids compounds: biological effects of some derivatives. *Poultry Sci.*, **44**, 357-94

Ridlehuber, J.M. and Gardner, H.K. (1954). Production of food-grade cottonseed protein by the liquid cyclone process. *J. Am. Oil Chem. Soc.*., **51**, 153-7

Robison, W.L. (1934). Cottonseed meal for pigs. *Ohio Agr. Exp. Sta. Bull.*, **534,**

Schaible, P.J., Moore, L.A. and Moore, J.M. (1934). Gossypol, a cause of discoloration in egg yolks. *Science*, **79**, 372

Sharma, M.P., Smith, F.H. and Clawson, A.J. (1966). Effect of levels of protein and gossypol and length of feeding period on the accumulation of gossypol in tissues of swine. *J. Nutr.*, **88**, 434-8

Smith, H.A. (1957). The pathology of gossypol poisoning. *Am. J. Pathol.*, **33**, 353-65

Smith, F.H. and Clawson, A.J. (1965). The effect of diet on the accumulation of gossypol in the organs of swine. *J. Nutr.*, **87**, 317-21

Spadaro, J.J. and Gardner, H.K. Jr. (1979). Food uses for cottonseed protein. *J. Am. Oil Chem. Soc.*, **56**, 422-4

Wallace, H.D., Cunha, T.J. and Combs, G.E. (1963). Low gossypol cottonseed meal as a source of protein for swine. *University of Florida Agr. Exptl. Sta. Bull.*, **556,** June 1955, Gainesville, Florida

Withers, W.A. and Brewster, F.J. (1913). Studies on cottonseed meal toxicity II. Iron as an antidote. *J. Biol. Chem.*, **15**, 161-6

Yatsu, L.Y., Hensarling, T.P. and Jacks, T.J. (1974). Extraction of lipids from cottonseed tissue. VI. Ultrastructural morphology of isolated pigment glands. *J. Am. Oil Chem. Soc.*, **51**, 548-50

Zatuchni, G.I. and Osborn, C.K. (1981). Gossypol: a possible male antifertility agent. Report of a workshop. *Research Frontiers in Fertility Regulation*, **1**, 1-14

11
Gossypol contraception and mechanism of action

S.P. XUE (SHIEH)

Gossypol is a yellowish polyphenolic compound found in the pigment glands of the seed, leaf, stem and root of the cotton plant, genus *Gossypium*, of the family Malvaceae. It was initially noted from its toxicological effects on non-ruminant animals when the livestock were fed with cottonseed meal as food supplement (Withers *et al.*, 1915). There was renewed interest in gossypol human physiology during 1956–1959, primarily because of the potential for using the high-protein cottonseed flour, Incaparina, as a protein supplement for malnourished children and pregnant women in developing countries. Results indicated that small amounts of gossypol in food was safe for human consumption (Bressani *et al.*, 1980). The elixir extracted from cotton root bark which contains a high concentration of gossypol has long been used traditionally in some countries as an abortifacient and menses inducer (Slocumb, 1980). Antitumour activity of gossypol on some ascites carcinoma and solid tumours was also cited (Vermel *et al.*, 1963). Much of the information indicated that the utilization of gossypol by humans around the world has a long history.

In the 1960s, Chinese workers discovered through mass investigation in some districts in China that cooking with crude cottonseed oil led to infertility in human males (Hubei provincial Hancuan 'Disease of Burning sensation', Treatment and Prevention group 1970). Large-scale animal experiments carried out in 1970s showed that the active ingredient associated with cottonseed oil which induced infertility was gossypol (National Coodinating Group on Male Antifertility Agents, 1978). Following an extensive series of studies using purified gossypol, gossypol–acetic acid and gossypol–formic acid on the antifertility effect, site and mechanism of action, pharmacokinetics, metabolism and toxicity in several species of animals (Wu, 1972; Wang and Lei, 1972; Jiangsu Provincial Cooperation Group on Male Contraception, 1972; Shangtung Provincial Herbaceous Contraceptive Group, 1972; Dai *et al.*, 1972, 1975; Xue *et al.*, 1973, 1975; Tang, 1980), clinical studies of gossypol as a male contraceptive agent were suggested. The first clinical trial of gossypol was started in 1972, and the above three types of gossypol tablet were tested in 14 districts of China. Over 10 000 men used the drugs for a period ranging from 6 months to 8 years, the overall efficacy is 99.07% as estimated by sperm examination. Besides an incidence of 0.75% hypokalaemic paralysis which may be related to dietary intake of potassium, no serious toxic side-effects were observed provided the dosage was kept at the antifertility level. The discovery of gossypol's antifertility effect has aroused worldwide attention and interest among andrologists and in the field of population and family planning, because it is a new non-steroid drug which has been tested on more than 10 000 subjects and for far longer periods than has any other agent. It constitutes a major lead in the search for male contraceptive agents from phenolic compounds, and represents the only approach to have a reasonable chance of being tested on a large-scale before the end of this decade.

CHEMISTRY, PHYSIOLOGICAL PROPERTIES AND METABOLISM OF GOSSYPOL

Gossypol exists mainly as the binaphthalene aldehyde form among its three tautomeric chemical structures (Fig. 11.1), with a molecular weight of 518.54, and an empirical formula $C_{30}H_{30}O_8$. Both the phenolic and carbonyl groups of gossypol are very reactive, they could react with acids, bases, oxygen and many other kinds of biochemical groups. Especially available are ε-amino groups of lysine, which bind, react and lead to a reduction in the availability of free protein and of protein quality (Lyman *et al.*, 1959). Gossypol can affect enzymes by reacting with the substrate or by combining with the enzyme itself thus inhibiting activity (Tankesly *et al.*, 1970; Abou-Donia, 1976), disturbing ion metabolism (i.e. depletion of intracellular potassium in some tissues), causing histological damage and

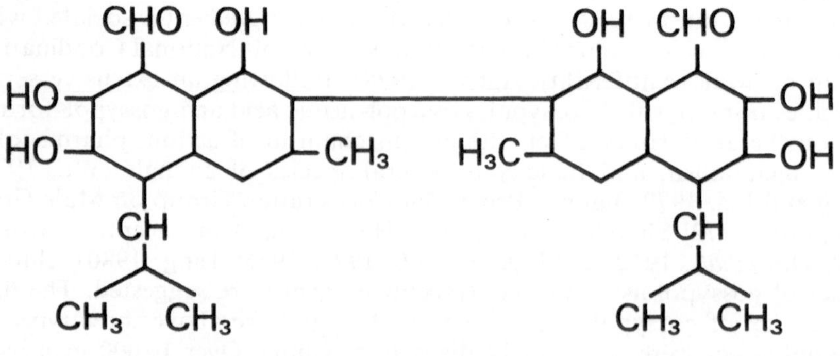

Fig. 11.1 Tautomeric structure of gossypol

inducing physiological toxic effects (Quan *et al.*, 1979). Gossypol might chelate ferrous ion, thereby interfering with the normal utilization of iron in blood in the synthesis of haemoglobin and lead to iron deficiency (Skutches *et al.*, 1973), haemolytic anaemia and malnutrition (Ridgon *et al.*, 1958). But the precise toxicological action is not yet clear.

Pharmacokinetic studies indicate that species differences exist between animals in the absorption, distribution, excretion and metabolism of gossypol within the body. The half-life of gossypol in the blood of mice and dogs after a single administration of [^{14}C]gossypol was longer than that in rats and monkeys (Tang *et al.*, 1980), and the accumulation of radioactive

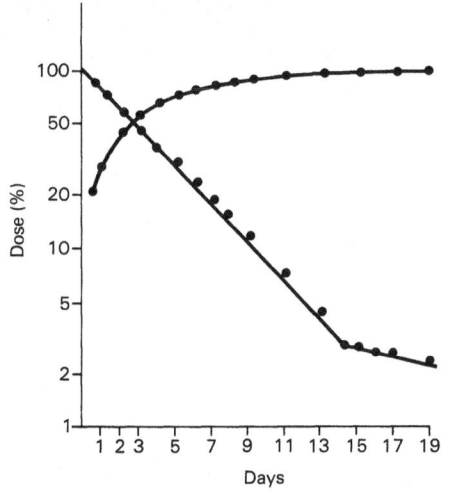

Fig. 11.2 Excretion of [^{14}C]gossypol from the rat body after a single oral dose of 20 μCi/ 7.5 mg. Half-excretion time = 60 h. (o) Total excretion; (0) Radioactivity in body

gossypol in tissues was also higher. This species difference with regard to the accumulation of gossypol in the blood and tissues might provide an explanation of the differences in toxic response in these animals. After a single oral dose of [^{14}C]gossypol to rats (20 μCi/7.5 mg/animal), the half-life for the elimination from the body was 60 h (Fig. 11.2), it took 19 days to eliminate 97.74% of the dose from the body (Xue *et al.*, 1975, 1979a,b). Excretion of gossypol has been shown to be mainly through the bile-faecal pathway. The amounts excreted in 19 days were 83.5% in the faeces, 11.7% in exhaled CO_2 and 2.5% in the urine (Xue *et al.*, 1979b). Whole-body autoradiography demonstrated that one to two days after oral administration, the radioactivity was located mainly in the gastrointestinal tract and liver. By day four there was a general increase in radioactivity in all tissues, and radioactivity in the main visceral organs rapidly reached a peak con-

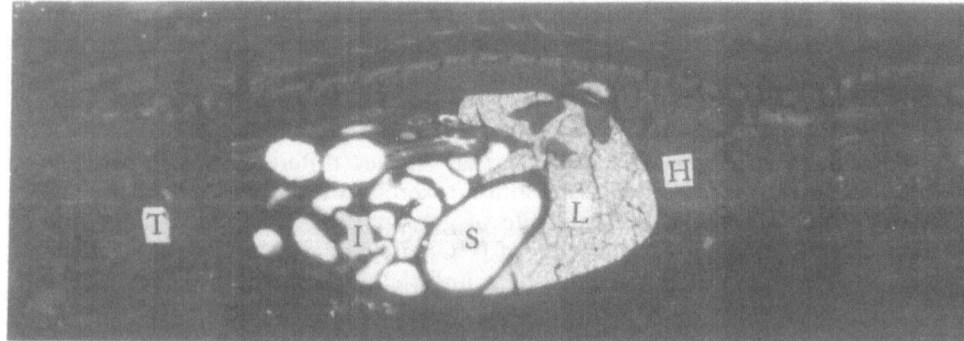

Fig. 11.3 Whole body autoradiograph showing the distribution of [^{14}C]gossypol (white area) in various tissues of rat one day after a single oral dose of labelled gossypol (20 μCi/7.5 mg). Note the high radioactivity in the gastrointestinal tract and liver, and the negligible amount in testis. H, heart; I, intestine; L, liver; S, stomach; T, testis; K, kidney

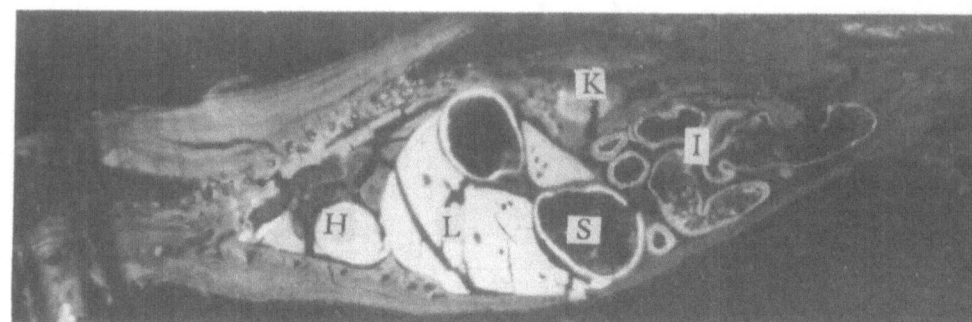

Fig. 11.4 Four days after a single oral dosing, note a general increase in the radioactivity in all tissues. Very low radioactivity could be detected in testis

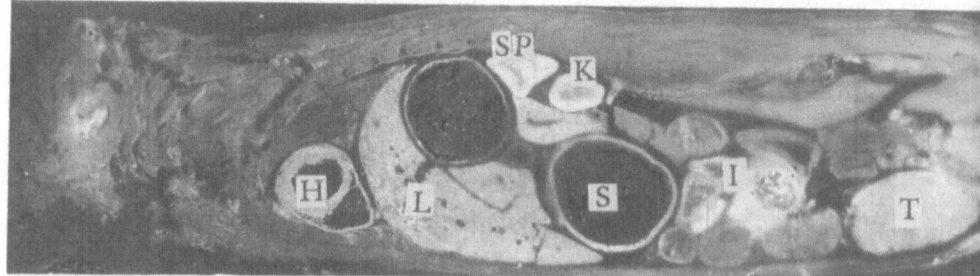

Fig. 11.5 High radioactivity in testis is shown in the whole body autoradiograph by day 9 after a single oral dose of labelled gossypol

centration by day 9 (Figs 11.3, 11.4 and 11.5). Two weeks after administration, the radioactivity in all tissues and organs was markedly decreased, and by day 19, most of the tissues had no detectable radioactivity (Xue *et al.*, 1979a). It is likely that continued administration would lead to accumulation in the body and toxic effects. The pattern of gossypol distribution in rats, mice, rabbits, dogs and monkeys was essentially similar, the highest concentrations of gossypol were found in the liver, followed by spleen, kidney, heart, lung, pancreas, muscle, adipose tissue, testis and brain (Table 11.1) (Xue *et al.*, 1979a,b). The low concentration of gossypol in the testis might be due to the blood–testis barrier, and in a similar manner, gossypol was undetectable in the brain and spinal cord apparently due to blood–brain barrier.

ANTIFERTILITY EFFECT OF GOSSYPOL AND ITS TARGET CELL TYPES

A large number of papers have reported the antifertility effect of gossypol in various species of animals including rats, mice, hamsters, guinea pigs, rabbits, dogs, pigs and monkeys (National Coordinating Group, 1978; Xue *et al.*, 1979c; Dai *et al.*, 1978; Chang *et al.*, 1980; Zatuchni and Osborn, 1981; Shantung Institute of Traditional Medicine and Chinese Academy of Medical Science, 1975). There are species differences between animals in terms of antifertility effect. These differences are mainly attributed to the differences in sensitivity to gossypol damage. Among them the golden hamster, rats, monkeys and humans are more sensitive to the antispermatogenic effect of gossypol, whereas rabbits, mice, dogs, guinea pigs and pigs seem to be insensitive. Toxic effects are usually manifested before the occurrence of damage to germinal epithelium. Quantitative determination and whole-body autoradiographic studies in rats revealed tissue and cell-type differences in response to gossypol. We found that even though the testis had a lower concentration of gossypol than many visceral organs (i.e. the peak concentration of liver, spleen, kidney, heart and testis are 1192, 716, 708, 398 and 372 d min^{-1} g^{-1} respectively, Table 11.1), it showed the most severe damage (Xue *et al.*, 1979b). The damage to testicular germ cells usually occurred before any toxic reaction could be detected in the somatic cells of organs such as liver, heart, and kidney as well as the interstitial and Sertoli cells in testis. The difference between somatic and germ cell response to gossypol and the fact that the testis was damaged at low dosage of gossypol suggests that the selective action of gossypol on the testis is not due to its local concentration but to a higher sensitivity and vulnerability of the germ cells to the drug (Xue *et al.*, 1979a,b, 1981).

Gossypol-acetic acid administered orally at 15–30 mg kg^{-1} body weight day^{-1} to male rats became infertile in approximately 4–5 weeks, the onset of infertility seemed to be dose related. The earliest damage was seen in the metamorphosing spermatids and pachytene spermatocytes 2–3 weeks after drug treatment (Xue *et al.*, 1979a, 1980), showing different degrees of pathological changes such as pyknosis, nuclear vacuolation, swelling or displace-

159

Table 11.1 The specific radioactivity in various tissues of rat following a single dose of [^{14}C]gossypol (20 µCi/7.5 mg)

Tissue	Specific radioactivity*						
	12 h	1 day	2 days	4 days	9 days	14 days	19 days
Heart	250	292	316	398	298	316	94
Liver	978	1192	970	400	287	67	70
Spleen	313	388	494	718	546	360	170
Lung	160	274	300	304	358	280	130
Kidney	314	420	536	708	360	100	86
Pancreas	192	232	244	348	268	110	72
Muscle	192	346	298	302	214	204	204
Testis	270	294	256	284	372	116	78
Gastro-tract content	2560	1760	520	562	206	148	38
Small intestine content	2770	2196	884	658	106	56	46
Large intestine content	3216	9256	1028	826	122	36	62
Adrenal	334	378	608	878	500	408	112
Thyroid	224	908	662	536	370	248	136
Pituitary	258	492	1272	1352	396	296	286
Hypothalmus	52	54	128	92	116	82	60
Medulla oblongata	34	70	86	110	132	76	30

* d min^{-1} g fresh tissue^{-1}, each value is an average of determinations from three animals. Quench corrections were made utilizing standard [^{14}C]hexadecane

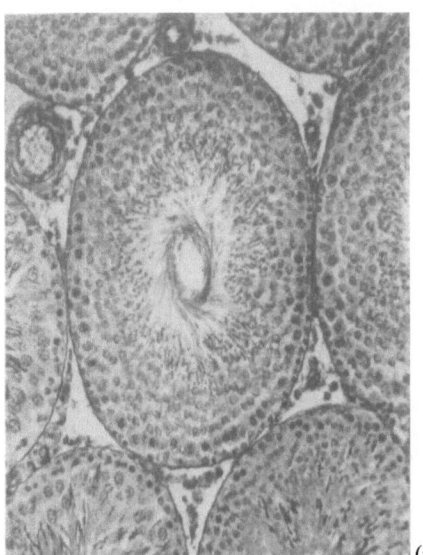 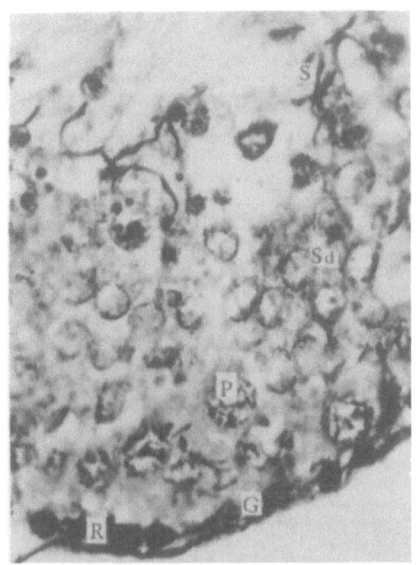

(a)　　　　　　　　　　　　　　　　　　　　(b)

Fig. 11.6 (a) Cross section of a stage VIII seminiferous tubule of normal rat testis, showing the normal structure of the germinal epithelium. G, spermatogonia; R, resting spermatocyte; Sd, spermatids; S, spermatozoa. PAS-haematoxylin. × 225 (b) Same stage of rat seminiferous tubule after gossypol treatment (30 mg kg^{-1} day^{-1}) for 3 weeks, showing vacuolation and karyorrhexis of spermatids (Sd); pyknosis or karyolysis of pachytene spermatocytes (P). Note a few cells are exfoliated from the germinal epithelium. PAS-haematoxylin. × 675

ment of head cap, karyorrhexis, and cytolysis. Exfoliated cells, ghost cells, multinucleated giant cells and necrotic spermatozoa with their heads and tails separated were seen in the lumen of the tubules (Fig. 11.6). By the end of 4–5 weeks, the severely damaged tubules become atrophic and depopulated to a marked degree, spermatids and spermatocytes of the mid- and late stages disappeared almost completely, and only a single layer of cells consisting of Sertoli cells and spermatogonia are left in the tubules (Fig. 11.7). Gossypol target cells were designated the spermatozoa, spermatids and spermatocytes of mid- and late stages based on the basis that: (1) they are the most susceptible and vulnerable to gossypol damage (i.e. the first to show a detectable change and the first to degenerate); (2) gossypol greatly inhibited the incorporation of labelled amino acids into these classes of cells; (3) calculated according to the kinetics of target cell types, the time span of onset of infertility obtained was in good agreement with the time calculated theoretically for chemical agents affecting testicular function (Xue *et al.*, 1979c, 1981, 1982).

The site of cellular damage and the sequence of pathological changes in testes of rhesus monkeys (Shantung Institute of Traditional Medicine and Chinese Academy of Medical Sciences, 1975; Bardin *et al.*, 1980) following the administration of gossypol were essentially identical with that of rats (Fig. 11.8). Hamsters also show a similar pattern of damage but appear to be more sensitive than rats to the effects of gossypol (Chang *et al.*, 1980).

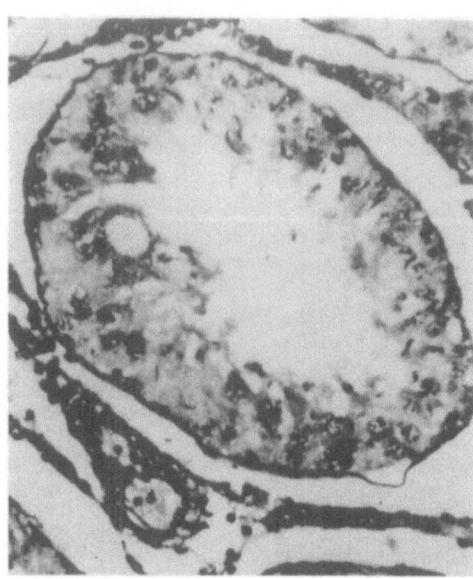

Fig. 11.7 Section of rat testis 4 weeks after gossypol treatment, showing the atrophic tubules with marked depopulation. PAS-haematoxylin. × 375

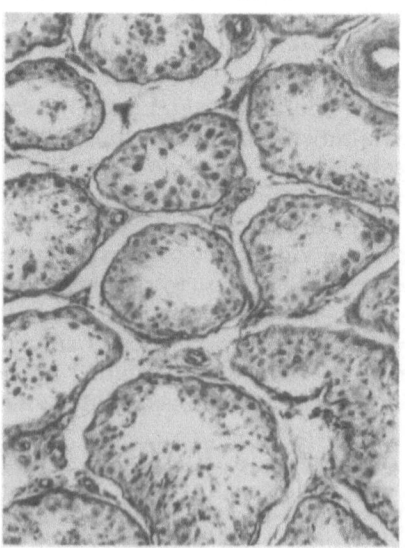

Fig. 11.8 Section of monkey testis 4 months after gossypol treatment ($4\,mg\ kg^{-1}\ day^{-1}$), showing the atrophic tubules with marked depopulation. PAS-haematoxylin. × 120

In human volunteers the testicular biopsies and exfoliated cell types found in semen were consistent with the pattern of cellular damage seen in rats and monkeys. This indicated that the target cell types and the site of gossypol action were exactly alike in rats, monkeys, and men (Xue, 1981).

No detectable damage to Leydig cells, Sertoli cells or the epididymal epithelium were observed in rats fed at antifertility dosages. Neither hormone levels, histochemical reactions nor morphology along the reproductive axis underwent significant changes (Xue *et al.*, 1979c; Xue, 1981). However, decrease in serum LH and testosterone levels in gossypol-treated rats have been reported recently by Hadley and some other workers (Hadley *et al.*, 1981).

Of the spermatogenic elements the spermatogonia are the least susceptible to gossypol, usually remaining unaffected and maintaining their abilities for mitosis (Xue *et al.*, 1979, 1981).

THE TARGET ORGANELLE AND SUBCELLULAR SITE OF ANTISPERMATOGENIC EFFECT OF GOSSYPOL

The target organelle

Since results of ultrastructural damage of rat testicular mitochondria following gossypol teatment were reported in 1973 (Xue *et al.*, 1973, 1979; Dai, 1973, 1978), similar mitochondrial and ultrastructural changes in rat testis (Hadley *et al.*, 1981; Hoffer, 1980) and human seminal (Hang *et al.*,

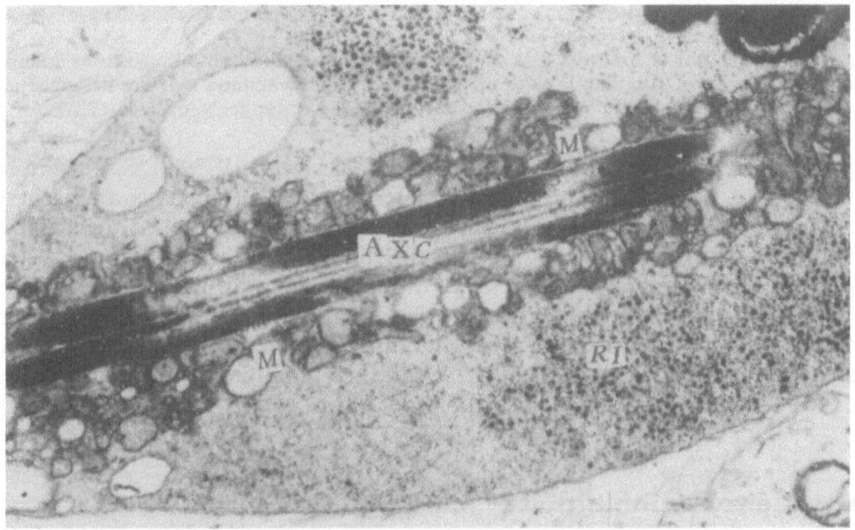

Fig. 11.9 Electron micrograph of a metamorphosing spermatid embedded in Sertoli cell cytoplasm from a rat after 6 weeks' treatment with gossypol, showing free ribosome granules (RI) and lysosome-like bodies (L) in residual cytoplasmic remnants (R) and derangement, swelling and vacuolation of the spiral sheath mitochondrial (M) × 19 800

1980) and testicular biopsy changes (Hei *et al.*, 1981) have been reported too. The damage to the germinal epithelium was found to begin with the spermiogenic spermatids around the seminiferous lumen and was characterized by prominent ultrastructural changes of mitochondria. Damage to the sperm tail spiral sheath mitochondria included derangement, swelling, cristae depletion, vacuolation and breakdown of the intact mitochondria (Fig. 11.9). The earliest sign of drug effect and the earliest organelle damage

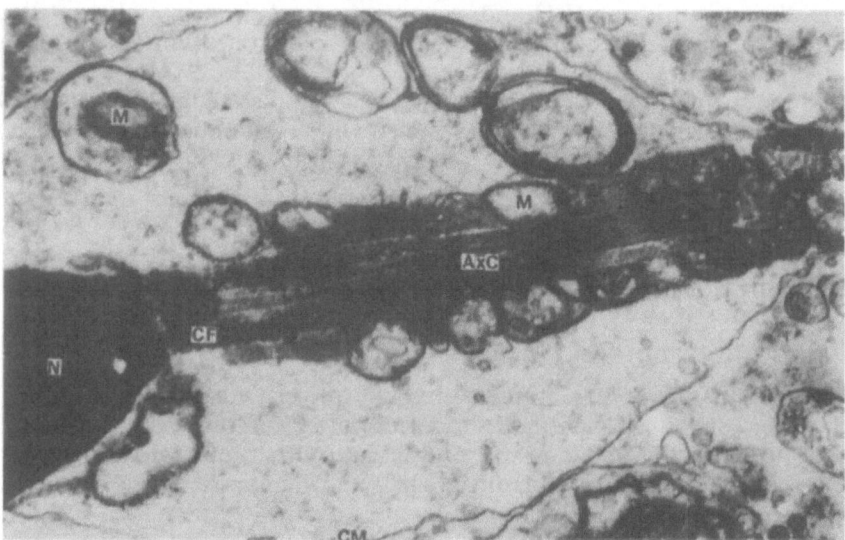

Fig. 11.10 Electron micrograph of a spermatozoon from a volunteer 30 days after administration of gossypol (20 mg/day). Note the spiral sheath mitochondria (M) are deranged and vacuolated. AXC, axial complex; AC, acrosome; CM, cell membrane; N, nucleus × 23 000

was observed in the germinal epithelium (Xue *et al.*, 1979c, 1982). Similar damage was observable in ejaculated spermatozoa 30–50 days after gossypol treatment (Fig. 11.10) (Hang *et al.*, 1980). With increased duration of drug administration, alteration in the spermatid head-cap acrosome system including the distortion and lysis of the acrosomal vesicles and granules, swelling and oedema of Golgi complex and pyknotic nucleus also were observed. No pathological damage could be detected in the Sertoli cell, except occasional, exhibition of some adaptive changes associated with the phagocytic activity (Xue *et al.*, 1982).

LDH-X enzyme inhibition

We found in 1977 that the mitochondrial marker enzyme LDH-X of human spermatozoa was markedly decreased after gossypol treatment (Chen *et al.*, 1978). The homogeneous blue–purple granules of LDH-X formazan in normal sperm mitochondria became coarse and decreased 30–50 days after

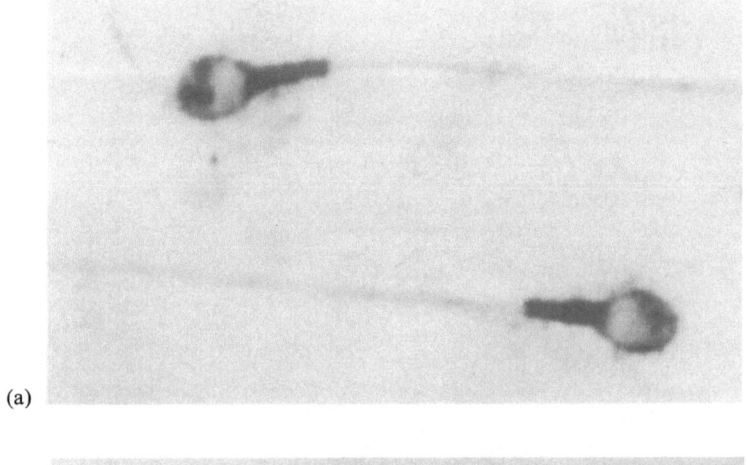

(a)

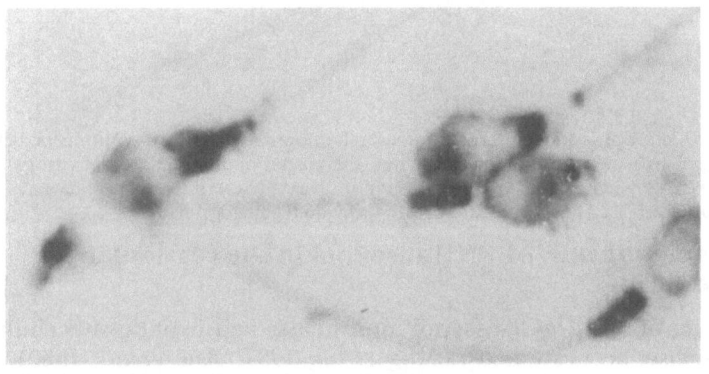

(b)

Fig. 11.11 (a) Spermatozoa from a volunteer before gossypol treatment, showing the LDH-X formazan deposits located homogeneously in the spiral sheath mitochondrial. Preston's method. × 2000. (b) Staining reaction of spermatozoa from a volunteer 50 days following gossypol treatment. Note that the formazan granules became coarse, unevenly distributed, lysed and decreased. Preston's method. × 2000

gossypol administration (Fig. 11.11). Six colour bands representing lactate dehydrogenase fractions (LDH-1, -2, -3, LDH-X, -4, -5) could be identified after electrophoretic separation on cellulose acetate strips prepared from the sperm homogenate of volunteers before treatment. The activity of LDH-X and LDH-1 decreased obviously (despite individual deviation) after gossypol treatment (Fig. 11.12). The mean amount of LDH-X as a percentage of the total LDH decreased from 42.6% before treatment to 31.1%, 26.3% and 10.2% respectively on days 30, 50 and 100 post-treatment (Chen et al., 1978; Xue et al., 1982). Lee and Malling (1981) also showed selective inactivation of LDH-X and LDH-5 from mouse and human by gossypol and regarded it as the target enzyme. Recently, we used [^{14}C]gossypol to test whether gossypol bound specifically to LDH-X. Preliminary results showed an electrophoretic pattern where [^{14}C]gossypol bound more heavily to LDH-4 than LDH-X.

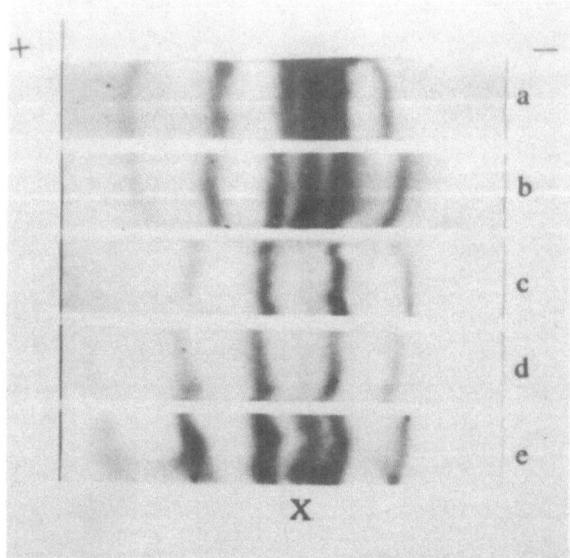

Fig. 11.12 Electrophoretic patterns of sperm homogenate LDH of volunteers before and after gossypol treatment, 6 bands represented the corresponding lactate dehydrogenase fractions (LDH-1, -2, -3, LDH-X, -4, -5). a,b, before treatment; c,d,e, after treatment. Note the inhibition of LDH-X (X) in c and d, and with individual deviation in e

High incorporation of [^{14}C]gossypol in the testicular mitochondria

The distribution of [^{14}C]gossypol in testicular and hepatic subcellular fractions has also been studied (Liang *et al.*, 1981; Xue *et al.*, 1982). Wistar adult male rats received an oral dose of 25μCi/1.95 mg [^{14}C]gossypol (specific activity 12.7μCi/mg) on the 1st and 4th day consecutively. Testis and liver were removed on days 7, 9 and 11 after treatment, and various subcellular fractions prepared for radioactivity determination by Beckman Liquid Scintillation Spectrometer. Additional intratesticular injection of [^{3}H]ouabain 1 h before death was performed in 7 animals for double tracing experiments. The results are shown in Tables 11.2, 11.3.

The distribution of [^{14}C]gossypol in all the five fractions reached their peak by day 9 (Table 11.2). The mitochondrial unit radioactivity was 2–3 times significantly higher than the other four subcellular fractions ($p < 0.001$–0.05). The high affinity of [^{14}C]gossypol for testicular mitochondria was reproducible and independent of dosage. The distribution of [^{14}C]gossypol in liver subcellular fractions had a different order with the highest radioactivity in the microsome and cell membrane fractions, followed by the mitochondrial fraction (Table 11.2). This result was similar to that found by Abou-Donia (1970). The deviation in intracellular distribution of [^{14}C]gossypol between hepatic and spermatogenic cells provide further evidence that the patterns of gossypol incorporation and intracellular localization are different according to their cellular structures and to different cell types.

Table 11.2 Distribution of [^{14}C]gossypol in testicular and hepatic subcellular fractions of rats

Organ	Dosage	Days after dosing	Radioactivity (d min^{-1} mg protein^{-1})*				
			Mitochondria	Nuclear fraction	Plasma membrane	Microsome	Soluble fraction
Testis	50 μCi/ 3.9 mg	7(4)* p**	692±129	170±27 p<0.05	224±24 p<0.05	98±15 p<0.01	45±8 p<0.01
		9(5) p**	1071±274	261±68 p<0.05	245±50 p<0.05	141±38 p<0.01	36±9 p<0.01
		11(4) p**	462±29	148±28 p<0.001	139±8 p<0.001	75±8 p<0.001	42±13 p<0.001
	25 μCi/ 1.95 mg	9(3) p**	311±21	71±5 p<0.01	98±1 p<0.01	68±28 p<0.01	15±4 p<0.001
Liver	20 μCi/ 1.56 mg	2(7) p**	665±194 p<0.05	520±141 p<0.05	1423±156 p<0.05	1708±448	443±48 p<0.05

* Expressed as mean value for animals indicated in ().
** p values expressed as the difference in radioactivity between mitochondria and the four subcellular fractions of testis and liver respectively

167

Table 11.3 The distribution of [^{14}C]gossypol and [^{3}H]ouabain in subcellular fractions of rat testes

Fraction	Radioactivity (d min^{-1} mg protein^{-1})									
	Mitochondria		Nuclear fraction		Plasma membrane		Microsome		Soluble fraction	
	^{3}H	^{14}C	^{3}H	^{14}C	^{3}H	^{14}C	^{3}H	^{14}C	^{3}H	^{14}C
Mean value	3668	481	1349	100	2038	164	835	79	2758	41
± SE (7*)	±373	±45	±171	±12	±245	±21	±112	±9	±396	±4
p**			<0.001	<0.001	<0.001	<0.001	<0.001	<0.001	<0.05	<0.001

* Number of animals

** p value represents difference in radioactivity of ^{14}C and ^{3}H respectively of mitochondria from those of the other four subcellular fractions

The double tracer experiments demonstrated that the distribution of [^{14}C]gossypol and [^{3}H]ouabain in mitochondria was the highest among the five subcellular fractions. These results suggest that the testicular mitochondria might be the gossypol sensitive target organelles and the mitochondrial protein (including Na-K-ATPase which binds to [^{3}H]ouabain) might be the binding site. Receptor assays for gossypol using [^{3}H]gossypol (specific activity 2 Ci/nmol) are now in progress to test this hypothesis.

Effect of gossypol on the respiration and oxidative phosphorylation of isolated rat testicular mitochondria

The effects of gossypol on the respiration and oxidative phosphorylation of isolated testicular mitochondria were determined by the Warburg manometric method and are shown in Fig. 11.13. Low concentrations of gossypol (20–40 μmol/l) stimulate mitochondrial respiration, but as gossypol concentrations increase the respiration declines sharply. Respiration was completely inhibited as the concentration reached 300 μmol/l. Inorganic phosphate (P_i) steadily decreased following the addition of gossypol, and oxidative phosphorylation was inhibited completely at about 80 μmol/l (Xue et al., 1982).

The functions of isolated mitochondria determined by the oxygen electrode polarographic method also gave a similar result. Figure 11.14 and Table 11.4 show that the rate of oxygen consumption decreased steadily with the increase in gossypol concentration, and was inhibited completely at a concentration of 300–400 μmol/l (Xue et al., 1982).

These results show that gossypol can uncouple oxidative phosphorylation and respiratory chain of testicular mitochondria, in a dose-dependent way. Similar results were obtained for the P/O value of testicular mitochondria isolated from rats that had been administered gossypol previously. The mean P/O ratio of the control group mitochondria was 3.75, whereas the groups treated with gossypol in vivo at dosages of 6, 10, and 15 mg decrease to 2.84, 2.60 and 2.58 respectively (Xue et al., 1982). The difference between the treated and control groups was highly significant ($p < 0.001$). In addi-

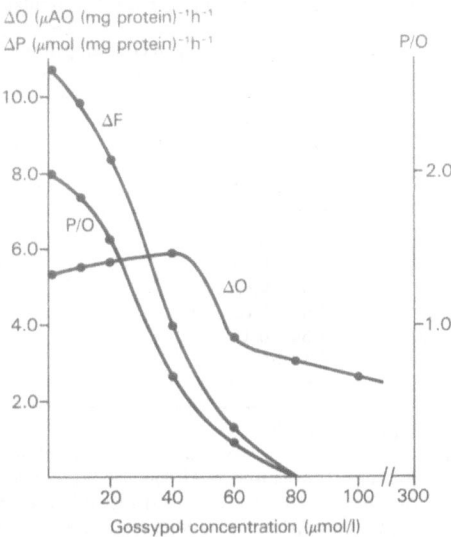

Fig. 11.13 Gossypol effect on the oxidative phosphorylation of isolated testicular mitochondria of rats. Each point represente mean values of three experiments each with three animals

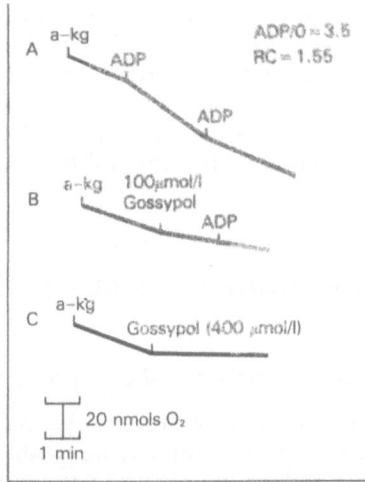

Fig. 11.14 Effect of gossypol on the respiration of isolated rat testicular mitochondria. Curve A shows a typical polarographic trace of oxygen consumption by mitochondria. Curve B shows the inhibition of mitochondrial respiration by gossypol (100 μmol/l). Curve C shows the complete inhibition of mitochondrial respiration at a final concentration of 400 μmol/l of gossypol. The inhibition both in B and C curves was not reversed by ADP. Numbers indicate nmol O_2 mg protein^{-1} min^{-1}, RC., respiratory control ratio: α-kg, α-ketoglutarate

Table 11.4   Effect of gossypol on the respiration of isolated rat testicular mitochondria

Gossypol concn (μmol/l)	Oxygen consumption (nmol O_2 mg protein^{-1} min$^{-1} \pm$ SE)*	
	Gossypol added before ADP**	Gossypol added after ADP**
0	8.05 ± 1.02	16.76 ± 1.49
2	10.48 ± 0.96	16.03 ± 0.25
5	9.37 ± 0.95	11.79 ± 0.90
10	6.58 ± 0.51	6.66 ± 0.14
40	5.07 ± 0.49	2.23 ± 0.47
100	4.02 ± 0.65	1.05 ± 0.11
200	1.60 ± 0.13	0.76 ± 0.23
300	0.53 ± 0.32	0.00 ± 0.00
400	0.00 ± 0.00	0.00 ± 0.00

* Data are mean values of 5 replicates $\pm$ SE
** Experiments were conducted at 30°C in 2 ml of reaction medium (pH7.5) in which α-ketoglutarate was used as substrate. Mitochondria (1.5 mg protein) were added, when a steady state of respiration was recorded, gossypol (in 0.5 mol/l NaOH solution, adjusted to pH7.5) and ADP (160 μmol/l) as phosphate receptor were added respectively to the table listed

tion, experiments on guinea pig renal cell mitochondria demonstrated that previous gossypol treatment *in vivo* would increase the sensitivity of isolated mitochondria to gossypol *in vitro*.

Abou-Donia (1974) reported that gossypol inhibited rat liver mitochondrial respiration *in vitro*. These results demonstrated further that gossypol could uncouple oxidative phosphorylation and respiratory chain in rat testicular mitochondria. But this does not mean that gossypol would affect hepatic cells *in vivo* at a concentration similar to that which caused germ cell damage, as the incorporation and intracellular distribution of gossypol are tissue specific. The concentration of gossypol in mitochondria of hepatic and testicular mitochondria are obviously different. Clearly under *in vivo* conditions the testicular mitochondria are vulnerable target organelles for gossypol.

THE MOLECULAR MECHANISM OF ANTIFERTILITY ACTION OF GOSSYPOL

Direct cytotoxic action of gossypol on spermatogenic cells

Gossypol has been shown to be a cytotoxic substance capable of reducing the activity of oxidative enzymes; interfering with oxidative metabolism (Myers *et al.*, 1966); uncoupling the respiratory chain and oxidative phosphorylation at high concentration (Abou-Donia, 1974; Xue *et al.*, 1982); reducing energy–linked enzyme activities (Adeyemo *et al.*, 1981; Burgos *et al.*, 1980; Kalla *et al.*, 1981; Tso *et al.*, 1982a); affecting Na-K-ATPase (Bi, 1980); blocking the action of proteolytic enzymes, pepsinogen and acrosin (Tanksly *et al.*, 1970; Tso, 1982b); and inactivating LDH-X, malate dehydrogenase and glutathione S-transferase (Lee *et al.*, 1981, 1982). Gossypol fed to male rats at antifertility dosages induced infertility but did not cause significant effects on the body weight, seminal vesicle and prostate weight, nor changes in the interstitiual cells of Leydig, libido and steroid hormone levels—plasma testosterone, dihydrotestosterone, serum LH and FSH (Bardin *et al.*, 1980; Xue *et al.*, 1979, 1981; Hoffer, 1980). No significant effect on the blood chemistry, bone marrow, serum sodium, calcium, chloride iron and seminal plasma fructose (National Coordinating Group, 1978). However, it is feasible to inhibit spermatogenesis by intereference with certain metabolic steps in mitochondria, thereby decreasing the incorporation of labelled amino acids with concomitant selective damage in target germ cells (Xue *et al.*, 1979c, 1980). In contrast to most sex hormone drugs, gossypol works locally at the level of the seminiferous tubules. A dose-dependent cytotoxic effect on the number of viable cells and mitotic index was demonstrated with both Chinese hamster ovary (CHO) cells and human lymphocytes after the cultures received treatment of gossypol (5 μg/ml) for various durations (Ye *et al.*, 1983). Cellular DNA, RNA and protein synthetic activities were also reduced, but did not seem to induce chromosome breakage. Inhibition of the motility of sea urchin (Adeyems *et al.*, 1981) and human spermatozoa (Kalla *et al.*, 1981; Tso *et al.*, 1982a) *in vitro* is due to the impairment of the ATPase activity in the sperm. The *in vitro* fertilization capacity of gossypol-treated human spermatozoa showed an obvious decrease in penetration rate into golden hamster ova (Young *et al.*, personal communication). Gossypol blocked acrosin activity of boar spermatozoa *in vitro* (Tso *et al.*, 1982b). All the data confirmed the direct effect of gossypol on sperm and spermatogenic cells. For this reason the use of gossypol as a vaginal spermicidal contraceptive has been suggested.

CONCLUDING REMARKS

Gossypol has been shown to be an effective male antifertility agent of relatively safety at the antifertility dosage. It has provided a new lead in the search for drugs for male fertility control from phenolic compounds, and represents the only approach to appear to have a reasonable chance to reach large-scale clinical tests in the near future. However, it possesses several disadvantages, especially hypokalaemia and the danger of sterility after long-term administration.

Gossypol damaged testicular mitochondrial ultrastructure, uncoupling mitochondrial respiration and oxidative phosphorylation, inhibited specifically mitochondrial energy-linked enzymes, ion-regulating enzymes and sperm marker enzyme LDH-X. The concomitantly high affinity of [^{14}C]gossypol for mitochondria suggests that testicular mitochondria might be the sensitive target organelle. On the basis of these findings, the author suggests that mitochondrial protein (enzyme) might be the binding and active site of gossypol thus impairing sperm motility and interrupting spermatogenesis.

Acknowledgements

This work was supported in part by grants from the Rockefeller Foundation given to the laboratory for gossypol animal study, Chinese Academy of Medical Sciences. I thank Mr Yao Heng-teh for typing the manuscript.

Reference

Abou-Donia, M.B. (1970), Metabolic fate of gossypol: the metabolism of ^{14}C-gossypol in rats. *Lipids*, **5**, 938

Abou-Donia, M.B. (1974). Gossypol: uncoupling of respiratory chain and oxidative phosphorylation. *Life Sci*, **14**, 1955–63

Abou-Donia, M.B. (1976). Physiological effects and metabolism of gossypol. In Gunther, F.A. (ed.) *Residue Reviews*, **61**, 126–52

Adeyemo, O. *et al.* (1981). Effect of gossypol on the production and utilization of ATP by sea urchin spermatozoa. *Biol. Bull.*, **161**, 333

Bardin, C.M. *et al.*, (1980). Toxicology, endocrine and histopathologic studies in small animals and Rhesus monkeys administered gossypol. Presented at *PARFR Workshop on Gossypol Program for Applied Research on Fertility Regulation*, 11 March, Chicago, Ill

Berardi, L.C. and Goldblatt, L.A. (1969). Gossypol. In Liener I.E. (ed.) *Toxic Constituents of Plant Foodstuffs*, pp. 211–266. (Academic Press: New York)

Bi, S.F. (1980). Gossypol effects on the activity of renal ATPase. *Scientia Sinica*, **9**, 914–19

Bressani, R. (1980). Human nutrition and gossypol. Presented at *PARFR Workshop on Gossypol Program for Applied Research on Fertility Regulation*, 11 March, Chicago, Ill

Burgos, M.H. *et al.* (1980). Gossypol inhibits motility of Arbacia sperm. *Biol. Bull.*, **159**, 467–8

Chang, M.C. *et al.* (1980). Effects of gossypol on the fertility of male rats, hamsters and rabbits. *Contraception*, **21**, 461–9

Chen, X.M. *et al.* (1978). The effect of gossypol on lactate dehydrogenase isoenzyme-X (LDH-X) of human spermatozoa. Abstract in *Symposium of Chinese Society of Anatomy*, p. 127. (Whole text in *Acta Acad. Med. Sinica* **5** (4), 223–6 (1983)

Dai, R.X. *et al.* (1972). A study of antifertility of cottonseed, Document of the *First National Conference on Gossypol*, Wuhan. *Acta Biol. Exp. Sin.*, **11**, 1–14, 1978

Dai, R.X. *et al.* (1978). Studies on the antifertility effect of gossypol 11. A morphological analysis of the antifertility effect of gossypol. *Acta Biol. Exp. Sin.*, **11**, 27–36

Hadley, M.A. *et al.* (1981). Effect of gossypol on the reproductive system of male rats. *J. Andrology*, **2**, 190

Hang, Z.B. *et al.* (1980). Electron microscopic observations of gossypol effects on the spermatozoa of healthy men. *Acta Anatomica Sinica*, **11**, 299–302

Hei, L.S. *et al.* (1981). Electron microscopic observations on the testicular biopsy tissues of tumour patients with gossypol treatment. *Chin. Med. J.*, **61**, 527–9

Hoffer, A.P. (1980). Light and electron microscopic studies on the effects of gossypol in the male rat. Presented at *PARFR Workshop on Gossypol, Program for Applied Research on Fertility Regulation*, 11 March, Chicago, Ill

Hubei Pronvical Hancuan 'Disease of Burning Sensation', Treatment and Prevention Group (1970). Collected materials about disease of burning sensation. Document of *Conference on Disease of Burning Sensation*, Hubei

Jiangsu Provincial Cooperation Group on Male Contraception (1972). Studies on Gossypol, Document of the *First National Conference on Male Antifertility Agents*, Wuhan

Kalla, N.R. *et al.* (1981a). Studies on the male antifertility agent-gossypol acetic acid 11. Effect of gossypol acetic acid on the motility and ATPase activity of human spermatozoa. *Andrologia*, **13** (2), 95–8

Kalla, N.R. *et al.* (1981b). Studies on the male antifertility agent–gossypol acetic acid 111. Effect of gossypol acetic acid on rat testis. *Andrologia*, **13**, 242–9

Lee, C.Y. and Malling, H.Y. (1981). Selective inhibition of sperm specific lactate dehydrogenase X by an antifertility agent, gossypol. *Fed. Proc.*, **40**, 718

Lee, C.Y. *et al.*, (1982). Enzyme inactivation and inhibition by gossypol. *Mol. Cell. Biochem.*, **47**, 65–70

Liang, D.C. *et al.* (1981). Studies on the distribution of ^{14}C-gossypol in subcellular fractions of rat testes and the site of gossypol action. *Acta Academia Medicinas Sinica*, **3**, 153–7

Lyman, G.M. *et al.* (1959). Reactions of proteins with gossypol. *Arch. Biochem.*, **84**, 486–97

Myers, B.D. *et al.* (1966). Effect of gossypol on some oxidative respiratory enzymes. *Plant Physiol.*, **41**, 787–91

National Coordinating Group on Male Antifertility Agents (1978). Gossypol, a new antifertility agent for males. *Chin. Med. J.*, **4**, 417–28

Päso, W. *et al.* (1980). Gossypol, a powerful inhibitor of human spermatozoa metabolism. *Lancet*, **1**, 885

Qian, S.Z. *et al.* (1979). The potassium depleting effect of gossypol on isolated rabbit heart and its possible mechanism. *Acta Pharm. Sin.*, **14**, 116–19

Ridgon, R.H. *et al.* (1958). Effect of gossypol in young chickens with the production of a ceriod-like pigment. *Am. Med. Assoc. Arch. Pathol.*, **65**, 228

Shantung Provincial Herbaceous Contraceptive Group (1972). The antifertility effect of cottonseed. Document of the *First National Conference on Male Antifertility Agents*. Wuhan

Shantung Institute of Traditional Medicine and Chinese Academy of Medical Sciences (1975). Studies on the antifertility effect and toxicity of gossypol in Rhesus monkeys. Document of the *4th National Conference on Male Antifertility Agents*, Suzhou

Skutches, C.L. *et al.* (1973). Effect of intravenous gossypol injection on iron utilization in swine. *J. Nutr.*, **103**, 851

Slocumb, J. (1980). Medical and sociological aspects of gossypol use among women in Southwest United States. Presented as *PARFR Workshop on Gossypol, Program for Applied Research on Fertility Regulation*, 11 March, Chicago, Ill

Tang, X.C. *et al.* (1980). Comparative studies on the absorption, distribution and excretion of ^{14}C-gossypol in four species of animals. *Acta. Pharm. Sin.*, **15**, 212–17

Tanksley, T.D. *et al.* (1970). Inhibition of pepsinogen activation by gossypol. *J. Biol. Chem.*, **245**, 6456

Tso, W.W. *et al.* (1982a). Effect of gossypol on boar spermatozoa adenosine triphosphate metabolism. *Arch. Androl.*, **9**, 319–31

Tso, W.W. *et al.* (1982b). Gossypol: An effective acrosin blocker. *Arch. Androl.*, **8**, 143–7

Vermel, E.M. *et al.* (1963). Antitumour activity of gossypol in experiments on transplantable tumors. *Voprosy Onkologii* (in Russian), **9**, 39

Wang, N.G. and Lei, H.P. (1979). Antifertility effect of gossypol acetic acid on male rats. Document of *2nd National Conference on Male Antifertility Agents*, Qingdao, 1973

Withers, W.A. *et al.* (1915). Gossypol—A toxic substance in cottonseed meal, A preliminary note. *Science*, **41**, 324

Wu, Xi-Rui (1972). Study of antifertility action of cottonseed and the effective component-gossypol. Document and Presentation at the *National Conference on Recent Advance of Family Planning Research*, Beijing

Xue (Shieh), S.P. *et al.* (1979a). The pharmacokinetics of ^{14}C-gossypol acetic acid in rats I. Whole body and micro-autoradiographic studies on the distribution and fate of ^{14}C-gossypol in the rat body. Document of *4th National Conference on Male Antifertility Agents*, Suzhou, 1975, *Acta Biol. Exp. Sin.*, **12**, 179–94

Xue (Shieh), S.P. *et al.* (1979b). The pharmcokinetics of ^{14}C-gossypol acetic acid in rats II. Quantitative studies on the kinetics of distribution, excretion and metabolism of ^{14}C-gossypol acetic acid in the rat body. Document of *4th National Conference on Male Antifertility Agents*, Suzhou, 1975, *Acta Biol. Exp. Sin.*, **12**, 275–87

Xue (Shieh), S.P. *et al.* (1979c). Antifertility effect of gossypol on the germinal epithelium of the rat testes. A cytological, autoradiographical and ultrastructural observation. Document of *2nd National Conference on Male Antifertility Agents*, Qingdao, 1973, *Sci. Sin.*, **9**, 915–28 (English edition **23**, 642, 1980)

Xue, S.P. (1981). Studies on the antifertility effect of gossypol. A new contraceptive for males. *Recent Advances in Fertility Regulation, Proceedings of a Symposium*, Beijing, September, 1980, pp. 122–46

Xue, S.P. *et al.* (1982). The subcellular site of the antispermatogenic effect of gossypol and its possible molecular mechanism of action. *Scientia Sinica, B series*, **12**, 1095–108

Ye, W.S. *et al.* (1983). Toxicity of a male contraceptive, gossypol, in mammalian cell culture. *In vitro*, **19**, 53-7.

Zatuchni, G.I. and Osborn, C.K. (1981). Gossypol: A possible male infertility agent, Report of a Workshop. *Research Frontiers in Fertility Regulation*, **1** (4), 1-15

12
Gossypol inhibition of boar spermatozoal enzymes

W.-W. TSO, C.-S. LEE and M.-Y.W. TSO

The antifertility effect of cottonseed oil in men was first observed in China in 1957 (Liu, 1957). Gossypol [1,1',6,6',7,7'-hexahydroxy-3,3'-dimethyl-5,5'-bis-isopropyl[2,2'binaphthalene]-8,8'-dicarboxaldehyde] a yellowish polyphenolic pigment, was later identified as the active antifertility ingredient in cottonseed oil (Dai et al., 1978; Wang et al., 1979) and clinically tested on more than 4000 healthy males with 99% infertility success (Dai et al., 1978; National Coordinating Group, 1978; Liu et al., 1981). The administered dose was 20 mg/day for the first 60–70 days, followed by a maintenance dose of about 60 mg/week. The antifertility effect was manifested by low sperm counts and a loss of motility in spermatozoa leading eventually to severe oligospermia and azoospermia in the tested human subjects. Morphologically, the spermatozoa from treated subjects showed defects in their ultrastructure, which included decondensation of the nucleus, loss of axial filaments, swelling of the mitochondria, absence of cristae in the mitochondria and degeneration of the acrosome and head cap (National Coordinating Group, 1978). In view of its small side-effects at the level prescribed and high recovery rate of the treated subjects after discontinuation of its administration, gossypol has been considered a very promising male contraceptive (Prasad and Diczfalusy, 1982).

Similar antifertility effects were observed in mammals, including hamster, rat, mouse, dog and monkey, with various degrees of sensitivity to gossypol. In vitro, gossypol inhibits spermatozoal motility and is spermicidal at high concentrations (Kalla and Vasudev, 1980; Kalla and Vasudev, 1981; Poso et al., 1980; Tso, 1980; Waller et al., 1980; Tso and Lee, 1981a). However, rabbit is an exception (National Coordinating Group, 1978; Chang et al., 1980). The sensitivity to antifertility action of gossypol in rats, furthermore, is strain specific.

The specific structure of the gossypol molecule appears to be important for its antifertility action. The gossypol molecule contains two aldehyde and six hydroxyl groups which are strongly acidic and react to form ethers, esters and ionic species at physiological pH. The aldehyde groups can react readily with amines to form Schiff bases. This high chemical activity of gossypol might be the cause of its many diversified interactions with cellular functions as listed below:

Inhibiting testicular steroidogenesis (Lin et al., 1981)

Weakening the depresser effect of acetylcholine, depressing intestinal contraction, and inhibiting the secretion of the salivary gland and the sweat gland (Ma et al., 1980)

Inducing spermatozoal and body potassium depletion and hypokalemia (Qian et al., 1979; Tso & Lee, 1982c)

Uncoupling respiratory chain and oxidation phosphorylation (Abou-Donia & Dieckert, 1974)

Reducing cellular ATP content (Ke & Tso, 1981; Tso et al., 1982)

Interfering the normal function of the electron transport chain segments (Tso & Lee, 1981b)

Reducing serum testosterone and LH levels (Hadley et al., 1981; Hiroshi et al., 1981)

Increasing the potential of the androgenicity of methyltestosterone (Haln et al., 1981) and

Inhibiting of herpes simplex virus 2 infection in human epithelial cells (Wichmann et al., 1982)

However, the antifertility effect of gossypol is highly structure-specific because changes in either the aldehyde or the hydroxyl group reduces its antifertility activity substantially (Wang et al., 1979).

The mechanism of gossypol's male contraceptive action is unknown. In spite of the recent reports on the reduction of testosterone and LH levels the primary target of the antifertility effect of gossypol is not associated with hormonal imbalance (Chang et al., 1982; Liu, G.Z. personal communication). Nevertheless, an endocrine imbalance at high levels of gossypol in some animal systems may bring about the disruption of spermatogenesis, thus leading to infertility.

On the other hand, the antifertility effect of gossypol may be due to inhibition on one or several key spermatozoal enzymes. The effect of gossypol in altering enzyme reactions has long been noted, for example, its inhibition of pepsin, trypsin, xanthine oxidase, succinate dehydrogenase from chicken liver homogenate, cytochrome oxidase and many others (Furguson et al., 1959; Myers and Throneberry, 1966; National Coordinating Group, 1978; Lee and Malling, 1981), and its stimulation effect on rat liver microsomal oxidases (Abou-Donia and Dieckert, 1974).

This study will describe gossypol's interaction with a number of important boar spermatozoal enzymes. Since gossypol is noted for its antimotility action on spermatozoa in vitro with a concomitant reduction in cellular ATP content, its interaction with some of the key enzymes related to the energy metabolism and to the fertilizing potential of spermatozoa will be reviewed.

THREE CLASSES OF GOSSYPOL INHIBITION

Boar ejaculated spermatozoa used in this study were collected as described in our previous publication (Tso and Lee, 1981a). The activities of 15 enzymes were assayed according to conventional methods in the presence of various concentrations of gossypol ranging from 0.1 to 300 μmol/l and the results were expressed as percentages of their corresponding controls. The inhibition profiles of the enzymes may be grouped into the following three classes according to their response to gossypol (Table 12.1).

Table 12.1 The effect of gossypol on several boar spermatozoal enzymes

Class	Enzyme	*Effective gossypol concentrations (μmol/l)**			
		Stimulation†	*Inhibition*▲		
			IC_{20}	IC_{50}	IC_{80}
I. Inert		—			
	Carnitine acetyltransferase	—	—	—	—
	Flagellar ATPase*	—	—	—	—
	Mitochondrial fragment ATPase*	—	—	—	—
II. Mild inhibitory (with occasional slight stimulation)					
	Citrate synthetase	—	200	300	—
	Hexokinase	—	100	100	200
	α-Ketoglutarate dehydrogenase	10(127%)	200	—	—
	Lactate dehydrogenase (total)	100(117%)	200	—	—
	NAD–malate dehydrogenase	—	100	200	300
	Succinate dehydrogenase	100(123%)	200	—	—
III. Strong inhibitory					
	Aconitase	10(110%)	20	40	60
	Acrosin	—	3	10	50
	Fumarase	—	40	50	80
	NAD–isocitrate dehydrogenase	—	20	100	—
	Lactate dehydrogenase-X	—	20	100	—
	Succinyl-CoA synthetase	—	20	60	200

* Data obtained from sonicated spermatozoa
† Maximum stimulation concentration; numerical values in brackets represent the activity as a percentage of control
▲ Concentration at 20, 50 or 80% activity of control

The inert class includes enzymes whose activities are not affected or are insignificantly affected by 300 μmol/l gossypol, the highest concentration used in our experiments, as shown in Fig. 12.1a for the case of carnitine acetyltransferase. The ATPases obtained from sonicated spermatozoa fall into this class. However, when intact cellular ATPase was studied with hypotonically treated spermatozoa, a substantial biphasic response of ATP-ase activity was observed, i.e. stimulation at low gossypol concentration (< 100 μmol/l) and inhibition at concentration above 100 μmol/l. This un-usual behaviour has been accounted for by the interaction of gossypol with the intact mitochondrial membrane (Tso *et al.*, 1982).

The mildly inhibited class includes a group of enzymes that are inhibited

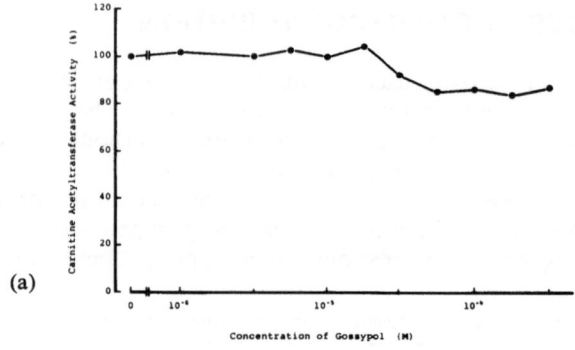

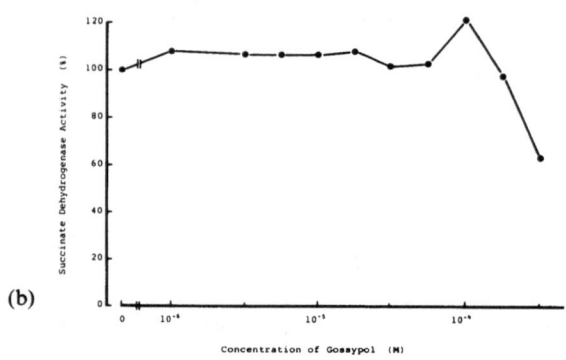

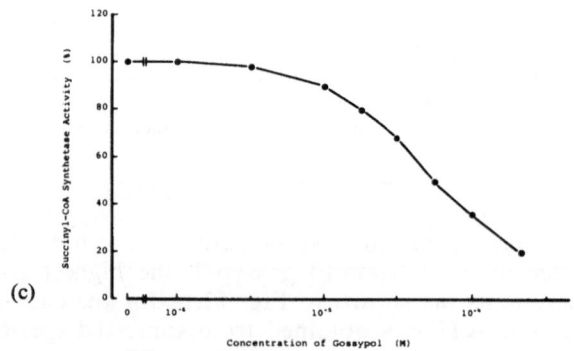

Fig. 12.1 Effect of gossypol on spermatozoal enzyme activities. The assays were done at 25°C with sonicated boar spermatozoal preparations (Tso and Lee, 1981). The activities of these enzymes were stable during the entire assay period (2-4 h). The control values for the three enzymes, carnitine acetyltransferase, succinate dehydrogenase and succinyl-CoA synthetase were: (a) 22.4 nmol CoA formed $\min^{-1}$ $(10^8$ sperm$)^{-1}$, (b) 33.4 nmol dichlorophenol-indo-phenol reduced $\min^{-1}$ $(10^8$ sperm$)^{-1}$ and (c) 3.02 nmol GDP formed $\min^{-1}$ $(10^8$ sperm$)^{-1}$ correspondingly

only at a relatively high gossypol concentration ($> 100 \, \mu$mol/l), as shown in Fig. 12.1b for the case of succinate dehydrogenase. This group also includes several enzymes that exhibit a slight stimulatory effect at preinhibitory concentrations. It is interesting to note that the total lactate dehydrogenase (LDH), unlike its gonad-specific isoenzyme LDH-X (see below), falls into this class.

The strongly inhibited class are enzymes whose activities are inhibited at gossypol concentrations lower than $100 \, \mu$mol/l as shown in Fig. 12.1c for the case of succinyl-CoA synthetase. Four tricarboxylic acid (TCA) cycle enzymes: aconitase, fumarase, NAD–isocitrate dehydrogenase and succinyl-CoA synthetase, one gonad-specific enzyme, lactate dehydrogenase-X, and one fertilization enzyme, acrosin are listed under this class.

ROLE OF THE SIX ENZYMES THAT ARE MOST SENSITIVE TO GOSSYPOL INHIBITION

Lactate dehydrogenase-X

The final step in anaerobic glycolysis is the reduction of pyruvate to lactate with a regeneration of NAD catalysed by lactate dehydrogenase (LDH). NADH is reoxidized anaerobically by this process. LDH also converts lactate back into pyruvate which is then channelled through the TCA cycle under aerobic conditions. LDH-X, unlike the other five common LDH isoenzymes, is found only in animal testes and spermatozoa following differentiation to the primary spermatocytes (Sarkar et al., 1978). With unique molecular properties and a wide substrate specificity (Blanco et al., 1976), LDH-X serves as a mitochondrial shuttle system (Calvin and Tubbs, 1978). Total LDH activity was relatively insensitive to gossypol with inhibitory concentration well above $180 \, \mu$mol/l whereas LDH-X inhibition by gossypol begins at $20 \, \mu$mol/l (Tso and Lee, 1982d). Of all the enzymes involved in energy metabolism, LDH-X is the most sensitive to gossypol. This gossypol effect may be significant in spermatogenesis and spermatozoal maturation which are energy-intensive processes.

The four enzymes in the tricarboxylic acid (TCA) cycle

All TCA cycle enzymes tested showed signs of inhibition at high gossypol concentration. The 50% inhibition in aconitase, fumarase, NAD–isocitrate dehydrogenase and succinyl-CoA synthetase was found at 40, 50, 100 and $60 \, \mu$mol/l gossypol respectively. Inhibition of aconitase activity leads to blockage in acetyl group metabolism, whereas fumarase inhibition slows down the conversion of various TCA cycle intermediates into malate resulting in a lower oxaloacetate content that leads to a further reduction of the acetyl group metabolism as shown in Fig. 12.2. All inhibitions on the TCA cycle enzymes lead to a decline in electron supply to the electron transport chain which in turn decreases ATP production. Furthermore, the effect of gossypol on succinyl-CoA synthetase, an enzyme that catalyses

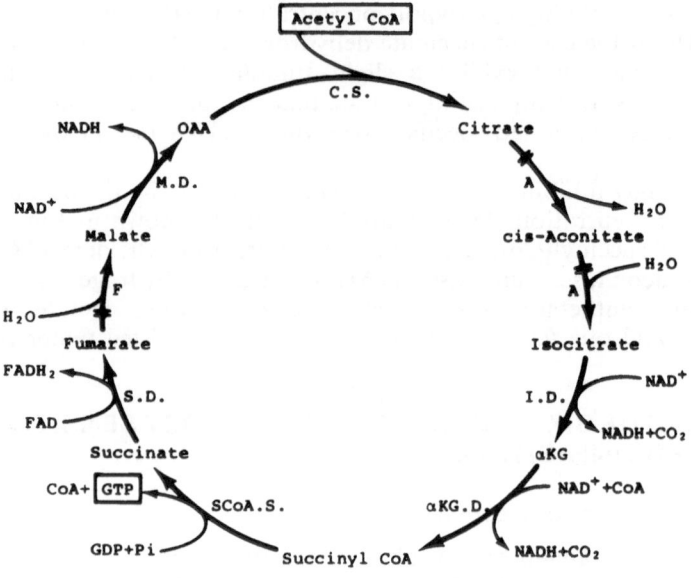

Abbreviations for enzymes:

C.S.	citrate synthetase
A	aconitase
I.D.	NAD-isocitrate dehydrogenase
αKG.D.	α-ketoglutarate dehydrogenase
SCoA.S.	succinyl-CoA synthetase
S.D.	succinyl dehydrogenase
F	fumarase
M.D.	malate dehydrogenase

Fig. 12.2 The enzymes in the tricarboxylic acid cycle. The strongly inhibited enzymes are marked with a // (see text for explanation)

substrate level phosphorylation in the TCA cycle, is likely to reduce further the ATP level in spermatozoa, which is important in sperm maturation and development (Dop *et al.*, 1977).

Acrosin

In addition to its inhibitory effect on spermatozoal energy metabolism, gossypol also exhibits significant effects on the vital function of the spermatozoa by reducing the fertilizing potential of the male gamete (Johnsen *et al.*, 1982). Spermatozoal acrosin, the trypsin-like proteolytic enzyme located exclusively within the acrosome in the head of the spermatozoa, causes a local hydrolysis of the zona pellucida glycoprotein of the egg, through which the spermatozoon penetrates to fertilize the egg. It is bound to the inner acrosomal membrane and is particularly sensitive to gossypol inhibition. The assay was done with TAME (p-toluenesulphonylarginine methyl ester) as substrate (Schleuning and Fritz, 1974) which is not hydrolysed by chymotrypsin. The inhibition threshold of gossypol in acrosin is 1 μmol/l and is by far the lowest yet observed among all enzymes. It is also lower than that for the antimotility effect. Therefore, micromolar concentrations of gossypol can effectively block fertilization and can be used as an ingredient in vaginal contraceptives (Tso and Lee, 1981a, 1982b).

DISCUSSION

It has been suggested that the chemically highly reactive aldehyde group of gossypol, interacts readily with the lysine residue of many proteins. Recently, studies in various biological systems have demonstrated that gossypol interferes with many enzymatic reactions (Furguson et al., 1959; Myers and Throneberry, 1966; National Coordinating Group, 1978). This broad interaction with many enzyme systems may give rise to the diversified nature of the gossypol effects from inhibiting herpes simplex virus 2 infection to weakening the depresser effect of acetylcholine (Wichmann et al., 1982; Ma et al., 1980). In this in vitro study, the interaction of gossypol with 15 spermatozoal enzymes may be classified into three groups according to their degree of inhibition. Eighty per cent of the enzymes, chosen only for their relatedness to the spermatozoal fertilization function, interact with gossypol at moderate concentrations (sum of the mildly inhibited and the strongly inhibited groups). This is consistent with the vast interaction of gossypol with proteinaceous molecules. However, there are three enzymes inert to gossypol. The inertness may be due to the non-existence, unavailability or inaccessibility of the lysine residue in the protein moiety or due to the modified lysine group, not being at the active site. This study offers no details of the inhibition.

The antimotility effect of gossypol in spermatozoa is caused by uncoupling the electron transport chain. Based on this and other observations, a suggestion has been made that energy deprivation is the primary consequence of the gossypol contraceptive effect (Kalla and Vasudev, 1981; Lee and Malling, 1981). The finding in this study that as many as four enzymes in the TCA cycle and the gonad-specific enzyme, LDH-X, are highly susceptible to gossypol inhibition, is in agreement with the above suggestion. There is, however, at present, no clear indication as to which enzyme inhibition is more directly related to gossypol contraception.

The target enzymes may be: (1) many enzymes in the energy-producing pathway except gonad-specific LDH-X, (2) both LDH-X and all the enzymes in (1), and (3) LDH-X alone. Apparently, (1) is unlikely, as this group of enzymes are not gonad-specific, and presumably all have similar susceptibility to gossypol (gossypol was first reported to be an uncoupler in sweet potato). As liver is the highest gossypol depot, cell mortality would be expected to be higher in liver cells if (1) is the case; however, of the 4000 clinical cases tested by the Shanghai group for contraception, none has been reported to exhibit liver malfunction (National Coordinating Group, 1978). Although it is difficult, based on the amount of data available at present, to differentiate whether the cause of contraception is an inhibition of enzymes in (2) or (3), a consideration that all the TCA cycle enzymes as well as LDH-X are inhibited to the same extent tends to suggest that contraception may be a consequence of inhibition of several enzymes with LDH-X as the key one.

All cells need a balance of energy metabolism but growing cells need more. We have shown recently in mouse implanted with ascites tumour cells, that administration of gossypol can selectively kill tumour cells (Tso, unpublished data). Apparently, in spermatogenesis, a sufficient energy balance is critically needed for the rapidly developing cells. In the presence of gossypol, the energy supply will be drastically reduced due to an inhibition of, not only, the TCA cycle enzymes but also of the gonad-specific LDH-X. This energy reduction might have an incompensatable effect on spermatogenesis and lead to infertility.

The suggestion proposed in this review that not only LDH-X alone, but also enzymes involved in energy metabolism are responsible for gossypol contraception is worthy of more consideration. It calls for the design of analogues which can work specifically on LDH-X alone. Unless this can be accomplished, other unwanted side-effects in various organs that originate from cellular energy deprivation may not be effectively prevented. While the investigation of gossypol's contraceptive mechanism is still in its infancy, hypotheses should not be prematurely abandoned.

Acknowledgements

We are grateful to the Agriculture and Fisheries Department of Hong Kong for supplying the boar semen. The research was supported in part by a grant from the Chinese Medicinal Material Research Centre of The Chinese University of Hong Kong and a research grant of the University of Hong Kong. Wung-Wai Tso was supported by a grant from the Population Council (number B82.59M). We thank Dr C.W. Bardin for helpful discussions during the preparation of this manuscript.

References

Abou-Donia, M.B. and Dieckert, J.W. (1974). Gossypol: uncoupling of respiratory chain and oxidative chain and oxidative phosphorylation. *Life Sci.*, **14**, 1955–63

Blanco, A., Burgos, C., Burgos, N.M.G.D. and Montamat, E.E. (1976). Properties of the testicular lactate dehydrogenase isoenzyme. *Biochem. J.*, **153**, 165–72

Calvin, J. and Tubbs, P.K. (1978). Mitochondrial transport process and oxidation of NADH by hypotonically-treated boar spermatozoa. *Eur. J. Biochem.*, **89**, 315–20

Chang, C.C., Gu, Z. and Tsong, Y.-Y. (1982). Studies on gossypol. I. Toxicity, antifertility, and endocrine analyses in male rats. *Int. J. Fert.*, **27**, 213–18

Chang, M.C., Zhi, P.C. and Saksena, S.K. (1980). Effects of gossypol on the fertility of male rats, hamsters and rabbits. *Contraception*, **21**, 461–9

Dai, R.X., Pang, S.N., Lin, X.K., Ke, Y.B., Liu, Z.L. and Dong, R.H. (1978). A study of antifertility effect of cottonseed. *Acta Biol. Exp. Sin.*, **11**, 10.

Dop, C.W., Hutson, S.M. and Lardy, H.A. (1977). Pyruvate metabolism in bovine epididymal spermatozoa. *J. Biol. Chem.*, **252**, 1303–8

Furguson, T.M., Couch, J.R. and Rigdon, R.H. (1959). Histopathology of animal reactions to pigment compounds: chickens. Conference on the *Chemical Structure and Reactions of Gossypol and Nongossypol Pigments of Cottonseed*. Proc. Nat'l Cottonseed, pp. 131–41.

Hadley, M.A., Lin, C.Y. and Dym, M. (1981). Effects of gossypol on the reproductive system of male rats. *J. Androl.*, **2**, 190–9

Haln, D.W., Rusticus, C., Probst, A., Homm, R. and Johnson, A.N. (1981). Antifertility and endocrine activities of gossypol in rodents. *Contraception*, **24**, 97–105

Hiroshi, H., Uehara, S., Negaike, F., Momono, K., Nori, R., Suzuki, M. and Lin, Y.C. (1981). Action mechanisms of gossypol on rats as male contraceptive agents: *in vivo* study. *Jpn J. Fertil. Steril.*, **26**, 35–9

Johnsen, O., Diaz, M. and Eliasson, R. (1982). Gossypol; a potent inhibitor of human sperm acrosomal proteinase. *Int. J. Androl.*, **5**, 636–40

Kalla, N.R. and Vasudev, M. (1980). Studies on the male antifertility agent, gossypol acetic acid: I. *In vitro* studies on the effect of gossypol acetic acid in human spermatozoa. *IRC Med. Sci. Biochem.*, **8**, 375–6

Kalla, N.R. and Vasudev, M. (1981). Studies on the male antifertility agent-gossypol acetic acid. II. Effect of gossypol acetic acid on the motility and ATPase activity of human spermatozoa. *Andrologia*, **13**, 95–8

Ke, Y.-B. and Tso, W.-W. (1982). Variations of gossypol susceptibility in rat spermatozoa during spermatogenesis. *Int. J. Fertil.*, **27**, 42–6

Lee, C.Y. and Malling, H.V. (1981). Selective inhibition of sperm-specific lactate dehydrogenase-X by an anti-fertility agent, gossypol. *Fed. Proc.*, **40**, 718

Lin, T., Murano, E.P., Osterman, J., Nankin, H.R. and Coulson, P.B. (1981). Gossypol inhibits testicular steroidogenesis. *Fertil. Steril.*, **35**, 563–6

Liu, B.S. (1957). Suggestions of feeding crude cottonseed oil for contraception. *Shanghai Acad. Med.*, **6**, 43

Liu, Z.Q., Liu, G.Z., Hei, L.S., Zhang, R.A. and Yu, C.Z. (1981). Clinical trial of gossypol as a male antifertility agent. In Chang, E.F., Griffin, D. and Woolman, A. (eds.) *Recent Advances in Fertility Regulation*, Proc. Symp. Beijing, (Geneva, Atar)

Ma, R., Jiang, G., Li, F. and Wu, X. (1980). The effects of gossypol on some functions of autonomic nervous system. *J. Wuhan Med. Coll.*, **1**, 65–7

Myers, B.D. and Throneberry, G.O. (1966). Effect of gossypol on some oxidative respiratory enzymes. *Plant Physiol.*, **41**, 787–91

National Coordinating Group on Male Antifertility Agents (1978). Gossypol—A new antifertility agent for males. *Chin. Med. J.* (Engl. Edn.), **6**, 417–28

Poso, H., Wichmann, K., Janne, J. and Luukkainen, T. (1980). Gossypol, a powerful inhibitor of human spermatozoa metabolism. *Lancet*, **1**, 885–6

Prasad, M.R.N. and Diczfalusy, E. (1982). Gossypol. *Int. J. Androl. Suppl.*, **5**, 53–70

Qian, S., Xu, Y., Chen, Z., Cao, L., Sun, S., Tang, X., Wang, X., Shen, L. and Zhu, M. (1979). The influence of gossypol on the potassium metabolism of rats and the effect of some possible contributing factors. *Acta Pharm. Sin.*, **14**, 513–20

Ridley, A.J. and Blasco, L. (1981). Testosterone and gossypol effects on human sperm motility. *Fertil. Steril.*, **36**, 638–42

Sarkar, S., Dubey, A.K., Banergi, A.P. and Shah, P.N. (1978). Patterns of lactate dehydrogenase isoenzymes during gonadogenesis in the rat. *J. Reprod. Fertil.*, **53**, 285–8

Schleuning, W.D. and Fritz, H. (1974). Characteristics of highly purified boar sperm acrosin. *Hoppe Seyler's Z. Physiol. Chem.*, **355**, 125–30

Shi, Q. and Zhang, Y. (1980). Studies in antifertility effect of gossypol. I. Effects of gossypol on androgen-dependent organs in mice and rats. *Acta Zool. Sin.*, **26**, 311–16

Tso, W.-W. (1980). Response of spermatozoa to gossypol, a male contraceptive. II Pan American Congress. *Andrology*, **100**

Tso, W.-W. and Lee, C.-S. (1981a). Effect of gossypol on boar spermatozoa *in vitro*. *Arch. Androl.*, **7**, 85–8

Tso, W.-W. and Lee, C.-S. (1981b). Variations of gossypol sensitivity in boar spermatozoal electron transport chain segment. *Contraception*, **24**, 569–76

Tso, W.-W. and Lee, C.-S. (1982a). Cottonseed oil as a vaginal contraceptive. *Arch. Androl.*, **8**, 11-14

Tso, W.-W. and Lee, E.-S. (1982b). Gossypol: an effective acrosin blocker. *Arch. Androl.*, **8**, 143-7

Tso, W.-W. and Lee, C.-S. (1982c). Potassium leakage: not a cause of gossypol induced anti-motility in spermatozoa. *Int. J. Androl.*, **5**, 317-24

Tso, W.-W. and Lee, C.-S. (1982d). Lactate dehydrogenase-X: an isoenzyme particularly sensitive to gossypol inhibition. *Int. J. Androl.*, **5**, 205-9

Tso, W.-W., Lee, C.-S. and Tso, M.-Y.W. (1982). The effect of gossypol on boar spermatozoa adenosine triphosphate metabolism. *Arch. Androl.*, **9**, 319-31

Waller, D.P., Zaneveld, L.J.D. and Fong, H.H.S. (1980). *In vitro* spermicidal activity of gossypol. *Contraception*, **22**, 183-7

Wang, Y.E., Luo, Y.G. and Tang, X.C. (1979). Studies on the antifertility actions of cotton-seed meal and gossypol. *Acta Pharmacol. Sin.*, **14**, 662-9

Wichmann, K., Vaheri, A. and Luukkainen, T. (1982). Inhibiting herpes simplex virus type 2 infection in human epithelial cells by gossypol, a potential spermicidal and contraceptive agent. *Am. J. Obstet. Gynecol.*, **142**, 593-4

13
Gossypol modulation of testosterone secretion and metabolism

G.F. PAZ and Z.T. HOMONNAI

PREVIOUS INVESTIGATIONS OF GOSSYPOL

Gossypol is a polyphenolic compound isolated from the seed of cotton plants, that exhibits male antifertility characteristics. Rats, hamsters, mice, dogs and monkeys, all show varying degrees of sensitivity to gossypol; whereas rabbits seem to be insensitive (National Coordinating Group, 1978; Chang et al., 1980). In rats, however, there appear to be strain differences in response to its antifertility action. An extensive study was performed in China, in which the treatment of human males with gossypol resulted in azoospermia (Zatuchni and Osborn, 1981; Prasad and Diczfalusy, 1982).

Gossypol has been shown to be a reversible contraceptive drug that causes azoospermia or severe oligozoospermia. Its mode of action seems to be by damaging spermatogenesis and sperm maturation (Prasad and Diczfalusy, 1982). Biochemically, gossypol interferes with many enzymatic reactions, including succinate dehydrogenase, cyctochrome oxidase, microsomal oxidase and uncoupling of oxidative phosphorylation (Tso and Lee, 1981). Gossypol inhibits Na-K-ATPase and other magnesium-dependent enzyme systems (Myers and Throneberry 1966) and selectively inhibits LDH-X of the sperm (Lee and Malling, 1981). Gossypol has been shown to have a direct effect on the spermatozoa, exhibiting spermicidal activity (Waller et al., 1981), possibly due to a direct effect of the drug on the mitochondria and/or pronounced depression of spermatozoal fructose utilization. Studies of the male endocrine system, following gossypol administration, showed controversial results. In men, testosterone levels and blood chemistry were normal, without any reported loss of libido or potency (Coutinho et al., 1981).

Bardin et al. (1981) found in the male rhesus monkey, which has proven to be resistant to gossypol, no changes in the levels of testosterone, or in gonadotropins and only slight changes in sperm quality.

Treatment of Cynomolgus monkeys with gossypol–acetic acid induced severe pathology in the semen. No change in serum testosterone, or in

Leydig cells, in response to endogenous LH (following LHRH administration) was noticed (Shandilya *et al.*, 1982). In rats, Hadley *et al.* (1981) showed that serum LH and testosterone were reduced and that Leydig cells from treated rats produced less testosterone than controls when incubated with LH.

Hahn *et al.* (1981) reported insignificant changes in the weights of accessory sex organs observed during the course of gossypol treatment of rats. This indicates that there is no interference with androgen synthesis in the testis.

GOSSYPOL AND LEYDIG CELLS

Mammalian Leydig cells are the principal cells which produce most of the androgens in males. Evidence for testosterone synthesis in the Leydig cells comes from studies of the histochemical localization of 3β-hydroxysteroid dehydrogenase in these cells or fluorescent peroxidase-labelled antibodies against testosterone (Bubenik *et al.*, 1979). The muscaline activity, i.e. libido, male accessory gland function and spermatogenesis, are all dependent on the procreate activities of these cells. A number of hormones are involved in the regulation of Leydig cell function, including LH, prolactin, oestrogen, glucocorticoids and somatotrophic hormone (Purvis and Hansson, 1981).

Leydig cells were described by their peculiar ultrastructure, which is consonant with the function of steroid synthesis. They contain large amounts of smooth endoplasmic reticulum, plentiful mitochondria, prominent Golgi complex, centrioles, and a number of lipid droplets. Studies have been performed on the energetic metabolism of testicular tissue, especially the tubular fraction, which has been shown to have extensive aerobic activity and glucose uptake. No attention has been devoted to the interstitial tissue, including the Leydig cells (Setchell, 1978).

Since gossypol affects enzyme activity in cells, it is logical to assume that gossypol may have a direct effect on the basal metabolism of Leydig cells and on the energy supply of these cells that support the major function in the biosynthesis of testosterone.

Lin *et al.* (1981) demonstrated clearly that gossypol, *in vivo* and *in vitro*, caused decreased testosterone production by Leydig cells. Thus, a possible direct effect of gossypol on the rat Leydig cells is strongly suggested.

Preparation of Leydig cells

To study the effect of gossypol on Leydig cells, various concentrations of gossypol were added to isolated rat interstitial cells and the cells' basic metabolism was measured. The interstitial cells (I-cells) were isolated from the testes of adult male Wistar rats following the method described by Dufau and Catt (1975). Each pair of testes was decapsulated and the tissue incubated in a 45 ml plastic centrifuge tube containing 7 ml of medium 199 plus Hepes [4'-(2-hydroxyethyl)-1-piperazine-ethanesulphonic acid],

1 mg/ml collagenase (Sigma, Type 1) and 1 mg/ml of bovine serum albumin (BSA). Incubation was performed by shaking the tubes in their long axis in a water thermostatted shaker at 34°C for 10 minutes. Afterwards saline solution was added up to 25 ml. The tubes were inverted gently several times and allowed to stand for 5 minutes at room temperature. The supernatants were transferred to clean tubes and centrifuged at 1700 g for 10 minutes. The sediment of cells was resuspended in medium 199–Hepes–BSA.

Gossypol-acetic acid was dissolved in dimethylsulphoxide (DMSO) in a stock solution of 50 mg/ml. Gossypol was prepared by dilution in DMSO; 10 μl was added to the cell suspensions and the tubes were incubated for 2 or 3 hours; suspensions were centrifuged and the supernatant used for the various estimations. Under the conditions of the experiment, a concentration of I-cells that ranged between 10 and 40 million/ml was optimium for *in vitro* studies, in the time range between 2 and 4 hours.

Effect of gossypol on glucose utilization

Table 13.1 shows the effect of increasing gossypol concentrations on the glucose utilization of the cells, determined using a Beckman glucometer. Gossypol decreased glucose utilization when added to final concentrations higher than 100 μg/ml. At 500 μg/ml gossypol abolished glucose utilization dramatically. A dose of 10 μg/ml of gossypol had no significant effect on glucose utilization.

Table 13.1 Effect of different doses of gossypol on glucose utilization of isolated interstitial cells from rats, incubated for 3 hours. The results are means of four runs. Characteristics of interstitial cells at zero time were: concentration, 15 millions/ml; 3βHSD stain, 65%; TBE-test, 90%

Gossypol (μg/ml)	Glucose utilization (μg glucose 10^{-6} cells h^{-1}).
Control (DMSO)	3.05
10	2.66
100	1.83*
250	1.16†
500	0.66‡

* Significantly decreased, $p < 0.02$
† Significantly decreased, $p < 0.001$
‡ Significantly decreased, $p < 0.005$

Effect of gossypol on oxygen consumption

Consumption of oxygen (ZO_2) by I-cells was assessed using a method described by Frenkel *et al.* (1973). It was found that I-cell concentrations higher than 6.8 million/ml were sufficient in order to measure accurately oxygen consumption. I-cells were incubated with constant stirring at 34°C in a glass chamber, one wall of which was the fluorocarbon polymer (Teflon) membrane of a polarographic oxygen electrode (pHM-71, Radiometer Copenhagen). The electrode was calibrated using the glucose oxidase peroxide method. The decay in oxygen tension in the suspension of I-cells was followed for 5 minutes (following temperature stabilization). Gossypol-acetic acid was injected into the cell suspensions through a special hole in the wall of the chamber or was added to the cells before starting the measurements.

Table 13.2 summarizes the effect of increasing doses of gossypol on ZO_2

Table 13.2 Effect of the time of incubation in the presence of gossypol on the oxygen consumption (ZO_2) of isolated interstitial cells, from four adult rats. Cell characteristics were: concentration, 9.1 millions/ml; 3β-HSD stain, 48%; TBE test, 92%. Individual numbers are mean of two measurements at each point.

Treatment Time (min)	ZO_2 ($\mu lO_2 10^{-6}$ cells h^{-1})			
	5	30	60	120
Gossypol ($\mu g/ml$)				
0 (DMSO)	3.05	2.95	2.45	2.30
10	2.95	2.75	2.27	2.25
50	2.37	1.40	1.37	1.12
100	1.15	0.86	0.76	0.72
500	0.64	0.57	0.55	0.55

of I-cells, as a function of incubation time. A slow decrease in ZO_2 after 2 hours of incubation in the presence of $10\,\mu g/ml$ of gossypol, was noticed (-25%). At higher doses ($50\,\mu g/ml$), a decrease in the ZO_2 was recorded after 30 minutes of incubation. Furthermore, concentrations of 100 and $500\,\mu g/ml$ of gossypol caused the decrease in ZO_2 even after 5 minutes. Thus, 30 minutes of incubation in the presence of gossypol was the appropriate period of incubation for studying the effect of gossypol on the ZO_2 of I-cells. Gossypol in doses higher than $10\,\mu g/ml$, significantly depressed I-cell oxygen consumption.

Effect of gossypol on testosterone secretion and cell characteristics

The effect of gossypol on testosterone secretion of isolated I-cells and cell characteristics are given in Table 13.3. The vitality of cells was measured by trypan blue exclusion test (TBE test). Aliquots of cell suspensions were taken for 3β-HSD histochemical staining, according to the method of Mendelson et al. (1975). Cell counts were performed by the haemocytometer method (Freund and Caroll, 1964). hCG (human chorionogonadotropin, Sigma, USA) was added to the cell suspensions to a final concentration of $25\,IU/ml$. I-cells responded well to hCG stimulation. Gossypol did not affect testosterone tonic secretion by I-cells, although cell vitality and

Table 13.3 Effect of gossypol on the characteristics of rat isolated interstitial cells (cell concentration, 9.5 millions/ml), and testosterone secretion *in vitro*, under different doses of gossypol. Numbers are mean of five runs.

Treatment	3β-HSD (% stained)	Trypan blue exclusion (% stained)	Testosterone secretion (ng 10^{-6} cells h^{-1})
(O) DMSO (10μl)	50	73	0.39*
hCG (25 IU/ml)	73	81	0.60†
Gossypol 10 (μg/ml)	45	74	0.46
Gossypol 50 (μg/ml)	39	68	0.46
Gossypol 500 (μg/ml)	5	34	0.34

* Mean of the five runs
† Significantly increased. $p < 0.001$

3β-HSD histochemical stain were depressed. In order further to explore these findings, the effect of gossypol in I-cells stimulated by hCG was studied. The results clearly demonstrate that hCG increased the vitality significantly ($p < 0.01$) and enhanced the staining response to 3β-HSD ($P < 0.0001$) of the I-cells incubated for 2 hours. Gossypol, in a low dose (50 μg/ml) abolished the hCG stimulatory effect on testosterone secretion. Vitality of the cells and their 3β-HSD were also depressed significantly. Increasing gossypol concentrations to 500 μg/ml caused total destruction of I-cells, vitality dropped by 60%, 3β-HSD was depressed dramatically and the cells stopped secreting testosterone, even in the presence of hCG.

Possible influence of pH

In order to rule out the possibility that gossypol–acetic acid kills the cells by its acidity effect, the pH of the incubation media was measured. Only minor changes were found. Thus, gossypol has been shown to have a direct inhibitory, lytic and antisteroidogenic effect on the endocrine function of the testicular I-cells.

POSSIBLE MECHANISMS OF GOSSYPOL ACTION

The present study shows clearly that gossypol acetic acid has a direct effect on isolated interstitial cells of rats. Gossypol depressed significantly the metabolic rate of the I-cells and demonstrated a toxic effect which can be explained on the basis of its direct effect on mitochondria of cells (Xue, 1981), and enzymatic inhibition on a large scale of enzymes (Myers and Throneberry, 1966, Lee and Malling, 1981). Gossypol is known to have some chelating activity, which may react with cations and affect cell activity.

In spite of the discrepancy in the literature on the effect of gossypol on androgen production, it is quite possible that in humans and monkeys, gossypol, in the doses administered, has no effect on the steroidogenic activity (National Coordinating Group, 1978; Coutinho *et al.*, 1981; Shandilya *et al.*, 1982), yet it is active in depressing spermatogenesis (Frick *et al.*, 1981; Wang *et al.*, 1979). In the rat, some authors showed inhibition of steroidogenesis *in vivo* (Lin *et al.*, 1981; Hadley *et al.*, 1981) and *in vitro* (Lin *et al.*, 1981). Others failed to show such a change *in vivo* (Kalla *et al.*, 1982; Hahn *et al.*, 1981). They even showed no change in male accessory sex gland weights or secretions.

We have shown a decrease in testosterone production of isolated I-cells only in the stimulated (hCG) phase. This result can explain the discrepancy between the various groups. When Leydig cells are stimulated by LH, gossypol inhibits steroidogenesis, but under non-stimulated conditions, the effect of gossypol is only mildly manifested. This, of course, cannot explain the *in vivo* situation where the Leydig cells are under a constant stimulatory effect of endogenous LH.

CONCLUDING REMARKS

Gossypol–acetic acid is a polyphenolic compound present in the seed of cotton plants. Its antifertility activity by inhibition of spermatogenesis was proven in a large group of animals, including man. In the present study, the direct effect of gossypol–acetic acid on collagenase isolated rat I-cells was investigated. It was shown that gossypol–acetic acid depressed significantly the metabolic rate of the cells. Glucose utilization was abolished by a starting dose of $100\,\mu g/ml$. Oxygen consumption of I-cells was reduced even at a smaller dose of gossypol ($50\,\mu g/ml$). At these doses, the vitality of the cells remained (proven by trypan blue exclusion test), 3β-HSD histochemical stain was slightly decreased. Increasing doses of gossypol caused a marked decrease in the vitality of I-cells and a dramatic drop in histochemical stain for 3β-HSD. The pH of the medium was not changed at any dose of treatment. Testosterone secretion of I-cells *in vitro* was significantly decreased only when I-cells were stimulated by hCG ($25\,IU$). In cultures of I-cells not stimulated by hCG, gossypol did not affect the tonic slow release of testosterone. Thus, gossypol–acetic acid has a direct inhibitory effect on isolated rat I-cells, depressing cell metabolism and endocrine function. The failure of some of the other groups to show such an effect, especially *in vivo*, can be attributed to differences in the dose of treatment and strain of animals (Zatuchni and Osborn, 1980).

Acknowledgements

The authors express their grateful appreciation for the excellent assistance of Mrs Ariela Carmon and Mr L. Fleisher. The study was partially supported by a grant from the Schrieber Foundation, Tel Aviv University Sackler Medical School.

References

Bardin, C.W., Sundaram, K.S. and Chang, C.C. (1981). Toxicology, endocrine and histopathology studies in small animals and rhesus monkeys administered gossypol. Presented

GOSSYPOL MODULATION OF TESTOSTERONE SECRETION

at *PARFR Workshop on Gossypol, Program for Applied Research on Fertility Regulation.* **1,** 1

Bubenik, G.A., Brown, G.M. and Grota (1979). Localization of immunoreactive androgen in testosterone tissue. *Endocrinology,* **96,** 63

Chang, M.C., Zhi, P.G. and Saksena, S.K. (1980). Effects of gossypol on the fertility of male rats, hamsters and rabbits. *Contraception,* **21,** 461

Coutinho, E., Segal and Melo, J.F. (1981). Biphasic action of gossypol in men. *Fertil. Steril.,* (in press)

Dufau, M.L. and Catt, K.J. (1975). Gonadotropic stimulation of interstitial cell function of rat testis *in vitro. Methods Enzymol.,* **39,** 252

Frenkel, G., Peterson, R.N. and Freund, M. (1973). Changes in the metabolism of guinea pig sperm from different segments of the epididymis. *Proc. Soc. Exp. Biol. (NY),* **143,** 1231

Freund, M., Caroll, B. (1964). Factors affecting hemocytometer counts of sperm concentration in human semen. *J. Reprod. Fertil.,* **8,** 149

Frick, J., Danner, Ch., Kohle, R. and Kunit C. (1981). Male fertility regulation. In Cotes-Prieto, J., Campos da Paz, A. and Neves-e-Castro, M. (eds.) *Research on Fertility and Sterility,* p. 291, (Lancaster: MTP)

Hadley, M.A., Lin, C.Y. and Dym, M. (1981). Effects of gossypol on the reproductive system of the male rats. *J. Androl.,* **2,** 190

Hahn, D.W., Rusticus, C., Probst, A., Hahn, R. and Johnson, A.N. (1981). Antifertility and endocrine activities of gossypol in rodents. *Contraception,* **24,** 97

Kalla, N.R., Foo, J.J.W., Sheth, A.R. (1982). Studies on the male antifertility agent gossypol acetic acid. V. Effect of gossypol acetic acid on the fertility of male rats. *Andrologia,* **14,** 492

Lee, C.Y. and Malling, H.Y. (1981). Selective inhibition of sperm-specific lactate dehydrogenase X by an antifertility agent, gossypol. *Fed. Proc.,* **40,** 718

Lin, J., Murono, E.P., Osterman, J., Nankin, H.R. and Couleson, P.B. (1981). Gossypol inhibits testicular steroidogenesis. *Fertil. Steril.,* **35,** 563

Mendelson, C., Dufau, M. and Catt, K. (1975). Gonadotropin binding and stimulation of cyclic adenosine 3′,5′-monophosphate and testosterone production in isolated Leydig cells. *J. Biol. Chem.,* **250,** 8818

Myers, B.D. and Throneberry, C.O. (1966). Effect of gossypol on some oxidative respiratory enzymes. *Plant Physiol.,* **41,** 787

National Coordinating Group on Male Antifertility Agents (1978). Gossypol. A new antifertility agent for males. *Chin. Med. J. (English edn),* **4,** 417

Prasad, M.R.N. and Diczfalusy, E. (1982) Gossypol. *Int. J. Androl. Suppl.,* **5,** 53

Purvis, K. and Hansson, V. (1981). Hormonal regulation of spermatogenesis. Regulation of target cell response. *Int. J. Androl. Suppl.* **3,** 85

Setchell, B.P. (1978). Metabolism in the testis. In *The Mamallian Testis,* p. 285. (Ithaca, NY: Cornell University Press)

Shandilya, L., Clarkson, T.B. Adams, M.R. and Lewis, J.C. (1982). Effects of gossypol on reproductive and endocrine functions of male Cynomolgus Monkeys *(Macaca fascicularis). Biol. Reprod.,* **27,** 241

Tso, W.W. and Lee C.S. Effect of gossypol on boar spermatozoa *in vitro. Arch. Androl.,* **7,** 85

Waller, D.P., Fong, H.H.S., Cordell, C.F. and Soejarto, D.D. (1981). Antifertility effects of gossypol and its impurities on male hamsters. *Contraception,* **23,** 653

Wang, Y., Luo, Y, and Tang, X. (1979). Studies on the antifertility action of cotton seed meal and gossypol. *Acta Pharm. Sin.,* **14,** 662

Xue, S.P. (1981). Studies on the antifertility effect of gossypol, a new contraceptive for males. In Chang, C.F., Griffin, D. and Wollman, A. (eds.) *Recent Advances in Fertility Regulation. Proc. Symp. Beijing,* Sept 1980 (Geneva: Atar).

Zatuchni, G.I. and Osborn, C.K. (1981). Gossypol: a possible male antifertility agent. Report of a workshop. *Res. Frontiers. in Fertil. Reg.,* **1,** 1

14
Gossypol inhibition of LDH-X

C.-Y.G. LEE, Y.S. MOON, A. DULEBA, A.F. CHEN and V. GOMEL

HISTORICAL BACKGROUND

Gossypol, a yellowish polyphenolic compound isolated from the cotton plant, was first identified in China as the active ingredient in crude cotton-seed oil causing the male antifertility effect (National Coordinating Group on Male Antifertility Agent, 1978). During the 1970s, animal experiments and clinical studies were initiated by Chinese scientists with the emphasis on the male antifertility effect, the site of action, pharmacokinetics as well as the toxicity of gossypol. The results seemed to suggest that the efficacy of gossypol as a male antifertility agent was as high as 99.89% among the 4000 volunteers who had been on the contraceptive pill for 6 months to 4 years. Moreover, the intake of this male contraceptive drug did not affect the sex hormonal levels and libido of the male individuals. The fertility was usually recovered for most of the volunteers three months after the discontinuation of treatment. The offspring of those who stopped using gossypol appeared to be normal after birth. Drug related side-effects include transient weakness, hypokalaemia, epigastric discomfort and nausea. The reports by Chinese scientists caused considerable excitement in the field of population research and family planning. Understanding the biochemical mechanism of this effective male contraceptive drug now becomes essential, since such investigation may eventually lead to the development of synthetic compounds exhibiting the desired antifertility effect but with far less toxicity in animals and in humans.

Long before the Chinese discovery, it was known that gossypol in cottonseed is poisonous to non-ruminant animals including humans (Abou-Donia, 1976). Despite the extensive research of the last several decades into gossypol toxicology, the mechanisms by which gossypol causes tissue damage are as yet poorly understood. The results of these investigations suggest gossypol toxicity may be associated with its binding to specific enzymes or proteins, or its interference with amino acid, protein or ion metabolism. Unfortunately, none of these observations is closely associated with any specific cytotoxicity to spermatogenic cells or its male antifertility effect. The understanding of gossypol's biochemical mechanism of action at molecular or enzyme levels will certainly make a far-reaching contribution to its development as a male contraceptive (Zatuchni and Osborn, 1981).

Recently, biochemical studies of gossypol were initiated in our laboratory in an attempt to elucidate its possible mechanism of action as a male antifertility agent (Lee and Malling, 1981; Lee *et al.*, 1982).

GOSSYPOL INACTIVATION OF LDH-X AND ITS IMPLICATIONS

Since little was known about the biochemical mechanisms of gossypol action as a male antifertility agent, three working hypotheses regarding its antifertility mechanisms were originally proposed. First, spermatogenesis is a well programmed event during which specific isoenzymes of certain enzymes are expressed to fulfil metabolic functions of certain spermatogenic cells (Goldberg, 1977). If any of the sperm- or testis-specific enzymes are selectively inhibited or inactivated by gossypol, their presence may lead to metabolic disturbance of some spermatogenic cells, but not other types of cells or tissues. Secondly, spermatogenic cells may have specific 'receptors' to gossypol. The binding of gossypol to certain spermatogenic cells may result in specific cytoxicity. Thirdly, since spermatogenic cells are rapidly dividing, gossypol may have a specific inhibitory effect on DNA/RNA or protein synthesis during the active mitosis or meiosis of spermatogenesis.

To test the first of these hypotheses, an initial biochemical study was conducted regarding the effect of gossypol on the activity of about 20 enzymes from mouse testis *in vitro* (Lee and Malling, 1981). Among the enzymes examined, isoenzymes of lactate dehydrogenase and malate dehydrogenase as well as glutathione *S*-transferase were shown to be significantly inactivated by low concentrations of gossypol in neutral, aqueous solution (Lee and Malling, 1981; Lee *et al.*, 1982).

Figure 14.1 shows that of the isoenzymes of lactate dehydrogenase, lactate dehydrogenase-X (LDH-X) from mouse and human was selectively inactivated by gossypol. The degree of enzyme inactivation depends on time, concentration of gossypol and enzyme as well as the order of assay component addition. If LDH was first mixed with gossypol, a significantly higher degree of enzyme inactivation was observed than when the enzyme was added to the assay solution containing premixed NADH, pyruvate and gossypol. By either procedure, LDH-X and LDH-5 were consistently inactivated faster than LDH-1.

Inactivation of LDH isoenzymes by gossypol is time-dependent. When 0.01 unit/ml of LDH-X was incubated with $10 \mu mol/l$ gossypol at room temperature in $50 mmol/l$ potassium phosphate (pH 7.0), 50, 35, and 20% of the initial enzyme activity was observed, respectively, after 5, 10 and 20 minutes of incubation. In the presence of the same concentration of LDH-X, the extent of time-dependent inactivation is gossypol-concentration dependent. After 20 minutes of pre-incubation of gossypol with 0.01 unit/ml LDH-X, the residual enzyme activity observed is 95, 70, and 21%, respectively, in the presence of 1, 5, and $10 \mu mol/l$ gossypol. The results of this study are presented in Fig. 14.2.

The degree of enzyme inactivation by gossypol is also enzyme-concentration dependent. When 0.4 unit/ml LDH-X was incubated with $10 \mu mol/l$

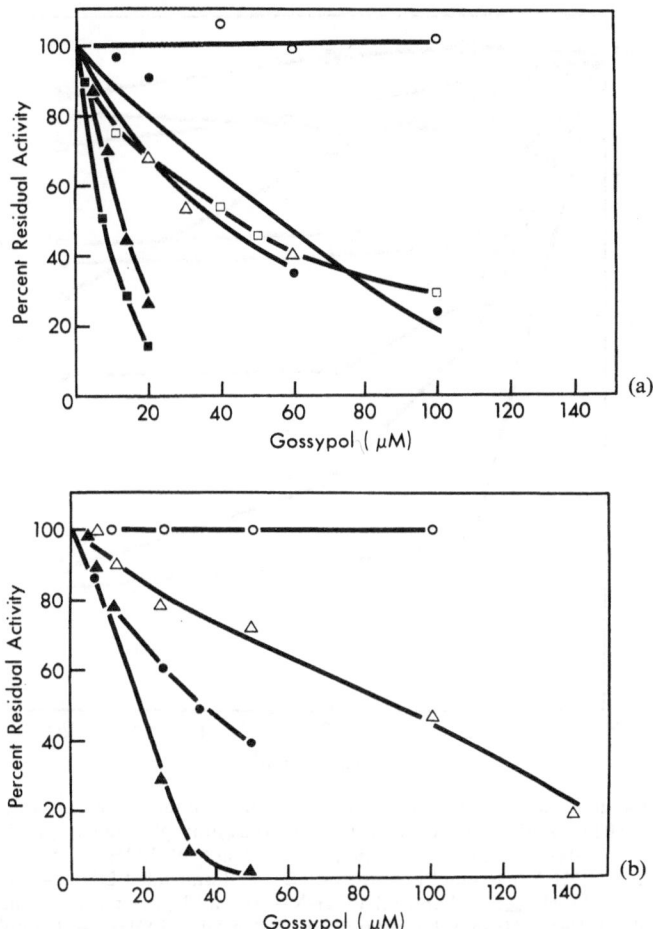

Fig. 14.1 (a) Activity of mouse lactate dehydrogenase isoenzymes in a mixture of NADH, pyruvate and gossypol (open symbols; ○: LDH-1, △: LDH-5 and □: LDH-X) and activity of mouse lactate dehydrogenase isoenzymes, when the enzyme was mixed with gossypol prior to the addition of NADH and pyruvate within 10 s before assay (closed symbol; ●: LDH-1, ▲: LDH-5 and ■: LDH-X). (b) Activity of human LDH-1 (○) and LDH-X (△) in a mixture of NADH, pyruvate and gossypol; and activity of human LDH-1 (●) and LDH-X (▲), when the enzyme was mixed with gossypol prior to the addition of NADH and pyruvate within 10 s before assay. Initial enzyme activity in each assay was about 0.01 unit/ml.

gossypol, more than 70% of the enzyme activity remained after 20 minutes of incubation. In contrast, on incubation of 0.01 unit/ml of LDH-X under the same conditions only 20% of the original activity remained (Fig. 14.2).

Inactivation of LDH-X by gossypol has been found to be irreversible since a further incubation with coenzyme or substrate failed to restore the original enzyme activity. On the other hand, the presence of NADH appeared partially to protect LDH-X from gossypol inactivation. In the absence of NADH, more than 80% of LDH-X activity was inactivated by

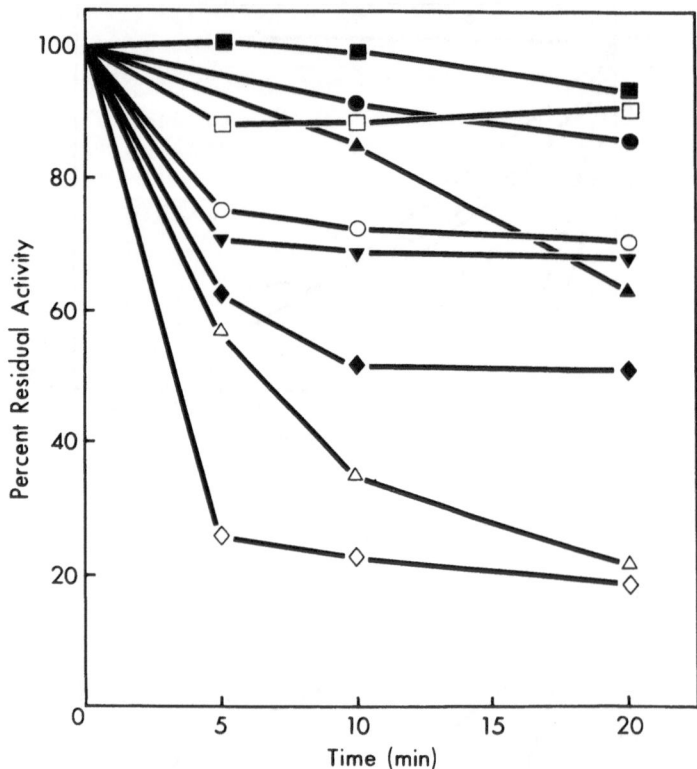

Fig. 14.2 Time-dependent inactivation of mouse LDH-X under different conditions of incubation; ■: 0.01 unit/ml LDH-X in 50 mmol/l potassium phosphate, pH 7.0 (control); □: 0.01 unit/ml LDH-X + 1 μmol/l gossypol; ○: 0.01 unit/ml LDH-X + 5 μmol/l gossypol; △: 0.01 unit/ml LDH-X + 10 μmol/l gossypol; ●: 0.01 unit/ml LDH-X + 5 μmol/l gossypol + 100 μmol/l NADH; ▲: 0.01 unit/ml LDH-X + 10 μmol/l gossypol + 100 μmol/l NADH; ▼: 0.4 unit/ml LDH-X + 10 μmol/l gossypol; ◆: 0.4 unit/ml LDH-X + 50 μmol/l gossypol; ◇: 0.4 unit/ml LDH-X + 100 μmol/l gossypol

10 μmol/l gossypol after 20 minutes of incubation. However, in the presence of 100 μmol/l NADH and 10 μmol/l gossypol, only 40% inactivation of LDH-X activity was observed after the same incubation time (Fig. 14.2).

Recently, we also found that the degree of LDH-X inactivation by gossypol is pH- and buffer-dependent. At a given pH, the relative potency of enzyme inactivated by gossypol varied more than 10-fold depending on the counter anions of the Tris buffer. The following counter ion order was observed: acetate > Cl⁻ > glycine > phosphate. In a given buffer, the degree of enzyme inactivation increases with pH from 7.0 to 8.0 as in the case of Hepes buffer.

These results suggest that gossypol is a selective inactivator of sperm-specific LDH-X from mouse and human. The degree of LDH-X inactivation was found to depend on gossypol concentration, even though it is always in great excess. This observation can be construed to suggest that minor active impurities in gossypol may be responsible for LDH-X inactivation in neutral aqueous solution. Based on the study of enzyme- and gossypol-dependent inactivation of LDH-X, it is estimated that the minor active components may amount to only 0.1–0.5% of the total gossypol in solution.

The fact that the enzyme inactivation is partially blocked by NADH indicates that the processes may be coenzyme binding site-directed. The irreversible inactivation of LDH-X could result from the covalent interaction between the active minor components of gossypol and the enzyme. To prove this point, currently, we are employing ^{14}C-labelled gossypol for further analysis.

It has been reported that LDH-X is not expressed until the spermatocytes have reached the pachytene stage, and is found only in spermatocytes, spermatids and spermatozoa (Goldberg, 1977). Although it has been demonstrated that several enzymes in mouse testis are inhibited or inactivated by gossypol (Lee et al., 1982), the selective inactivation of LDH-X in the present study may contribute to its cytotoxicity on spermatogenic cells and to the male infertility. Recently, it has been reported that gossypol inhibits the uptake of sugar and lactate by human spermatozoa (Pösö et al., 1980). This evidence also supports the assertion that LDH-X inactivation by gossypol may interfere with the metabolism of spermatogenic cells in testis. Understanding of the functional role of LDH-X in spermatogenic cells may lead to a better understanding of the biochemical mechanism of action of gossypol on male infertility.

STABILITY OF GOSSYPOL

Since gossypol is a polyphenolic compound, a high degree of instability would be expected in aqueous solution. The decomposition of gossypol may easily occur via air oxidation, alcohol–aldehyde dismutation or chelation/oxidation by metal ions such as Fe^{3+} (Abou-Donia, 1976).

The minor active components of gossypol that putatively irreversibly inactivate LDH-X may arise from either the impurities present in the original gossypol sample, the decomposition products or minor tautomeric forms of gossypol. In view of the instability of gossypol, it is consistent that the minor decomposition products of gossypol could be responsible for the inactivation of LDH-X in aqueous solution. Therefore, the decomposition or the metabolic fate of gossypol may play a key role in its physiological actions. Based on this assumption, the stability of gossypol in aqueous solution was investigated in an attempt to find minor gossypol components that inactivate LDH-X. Factors which affect the stability of gossypol in solutions were elucidated in detail by thin-layer chromatography, high-pressure liquid chromatography and by UV/visible spectrophotometry.

In absolute ethanol, gossypol exhibits high solubility, but undergoes gradual spectral changes with time either in the presence or absence of oxygen. On thin-layer chromatography (on polyamide plates using a solvent system: benzene–acetic acid–H_2O (57: 28: 15 by vol.), two additional UV-

197

positive spots appear on thin-layer plates with R_f values of 0.6 and 0.4, respectively (instead of 0.75 for gossypol) after 96 h incubation in absolute ethanol. The gradual transformation of gossypol in ethanol is not oxygen-dependent and is accompanied by a shift in λ_{max} from 238 nm to 259 nm and a decrease in absorbance at 370 nm.

pH- and time-dependent stability of gossypol in aqueous solution was also studied by high pressure liquid chromatography (HPLC) (C_{18} reversed-phase column, 2.3 × 250 mm, 10 μm particle size, Altex). At pH 4.5 in 0.05 mol/l citrate buffer, gossypol is stable indefinitely as judged from tracings by HPLC. The rate of gossypol decomposition is slow at pH 7.0 and faster at higher pH. Typical tracings from HPLC are presented in

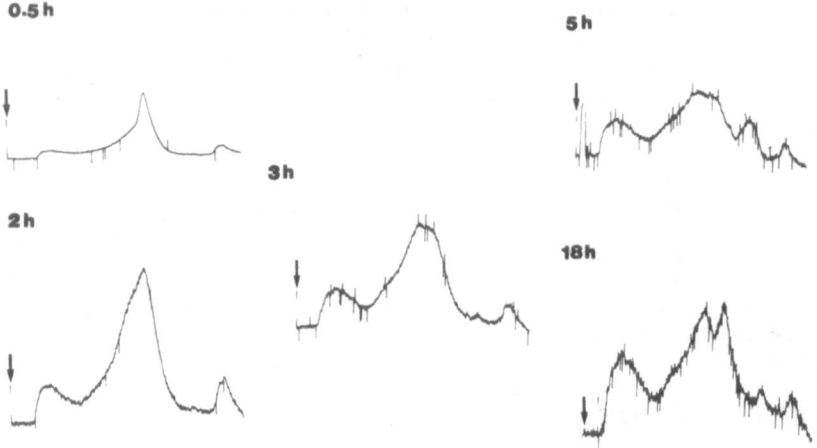

Fig 14.3 Decomposition of gossypol in 0.05 mol/l sodium bicarbonate, pH 8.5, as a function of time, when analysed by HPLC. Solvent system used and conditions: 40% CH_3CN in 0.01% acetic acid for 1 min, 70% CH_3CN in 0.01% acetic acid for 4 min linear gradient, 100% CH_3CN in 0.01% acetic acid for 3 min linear gradient, and 100% CH_3CN in 0.01% acetic acid for three isocratic conditions

Fig. 14.3 to demonstrate the time-dependent decomposition of gossypol in aqueous solution.

The instability of gossypol in aqueous solution is also confirmed by thin-layer chromatography and UV/visible spectrophotometry. Generally speaking, in oxygenated neutral aqueous solution, gossypol exhibits a marked decrease in absorbance at λ_{max} 238 and 370 nm and a concomitant increase in absorbance at λ_{max} 315 nm. In the absence of oxygen, no apparent changes in UV spectra of gossypol were observed with time. Similarly, by thin-layer chromatography, one can show the appearance of three additional UV-positive spots on thin-layer plates with R_f values of 0.1, 0.2, and 0.65, respectively upon incubation in oxygenated phosphate buffer at pH 7.0 for 96 h. It was noted that the R_f values of these three UV-positive spots are not identical to those observed for gossypol in absolute ethanol. This clearly indicates the difference in pathways of 'decomposition' between that in ethanol and in aqueous solution. In the oxygen-free aqueous solution, gossypol remains stable without apparent decomposition.

In summary, it is apparent that the decomposition of gossypol in aqueous solution is pH- and oxygen-dependent. Such decomposition processes may also occur *in vivo* after the drug intake. The instability of gossypol in oxygenated aqueous solution raises questions regarding the actual active ingredients in 'gossypol' that cause the male antifertility action in animals and in humans. In view of the observation that the sperm- and testis-specific LDH-X are selectively inactivated by gossypol containing minor components in aqueous solution, the metabolic fate of gossypol *in vivo* becomes esential before the question about the antifertility action of this agent can be answered.

References

Abou-Donia, M.B. (1976). Physiological effect and metabolism of gossypol. *Residual Reviews*, Vol. **61**, pp. 126-160 (New York; Springer-Verlag)

Goldberg, E. (1977). Isozymes in testes and spermatozoa. In Rattazzi, M.C., Scandalios, J.G. and Whitt, G. (eds) *Isozymes: Current Topics in Biological and Medical Research*, Vol. 1, pp. 79-124. (New York: Alan R. Liss)

Lee, C.Y. and Malling, H.V. (1981). Selective inhibition of lactate dehydrogenase-X by a male antifertility agent-gossypol. *Fed. Proc.*, **40**, 2790

Lee, C.Y., Moon, Y.S., Yuan, J.H. and Chen, A.F. (1982). Enzyme inactivation and inhibition by gossypol. *Mol. Cell. Biochem.* **47**, 65-70

National Coordinating Group on Male Fertility. (1978) *Chinese Med. J.*, **4**, 417-28

Pöso, H. Wichmann, K., Jänne, J. and Luuk-kainen, T. (1980). Gossypol, a powerful inhibitor of human spermatozoal metabolism. *Lancet*, **1**, 885

Zatuchni, G.I. and Osborn, C.K. (1981). Gossypol: a possible male antifertility agent-Report of a workshop. In Zatuchni, G.I. (ed.) *Frontiers in Fertility Regulation*, Vol. 1, pp. 1-15. (Northwestern University press: Evanston, Ill.)

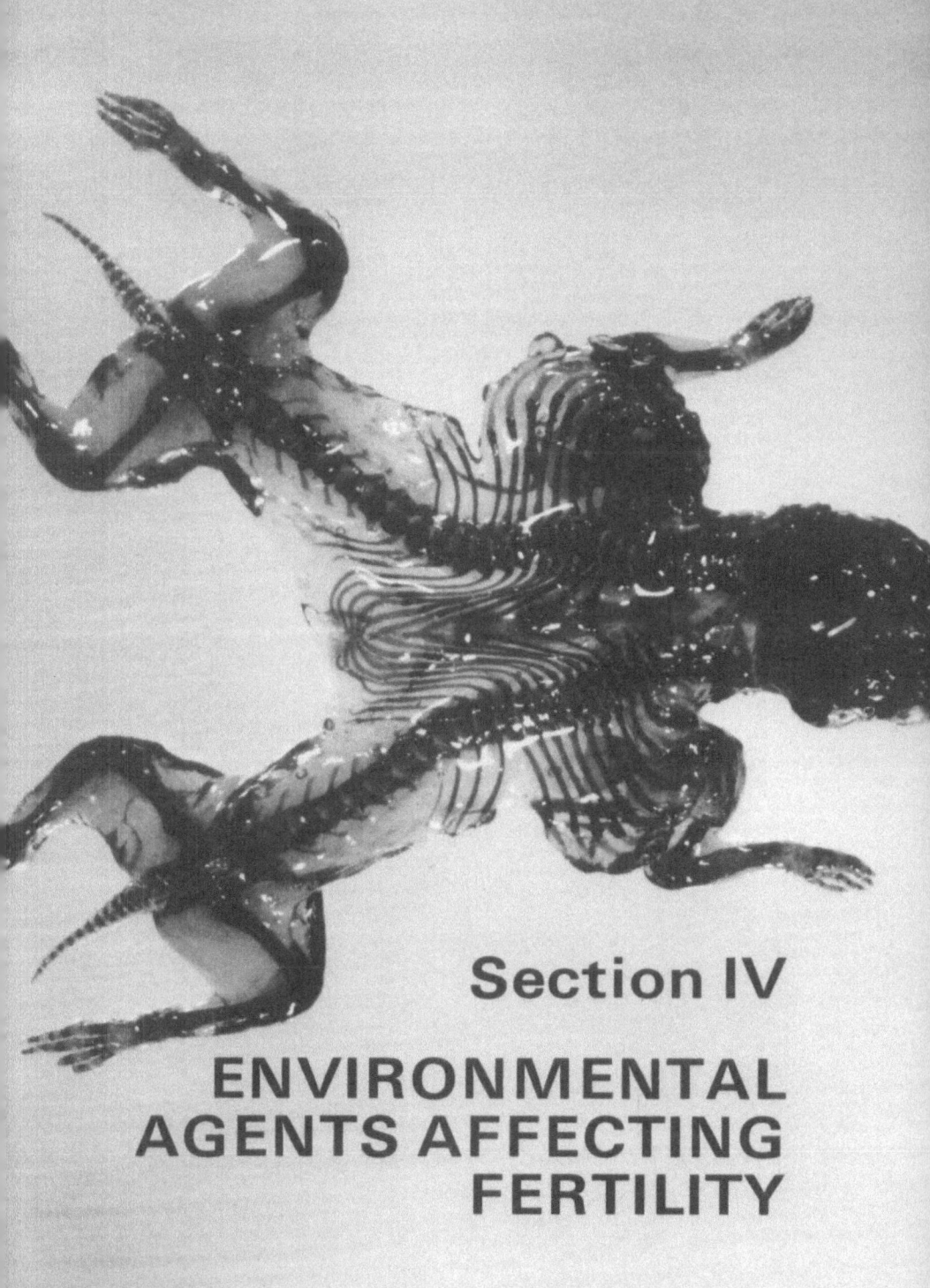

Section IV
ENVIRONMENTAL AGENTS AFFECTING FERTILITY

15
Environmental chemical effects on testicular function

I.P. LEE and L.L. RUSSELL

INTRODUCTION

Over the past few decades, the increasing use and production of chemicals in agriculture, industry and medicine have greatly benefited quality of health and as a consequence, have extended longevity of man. Thousands of new compounds are used to control infections, pests and parasites and to manufacture goods. However, some compounds may be more detrimental than beneficial to health. The advent of new chemicals and their potential toxic effects has become a major health concern. In particular, there has been increasing concern that environmental chemicals may cause germ cell damage, infertility, fetal malformation, and heritable genetic diseases. Indeed, the evidence for chemically induced germ cell damage and infertility appears to be on the increase, especially in man. For example, in the United States approximately 6 954 000 couples are involuntarily infertile, 3 000 000 of which have at least one partner who is sterile (Mosher, 1980, Placek and Cynamon, 1980). In addition, many contend that average sperm count of population with fewer than 25 million/ml varied from 20 to 30% (MacLeod and Wang, 1979; Dougherty et al., 1981).

Recently in the United States, some male workers occupationally exposed to 1,2-dibromo-3-chloropropane (DBCP) became sterile, evidencing oligospermia, azoospermia and germinal aplasia. Workers in battery plants in Bulgaria, lead mine workers in the state of Missouri, and workers handling organic solvents in Sweden have been found to have low sperm counts, abnormal sperm and varying degrees of infertility. Hexafluoroacetone, phthalate esters, kepone, borax, cadmium, lead, methylmercury, diethylstilboestrol (DES) and many cancer chemotherapeutic agents have been shown to be toxic to male and female reproductive systems. Furthermore, in the United States, there are approximately 600 000 spontaneous abortions per 3 000 000 births per year. Of those born alive, about 10% are premature, approximately 13% have a low birth weight and 3 to 7% have birth defects. Of the 150 000 babies born with a birth defect per year, 5% of the defects are thought to be due to gene mutations, 15% to intrauterine infections, 20% to multifactorial causes and the cause(s) of 60% of all birth defects are presently unknown (Nelson, 1977; Fabro, 1983). It is speculated, however, that a signficant percentage of birth defects may be attributed to environmental factors.

Epidemiologically, the aetiology of male infertility is difficult to identify to any single compound because of the frequency of exposure to other chemicals and other important factors (e.g. genetic, physiological, nutritional and health state of individuals, etc.), which affect germ cell differentiation and reproductive organ function. Given these complexities, molecular, biochemical and physiological bases of reproductive processes in

Table 15.1 Adverse reproductive effects of environmental chemicals in man

Chemicals	Effects	References
Lead	Asthenospermia, hypospermia, and teratospermia	Lancranjan et al. (1975)
Kepone	Reduced sperm motility and reproductive failure	Longford (1978), Taylor et al. (1978)
Ethanol	Testicular atrophy, azoospermia	Turner et al. (1977)
Carbon disulphide	Asthenospermia, hypospermia, teratospermia, reduced libido, impotence	Lancranjan et al. (1972)
Carbon dibromide	Decreased fertility	Wong et al. (1979)
DBCP (1,2-dibromo-3-chloropropane)	Azoospermia, oligospermia, testicular atrophy, infertility, impotence	Whorton et al. (1977), Whorton et al. (1979), Potashnick et al. (1978)
Boron	Reduced libido, infertility, oligospermia	Tarasenko et al. (1972)
Pesticide (mixture)	Impotence	Espir et al. (1970)
DES	Gynaecomastia	Pacynski et al. (1971)
PBB (polybrominated biphenyl)	Reduced libido	Rosenman et al. (1979)

Source: Sullivan and Barlow (1979)

both experimental animals and man need to be investigated more extensively in order to identify pertinent animal data which can be 'extrapolated' to that of man.

There are numerous test systems for assessing potentially toxic chemicals on reproductive organs of laboratory animals. Some of these test systems have been developed primarily to investigate physiological and biochemical mechanisms of action, while others have been developed primarily as test systems for routine screening of potentially hazardous toxic chemicals to animals and human population. This chapter lists the environmental chemicals which have been shown to affect male reproductive function (Table 15.1) and considers the various laboratory tests which may serve as useful indicators of reproductive toxicity in laboratory animals.

ASSESSMENT OF TESTICULAR DAMAGE AND MALE FERTILITY

Experimental design (Selection of species, doses, route of exposure, duration of exposure and end-point measurements, and statistics)

The ultimate objective of reproductive toxicity testing is to assess the toxic effects of experimental data pertinent to man. To accomplish this objective, one must consider the selection of species, number of animals, route of administration, duration of exposure, pharmacokinetic parameters governing chemical absorption, distribution, activation and detoxification. The most ideal species for toxicological testing is one with pharmacokinetic and pharmacodynamic properties similar to those of man, as well as similar manifestations of target organ toxicity. All of these parameters are important considerations in selecting the species and strains to be used for testing a particular chemical. However, those data may not be readily available for a test chemical and the selection of a species then becomes a difficult task. There does not appear to be an ideal laboratory species other than the subhuman primates. However, mice, rats and rabbits have been widely used for routine toxicity studies and these animal species are readily available, inexpensive, easy to maintain and they can be bred with ease in laboratories. Although subhuman primates are ideal because of their physiological similarities to man (in particular the spermatogenic cells and the spermatogenic cycle of the baboon closely resemble those of man), costs and availability are impractical for routine fertility tests.

Dosage is a primary consideration in designing a reproductive toxicity test. At least three dose levels are normally used, in addition to a control and vehicle control. As a preliminary screen, a single maximally tolerated dose of a test chemical (not exceeding LD_{10}) should be administered, as well as *in vivo* fertility tests in excess of the entire duration of spermatogenic cycles (e.g. 70 day period for CD-rats), along with testicular weight, morphological evaluation and other *in vitro* tests. If a test dose is positive, subsequent doses should be reduced to determine the no-effect dose, the threshold dose for both single and multiple doses and the minimum effective dose for subchronic and chronic studies. For both subchronic and chronic studies, the design of such experiments should be based on the anticipated amounts and patterns of consumption or exposure of a chemical in man. The route of administration of the test dose should also parallel the human experience, and the purity of the test compound should be carefully determined and maintained. The value of rather simple pharmacokinetic parameters, such as rate of absorption, volume of distribution, biological half-life and routes of biotransformation, should be determined.

The end-points of a reproductive test include serial mating studies of the male following either a single dose or multiple doses, for one generation or multigeneration studies. In addition, a variety of *in vitro* tests are carried out to understand possible mechanisms of reproductive toxicity.

Statistical analysis of one generation, dominant lethal studies or multigeneration studies are straightforward, and simple statistical techniques may satisfy most criteria for statistical analysis. For satisfactory interpretation of experiments involving fertility and dominant lethality assessments, an adequate number of animals must be used to provide statistically meaningful data. The number of animals to be exposed in each dose group depends on a number of factors: the reproductive effects to be measured, the reproducibility of the effects in an experimental system and the incidences of spontaneous occurrences of any effect and the sensitivity of the experiments (e.g. 10 males/treatment group with 1 female/male per week).

Determination of the size and weight of the testis and testis morphology

The initial means for evaluating testicular function in experimental animals is through measurement of its testis size and weight, as well as thorough histological examination. If these determinations are negative, then there is low probability that the testis is affected by a particular chemical, although biochemical and genetic abnormalities may well not be adequately assessed by these methods. Positive findings, on the other hand, indicate that other types of evaluation such as those described in subsequent sections of this chapter may shed more light on the mechanistic processes involved.

Volume of the excised testis may be determined by water displacement, dimensions by measurement of its long and short axes, and weight by an appropriate balance. Weight measurements are the most common type of determination and they are considered one of the important indicators of testicular damage. Accessory sex glands may be taken at the same time and weighed as an indirect indication of androgen status.

Histological examination may proceed from one of two basic methodologies. Paraffin-processed tissues for light microscopy traditionally have been used to evaluate testicular structure. The advantage of processing tissue in this manner is that large areas of the testis may be examined with the light microscope with relative ease. However, cytological structure is poorly preserved with most light microscope fixatives, while the testis fixed with glutaraldehyde allows the investigator critically to examine well-fixed specimens and pinpoint specific cytological features. In addition, plastic embedded tissues may be sectioned for electron-microscopic observation for further cytological examination. Several reviews of testis structure and spermatogenesis are available (Roosen-Runge, 1962, 1973; Steinberger, 1975; Ewing et al., 1980, Russell, 1980, 1983). Especially valuable in any analysis of testis morphology is knowledge of the spermatogenic cycle and its timing for the various species under consideration (Leblond and Clermont, 1952, for the rat). The complexities of testis structure are emphasized in ultrastructural studies where both Sertoli cells and germinal cells are seen in intimate and elaborate relationships (Russell, 1980). The detailed structure of spermatozoa should be evaluated by ultrastructural analysis.

Having encountered subtle changes in testicular structure, it is frequently necessary for the investigators to quantify the changes and subject them to statistical analysis. The quantitative expression of testicular weight and tubular diameter are relatively straightforward techniques (tubular diameter must be measured in round tubular cross-sections) and may yield valuable information. Cell counts, while desirable, must be undertaken with extreme caution to ensure meaningful data. For example, cell counts must be made in tubules which are round cross-sections. Counts of one cell type in a particular stage from a treated animal must be compared with counts in the same stage from control animals. A reference and/or correction factor is necessary from which to base cell counts since tubular shrinkage may affect the counts. The most reliable reference appears to be the Sertoli cell nucleolus (Russell and Clermont, 1977) from which the data can be expressed as a ratio of germ cells to Sertoli cells.

Germ cells, once committed to the spermatogenic process, rarely pause in their development but proceed at a predetermined rate until they are released as spermatozoa. Chemicals which affect spermatogenesis usually cause cells to degenerate along this pathway. Here degenerating cells are readily identified in plastic sections. The cytological characteristics allow the particular state of germ cell development at the time of germ cell arrest to be determined and this knowledge provides insight into the mechanism of action of a particular agent. This is possible since the processes taking place *in specific* germ cells at specific steps in their development are relatively well known. Degenerating cells may be quantitated in a similar way as described above for viable cells. More detailed information relating to quantitation of spermatogenesis and the general evaluation of the morphology of the testis has been provided (Russell, 1983).

Biochemical and cytogenetic assessment of spermatogenic cells

Studies of genetic toxicity and mutagens have become increasingly important in the toxicological evaluation of both drugs and environmental chemicals. Several short-term tests such as the inhibition of DNA synthesis (DSI), unscheduled DNA synthesis (UDS), determination of DNA breaks, chromosomal analysis of spermatogonia, spermatocytes, sperm and sister chromatid exchange (SCE) have been developed to identify genotoxins.

Inhibition of DNA, RNA and protein synthesis in spermatogenic cells have been used to determine cytotoxicity of various chemotherapeutic agents as well as environmental chemicals (Lee and Dixon, 1972a, 1973, 1978; Sieber and Adamson, 1975; Lucier *et al.*, 1977). Furthermore, inhibition of testicular DNA synthesis may be used as a preliminary screening assay for genetic toxicity (Friedman and Staub, 1976; Seiler, 1977; Lambert and Eriksson, 1979). However, inhibition of DNA synthesis can occur with non-chemical mutagens or carcinogens. Inhibition of DNA synthesis can occur indirectly, for example, via metabolic inhibition. (Werkheiser, 1963).

DNA damage is caused by chemical mutagens and carcinogens. Consequently, eukaryotic DNA damage leads to DNA strand breaks mediated by alkylation, inter- and intra-crosslinks on DNA strands, protein–DNA cross links, intercalation, formation of adducts, apurinic and apyrimidinic sites. Most of these primary lesions do not represent breakage in the DNA molecule. The lesions handled by the DNA repair enzymes and misrepair of DNA may result in chromosomal aberrations (Evans *et al.*, 1977). The regions can also disturb DNA synthesis in S-phase of the cell cycle and may cause misreplication. The induction of chromosomal aberration in germ cells by a test chemical is therefore considered as a reliable indication of mutagenic exposure. Although there is no absolute proof that DNA repair is directly involved in the production of chromosome breaks or SCE, the general consensus is that double-strand breaks are the basis of chromosome breaks. DNA repair can also change a single-strand break into a double-strand break causing chromosomal aberrations (Bender *et al.*, 1974, Painter, 1982). SCE represents interchange of DNA strands between replication products at homologous loci. SCE is detected in metaphase and is thought to involve DNA breakage and reunion. Biological significance is not known, however, SCE has been used extensively to evaluate potential mutagens (Allen and Latt, 1976; Latt *et al.*, 1982).

Therefore, DSI, UDS, detection of DNA breaks, chromosomal analysis and SCE in germ cells following exposure to test chemicals may serve as reliable screening tests for genotoxicants.

Experimental procedures

Determination of DNA, RNA, and protein synthesis in spermatogenic cells. The rate of spermatogenic cell DNA, RNA and protein synthesis can be measured at various times after the last dose of a test chemical (Lee and Dixon, 1972). Either ^{3}H- or ^{14}C-radiolabelled thymidine, uridine and L-leucine with high specific activities can be used. Incorporation of DNA, RNA and protein substrates into spermatogenic cells is determined 24 h after the treatment with radiolabelled substrate and then every 5 days thereafter for a total of 30 days or longer. The spermatogenic cells are separated by unit gravity sedimentation cell separation technique (Lam *et al.*, 1970; Lee and Dixon, 1972b; Meistrich, 1972; Preslow *et al.*, 1974; Romrell *et al.*, 1976). After the cell separation, the acid insoluble (5% trichloroacetic acid) fraction is subject to alkaline digestion at 60°C for 120 min. The radioactivity is then determined with a liquid-scintillation spectrometer (Lee and Dixon, 1972a). In addition, immediate and delayed effects of a test chemical on the spermatogenic cell DNA synthesis by the use of double labelling techniques can also be measured (Lambert and Ericksson, 1979). Acid-insoluble radioactivities can be expressed either per cell or per unit weight of DNA, RNA or protein respectively.

UDS measurement. UDS in mouse spermatogenic cells can be determined either *in vitro* or *in vivo* following exposure to a test chemical (Lee and Suzuki, 1981; Schmid *et al.*, 1978; Sega *et al.*, 1976), as described earlier in this chapter. Spermatogenic cells are isolated by digesting minced seminiferous tubules in CTC solution (collagenase-trypsin-chicken serum, 0.1:0.25:10%, w/v/v) for 17 min at 32°C. At the end of digesion, fetal calf serum is added to stop trypsin action. The suspension is then filtered through four layers of Kodak lens paper to remove tubular fragments. The filtrate is then centrifuged at $100\,g$ for 10 min. Spermatogenic cells are resuspended and loaded onto albumin gradient (3% in RPMI 1620 medium) and centrifuged at $20\,g$ for 10 min. The supernatant is decanted and the sedimented cells are resuspended in RPMI 1620 medium fortified with 10% calf serum and antibiotics. Hydroxyurea is added to the cell suspension to give a final concentration of $20\,mmol/10^{-6}$ spermatogenic cells. After 30 min incubation at 32°C, $0.4\,\mu Ci$ [^{3}H]thymidine (sp. activity: 40–60 Ci/mmol) is added and incubated for 1, 2 and 4 h. The reaction is stopped by the addition of unlabelled thymidine (1 nmol/ml) and 5×10^6 cells are immediately filtered (Celotate 25 mm, Millipore). The filter is washed with cold PBS containing unlabelled thymidine, precipitated with trichloroacetic acid (5%), and washed with ethanol and dried. The filters are digested with 0.5 ml of NCS solubilizer at 60°C in an oven for 2 h. The net UDS activity in spermatogenic cells are calculated as follows: Net UDS = Total DPM (MMS + HU) − DPM (HU control).

UDS activity in various stages of spermatogenic cells following chemical exposure can be monitored indirectly in ejaculated spermatozoa. Rabbits can be conveniently utilized for sperm collection using an artificial vagina.

At various times after treatment with test chemicals, $2\,\mu Ci$ of [^{3}H]thymidine is administered intratesticularly in $20\,\mu l$ volume. Sperm heads are isolated from the ejaculate (Lee *et al.*, 1977) and washed. Sperm heads ($10^7/ml$) are mixed with 1 ml of 1% sodium dodecyl sulphate solution containing 10 mmol/l dithiothreitol and incubated for 1 h at 37°C and radioactivity is determined in a liquid–scintillation spectrometer. Similar studies can also be done with rodents (Sega *et al.*, 1976).

Chromosomal analysis. Most of the cytogenetic studies on spermatocytes and spermatozoa are performed with mice (Hoo and Bowles, 1971; Adler, 1982; Leonard, 1975), the Chinese hamster (Kamiguci *et al.*, 1976) and man (Martin *et al.*, 1982; Yanagimachi *et al.*, 1976). At appropriate times after the treatment with a test chemical, chromosomes can be prepared from mitotic spermatogonia, meiotic spermatocytes and a mitotic single cell embryo by colchicine treatment of animals $3.5 - 5\,h$ prior to sampling of testes or collection of one cell embryo from oviducts. Colchicine is given at 4 mg/kg for mice and rats and 10 mg/kg for Chinese hamsters. Testes are removed from the animal, decapsulated and placed in a vial containing sodium citrate for 20 min. The washed tubules are immersed in cold fixative (glacial acetic acid–methanol, 1:3, v/v) which is changed after 10 min. The fixed tubules are transferred to a centrifuge tube containing 5 ml of 50% acetic acid and pipetted vigorously until the cells are released from the tubules. The cell suspension is centrifuged at 1500 r.p.m. for 10 min; 0.5–3 ml of fixative is added and cells are resuspended. Three to four drops of the cell suspension are placed on the alcohol (70%)-wet slides and flame dried. Slides are stained in 5% Giemsa solution at pH 6.8 for 10 min, rinsed in acetone, acetone–xylene (1:1, v/v) and xylene before mounting. The spermatocyte preparation is stained in 2% orcein (50% acetic acid) for 30 min, in 70% ethanol for 30 s, dried in 90% and 98% ethanol, and rinsed in xylene before mounting.

Direct chromosomal analysis of sperm is not possible and, therefore, males treated with a test chemical are mated with syngeneic females and male sperm chromosomes are observed in one-cell embryos at metaphase, in which female chromosomes may be simultaneously observed. A new technique has been developed to avoid dispersion, overlap and loss of sperm–egg chromosomes due to sudden rupture of the cell membrane (Kamiguchi *et al.*, 1976). One-cell embryos from either mouse or Chinese hamster are recovered from the ampulla region of oviducts and denuded with 0.5% trypsin in phosphate-buffered saline for 1.5 min. The denuded embryos are subjected to 30% calf serum for 60 min at 37°C. This long duration of hypotonic treatment is important for disintegration of the intracellular spindles and microtubules and allows chromosomes to be dispersed within the ooplasm. The denuded embryo is placed in a solution of methanol–glacial acetic acid–water (5:1:4, by vol.) for 5 min to dissolve the zona pellucida. The embryo is gently pipetted into a Spemann pipette and then released onto a glass slide. While the fixative spreads, a single–cell embryo sticks to the slide near the tip of the pipette. The slide is immediately placed in a jar containing the same fixative for at least 20 min. Subsequently, the slide is dipped into another fixative containing absolute methanol–glacial acetic acid-distilled water (3:3:1, by vol.). Adequate humidity in the air is essential for even spreading of chromosomes within the ooplasm of embryo.

SCE. Male mice, 3–5 months of age are given 0.2 ml of 14 hourly injections of 10 mmol/l BrdU in 5 mmol/l deoxycytidine (or a 50 mg BrdU tablet can be implanted in the abdominal cavity). The use of the deoxynucleoside is to replenish the nucleoside pool *in vivo* to reduce BrdU toxicity. Spermatogonial, or meiotic spermatocytes are prepared at 3–19 h, 6-72 h or 3-15 day, respectively, following the last administration of BrdU. The optimum yield of second division spermatogonial cells for SCE analysis is carried out as a function of time after test compound treatment (e.g. 32 h after the treatment with the chemical). Spermatogonial cell chromosomes are prepared according to the method of Meredith (1969). Seminiferous tubules are prepared in sodium citrate solution as described above. The fixed tubular fragments are resuspended in a small volume of 60% glacial acetic acid, and the suspension is flushed with a siliconized Pasteur pipette in order to release cells from the tubules. Spermatogonial cells are applied dropwise to prewarmed (60°C) slides. Meiotic chromosomes are prepared according to the method of Evans *et al.* (1964). Seminiferous tubules are dissected out and immersed in isotonic sodium citrate solution. A tubule is held with a forcep at one end and gently squeezed over the entire length with another pair of forceps in isotonic sodium citrate solution. After approximately 10 min, the dispersed meiotic spermatocytes are centrifuged and dispersed gently. Approximately 2 ml of hypotonic 1% sodium citrate is added and permitted to stand for 10 to 12 min. Spermatocytes are then fixed at least twice in acetic-methanol (1:3, v/v) solution and applied dropwise to a clean slide at room temperature. Slides are stained with 0.5 µg/ml 33258 Hoechst (Latt, 1973). Slides are examined directly by fluorescence microscopy.

Physiological assessment of testicular function

Leydig cell function

Leydig cells are the source of testicular testosterone which regulates spermatogenesis, epididymal sperm maturation, accessory sex organ development and function and regulates sexual behaviour in adults. The steroidogenic function of Leydig cells has been thoroughly reviewed previously (Christiansen, 1975; Christiansen and Gillim, 1969; Hall, 1970; Ewing and Brown, 1977). Thus, environmental chemicals that may inhibit testosterone biosynthesis and/or secretion or alter LH receptors may have profound detrimental effects on the complex processes of generating functional spermatozoa and maintaining a functional male reproductive system. Although the *in vivo* assessment of Leydig cell function is difficult, *in vitro* testicular perfusion technique has been perfected to a point where it clearly mimics *in situ* testosterone secretion and determines the site of inhibition of androgen biosynthetic pathways (Ewing et al., 1981). In addition, the nature of xenobiotic metabolism in Leydig cells can be determined using the isolated perfused testis (Lee and Nagayama, 1980).

Experimental procedure

The perfusion technique was described originally by Van Demark and Ewing (1963) and Ewing et al. (1975) and modified by Lee and Nagayama in 1980. Adult rats weighing 250–300 g are killed by cervical dislocation. The testes are immediately removed and placed in a prechilled beaker containing 0.15 mol/l phosphate–buffered saline (pH 7.4). This procedure is necessary to prevent thrombi and to minimize cellular damage. The testis is placed under a stereomicroscope, and the testicular artery is cannulated through a small incision with a 80 μm tip glass capillary which is secured with a silk suture. This procedure takes approximately 5 min for each testis. The isolated testis is then placed in a perfusion chamber with a constant temperature of $32 \pm 0.5°C$ which was designed and constructed at the National Institute of Environmental Health Science. The testis is perfused with an oxygenated Krebs–Ringer bicarbonate solution containing bovine serum albumin fraction V (3%), glucose (100 mg%) and either rat washed red blood cells (Hct 25) or Oxypherol (GCC-3012) synthetic O_2 carrier (Alpha Therapeutic Corporation, 5555 Valley Blvd, Los Angeles, CA). The testis is perfused with this medium at a flow rate at $13.3 \, ml \, g^{-1} \, h^{-1}$ in a humidified perfusion chamber using an Ismatiec GJ-4, a multichannel pulse-free precision pump (Ismatec, Zurich, Switzerland). Ovine LH-S19 (NIH) is infused into the arterial cannula to achieve a final concentration of LH at 10 and 100 ng/ml of perfusion medium, respectively. These LH concentrations are necessary to achieve the maximal rate of testosterone secretion. The pH of the perfusion medium is maintained at 7.4 by exposing the medium to a gas mixture (O_2/CO_2, 95:5). In each experiment, 6 to 8 testes can be perfused simultaneously, and the effluent is collected at the desired time interval to determine the rate of steroid metabolism and secretion. Either steroid metabolites or xenobiotic metabolites can be isolated from the effluent medium and subjected to quantitative and qualitative analysis, using gas chromatography, high performance liquid chromatography or GC–mass spectrometry (Ewing *et al.*, 1975; Chubb and Ewing, 1981; Lee *et al.*, 1980, 1983).

Blood–testis barrier

Physiological evidence for the existence of a blood–testis barrier (BTB) has been clearly demonstrated previously (Setchell *et al.*, 1969, Setchell and Waites, 1970; Tuck *et al.*, 1970; Okumura *et al.*, 1975; Dixon and Lee, 1980; Hinton and Howards, 1982). These studies demonstrated that the BTB excluded immunoglobulins, albumin, inulin and other chemicals from the seminiferous tubules and suggested the existence of a barrier protecting the seminiferous tubules. Permeability studies with non-electrolytes with various molecular sizes, barbiturates with various lipid solubilities and sulphonamides with various pK_a values demonstrated that the major transport process of chemicals across the BTB depends on their lipid solubility and molecular size. Transfer rates of all chemicals tested correlated well with partition coefficients and, in general, obeyed simple diffusion kinetics. Thus, the rates of permeability into seminiferous tubules can now be predicted on the basis of partition coefficients. Therefore, the transport rate of a chemical can now be predicted and transport rate constants may be used as an indicator for testicular damage since the BTB is apparently a complex multicellular system composed of both myoid cells surrounding the seminiferous tubules and several highly organized layers of spermatogenic cells within the tubules. This system restricts the permeability of many foreign and endogenous macromolecules to male germ cells.

Experimental procedures

Eighteen to 20 h before cannulation of the rete testis, rats are anaesthetized with ether, abdominal incisions are made and the efferent ducts are ligated. This procedure is necessary to facilitate the cannulation of the rete testis for the collection of fluid. It has been reported that the ligation (24 h) of the efferent ducts has little effect on capillary blood flow or permeability as assessed by studies of testicular vascular function (Setchell and Waites, 1970). Ligation of efferent ducts for as long as 30 h failed to alter the rate of rete testis fluid secretion (Setchell, 1970; Tuck *et al.*, 1970). Animals are anaesthetized with Inactin (100 mg/kg body weight, Henley, Inc., New York, NY), and the testis and epididymis are exposed through a scrotal incision and positioned. A 32-gauge needle is inserted through the tunica albuginea at the side of the avascular area of the testis and is advanced until the tip of the needle penetrates the rete testis. After removal of the needle, polyethylene tubing (PE-10, o.d 0.024 in and i.d. 0.011 in from Clay Adams, Parsippany, NJ) with a sharp tip is inserted into the same hole and passed into the punctured rete testis. Instantaneous adhesive (Eastman 910 from Eastman Kodak Co., Rochester, NY) is used to seal the area around the point of insertion to secure the tubing. During the collection period, rats are kept warm under a heat lamp and the testes are moistened continuously with saline. A stable flow rate of rete testis fluid ranging from 30 to $90 \mu l h^{-1}$ testis^{-1} is achieved 60-90 min after cannulation. Plasma concentrations of chemicals should be maintained by a suitable combination of priming injections and continuous i.v. infusion using an infusion pump (e.g. Harvard pump). Transport rate is derived from $K = -1/t$. In (Cp-Crtf/Cp), where Cp is unbound plasma concentration of a chemical, and Crtf is unbound chemical concentration in rete-testis fluid. When In (Cp-Crtf/Cp) is plotted against time, a straight line is achieved and the slope represents the transfer rate constant.

Analysis of sperm

One of the important assessements of testicular function and male fertility is to determine sperm counts in the testis, epididymis and ejaculated semen. Sperm counts in the male reproductive tract reflect the normalcy of testicular function, as sperm production is the end-product of spermatogenesis. Sperm production is influenced by nutritional and hormonal status, age, drugs and environmental chemicals. Sperm motility and morphology also reflect the normalcy of sperm metabolism and spermatogenesis, respectively. Therefore, reduced numbers of motile sperm and increased numbers of misshapen sperm morphology indicate both cytotoxicity and genotoxicity (Katz and Overstreet, 1981; Overstreet *et al.*, 1979; MacLoed and Gold, 1951; Belsey *et al.*, 1980; Eliasson, 1975). Furthermore, *in vitro* fertilization tests also encompass epididymal function.

In recent years, *in vitro* fertilization techniques utilizing mice, rats, hamsters and rabbits have led, to an increased understanding of the basic biological mechanisms of fertilization. These advances also make it possible to study the effects of environmental chemicals on fertilization processes *in vitro*. Indeed, there is growing evidence from animal studies that certain chemicals may inhibit the fertilizing ability of sperm with no marked effects on any of the semen criteria (Tsunoda and Chang, 1976; Carroll and Levitan, 1978). With *in vitro* fertilization methods, it is now possible to identify chemicals which affect sperm. *In vitro* fertilization can also be coupled with preimplantation embryo culture, the transfer of blastocysts to pseudopregnant recipients and the evaluation of pregnancy outcome to identify critical developmental targets of environmental chemicals. Male and female germ cells can be exposed to environmental chemicals either *in vitro* or *in vivo* and can then be used for *in vitro* fertilization. In an attempt to evaluate human sperm with respect to fertilizability and the state of sperm chromosomes, human sperm penetration of zona free hamster eggs has been studied (Hall, 1981; Yanagimachi *et al.*, 1976; Rogers *et al.*, 1979). This *in vitro* method should be useful in determining how the chemicals interfere with the events surrounding fertilization and in identifying those potentially toxic chemicals which may affect human sperm. Human sperm chromosome studies were possible using the human sperm denuded-hamster egg test system which was discussed earlier in the chapter (Yanagimachi *et al.*, 1976; Martin *et al.*, 1982).

Therefore, sperm counts, morphology and *in vitro* fertilization tests are all important test systems towards assessing spermatogenesis and epididymal function.

Experimental procedures

Sperm counts. Sperm enumeration methods from testis, epididymis, vas deferens and ejaculated semen have been published (Robb *et al.*, 1978; Amann *et al.*, 1974; Johnson *et al.*, 1981). However, these methods have recently been modified to improve consistency. Following treatment with test chemicals, mice or rats are killed and the testes and epididymides are removed and weighed. The tunica albuginea is removed and the bundles of seminiferous tubules are minced in a 20 ml capacity vial containing 5 ml of CTC (collagenase–trypsin–chicken serum, 0.2%:0.2%:10%, w/v/v) in phosphate-buffered saline (PBS) (pH 7.4). After mincing, an additional 5 ml of CTC solution is added to the vial. Caput plus corpus, and cauda epididymides are also placed in a vial containing 5 ml CTC solution and minced

Table 15.2 Recovery of sperm numbers in testes, caput plus corpus epididymides and cauda epididymides*

Methods†	Testis	Caput and corpus (10⁸ SPZ/g testis)	Cauda
Homogenization	0.17 ± 0.01 (37)	4.75 ± 0.58 (20)	10.6 ± 0.94 (20)
Homogenization + CTC	0.87 ± 0.015 (26)‡	5.62 ± 0.26 (20)‡	11.28 ± 1.08 (20)
CTC + homogenization	1.38 ± 0.05 (11)‡	6.38 ± 0.21 (17)‡	11.74 ± 0.88 (17)

* Mean ± SE; the numbers in the parentheses represent the number of animals
† Sperm isolation methods refer to the method of sperm isolation in p 211
‡ Significantly different from that of the homogenization method (Robb *et al.*, 1978) at $p < 0.01$–0.05

with scissors. At the end of mincing, an additional 5 ml of CTC solution is added to each vial. Vials are then incubated at room temperature for 3–4 h at 400 r.p.m. At the end of CTC digestion, the contents are homogenized with an equal volume of 0.15 mol/l KCl in 10 mmol/l Hepes (4-2-hydroxyethyl-1-piperazine-ethanesulphonic acid, pH 7.4) containing 0.3 mol/l $MgCl_2$, 0.05% sodium azide and Triton X-100 (0.5%) for 2 min at 10 000 r.p.m. using a semimicro-Eberbach homogenizer. The sperm suspension is mixed well and sperm heads are enumerated using a Makler counting chamber. CTC digestion of caput and corpus epididymal fragments are necessary to inhibit agglutination of sperm with epididymal epithelial cells and to give more reproducible sperm counts. The typical distribution of sperm counts in adult Sprague–Dawley rats is shown in Table 15.2. Studies with chemotherapeutic agents demonstrated that antispermatogenic effects and sperm counts are best correlated with either testicular or caput epididymal sperm numbers whereas that of cauda epididymides showed the least correlation (Bechter *et al.*, 1983).

Sperm morphology. Thirty five days following treatment of adult mice with test chemicals, animals are killed to collect cauda epididymal sperm by mincing cauda epididymis in a Petri dish containing PBS and pipetted vigorously several times to obtain enough sperm (these sperm correspond to the late spermatogonial cells at the time of treatment). The cell suspension is transferred to a test-tube and stored at 4°C until examination. The sample can be kept in this condition for more than 24 h. The cell suspension is then stained with 0.1% eosin-Y and smeared on the slide and sealed with a cover slip. Spermatozoa are examined at 400 or 1000 times magnification using bright field with a green filter (Mori, 1961; Krzanowska, 1971; Wyrobek and Bruce, 1978). Criteria for morphological abnormality of mouse sperm based on various shape changes as compared to that of control can be easily scored (Wyrobek and Bruce, 1978).

In vitro fertilization. Cauda epididymides are dissected from selected laboratory animals, and 1-2 cm long tubules are carefully teased out under a stereomicroscope (× 60 magnification). Tubular segments are transferred to a Petri dish containing modified Tyrode's solution containing 154 μmol/l pyruvate and 1% bovine serum albumin (BSA) in 100 ml of the medium. Cauda epididymal sperm are released from the tubules by gently pressing from one end of tubule over the entire length of the tubule with a bent forcep under a stereomicroscope. Sperm suspension is then transferred to a Petri dish containing 1 ml of the medium under paraffin oil equilibrated with 5% CO_2-air. The Petri dish is then placed on a warm plate (30°C) and covered with an inverted glass funnel connected to a 5% CO_2-air supply. The pH of the medium should be maintained between 7.2 and 7.4. After 20 min, the sperm suspension is further diluted with modified Tyrode's solution to give $1-2 \times 10^6$ sperm/ml. The final sperm suspension is transferred to a jar, constantly gassed with 5% CO_2-air, and maintained at 37°C for 1 h for sperm capacitation. Adult females, usually female mice, are superovulated by treating the animals with 10 IU PMSG and 10 IU hCG intraperitoneally 48 h apart. The animals are killed 12-14 h after the hCG treatment. Ova are flushed from ampulla of the oviduct with a blunt 30 gauge needle attached to a 10 ml syringe containing modified Tyrode's solution at 23-25°C. Collected ova are treated with 0.1% hyaluronidase in the medium. Cumulus and corona cells are removed within 15 min, and the ova are then washed twice in fresh medium and 20 ova are added to the dish containing capacitated sperm under oil and constantly gassed with 5% CO_2-air in a jar at 37°C.

The fertilization process is allowed to proceed for 5 h prior to examination for fertilization. Further details of *in vitro* fertilization of human and laboratory animals have been described previously by many investigators (Miyamoto and Chang, 1972; Kaufman, 1973; Pavlok and McLaren, 1972; Fraser and Drury, 1975; Martin *et al.*, 1982).

Serial mating, dominant lethality and multigeneration studies

The serial mating technique using experimental mice (Hershberger *et al.*, 1969) and rats (Jackson *et al.*, 1961) assesses the biological function of spermatozoa and produces fertility patterns which are inversely related in time to the phase of spermatogenesis damaged by the test chemicals. For example, toxic effects on spermatozoa appear first and those due to interference with spermatogonia and stem cells appear last. The successful application of this method depends upon the fact that in the mouse and rat, spermatogenesis and spermiation proceed continuously without regard to frequency of mating. Chemical treatment does not affect libido and the capacity to copulate. Thus, the relationship between the fertility and the type of spermatogenic stage affected by the test chemical can be readily estimated. In addition, this technique is convenient in assaying dominant lethal mutations in mice or rats. Dominant lethal mutations are useful indicators of major genetic damage which have been used to measure effects of chemical mutagens in experimental animals (Bateman, 1960; Cattanach et al., 1968; Ehling et al., 1968; Epstein and Shafner, 1968; Generoso, 1969; Rohrborn, 1968). Dominant lethal mutation data in experimental animals may appropriately be extrapolated to man, as most human mutations are due to dominant autosomal traits. The genetic basis for dominant lethality is the induction of chromosomal damage and rearrangements, such as translocations by chemical mutagens, resulting in non-viable embryos.

In multigeneration reproduction studies with mice and rats, experiments are designed to assess the effects of chronic exposure to low levels of a test chemical on the reproductive capacity of the parents and on the growth, survival and reproductive capacity of the progeny. Some experiments may begin at the time of organogenesis (during pregnancy) to include effects of chemicals on organ differentiation and development.

Experimental procedures

Male fertility and dominant lethality in rodents can be assayed following acute, subacute, or chronic administration of test chemicals, either orally or via any parenteral route, including inhalation, with a highest non-toxic dose.

Each dose level should have 10 to 20 mature adult male mice or rats of a highly fertile strain of 8–10 weeks of age for the serial mating or dominant lethal studies. Special inbred strains of mice or rats may be chosen for special objectives in mutagenicity testing. Before treatment of test chemicals, each male animal is permanently marked and housed with a single virgin female for a period of 7 days. This duration ensures that the female animal would experience at least one oestrous cycle. Female is examined for vaginal plug or vaginal sperm to ensure that either a test chemical or other factors did not interfere with either ejaculation, mating capability or libido. After 7 days, the female animals are removed from the males and replaced with a virgin female. Pretreatment mating studies are carried out for 2–3 weeks to establish reproductive capacity of each male prior to treatment. At the end of the pretreatment mating period, a test chemical is administered at a dose equal to or less than the LD_{10} dose as a preliminary study and males are allowed to mate serially for 10 weeks. Nine days after removal of females from males, the female animals are killed to enumerate total implants, dead implants, resorption sites and corpora lutea. Early resorption sites can be conveniently identified by immersion of uteri in 10% ammonium sulphide solution for 15 min. Ambiguous resorption sites can now become visible as black spots. The test can be considerably modified and simplified to make it more suitable for routine practice by omitting corpora lutea counts which are notoriously laborious and inaccurate in rodents. Preimplantation loss can be assessed indirectly by the ratio of total number of implants in test animals to those in controls. Thus, dominant lethal mutations are measured directly by enumeration of early fetal deaths and indirectly by preimplantation losses, as measured by reduction in the

Table 15.3 Duration in days of stages of spermatogenic cycle, and ductular transit time

Spermatogenic phases	Mouse	Rat	Man
Mitotic Phase	6	7	8
Meiotic phase	12.7	14.9	23.2
Spermiogenic phase	14	20.6	23.0
Seminiferous epithelial cycle	8.7	12.9	16.0
Ductular transit time	8	14	21

From Jackson (1966); Oakberg and DiMinno (1960); Rowley *et al.* (1970)

number of total implants in the test compared with controls. Also the serial mating technique allows determination of effects of chemicals on pregnancy rates. Fertility or dominant lethal profiles can be drawn from these data. The ordinate expresses either the percentage of the males determined to be fertile or the percentage of dead implants as function of the days long enough to encompass the entire duration of spermatogenesis (Jackson *et al.*, 1961; Hershberger *et al.*, 1969; Lee and Dixon, 1972a, 1973; Lee *et al.*, 1978; Epstein and Shafner, 1968; Ehling *et al.*, 1968). The duration of various stages of spermatogenesis in mice, rat and man are shown in Table 15.3.

For multigeration studies, it is very common to use three generation studies. In this assay, groups of test animals (usually rats) are exposed to the test chemical, usually in the diet or in drinking water, continuously through three generations. A typical scheme for such study is shown in Fig. 15.1. The purpose of conducting the study for more than one generation is

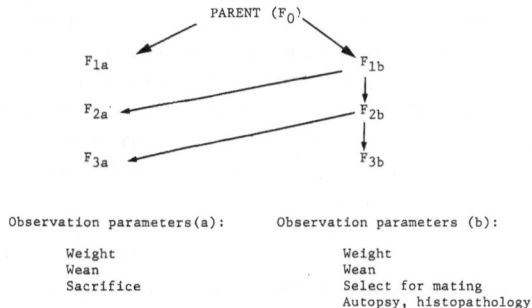

Fig. 15.1 Scheme for a three generation reproduction study

to test for cumulative and comprehensive mutagenic and toxic effects. Mutagenic and toxic effects may be detected in the second and third generation, although the system is now regarded as insensitive for mutagenicity (USFDA, 1970).

The parent animals (F_0) for three generation studies consist of at least 10 males and 10 females per dose group. After two matings, producing F_{1a} and F_{1b} generations, the parents are used for other end-point measurements. The F_{1a} generation is killed and autopsied at weaning. The F_{1b} generation is also killed, except for 10 males and 10 females taken at random from each group. These animals are mated twice to produce the F_{2a} and F_{2b} generations and are then killed and autopsied. The procedure followed with the F_2 generations is the same as that for the F_1 groups. The resulting F_{3a} and F_{3b} generations are killed and autopsied at weaning and examined histopathologically. Detailed protocol for multigeneration studies have been reported previously (USFDA, 1970; Wills *et al.*, 1981; Truhaut *et al.*, 1979; Groot *et al.*, 1974). A distinct advantage of the three generation test is that it gives an overall view of reproductive function which is not achieved by a single specific test. A one-generation reproduction study gives information on the fertility and pregnancy rates of the first parental generation (F_0) only. Observations of the F_1 generation would determine the effects of a test chemical on the uterine environment and on lactation, as well as on postweaning growth and development. The F_1 generation which have been exposed continuously to a test chemical from the time of conception could reveal changes during the periods of organogenesis and neonatal and postnatal development of reproductive systems. The accumulation of a potentially toxic chemical would be determined by the reproductive performance of the F_1 generation and by observation of the growth and development of the F_2 generation. F_2 generation reproductive studies are performed to determine if any effect would manifest itself in a F_3 generation which did not appear in an earlier generation.

CONCLUDING REMARKS

In this chapter, an attempt has been made to review and present some of the methodology used to assess male reproductive toxicity. An ultimate objective of laboratory testing is to extrapolate the animal data to man accurately to predict human reproductive risk. However, male reproductive processes are biologically complex and as a consequence, current reproductive test systems, especially *in vitro* testing, are inexact. Extrapolation of such data to man may be uncertain. Therefore, there is a greater need for the acquisition of comparative pharmacokinetic and pharmacodynamic factors toward various classes of toxic chemicals in animal species and man. Such information is necessary in order to select and design test systems that will best serve to predict human reproductive risks. In contrast to the *in vitro* test systems, *in vivo* serial mating and multigeneration studies, along with morphological evaluation are the simplest and most useful approaches towards assessing the overall functions of the male reproductive system.

Rapid research advances in molecular biology, biochemistry, physiology and other related basic areas will not only aid in clarifying male reproductive processes, but more reliable and relevant reproductive toxicity tests will result and prevail.

References

Adler, I.D. (1982). Male germ cell cytogenetics. In Hsu, T.C. (ed.) *Cytogenetic Assay of Environmental Mutagens* pp. 249–276 (Totowa, NJ: Allenheld, Osmun Publishers)

Allen J.W. and Latt, S.A. (1976). *In vivo* BrdU-33258 Hoechst analysis of DNA replication kinetics and sister chromatid exchange formation in mouse somatic and meiotic cells. *Chromosoma*, **58**, 325–40

Amann, R.P., Kavanaugh, J.F., Griel, L.C. Jr. and Voglmayr, T.K. (1974). Sperm production of Holstein bulls determined from testicular spermatid reserves after cannulation of rete testis or vas deferens and by daily ejaculation. *J. Dairy Sci.*, **57**, 93–9

Bateman, A.J. (1960). The induction of dominant lethal mutations in rats and mice with triethylenemelamine (TEM). *Genet. Res.*, **1**, 381–92

Bechter, R., Lee, I.P., Ettlin, R.A. and Dixon, R.L. (1984). Assessment of testicular toxicity associated with procarbazine: A multidisciplinary approach. *Toxicol. Appl. Pharmacol.* (in press)

Belsey, M.A., Eliasson, R., Gallegos, A.J., Moghissi, K.S., Paulsen, C.A. and Pradad, M.R.N. (1980). *Laboratory Manual for the Examination of Human Semen and Semen-cervical Mucus Interaction*, pp. 1–43 (Singapore: Press Concern)

Bender, M.A., Griggs, H.G. and Bedford, J.S. (1974). Mechanism of chromosomal aberration production III. Chemical and ionizing radiation. *Mutat. Res.*, **23**, 197–212

Carroll, E.J. and Levitan, H. (1978). Fertilization in the sea urchin, *Strongylocentratus purpuratus* is blocked by fluorescein dyes. *Dev. Biol.*, **63**, 432–40

Cattanach, B.M., Pollard, C.E. and Isaacson, J.H. (1968). The effects of cytoxan on the chromosomes of mouse bone marrow. *Mutat. Res.*, **8**, 623–8

Christiansen, A.K. (1975). Leydig cells. In Greep, R.O. and Astwood, E.B. (eds.) *Handbook of Physiology*, Vol. 7, Pt. 1, pp. 57–94 (Washington: American Physiological Society)

Christiansen, A.K. and Gillim, S.W. (1969). The correlation of fine structure and function in steroid-secreting cells, with emphasis on those of the gonads. In McKerns, K.W. (ed.) *The Gonads*, pp. 415–488 (New York: Appleton-Century-Crofts)

Chubb, C. and Ewing, L.L. (1981). Steroid secretion by sexually immature rat and rabbit testes perfused *in vitro. Endocrinology*, **109**, 1999–2015

Dixon R.L. and Lee, I.P. (1980). Pharmacokinetic and adaptation factors in testicular toxicity. *Fed. Proc.*, **39**, 66–72

Dougherty, R.C., Whitaker, M.J., Tang, S.Y., Bottcher, R., Keller, M. and Kuel, D.W. (1981). Sperm density and toxic substances: A potential key to identification of environmental health hazards. In McKinney, J.D. (ed.) *The Chemistry of Environmental Agents as Potential Human Hazards*, pp. 263–278 (Ann Arbor, MI: Ann Arbor Sci. Publishers)

Ehling, U.H., Cumming, R.B. and Malling, H.V. (1968). Induction of dominant lethal mutations by alkylating agents in male mice. *Mutat. Res.*, **5**, 417–28

Eliasson, R. (1975). Analysis of semen. In Behman, S.J. and Kistnes, R.W. (eds.) *Progress in Infertility*, pp. 691–713 (Boston: Little Brown)

Epstein, S. and Shafner, H. (1968). Chemical mutagens in the human environment. *Nature (Lond.)*, **219**, 385–7

Evans, E.P., Breckon, G. and Ford, C.E. (1964). An air-drying method for meiotic preparations from mammalian testes. *Cytogenetics*, **3**, 289–94

Evans, L.A., Kevin, M.J. and Jenkins, E.C. (1977). Human sister chromatid exchange caused by methylazoxymethanol acetate. *Mutat. Res.*, **56**, 51–8

Ewing, L.L. and Brown, B.L. (1977). Testicular steroidogenesis. In Johnson, A.J., Gomes, W.R. and Van Demark, N.L. (eds.) *The Testis*, Vol. 4, pp. 239–87 (N.Y.: Academic Press)

Ewing, L.L., Brown, B.L., Irby, D.C. and Hardines, I. (1975). Testosterone and 5α-reduced androgen secretion by rabbit testis-epididymides perfused *in vitro. Endocrinology*, **96**, 610–17

MALE FERTILITY AND ITS REGULATION

Ewing, L.L., Davis, J.C. and Zirkin, B.R. (1980). Regulation of testicular function: A spatial and temporal view. In Greep, R.O. (ed.) *Reproductive Physiology III*, Vol. 22, pp. 41-115 (Baltimore: University Park)

Ewing, L.L., Zirkin, B.R. and Chubb, C. (1981). Assessment of testicular testosterone production and Leydig cell structure. *Environ. Health Pers.*, **38**, 19-27

Fabro, S. (1983). Reproductive toxicology: State of the art, 1982. *Am. J. Ind. Med.*, **4**, 391-3

Fraser, L.R. and Drury, L.M. (1975). The relationship between sperm concentration and fertilization *in vitro* of mouse eggs. *Biol. Reprod.*, **13**, 513-18

Friedman, M.A. and Staub, J. (1976). Inhibition of mouse testicular DNA synthesis by mutagens and carcinogens as a potential simple mammalian assay for mutagenesis. *Mutat. Res.*, **37**, 67-76

Generoso, W.M. (1969). Chemical induction of dominant lethals in female mice. *Genetics*, **61**, 461-70

Groot, A.P., Til, H.P. and Feron, V.J. (1974). Two-year feeding and multigeneration studies in rats on five chemically modified starches. *Food Cosmet. Toxicol.*, **12**, 651-63

Hall, J. (1981). Relationship between semen quality and human sperm penetration of zona-free hamster ova. *Fertil. Steril.*, **35**, 457-63

Hall, P.F. (1970). Endocrinology of the testis. In Johnson, A.J., Gomes, W.R. and VanDemark, N.L. (eds.) *The Testis*, Vol. 2, pp. 1-72 (New York: Academic Press)

Hershberger, L.G., Hansen, D.M. and Hansen, L.M. (1969). Effects of antifertility agents on male mice, as determined by a serial mating method. *Proc. Soc. Exp. Biol. Med.*, **131**, 667-72

Hinton, B.T. and Howards, S.S. (1982). Micropuncture and microperfusion techniques for the study of testicular physiology. *Ann. New York Acad. Sci.*, **383**, 29-43

Hoo, S.S. and Bowles, B. (1971). An air-drying method for preparing metaphase chromosome from the spermatogonial cells of rats and mice. *Mutat. Res.*, **13**, 85-8

Jackson, H. (1966). In Jackson, H. (ed.) *Antifertility Compounds in the Male and Female, Spermatogenesis*, pp. 5-20 (Springfield: Charles C. Thomas)

Jackson, H., Fox, B.W. and Craig, A.W. (1961). Antifertility substances and their assessment in the male rodent. *J. Reprod. Fertil.*, **2**, 447-65

Johnson, L., Petty, C.S. and Neaves, W.B. (1981). A new approach to quantification of spermatogenesis and its application to germinal cell attrition during human spermiogenesis. *Biol. Reprod.*, **25**, 217-26

Kamiguchi, Y., Funaki, K. and Mikamo, K. (1976). A new technique for chromosome study of murine oocytes. *Proc. J. Acad.*, **52**, 316-19

Katz, D.F. and Overstreet, J.W. (1981). Sperm motility assessment by videomicrography. *Fertil. Steril.*, **35**, 188-93

Kaufman, M. (1973). Timing of the first cleavage division of the mouse and the duration of its component stages: a study of living and fixed eggs. *J. Cell Sci.*, **12**, 799-808

Krzanowska, H. (1971). Influence of Y chromosome on fertility in mice. In Beattey, R.A. and Glue cksohn-Waelsch, S. (eds.) *The Genetics of the Spermatozoon: Proc. International Symp.*, Edinburgh, UK, pp. 370-386, Department of Genetics, University of Edinburgh

Lam, D.M.K., Furrer, R. and Bruce, W.R. (1970). The separation, physical characterization and differentiation kinetics of spermatogonial cells of the mouse. *Proc. Natl. Acad. Sci. USA*, **65**, 192-9

Lambert, B. and Eriksson, G. (1979). Effects of cancer chemotherapeutic agents on testicular DNA synthesis in the rat. *Mutat. Res.*, **68**, 275-89

Latt, S.A. (1973). Microfluorometric analysis of deoxyribonucleic acid replication kinetics and sister chromatid exchanges in human chromosomes. *J. Hist. Chem. Cytochem.*, **22**, 478-91

Latt, S.A., Schreck, R.R., Loveday, K.S. and Shuler, C.F. (1982). Sister chromatid exchange analysis: Methodology, application, and interpretation. In Hsu, T.C. (ed.) *Cytogenetic Assay of Environmental Mutagens*, pp. 29-80 (Totowa: Allanheld, Osmun Publishers)

Leblond, C.P. and Clermont, Y. (1952). Definition of the stage of the cycle of the seminiferous epithelium in the rat. *Ann. NY Acad. Sci.*, **55**, 548-73

Lee, I.P. and Dixon, R.L. (1972a). Antineoplastic drug effects on spermatogenesis studied by velocity sedimentation cell separation. *Toxicol. Appl. Pharmacol.*, **23**, 20-41

Lee, I.P. and Dixon, R.L. (1972b). Effects of procarbazine on spermatogenesis determined by velocity sedimentation cell separation technique and serial mating. *J. Pharmacol. Exp. Ther.*, **181**, 219-26

Lee, I.P. and Dixon, R.L. (1973). Effects of cadmium on spermatogenesis studied by velocity sedimentation cell separation and serial mating. *J. Pharmacol. Exp. Ther.*, **187**, 641-52

Lee, I.P., Mukhtar, H., Suzuki, K. and Bend, J.R. (1983). Metabolism of benzo(a)pyrene 4,5-oxide by isolated perfused rat testis. *Biochem. Pharmacol.*, **32**, 159-61

Lee, I.P. and Nagayama, J. (1980). Metabolism of benzo(a)pyrene by the isolated perfused rat testis. *Cancer Res.*, **40**, 3297-303

Lee, I.P., Schmid, B. and Zbinden, G. (1977). A simplified method for the isolation of sperm heads from the caput epididymis of rodents and from ejaculated rabbit seminal plasma. *Exp. Cell Biol.*, **45**, 48-59

Lee, I.P., Sherins, R.J. and Dixon, R.L. (1978). Evidence for induction of germinal aplasia in male rats by environmental exposure to boron. *Toxicol. Appl. Pharmacol.*, **45**, 577-90

Lee, I.P. and Suzuki, K. (1981). Strain difference in DNA repair activity in prespermiogenic cells of CD-1 mice. *Mutat. Res.*, **80**, 201-11

Leonard, A. (1975). Tests for heritable translocations in male mammals. *Mutat. Res.*, **31**, 291-8

Lucier, G.W., Lee, I.P. and Dixon, R.L. (1977). Effects of environmental agents on male reproduction. In Gomes, W.R. (ed.) *The Testis*, pp. 578-604 (New York: Academic Press)

Macleod, J. and Gold, R.Z. (1951). The male factor in fertility and infertility. II. Spermatozoan counts in 1000 men of known fertility and in 1000 cases of infertile marriage. *J. Urol.*, **66**, 436-49

MacLeod, J. and Wang, Y. (1979). Male fertility potential in terms of semen quality: A review of the past and a study of the present. *Fertil. Steril.*, **31**, 103-16

Martin, R.H., Lin, C.C., Balkan, W. and Burns, K. (1982). Direct chromosomal analysis of human spermatozoa: Preliminary results from 18 normal men. *Am. J. Human Genet.*, **34**, 459-68

Meistrich, M.L. (1972). Separation of mouse spermatogenic cells by velocity sedimentation. *J. Cell Physiol.*, **80**, 299-312

Meredith, R. (1969). A simple method for preparing meiotic chromosomes from mammalian testis. *Chromosoma*, **26**, 254-8

Miyamoto, H. and Chang, M.C. (1972). Development of mouse eggs fertilized *in vitro* by epididymal spermatozoa. *J. Reprod. Fertil.*, **30**, 135-7

Mori, A. (1961). Difference in sperm-morphology in different strains of mice. *Tohoku J. Agr. Res.*, **12**, 107-18

Mosher, W.D. (1980). Reproductive impairments among currently married couples: United States, 1976. In Advanced Data from Vital and Health Statistics of the National Center for Health Statistics. US Department of Health, Education, and Welfare

Nelson, N. (1977). Human health and the environment: Some research needs. US Department of Health, Education, and Welfare Publication No 77-1277

Oakberg, E.F. and DiMinno, R.L. (1960). X-ray sensitivity of primary spermatocytes of the mouse. *Int. J. Radiat. Biol.*, **2**, 196-209

Okumura, K., Lee, I.P. and Dixon, R.L. (1975). Permeability of selected drugs and chemicals across the blood-testis barrier of the rat. *J. Pharmacol. Exp. Ther.*, **194**, 171-81

Overstreet, J.W., Katz, D.F., Hanson, F.W. and Foneca, J.R. (1979). A simple inexpensive method for objective assessment of human sperm movement characteristics. *Fertil. Steril.*, **31**, 162-72

Painter, R.B. (1982). DNA repair. In Hsu, T.C. (ed.) *Cytogenetic Assays of Environmental Mutagens* (Totowa: Allanheld, Osmun Publisher)

Pavlok, A. and McLaren, A. (1972). The role of cumulus cells and the zona pellucida in fertilization of mouse eggs *in vitro*. *J. Reprod. Fert.*, **29**, 91-7

Placek, P.J. and Cynamon, M.L. (1980). NCHS data on voluntary and involuntary infertility, with synthetic estimation application. Working paper series, No 1, Oct. 1980. Division of vital statistics, US Department of Health and Human services

Preslow, T.G. II, Saclise, M.M. and Weir, E.E. (1974). Separation of hamster testicular cells in successive stages of differentiation by velocity sedimentation in isokinetic gradient of ficoll in tissue culture medium. *Am. J. Pathol.*, **74**, 83-94

Robb, G.W., Amann, R.P. and Killian, G.J. (1978). Daily sperm production and epididymal sperm reserves of pubertal and adult rats. *J. Reprod. Fertil.*, **54**, 103-7

Rogers, B.J., Van Campen, H., Ueno, M., Lambert, H., Bronsen, R. and Hale, R.W. (1979).

Analysis of human spermatozoa fertilizing ability using zona-free ova. *Fertil. Steril.*, **32**, 664-70

Rohrborn, G. (1968). Mutagenicity tests in mice. I. The dominant lethal method and the control problem. *Humangenetik*, **6**, 345-98

Romrell, L.J., Belve, A.R. and Fawcett, D.W. (1976). Separation of mouse spermatogenic cells by sedimentation velocity: a morphological characterization. *Dev. Biol.*, **49**, 119-31

Roosen-Runge, E.C. (1962). The process of spermatogenesis in mammals. *Biol. Rev.*, **37**, 343-77

Roosen-Runge, E.C. (1973). Germinal-cell loss in normal metazoan spermatogenesis, *J. Reprod. Fertil.*, **35**, 339-48

Rowley, M.J., Teshima, F. and Heller, C.G. (1970). Duration of transit of spermatozoa through the human male ductular system. *Fertil. Steril.*, **21**, 390-6

Russell, L.D. and Clermont, Y. (1977). Degeneration of germ cells in normal, hypophysectomized and hormone-treated hypophysectomized rats. *Anat. Rec.*, **187**, 347-66

Russell, L.D. (1980). Sertoli-germ cell interrelations: A review. *Gamete Res.*, **3**, 179-202

Schmid, B., Lee, I.P. and Zbinden, G. (1978). DNA repair processes in germ cells demonstrated in ejaculated sperms of rabbits treated with methyl methane sulfonate. *Arch. Toxicol.*, **40**, 37-43

Sega, G.A., Owen, J.G. and Cummings, R. (1976). Studies on DNA repair in early spermatid stage of male mice after *in vivo* treatment with methyl, ethyl, propyl, isopropyl methane sulfonate. *Mutat. Res.*, **36**, 193-212

Sieber, S. and Adamson, R.H. (1975). Toxicity of antineoplastic agents in man: Chromosome aberration, antifertility effects, congenital malformations, carcinogenic potential. *Adv. Cancer Res.*, **22**, 57-155

Seiler, J.P. (1977). Inhibition of testicular DNA synthesis by chemical mutagens and carcinogens. Preliminary results in the validation of a novel short term test. *Mutat. Res.*, **46**, 305-10

Setchell, B.P. (1970). The secretion of fluid by the testes of rats, rams and goats, with some observations on the effect of age, cryptorchidism and hypophysectomy. *J. Reprod. Fertil.*, **23**, 79-85

Setchell, B.P., Voglmayr, J.R. and Waites, G.M.H. (1969). A blood-testis barrier restricting passage from blood into rete testis fluid but not into lymph. *J. Physiol. (Lond.)*, **200**, 73-85

Setchell, B.P. and Waites, G.M.H. (1970). Changes in the permeability of the testicular capillaries of the blood testis barrier after injection of cadmium chloride in the rat. *J. Endocrinol.*, **47**, 81-6

Steimberger, E. (1975). Hormonal regulation of the seminiferous tubules. In French, F.S., Hansson, V., Ritzen, E.M. and Hayfeth, S.N. (eds.) *Hormonal Regulation of Spermatogenesis*, pp. 337-52. (N.Y.: Plenum Press)

Sullivan, F.M. and Barlow, S.M. (1979). Congenital malformations and other reproductive hazards from environmental chemicals. *Proc. R. Soc. Lond. (Biol.)*, **205**, 91-110

Truhaut, R., Coquet, B., Fouillet, X., Galland, D., Guyot, D., Long, D. and Rouaud, J.L. (1979). Two-year oral toxicity and multigeneration studies in rats on two chemically modified maize starches. *Food Cosmet. Toxicol.*, **17**, 11-17

Tsunoda, Y. and Chang, M.C. (1976). Fertilizing ability *in vivo* and *in vitro* of rats and mice treated with α-chlorohydrin. *J. Reprod. Fertil.*, **46**, 401-6

Tuck, R.R., Setchell, B.P., Waites, G.M.H. and Young, J.A. (1970). The composition of fluid collected by micro-puncture and catheterization from the seminiferous tubules and rete testis of the rat. *Plugers Arch. Eur. J. Physiol.*, **318**, 225-43

US Food and Drug Administration (USFDA) (1970). Advisory Committee on Protocols for safety evaluation of food additives and pesticide residues. *Toxicol. Appl. Pharmacol.*, **16**, 264-96

VanDemark, N.L. and Ewing, L.L. (1963). Factors affecting testicular metabolism and function. I. A simplified perfusin technique for short term maintenance of rabbit testis. *J. Reprod. Fertil.*, **6**, 1-24

Werkheiser, W.C. (1963). Biochemical, cellular, and pharmacological action and effects of the folic acid antagonists. *Cancer Res.*, **23**, 1277-85

Wills, J.H., Groblewski, G.E. and Coulston, F. (1981). Chronic and multigeneration toxicities of small concentrations of cadmium in the diet of rats. *Ecotoxicol. Environ. Safety*, **5**, 452–64

Wyrobek, A.J. and Bruce, W.R. (1978). The induction of sperm shape abnormalities in mice and humans. In Hollaender, A. and de Serre, F.J. (eds) *Chemical Mutagens. Principles and Methods for their Detection*, Vol. 5, pp. 257–285 (New York and London: Plenum Press)

Yanagimachi, R., Yanagimachi, H. and Rogers, B.J. (1976). The use of zona–free ova as a test–system for the assessment of the fertilizing capacity of human spermatozoa. *Biol. Reprod.*, **15**, 471–6

16
Consequences to the progeny of paternal drug exposure

B. ROBAIRE, J.M. TRASLER and B.F. HALES

INTRODUCTION

Parental effects on progeny—maternal vs. paternal

Over the past 30 years evidence has accumulated demonstrating that drugs administered to the mother or environmental chemicals to which she is exposed during pregnancy can alter the pregnancy outcome (Aranda *et al.*, 1983; Schardein, 1976). These effects range from spontaneous abortions or stillbirths to major malformations evident at birth or delayed effects only evident many years later. Even for maternally administered drugs, the association between the drug and adverse pregnancy outcome has been made only in instances where a high incidence of a rare malformation or effect is induced. The specific effect of a drug given to the mother is dependent upon the timing of exposure to the drug during gestation. Drugs given early during pregnancy may result in spontaneous abortions; drugs given during organogenesis may produce major anomalies whereas drugs given late in pregnancy may lead to perinatal trauma.

Little attention has been given to the possibility of paternally mediated drug adverse effects on the progeny. Recently a number of studies have attempted to ascertain whether drugs administered to the father, or to which he is exposed, can have direct effects on the outcome of his progeny. The purpose of this review is to outline the potential sites of action of drugs in the father that could result in an adverse effect on his progeny and to attempt to integrate some of the existing literature in this context.

Mechanisms of paternally-mediated adverse pregnancy outcome

The conceptus may be exposed to drugs if the mother absorbs chemicals from the father's work clothes or other articles brought to the home. In this case, the paternal role in any potential adverse pregnancy outcome is clearly indirect. However, the father may more directly expose the conceptus to drugs via the semen. A wide range of compounds has been shown to enter semen. Unlike most other mammals, man continues to have intercourse throughout pregnancy. It has long been established that drugs are well absorbed after intravaginal administration (Benziger and Edelson, 1983). Thus, drugs in seminal fluid may be absorbed by the mother and affect the conceptus at any time during pregnancy from fertilization on.

Alternatively, drugs taken by the father may have an effect on the quantity and/or the quality of the spermatozoa produced. Effects on spermatozoal numbers can be mediated by alterations of the hypothalamo-pituitary-testicular axis or by direct cytotoxic effects in the testis. Effects on spermatozoal quality can range from alterations in morphology and motility (Lobl and Mathews, 1978) to more subtle alterations of the genome (Ehling, 1980).

Types of effects on pregnancy outcome

Adverse effects of paternal drug exposure can range from the extreme of infertility to delayed effects in offspring which are apparently normal at birth. Such effects include decreased litter size due to a decrease in the rate of fertilization or to pre- or post-implantation death. In addition, structural malformations or altered sex ratios may be apparent at parturition whereas heritable chromosomal abnormalities or behavioural effects may not be apparent until later in life.

DRUGS IN SEMEN

In most mammals semen is composed of secretions arising from a number of tissues. In species having seminal vesicles, such as the rat, rabbit and man, the secretions from this tissue comprise somewhat more than 50% of the semen volume. The prostate provides about 30% of seminal volume while the germ cells and the fluid bathing them, coming from the epididymis and the vas deferens, account for only approximately 10% of seminal volume. More than 100 chemicals have been identified in semen and it is apparent that this biological fluid is extremely complex (Mann and Lutwak-Mann, 1981; White and MacLeod, 1963). Though it has been hypothesized for many years that drugs taken by a man can potentially enter his semen, it is only in the last 15 years that the ability of drugs and endogenous chemicals to cross different regions of the male reproductive tract has been investigated.

Drug entry points into the male reproductive tract

The blood–testis barrier was first demonstrated in 1970 by Dym and Fawcett. At that time it was clearly shown that labelled lanthanum could not cross from the basal compartment to the adluminal compartment of seminiferous tubules. Tight junctions were found between projections from adjacent Sertoli cells. A number of studies by Setchell and his colleagues (1975) were able to establish that there was a barrier that was biochemically selective within the tubules and that could exclude certain materials from reaching the rete testis fluid.

It was not until recently that a clear demonstration of the existence of a similar barrier in the ductule system extending from the testis was established. The physiological aspects of this blood–epididymis barrier are discussed in Chapter 25. The presence of a physical barrier as assessed by the inability of lanthanum to cross the epididymal epithelium into the luminal compartment is now also established (Hoffer et al., 1983). It is not yet clear, however, whether the vas deferens also has a similar barrier.

There have been very few studies where the ability of specific drugs to cross the blood–testis or-epididymis barriers was assessed. In micropuncture studies from Howards' laboratory (Forrest et al., 1981) it was shown that cytotoxic agents such as cyclophosphamide will penetrate the lumen.

By collecting fluid from the prostate and the seminal vesicles, it has not been possible to demonstrate this type of tight junction between epithelial cells. The entry of drugs into semen is postulated to occur primarily via passage from the capillaries into ducts in these two tissues. The presence of numerous drugs has been demonstrated in prostatic secretions (Borski et al., 1954). An experiment in our laboratory assessed the time-course of entry of ^{14}C-labelled cyclophosphamide into seminal vesicle fluid after intravenous administration in rats. After a bolus injection of 50 μCi of cyclophosphamide into the jugular vein, serial samples of blood and seminal vesicle fluid were collected (Table 16.1). It is apparent from these results that labelled drug does penetrate into the lumen of the seminal vesicles, peaks at approximately 30 min and reaches, within 2 h, equilibrium with blood concentrations.

Table 16.1 Time-course of the entry of ^{14}C from intravenously administered cyclophosphamide into rat seminal vesicle fluid

	[^{14}C] Cyclophosphamide	
Time (min)	Seminal vesicle fluid ($10^{-4} \times DPM \ g^{-1}$)	Ratio of label in seminal vesicle fluid/plasma
0	5.0± 0.6*	0.04±0.01
10	16.6± 1.3	0.28±0.05
30	45.1± 4.5	0.81±0.05
60	46.9± 9.0	0.81±0.05
90	51.0± 5.6	1.10±0.17
120	47.7±11.8	0.93±0.07

*Values represent means ±SEM (n=4)

Chemicals in semen – endogenous and foreign

Extensive studies by White and Macleod (1963) and Mann and Lutwak-Mann (1981) have attempted to describe the chemical and biochemical composition of semen from a number of species. The pattern and concentrations of chemicals, hormones and enzymes found in semen differ markedly from those of serum. This indicates that the selective barriers at work in the testis and epididymis must contribute to the final chemical make-up of semen. In addition, it is likely that there are active transport processes in the prostate and/or seminal vesicles. The extremely high concentration of prostaglandins in semen, derived from the seminal vesicles, has been proposed to stimulate contraction of the uterus after intercourse and thus facilitate sperm transport to the egg. In this instance endogenous substances, prostaglandins, may be viewed functionally as 'drugs'.

There are a number of examples of xenobiotic chemicals or drugs given to the male that do enter semen. In an effort to develop better therapeutic approaches to prostatitis, the concentrations of a large number of antimicrobial agents have been measured in different fractions of split ejaculates (Eliasson and Dornbusch, 1977, 1980). These split ejaculate fractions can be used to indicate the entry point(s) of a drug into the semen. Metronidazole, trimethoprim-sulphamethoxazole, deoxycycline, erythromycin and pivampicillin have all been shown to enter semen via both the prostate and seminal vesicle fluid (Eliasson and Dornbusch, 1977, 1980; Malmborg, 1978).

The ability of the male reproductive system to concentrate drugs varies greatly. Some compounds such as the antimicrobial, thiamphenicol, are concentrated in semen relative to serum 24 hours after injection (Plomp et al., 1978). Others, such as amphetamine (Smith, 1981), attain concentrations similar to those in serum and still others, such as diphenylhydantoin (Cohn et al., 1982; Swanson et al., 1978), are found in semen in concentrations consistently lower than those in serum, even after prolonged exposure.

Many drugs that are found in semen can be readily absorbed by the vagina and some can affect both the female partner and the progeny. Vinblastine in semen has been associated with vulvovaginitis in women (Paladine et al., 1975). Pretreatment of male rats with high doses of oestradiol results in uterine hypertrophy and hyperplasia in the female partner (Ericsson and Baker, 1966). For a drug to have a direct effect on the conceptus, the drug concentration in semen must be extremely high, the drug should be very potent and/or the conceptus must be directly exposed to the drug. These conditions seem essential because the volume of semen in most mammals is very low.

Evidence indicating that short-term paternal exposure to methadone or morphine results in an increased perinatal mortality and decreased birth weight in the offspring has accumulated (Smith and Joffe, 1975; Soyka et al., 1978). Because of the short exposure time they have hypothesized that the effects of these drugs cannot be mediated by altering spermatogenesis or sperm maturation but rather are mediated directly by their presence in semen. An unequivocal substantiation of this hypothesis would require artificial insemination followed by mating with a drug-treated vasectomized animal.

Thalidomide has been shown to enter semen and there is evidence suggesting an effect on progeny (Lutwak-Mann, 1964; Lutwak-Mann et al., 1967). When male rabbits treated with thalidomide were mated with untreated females the resulting progeny had a higher neonatal mortality rate, lower birth weights and a higher incidence of birth defects.

In our laboratory, studies have been initiated to determine whether cyclo-

Table 16.2 Effects on the progeny of acute treatment of male rats with cyclophosphamide (CPA)

Treatment group	Pre-implantation loss* (% litter)	Resorptions (% litter)	Abnormal fetuses (% of total)
Saline	7.8±3.0†	6.4±2.5	0.5
CPA: 10 mg/kg	9.3±4.0	8.5±2.0	0.7
30 mg/kg	11.7±4.5	6.8±2.4	0.7
100 mg/kg	15.7±3.9‡	7.5±2.2	0

* Pre-implantation loss refers to the number of corpora lutea minus the number of implantations per pregnant female.
† Mean ± SEM (n is between 11 and 14)
‡ $p \leqslant 0.05$, Mann–Whitney U Test

phosphamide given to adult male rats within 12 hours of breeding can result in an altered pregnancy outcome (Table 16.2). Though there were no effects on numbers of resorptions, litter size or numbers of abnormal fetuses, there was a significant increase in pre-implantation loss. This would be consistent with a direct effect of cyclophosphamide or its metabolites in seminal fluid on fertilization or on the conceptus.

EFFECTS OF DRUGS ON SPERMATOGENESIS— QUANTITATIVE ASPECTS

The relationship of spermatozoal numbers to infertility and/or adverse pregnancy outcome is still imperfectly understood. Men with sperm counts less than 10^7/ml have been reported capable of fathering children, but few follow-up studies have been done to see whether the frequency of adverse pregnancy outcome is greater than among men with normal counts (Barfield et al., 1979). A significant correlation has been made, however, between sperm count and number of living children (Bostofte et al., 1982a).

One of the two major ways drugs may alter spermatozoal numbers is by modulating the activity of the hypothalamo-pituitary-testicular axis. Chemicals capable of acting via this route include analogues of gonadotropin releasing hormone (GnRH) and steroids as well as alcohol, diphenylhydantoin, cannabinoids and cimetidine. The second major way drugs may decrease spermatozoal numbers is by a direct cytotoxic effect on germ cells in the testis. Examples of drugs acting directly on germ cells include inhibitors of mitosis and/or meiosis such as the anticancer drugs and dibromochloropropane.

Modulators of the hypothalamo-pituitary-testicular axis

Spermatogenesis in the seminiferous tubules is directly regulated by testosterone (Robaire and Zirkin, 1981). Follicle stimulating hormone (FSH) also plays a role in controlling spermatogenesis during puberty and at least in some circumstances in the adult (Ewing and Robaire, 1978). The high local concentration of testosterone required for spermatogenesis is secreted by interstitial Leydig cells, which are regulated by luteinizing hormone (LH). The pituitary secretion of both LH and FSH is under the positive control of GnRH and the negative control (negative feedback) of steroids. Exogenously administered compounds, identical to or analogues of these hormones, will interfere with the fine regulation of this axis and can result in decreased spermatogenesis in an otherwise normal individual.

High doses of GnRH and its analogues have been reported to induce testicular and prostatic involution (Sandow et al., 1980). This 'shut-down' of spermatogenesis has been suggested as a therapeutic measure to protect the spermatogonial stem cells from potentially irreversible damage when anti-mitotic agents are administered (Glode et al., 1981). Such GnRH analogues alone or in combination with androgens have also been tested as potential male contraceptives (Heber and Swerdloff, 1980; Linde et al., 1981).

In one study, despite the production of testicular involution in rats after chronic administration (4-16 weeks) of high doses of a GnRH analogue (Buserelin), reproductive performance in terms of mean litter size was not affected (Sandow et al., 1980). However, no direct quantitative analyses of spermatozoal production rate or spermatozoa in the female reproductive tract were done. Thus, no definitive conclusion about the relationship between GnRH analogues, sperm count and fertility can yet be made.

Peripheral administration of steroids—androgens, progestagens, oestrogens-inhibits gonadotropin (FSH and LH) release from the pituitary by affecting pituitary and/or hypothalamic function (GnRH release). The resulting decrease in intratesticular testosterone, without necessarily a concomitant decrease in serum testosterone, has led to the proposition that such steroids could be used as male contraceptives (Ewing et al., 1973). Presently, the goal for any male contraceptive is to produce a complete shut-down of spermatogenesis, i.e. azoospermia (Schaffenburg et al., 1981).

Though in the rabbit (Ewing et al., 1973) an optimum dose of testosterone can suppress LH, intratesticular testosterone and hence spermatogenesis without itself maintaining spermatogenesis, such a situation cannot be produced in the rat, monkey or man (Robaire et al., 1979; Ewing et al., 1976; Swerdloff et al., 1978). Combinations of testosterone with other steroids are being tested as male contraceptives but it does not appear that it will be possible to guarantee azoospermia in all individuals. The consequences of contraceptive failure, i.e. fertility rate and pregnancy outcome, must be better evaluated. If, as is likely, azoospermia is not attained and maintained in 100% of the patients treated then the fate of any resulting progeny is critical. In one of the few reports to date, Barfield et al., (1979) claimed that of the six pregnancies occurring in partners of men treated with medroxyprogesterone acetate or testosterone (sperm counts less than 10^7/ml, five less than 10^6/ml) and carried to term, all the progeny were normal. However, this study was not designed to evaluate pregnancy outcome.

One recent study (Lobl et al., 1983) has indicated that testosterone—oestradiol treatment of male rhesus monkeys resulted in a reversible state of infertility. There were no significant concomitant side-effects. During the treatment period when infertility was attained, spermatozoal numbers did not decrease to zero (Table 16.3). Interestingly, the percentages of motile spermatozoa and normal morphology of the remaining spermatozoa were significantly lower in steroid-treated than in control monkeys. In post-treatment monkeys the spermatozoal number and motility returned to control values but the percentage normal morphology was still significantly decreased. Because there was no evidence of prolonged oestrous cycles in female rhesus monkeys impregnated by sterile, oligozoospermic rhesus males there probably was no increased incidence of early fetal resorption. Thus the abnormal spermatozoa in steroid-treated oligozoospermic male monkeys may not be able to fertilize an oocyte. More detailed studies with larger numbers of subjects are necessary to evaluate potential effects on pregnancy outcome.

Prostaglandins are another group of chemicals that may alter fertility by

Table 16.3 The effect of testosterone–oestradiol (T-E$_2$) treatment of male rhesus monkeys on spermatozoal numbers, motility and morphology of ejaculated spermatozoa*

	Control	T-E$_2$ treated
Spermatozoa/ejaculate $\times 10^6$	1046 ± 102†	74 ± 28‡
Motile spermatozoa (%)	82 ± 3	18 ± 6‡
Normal morphology (%)	75 ± 4	11 ± 4‡

* Data adapted from Lobl et al., (1983)
† Values represent mean $\pm$ SEM (n = 10)
‡ $p \leqslant 0.01$

influencing the hypothalamo-pituitary-testicular axis. These compounds cause a decrease in blood levels of testosterone, LH and FSH. Subcutaneous injections of prostaglandin F$_{2\alpha}$ or E$_1$ caused a 50% reduction in fertility rate in rats, and affected significantly spermatozoal density, motility and morphology and vas deferens contractility (Chinoy and Chinoy, 1981).

Ethanol and/or its metabolites can inhibit steroidogenesis in the testis (Cicero et al., 1981). There have been some studies on the effect of paternal alcohol consumption on the progeny. In one such study (Mankes et al., 1982) the inclusion of 20% ethanol in the drinking water of male rats for 60 days before mating resulted in decreased litter sizes, increased resorptions, decreased pup-weights and increased incidences of soft tissue anomalies (microcephalus, cranial fissure and hydronephrosis). However, earlier studies did not report an increase in anomalies among the offspring of alcoholic male guinea pigs (Stockard, 1913). In addition to affecting steroidogenesis, ethanol has been reported to be positive as a dominant lethal mutagen (Badr and Badr, 1975).

Recent studies have provided evidence that perinatal exposure of rodents to a number of drugs, including cannabinoids and cimetidine, can alter pituitary-testicular function in the male and may suppress adult copulatory activity (Dalterio et al., 1982; Dalterio and Bartke, 1979; Anand and Van Thiel, 1982). Male mice exposed to cannabinoids impregnate significantly fewer females than control males (Dalterio *et al.*, 1982). The percentage of pregnancies with pre- and postnatal fetal loss was increased. This reduction in fertility is associated with chromosomal aberrations, both in the primary spermatocytes of the treated males and in some of their F_1 male progeny. Thus, the role of the altered pituitary and gonadal endocrine function in mediating this effect is not clear.

Cytotoxic agents—inhibitors of mitosis and/or meiosis

Cancer chemotherapeutic drugs primarily affect rapidly dividing cells by interfering with DNA synthesis or cell replication. As the testis is a major site of mitotic and meiotic activity these drugs frequently produce germinal aplasia with resulting azoospermia. Some of these drugs arrest spermatogenesis at specific stages; these studies have been well reviewed by Jackson (1964). In one retrospective study (Chapman *et al.*, 1979) of 74 male patients receiving cyclical combination chemotherapy (nitrogen mustard, vinblastine, procarbazine and prednisolone, MOPP) for advanced Hodgkin's disease, all were azoospermic after therapy. With a median follow-up period of 27 months, only four of the 74 patients' testes regained spermatogenic activity. There are indications that a higher percentage of patients can regain the ability to produce spermatozoa after such therapy if it is given before or during puberty.

Both alkylating agents and antimetabolites may also produce mutations in germ cells. In fact, the effects of these drugs on resultant progeny are probably mediated via effects on the spermatozoal genome.

Exposure of male pesticide workers to dibromochloropropane, a nematocide, has been associated with a reduction in sperm counts and adverse effects on fertility (Whorton *et al.*, 1979). In the dibromochloropropane-exposed group, 13.1% were azoospermic, 16.8% oligozoospermic and 15.8% had low 'normal' sperm counts (20–39 million sperm/ml). In the control group, 2.9% were azoospermic, none were severely oligozoospermic and 5.7% were mildly oligozoospermic. One year after termination of dibromochloropropane exposure (Whorton and Milby, 1980), 11 of 12 azoospermic men were still azoospermic; of the nine oligozoospermic men, eight had improved sperm counts and had fathered four children (three normal, one with several defects). The design and numbers involved in this study do not permit any conclusion with respect to pregnancy outcome. One study in Israel (Kharrazi *et al.*, 1980) did report increased fetal loss in wives of men exposed to dibromochloropropane. Dibromochloropropane lesions are similar to those produced by alkylating agents.

From the above studies it would appear that most agents that decrease the number of germ cells in semen will also alter the remaining germ cells. This effect may be indirect—reduced seminiferous tubular activity may cause production of abnormal germ cells; alternatively it may be direct—alterations of the germ cells. To resolve the question of the relationship between low sperm number and progeny outcome, an experimental paradigm in which only the number of germ cells is decreased and pregnancy outcome is evaluated is essential.

EFFECTS OF DRUGS ON SPERMATOGENESIS—QUALITATIVE ASPECTS

Altered spermatozoal genome

Paternal exposure to drugs and/or chemicals can alter the genetic material in spermatozoa which could in turn have adverse effects on the fetus. The available mammalian test systems detect genetic damage to a limited degree. Information gained from such test systems can be used to elucidate the mechanism of such genetic effects and to study the factors that modulate their expression in the progeny.

Test systems for measuring germ cell damage

Cytogenetic, dominant lethal, heritable translocation and specific locus mutation studies are those most widely used to look at chromosomal damage and its heritability in the progeny of the treated male. A dominant lethal mutation induced in the germ cells by the treatment of the male, is usually characterized by death of the fertilized egg at or around the time of implantation (Bateman and Epstein, 1971). The heritable translocation test measures transmissible chromosomal aberrations and is based on the induction of balanced reciprocal translocations in the germ cells of treated animals (Generoso *et al.*, 1980). The specific locus mutation assay detects chemically induced visible recessive mutations (Ehling, 1978). Treated wild-type males are mated with females which carry recessive alleles coding for visible markers such as coat colour. Genetic mutations in the spermatozoa of the treated animals at any of the chosen loci are observed in the first generation offspring.

Studies using the test systems described above have shown that different alkylating agents have effects on the genetic material at different stages during spermatogenesis (Jackson, 1964). This germ cell specificity overlaps among the tests used. Most of the experimental evidence showing the existence of drug-induced heritable alterations in the genome in mammalian systems has come from studies with antineoplastic agents. Procarbazine, a methylhydrazine derivative used in Hodgkin's disease, has been found after treatment of the male mouse to cause dominant lethal mutations when spermatids and spermatocytes were sampled and a failure of fertilization when spermatogonia were sampled (Ehling, 1974). Cytogenetic analyses revealed chromosomal abnormalities after exposure of spermatogonial stages to procarbazine (Adler, 1982); that such abnormalities can be found in the progeny has been shown using the specific locus mutation test (Ehling and Neuhauser, 1979). The specific locus mutation test also demonstrates that procarbazine can cause chromosomal alterations in the progeny after exposure of post-spermatogonial stages. Mitomycin C is an antibotic which, when metabolized, becomes an alkylating agent. Like procarbazine, it has been shown to produce heritable chromosomal effects by acting on spermatogonia (Ehling, 1974). A commonly used chemotherapeutic and immunosuppressive agent, cyclophosphamide, induced heritable translocations after exposure of the male during the development of spermatocytes, spermatids and spermatozoa (Sotomayor and Cumming, 1975).

Methyl methanesulphonate is an alkylating agent that has not found wide clinical use but has been studied in all of these systems. It is an example of an agent that induces dominant lethal mutations and heritable genetic defects in the germ cells of the male rodent treated during the development of spermatids and spermatozoa but not spermatogonia (Ehling et al., 1968; Ehling, 1978; Lang and Adler, 1977).

Mechanisms of genetic damage

Postulated mechanisms of drug-induced genetic damage include alterations in either the DNA or proteins of chromosomes. In an investigation of the cytogenetic effects of methyl methanesulphonate, mitotic chromosomes of the first cleavage division were examined (Brewen et al., 1975). This group found a close correlation between the frequency of cytologically visible chromosomal aberrations and the previously published frequency of dominant lethal mutations. This was one of the first studies with chemical mutagens to suggest that dominant lethal mutations may be due to chromosomal aberrations. Ethyl methanesulphonate, another alkane sulphonic acid, acts at the same germ cell stages as does methyl methanesulphonate (Cattanach et al., 1968; Ehling et al., 1968). One group has tried to look more carefully at the site of action of ethyl methanesulphonate on the chromosomes (Sega and Owens, 1978). They found that the ethylation of sperm DNA did not increase in germ cell stages that were most sensitive to ethyl methanesulphonate, whereas the ethylation of the mouse sperm chromosomal protein, protamine, did. The authors suggested that alkylation of protamine may in turn lead to stresses in the chromatin structure which might eventually cause chromosomal breakage and chromosomal abnormalities that could be picked up in the progeny. Another mechanism of action that should be considered for drugs that have been reported to cause heritable effects through their action on spermatozoa, is instead, that these drugs have a direct effect through their presence in semen. In one example of a study that lends itself to such different interpretations, methyl methanesulphonate was found to produce widely differing incidences of dominant lethal mutations in the progeny of females mated to males in the first week after paternal treatment, when spermatozoa would have been exposed (Ehling et al., 1968).

Modulators of genetic damage

Some of the factors that can modulate genetic damage include the dosing schedules and DNA repair mechanisms in both the male germ cells as well as in the egg after fertilization. Most of the studies described so far involve administration of an acute dose whereas humans are often exposed over longer periods of time. The two alkylating agents, cyclophosphamide and triethylenemelamine, when administered to male rats five days a week over a ten week period, produced dominant lethal mutations (Moreland et al., 1981). Further studies that tested heritability in the progeny showed that chronic low dose triethylenemelamine, over a four to six week period, caused the induction of more translocations in the progeny than did an acute dose (Generoso et al., 1978; Sheu et al., 1978). The authors interpreted their data to suggest that prolonged therapy may cause the accumulation of chromosomal abnormalities in the progeny.

Although chronic dosage may cause cumulative effects, one study has shown that a single dose of procarbazine can produce more heritable chromosomal aberrations, as tested by the specific locus assay, than can the fractionation of that same dose over a number of days (Ehling, 1980). This fractionation effect has also been found for the alkyl nitrosourea, ethyl nitrosourea (Russell et al., 1982). These findings suggest the importance of repair processes in modulating the eventual damage found in the progeny. Investigators have used unscheduled DNA synthesis to estimate repair processes in germ cells (Sega and Sotomayor, 1982). The last scheduled DNA synthesis during spermatogenesis occurs in the meiotic prophase in spermatocytes. Germ cell damage in stages subsequent to meiotic prophase can be detected by the incorporation of tritiated thymidine. Unscheduled DNA synthesis has been found in meiotic and postmeiotic stages up to 'mid-spermatids' after treatment with ethyl methanesulphonate, methyl methanesulphonate and cyclophosphamide (Sega, 1974; Sega et al., 1976; Sotomayor et al., 1978). No unscheduled DNA synthesis has been found in late spermatids and spermatozoa, when the chromatin is more condensed, even though the DNA can still be alkylated at this time (Sega and Owens, 1978). Unscheduled DNA synthesis gives us no idea of the heritability of chemically induced effects on the spermatozoa, but is detected at doses lower than those needed to induce dominant lethal mutations or translocations (Sega et al., 1976). Using a number of alkylating agents, Sotomayor and his collaborators (1982) have been unable to correlate the induction of unscheduled DNA synthesis with drug-induced heritable chromosomal abnormalities. This lack of correlation may be explained by mutagen effects on repair processes or by strain differences in the animals used. Support for the latter suggestion has come from studies with methyl methanesulphonate where a variation in the amount of unscheduled DNA synthesis between strains of mice has been found (Lee and Suzuki, 1981). There is also evidence that damage induced in spermatozoa may be repaired in the egg (Generoso et al., 1979). Male mice were treated with different alkylating agents; chromosomal damage at the first cleavage division and the frequency of dominant lethal mutations were studied. It was found that the frequency of dominant lethal mutations after the treated males were mated with female mice from different strains depended on the strain of the female. The dominant lethal mutation and chromosomal aberration frequencies were similar; this would suggest that repair must take place between sperm entry and the first cleavage division.

It is thus clear that a number of agents can alter the genome of spermatozoa and consequently result in abnormalities in the progeny. The mechanisms involved in such alterations are still poorly understood, however, it would appear that changes in the DNA and the proteins of the chromosomes are likely.

Altered spermatozoal appearance and function

Cytology and morphology

In addition to alterations in the chromosomal genetic message, a number of physical changes may be induced that produce aberrant spermatozoa. Such changes can range from Y chromosome nondisjunction to alterations in cellular DNA content measured by flow cytometry or abnormally shaped spermatozoa.

Presently it is not possible chemically to decondense spermatozoal chromatin and perform chromosomal analyses. However, Y chromosome non-disjunction (aneuploidy) can be monitored directly in the spermatozoa by quantifying the number of spermatozoa with two fluorescent bodies (YFF). Kapp (1979) has suggested that an increase in YFF sperm is correlated with exposure to radiation, adriamycin or dibromochloropropane. To date, however, an increase in the number of XYY offspring produced by males exposed to these drugs has not been demonstrated.

An assessment of sperm abnormality is probably also possible using DNA flow cytometry. This technique has shown abnormal DNA patterns in testicular biopsy specimens from some oligozoospermic or azoospermic men (Clausen and Äbyholm, 1980). A small percentage of the spermatozoa from normal donors are not haploid. Yet, no one has reported a study of the relationship between abnormal DNA patterns on flow cytometry with adverse pregnancy outcome.

Grossly abnormal spermatozoa may have a variety of shapes. They may, for example, be amorphous, have markedly altered head shapes or possess two tails. The number of abnormal spermatozoa found is both species and strain specific. Many mouse strains have frequencies of abnormal spermatozoa in the range of 1-4% whereas men have from 10-50% of abnormal forms in semen samples. Consequently, it is much easier to detect chemical induction of sperm abnormalities in animal species with a low normal incidence than in the human. Experiments with mice have revealed that sperm abnormalities are most prevalent 35 days after exposure to drugs such as benzo(α)pyrene, lead acetate, procarbazine and methyl methanesulphonate (Wyrobek and Bruce, 1975). Thus, the period of maximum sensitivity corresponds to a time when the cells are exposed as late spermatogonia or as primary spermatocytes, a time of maximum mitotic and meiotic activity. Induced abnormalities in spermatozoa may be transmitted to the progeny (Wyrobek and Bruce, 1975). Sperm shape is genetically controlled and can be modified by alterations in DNA. The possibility that abnormal spermatozoa can reach an egg and then fertilize it may be reduced relative to normal spermatozoa. In one study spermatozoa with severe abnormalities were either not found in the oviduct or their proportion was greatly reduced (Krzanowska, 1974). In man a higher incidence (greater than 60%) of abnormal spermatozoa has been associated with a lower number of live births as well as with a higher number of spontaneous abortions (Bostofte *et al.*, 1982b; Furuhjelm *et al.*, 1962).

Two of the clearest examples in man of the association between abnormal spermatozoal morphology and paternally mediated adverse pregnancy outcome are lead (Lancranjan *et al.*, 1975) and cigarette smoking (Evans *et al.*, 1981). An increased incidence of teratospermia has been reported in workmen with long-term lead exposure. Lead acetate can also cause sperm-shape abnormalities in mice (Wyrobek and Bruce, 1975). Several studies have found an association between adverse pregnancy outcome, including Wilm's tumour in the offspring, and paternal lead exposure (Kantor *et al.*, 1979). In another study, only maternal or only paternal exposure to lead acetate for 60 days prior to mating significantly altered the learning ability of offspring (Brady *et al.*, 1975).

Unlike the effects of maternal cigarette smoking, paternal smoking does not seem to be associated with a decreased birth weight of the progeny; in one study there was an increase in perinatal mortality and malformations if the father smoked, regardless of the smoking status of the mother (Mau and Netter, 1974).

Motility

The mechanism by which spermatozoa acquire motility in the epididymis and the biochemical regulation of this motility are still poorly understood. A large variety of drugs has been shown to interfere with normal motility. These drugs include agents that can modify the genome, inhibit glycolysis, act as local anaesthetics and/or modify surface membrane proteins (Fiscor and Ginsberg, 1980; Hong *et al.*, 1982; Peterson and Freund, 1975). It would not be expected that an agent whose sole effect is to reduce sperm motility would cause abnormal progeny since the need for motility is primarily associated with the fertilization process. Indeed, none of the drugs that have been shown to alter primarily motility have been associated with paternally mediated teratogenicity.

Maturation

Over the last 15 years, it has been established that spermatozoa gain their ability to fertilize eggs during their passage through the epididymis (Orebin-Crist *et al.*, 1975). An interesting observation is that, in non-drug-treated rabbits, ova fertilized by spermatozoa from the lower corpus epididymis were delayed in their development compared to those fertilized by distal cauda or ejaculated spermatozoa (Orgebin-Crist, 1969). In addition, these 'newly matured' spermatozoa produced a higher incidence of pre-implantation death. A role for non-genetic spermatozoal material in supporting early embryonic development has been suggested by other investigators (Hoppe and Illmensee, 1982). Though no drug effects on pregnancy outcome are known to be mediated via the epididymis, there has been little effort to study this possibility.

237

MISCELLANEOUS

Two environmental workplaces have been associated with paternally mediated adverse pregnancy outcome: polyvinyl chloride production plants and hospital operating rooms. Because of the lack of available knowledge about the chemicals involved and the mechanisms mediating these effects, it is most appropriate to discuss them separately.

Vinyl chloride

An association between exposure of men to vinyl chloride in the workplace and fetal loss in their wives has been reported (Infante *et al.*, 1976). In an epidemiological study of the distribution of congenital anomalies in Ohio residents from three communities with polyvinyl chloride production facilities, the occurrence of malformations was much greater than expected. Significant excesses were observed for defects of the central nervous system, upper alimentary tract, genital organs and feet. Vinyl chloride is mutagenic and has been reported to cause an increased frequency of chromosomal aberrations in the lymphocytes of exposed workers (Ducatman *et al.*, 1975). In two case-control studies, however, no association between workplace exposure or proximity to polyvinyl chloride plants and central nervous system defects were found (Edmonds *et al.*, 1975, 1978).

Anaesthetic gases

In some studies, exposure of male personnel to anaesthetic gases was associated with an increased risk of adverse pregnancy outcome among the unexposed wives (Cohen, 1974; Cohen *et al.*, 1975), whereas in others this association was not found (Knill-Jones *et al.*, 1975; American Society of Anesthesiology, 1974). No significant differences were found in sperm concentration or morphology between anaesthesiologists with a minimum of one year in hospital operating rooms and beginning medical residents in anaesthesiology (controls) (Wyrobek *et al.*, 1981). However, in an animal study, exposure of mice to chloroform, trichloroethylene and enflurane significantly increased the levels of morphologically abnormal epididymal spermatozoa 28 days later (Land *et al.*, 1981). Exposure of male rats or mice to halothane for 12–17 weeks did not impair fertility and did not significantly affect embryonic development and fetal viability (Pope and Persaud, 1982; Wharton *et al.*, 1978). Extrapolation from rodents to man is uncertain but it seems likely that halothane is not the cause of the congenital abnormalities and spontaneous abortions reported to occur in operating room personnel.

CONCLUDING REMARKS

The role of the father in mediating drug-induced abnormal outcome of progeny is now becoming well established. In the present review we have attempted to highlight some of the clearest evidence for this process and to integrate this information in a systematic manner. There are numerous drugs that can or do act at more than one site in this scheme and we have tried to indicate this whenever possible. In assessing future evidence for drug-induced paternally mediated adverse pregnancy outcome, this scheme should be helpful as it permits delineation of the site(s) of action of such drugs

Acknowledgements

BFH is a Scholar and JMT a Fellow of the Medical Research Council of Canada. This work was supported by the National Foundation March of Dimes, the Medical Research Council of Canada and the Fraser Memorial Fund of the Royal Victoria Hospital. We acknowledge the excellent secretarial assistance of Ms S. Bluszyld.

References

Adler, I.-D. (1982). Male germ cell cytogenetics. In Hsu T.C. (ed.) *Cytogenetic Assays of Environmental Chemicals*, pp. 249-76 (Totowa, NJ. Allanheld, Osmun)

American Society of Anesthesiologists, Ad Hoc Committee (1974). Occupational disease among operating room personnel: a national study. *Anesthesiology*, **41**, 321-40

Anand, S. and Van Thiel, D.H. (1982). Prenatal and neonatal exposure to cimetidine results in gonadal and sexual dysfunction in adult males. *Science*, **218**, 493-4

Aranda, J.V., Hales, B.F. and Gibbs, J. (1983). Developmental pharmacology. In Fanaroff, A.A. and Martin, R.J. (eds.) *Behrman's Neonatal-Perinatal Medicine Diseases of the Fetus and Infant*. Chap. 12, pp. 150-73 (Saint Louis: C.V. Mosby)

Badr, R. and Badr, F. (1975). Induction of dominant lethal mutation in male mice by ethyl alcohol. *Nature*, **253**, 134-6

Barfield, A., Melo, J., Coutinho, E., Alvarez-Sanchez, F., Faundes, A., Brache, V., Leon, P., Frick, J., Bartsch, G., Weiske, W.-H., Brenner, P., Mishell, D., Jr, Bernstein, G. and Ortiz, A. (1979). Pregnancies associated with sperm concentrations below 10 million/ml in clinical studies of a potential male contraceptive method, monthly depot medroxyprogesterone acetate and testosterone esters. *Contraception*, **20**, 121-7

Bateman, A.J. and Epstein, S.A. (1971). Dominant lethal mutations in mammals. In Hollaender, A. (ed.) *Chemical Mutagens—Principles and Methods for their Detection*. Vol. 2, pp. 541-568. (New York and London: Plenum)

Benziger, D.P. and Edelson, J. (1983). Absorption from the vagina. *Drug Metabolism Reviews*, **14**, 137-68

Borski, A.A., Pulsaki, E.J., Kimbrough, J.C. and Fusillo, M.H. (1954). Prostatic fluid, semen and prostatic tissue concentrations of the major antibiotics following intravenous administration. *Antibiot. Chemother.*, **4**, 905-10

Bostofte, E., Serup, J. and Rebbe, H. (1982a). Relation between sperm count and semen volume, and pregnancies obtained during a twenty-year follow-up period. *Int. J. Androl.*, **5**, 267-75

Bostofte, E., Serup, J. and Rebbe, H. (1982b). Relation between morphologically abnormal spermatozoa and pregnancies obtained during a twenty-year follow-up period. *Int. J. Androl.*, **5**, 379-86

Brady, K., Herrara, Y. and Zenick, H. (1975). Influence of parental lead exposure on subsequent learning ability of offspring. *Pharmacol. Biochem. Behav.*, **3**, 561-5

Brewen, J.G., Payne, H.S., Jones, K.P. and Preston, R.J. (1975). Studies on chemically induced dominant lethality I. The cytogenetic basis of MMS-induced dominant lethality in post-meiotic male germ cells. *Mutat. Res.*, **33**, 239-50

Cattanach, B.M., Pollard, C.E. and Isaacson, J.H. (1968). Ethyl methanesulfonate-induced chromosome breakage in the mouse. *Mutat. Res.*, **6**, 297–307

Chapman, R.M., Sutcliffe, S.B., Ress, L.H., Edwards, C.R.W. and Malpas, J.S. (1979). Cyclical combination chemotherapy and gonadal function. Retrospective study in males. *Lancet*, **1**, 285–9

Chinoy, N.J. and Chinoy, M.R. (1981). Infertility induced by prostaglandins in albino rats by adrenergic block in the vas deferens. *Int. J. Fertil.*, **26**, 1–7

Cicero, T.J., Newman, K.S. and Meyer, E.R. (1981). Ethanol-induced inhibitions of testicular steroidogenesis in the male rat: mechanism of actions. *Life Sci.*, **28**, 871–7

Clausen, O.P.F. and Åbyholm, T. (1980). Deoxyribonucleic acid flow cytometry of germ cells in the investigation of male infertility. *Fertil. Steril.*, **34**, 369–74

Cohen, E.N. (1974). Occupational disease among operating room personnel: A National Study. *Anesthesiology*, **41**, 321–40

Cohen, E.N., Brown, B.W., Bruce, D.L. Cascorbi, H.F., Corbett, T.H., Jones, T.W. and Whitcher, C.E. (1975). A survey of anesthetic health hazards among dentists. *J. Am. Dent. Assoc.*, **90**, 1291–6

Cohn, D.F., Homonnai, Z.T. and Paz, G.P. (1982). Diphenylhydantoin excretion in the semen of treated epileptics. *Isr. J. Med. Sci.*, **18**, 509–11

Dalterio, S., Badr, F., Bartke, A. and Mayfield, D. (1982). Cannabinoids in male mice: effects on fertility and spermatogenesis. *Science*, **216**, 315–6

Dalterio, S. and Bartke, A. (1979). Perinatal exposure to cannabinoids alters male reproductive function in mice. *Science*, **205**, 1420–2

Ducatman, A., Hirschorn, K. and Selikoff, I.J. (1975). Vinyl chloride exposure and human chromosome aberrations. *Mutat. Res.*, **31**, 163–8

Dym, M. and Fawcett, D.W. (1970). Observations on the blood–testis barrier in the rat and the physiological compartmentation of the seminiferous epithelium. *Biol. Reprod.*, **3**, 308–26

Edmonds, L.D., Anderson, C.E., Flynt, J.W. Jr and James, L.M. (1978). Congenital central nervous system malformations and vinyl chloride monomer exposure: a community study. *Teratology*, **17**, 137–49

Edmonds, L.D., Falk, H. and Nissim, J.E. (1975). Congenital malformations and vinyl chloride. *Lancet*, **2**, 1098

Ehling, U.H. (1974). Differential spermatogenic response of mice to the induction of mutations by antineoplastic drugs. *Mutat. Res.*, **26**, 285–95

Ehling, U.H. (1978). Specific-locus mutations in mice. In Hollaender, A. and deSerres, F.J. (eds.) *Chemical Mutagens—Principles and Methods for their Detection*, Vol. 5, pp. 233–56 (New York: Plenum).

Ehling, U.H. (1980). Induction of gene mutations in germ cells of the mouse. *Arch. Toxicol.*, **46**, 123–38

Ehling, U.H., Cumming, R.B. and Malling, H.V. (1968). Induction of dominant lethal mutations by alkylating agents in male mice. *Mutat. Res.*, **5**, 417–28

Ehling, U.H. and Neuhauser, A. (1979). Procarbazine-induced specific-locus mutations in male mice. *Mutat, Res.*, **59**, 245–56

Eliasson, R. and Dornbusch, K. (1977). Levels of trimethoprim and sulphamethoxazole in human seminal plasma. *Andrologia*, **9**, 195–202

Eliasson, R. and Dornbusch, K. (1980). Secretion of metronidazole into the human semen. *Int. J. Androl.*, **3**, 236–42

Ericsson, R.J. and Baker, V.F. (1966). Transport of oestrogens in semen to the female rat during mating and its effect on fertility. *J. Reprod. Fertil.*, **12**, 381–4

Evans, H.J., Fletcher, J., Torrance, M. and Hargreave, T.B. (1981). Sperm abnormalities and cigarette smoking. *Lancet*, **1**, 627–9

Ewing, L.L. and Robaire, B. (1978). Endogenous antispermatogenic agents: prospects for male contraception. *Ann. Rev. Pharmacol. Toxicol.*, **18**, 167–87

Ewing, L.L., Schanbacher, B., Desjardins, C. and Chaffee, V. (1976). The effect of subdermal testosterone filled polydimethylsiloxane implants on spermatogenesis in rhesus monkeys (*Macaca mulata*). *Contraception*, **13**, 583–96

Ewing, L.L., Stratton, L.G. and Desjardins, C. (1973) Effect of testosterone polydimethylsiloxane implants upon sperm production, libido and accessory sex organ function in rabbits. *J. Reprod. Fertil.*, **35**, 245–53

Fiscor, G. and Ginsberg, L.C. (1980). The effect of hydroxyurea and mitomycin C on sperm motility in mice. *Mutat. Res.*, **70**, 383-7

Forrest, J.B., Turner, T.T. and Howards, S.S. (1981). Cyclophosphamide, vincristine, and the blood testis barrier. *Invest. Urol.*, **18**, 443-4

Furuhjelm, M., Jonson, B. and Lagergren, C.-G. (1962). The quality of human semen in spontaneous abortion. *Int. J. Fertil.* **7**, 17-21

Generoso, W.M., Bishop, J.B., Gosslee, D.G., Wewell, G.H., Sheu, C-J. and von Halle, E. (1980). Heritable translocation test in mice. *Mutat. Res.*, **76**, 191-215

Generoso, W.M., Cain, K.T., Huff, S.W. and Gosslee, D.G. (1978). Heritable translocation test in mice. In Hollaender, A. and de Serres, F.J. (eds.) *Chemical Mutagens—Principles and Methods for Their Detection*, Vol. 5, pp. 55-77 (New York: Plenum)

Generoso, W.M., Cain, K.T., Krishna, M. and Muff, S.W. (1979). Genetic lesions induced by chemicals in spermatozoa and spermatids of mice are repaired in the egg. *Proc. Natl. Acad. Sci. USA*, **76**, 435-7

Glode, L.M., Robinson, J. and Gould, S.F. (1981). Protection from cyclophosphamide-induced testicular damage with an analogue of gonadotropin-releasing hormone. *Lancet*, **1**, 1132-4

Heber, D. and Swerdloff, R.S. (1980). Male contraception: synergism of gonadotropin-releasing hormone analog and testosterone in suppressing gonadotropin. *Science*, **209**, 936-8

Hoffer, A.P., Hinton, B., Lisser S. and Weston, S. (1983). The effects of gossypol on the blood-testis and blood-epididymis barrier in rats. *J. Androl.*, **4**, 36

Hong, C.Y., Chaput de Saintonge, D.M. and Turner, P. (1982). Effects of chlorpromazine and other drugs acting on the central nervous system on human sperm motility. *Eur. J. Clin. Pharmacol.*, **22**, 413-6

Hoppe, P.C. and Illmensee, K. (1982). Full-term development after transplantation of parthenogenetic embryonic nuclei into fertilized mouse eggs. *Proc. Natl. Acad. Sci. USA*, **79**, 1912-16

Infante, P.F., Wagoner, J.K. and Waxweiler, R.J. (1976). Carcinogenic, mutagenic and teratogenic risks associated with vinyl chloride. *Mutat. Res.*, **41**, 131-42

Jackson, H. (1964). The effects of alkylating agents on fertility. *Br. Med. Bull.*, **20**, 107-14

Kantor, A.F., Curnen, M.G.M, Meigs, J.W. and Flannery, J.T. (1979). Occupations of fathers of patients with Wilm's Tumour. *J. Epidemiol. Community Health*, **33**, 253-6

Kapp, R.W., Jr (1979). Detection of aneuploidy in human sperm. *Environ. Health Perspec.*, **31**, 27-31

Kharrazi, M., Potashnik, G. and Goldsmith, J.R. (1980). Reproductive effects of dibromo-chloropropane. *Isr. J. Med. Sci.*, **16**, 403-6

Knill-Jones, R.P., Newnann, B.J. and Spence, A.A. (1975). Anesthetic practice and pregnancy. Controlled study of male anesthetists in the United Kingdom. *Lancet*, **2**, 807-9

Krzanowska, H. (1974). The passage of abnormal spermatozoa through the uterotubal junction of the mouse. *J. Reprod. Fertil.*, **38**, 81-90

Lancranjan, I., Popescu, H.J., Găvănescu, O., Klepsch, I. and Serbănescu, M. (1975). Reproductive ability of workmen occupationally exposed to lead. *Arch. Environ. Health*, **30**, 396-401

Land, P.C., Owen, E.L. and Linde, H.W. (1981). Morphologic changes in mouse spermatozoa after exposure to inhalational anesthetics during early spermatogenesis. *Anesthesiology*, **54**, 53-6

Lang, R. and Adler, I.-D. (1977). Heritable translocation test and dominant lethal assay in male mice with methyl methanesulfonate. *Mutat. Res.*, **48**, 75-88

Lee, I.P. and Suzuki, K. (1981). Differential DNA-repair activity in prespermiogenic cells of various mouse strains. *Mutat. Res.*, **80**, 201-11

Linde, R., Doelle, G.C. Alexander, N., Kirchner, F., Vale, W., Rivier, J. and Rabin, D. (1981). Reversible inhibition of testicular steroidogenesis and spermatogenesis by a potent gonadotropin-releasing hormone agonist in normal men. *N. Eng. J. Med.*, **305**, 663-7

Lobl, T.J., Kirton, K.T., Forbes, A.D., Ewing, L.L., Kemp, P.L. and Desjardins, C. (1983). Contraceptive efficacy of testosterone-estradiol implants in male rhesus monkeys. *Contraception*, **27**, 383-9

Lobl, T.J. and Mathews, J. (1978). Effect of 1-(2, 4-dichlorobenzyl)-indazole-3-carboxylic acid on sperm tails in rhesus monkeys, *J. Reprod. Fertil.*, **52**, 275-8

Lutwak-Mann, C. (1964). Observations on progeny of thalidomide-treated male rabbits. *Br. Med. J.*, **1**, 1090–1

Lutwak-Mann, C., Schmid, K. and Keberle, H. (1967). Thalidomide in rabbit semen. *Nature*, **214**, 1018–20

Malmborg, A.S. (1978). Antimicrobial drugs in human seminal plasma. *J. Antimicrob. Chemother.*, **6**, 483–5

Mankes, R.F., LeFevre, R., Benitz, K.F., Rosenblum, I., Bates, H., Walker, A.I.T. and Abraham, R. (1982). Paternal effects of ethanol in the Long-Evans rat. *J. Toxicol. Environ. Health*, **10**, 871–8

Mann, T. and Lutwak-Mann, C. (1981). Male reproductive function and semen. Themes and Trends in Physiology, Biochemistry and Investigative Andrology. (Berlin: Springer-Verlag)

Mau, G. and Netter, P. (1974). Die auswirkungen des väterlichen zigarettenkonsums auf die perinatale sterblichkeit und die mibbildungshäufigkeit. *Dtsch. Med. Wschr.*, **99**, 1113–8

Moreland, F.M., Sheu, C.W., Springer, J.A. and Green, S. (1981). Effects of prolonged chemical treatment with cyclophosphamide and 6-mercaptopurine in the dominant lethal test system. *Mutat. Res.*, **90**, 193–9

Orgebin-Crist, M.C. (1969). Studies on the function of the epididymis. *Biol. Reprod.*, **1**, 155–75

Orgebin-Crist, M.C., Danzo, B.J. and Davies, J. (1975). Endocrine control of the development and maintenance of sperm fertilizing ability in the epididymis. In Greep,. R.O. and Astwood, E.B. (eds.) *Handbook of Physiology.* Sect. 7, Vol. 5, pp. 319–38. (Washington: American Physiological Society)

Paladine, W.J., Cunningham, T.J., Donavan, M.A. and Dumper, C.W. (1975). Possible sensitivity to vinblastine in prostatic or seminal fluid. *N. Engl. J. Med.*, **292**, 52

Peterson, R.N. and Freund, M. (1975). The inhibition of the motility of human spermatozoa by various pharmacologic agents. *Biol. Reprod.*, **13**, 552–6

Plomp, T.A., Mattelaer, J.J. and Maes, R.A.A. (1978). The concentration of thiamphenicol in seminal fluid and prostatic tissue. *J. Antimicrob. Chemother.*, **4**, 65–71

Pope, W.D.P. and Persaud, T.V.N. (1982). Fertility and reproduction after male rat exposure to halothane. *Exp. Pathol.*, **22**, 59–62

Robaire, B., Ewing, L.L., Irby, D.C. and Desjardins, C. (1979). Interactions of testosterone and estradiol-17β on the reproductive tract of the male rat. *Biol. Reprod.*, **21**, 455–63

Robaire, B. and Zirkin, B.R. (1981). Hypophysectomy and simultaneous testosterone replacement: Effects on male rat reproductive tract and epididymal Δ^4-5α-reductase and 3α-hydroxysteroid dehydrogenase. *Endocrinology*, **109**, 1225–33

Russell, W.L., Hunsicker, P.R., Carpenter, D.A., Cornett, C.V. and Guinn, G.M. (1982). Effect of dose fractionation of the ethylnitrosourea induction of specific locus mutations in mouse spermatogonia. *Proc. Natl. Acad. Sci. USA*, **79**, 3592–3

Sandow, J., Rechenberg, W.V., Baeder, C. and Engelbart, K. (1980). Antifertility effects of an LHRH analogue in male rats and dogs. *Int. J. Fert.*, **25**, 213–21

Schaffenburg, C.A., Gregoire, A.T. and Gueriguian, J.L. (1981). Guidelines for the clinical testing of male contraceptive drugs. *J. Androl.*, **2**, 225–8

Schardein, J.L. (1976). *Drugs as Teratogens.* (Cleveland: CRC Press)

Sega, G.A. (1974). Unscheduled DNA synthesis in the germ cells of male mice exposed *in vivo* to the chemical mutagen ethyl methanesulfonate. *Proc. Natl. Acad. Sci. USA*, **71**, 4955–9.

Sega, G.A., Owens, J.G. and Cumming, R.B. (1976). Studies on DNA repair in early spematid stages of male mice after *in vivo* treatment with methyl-, ethyl-, propyl- and isopropyl methanesulfonate. *Mutat. Res.*, **36**, 193–212

Sega, G.A. and Owens, J.G. (1978). Ethylation of DNA and protamine by ethyl methanesulfonate in the germ cells of male mice and the relevancy of these molecular targets to the induction of dominant lethals. *Mutat. Res.*, **52**, 87–106

Sega, G.A. and Sotomayor, R.E. (1982). Unscheduled DNA synthesis in mammalian germ cells—Its potential use in mutagenicity testing. In de Serres, F.J. and Hollaender, A. (eds.) *Chemical Mutagens—Principles and Methods for their Detection.* Vol. 7, pp. 421–45 (New York: Plenum)

Setchell, B.P. and Waites, G.M.H. (1975). The blood-testis barrier. In Greep, R.O. and Astwood, E.B. (eds.) *Handbook of Physiology*, Sect. 7, Vol. 5, pp. 143–72 (Washington: American Physiological Society)

Sheu, C.W., Moreland, F.M., Oswald, E.J., Green S. and Flamm, W.G. (1978). Heritable translocation test on random-bred mice after prolonged triethylenemelamine treatment. *Mutat. Res.*, **50**, 241–50

Smith, D.J. and Joffe, J.M. (1975). Increased neonatal mortality in offspring of male rats treated with methadone or morphine before mating. *Nature (London)*, **253**, 202–3

Smith, F.P. (1981). Detection of amphetamine in bloodstains, semen, seminal stains, saliva, and saliva stains. *Forensic Science*, **17**, 225–8

Sotomayor, R.E. and Cumming, R.B. (1975). Induction of translocations by cyclophosphamide in different germ cell stages of male mice: cytological characterization and transmission. *Mutat. Res.*, **27**, 375–88

Sotomayor, R.E., Sega, G.A. and Cumming, R.B. (1978). Unscheduled DNA synthesis in spermatogenic cells of mice treated *in vivo* with the indirect alkylating agents cyclophosphamide and mitomen. *Mutat. Res.*, **50**, 229–40

Soyka, L.F., Peterson, J.M. and Joffe, J.M. (1978). Lethal and sublethal effects on the progeny of male rats treated with methadone. *Toxicol. Appl. Pharmacol.*, **45**, 797–807

Stockard, C.R. (1913). The effect on the offspring of intoxicating the male parent and the transmission of the defects to subsequent generations. *Am. Nat.*, **47**, 641–82

Swanson, B.N., Leger, R.M., Gordon, W.P., Lynn, R.K. and Gerber, N. (1978). Excretion of phenytoin into semen of rabbits and man. Comparison with plasma levels. *Drug Metabol. Dispos.*, **6**, 70–4

Swerdloff, R.S., Palacios, A., McClure, R.D., Campfield, L.A. and Brosman, S.A. (1978). Male contraception: clinical assessment of chronic administration of testosterone enanthate. *Int. J. Androl. Suppl.*, **2**, 731–45

Wharton, R.S., Mazze, R.I., Baden, J.M., Hitt, B.A. and Dooley, J.R. (1978). Fertility, reproduction and postnatal survival in mice chronically exposed to halothane. *Anesthesiology*, **48**, 167–74

White, I.G. and Macleod, J. (1963). Composition and physiology of semen. In Hartman, C.G. (ed.) *Mechanisms Concerned with Contraception*, pp. 136–172 (New York; MacMillan)

Whorton, M.D. and Milby, T.H. (1980). Recovery of testicular function among DBCP workers. *J. Occup. Med.*, **22**, 177–9

Whorton, M.D., Milby, T.H., Krauss, R.M. and Stubbs, H.A. (1979). Testicular function in DBCP exposed pesticide workers. *J. Occup. Med.*, **21**, 161–6

Wyrobek, A.J., Brodsky, J., Gordon, L., Moore, D.H., II, Watchmaker, G. and Cohen, E.N. (1981). Sperm studies in anesthesiologists. *Anesthesiology*, **55**, 527–32

Wyrobek, A.J. and Bruce, W.R. (1975). Chemical induction of sperm abnormalities in mice. *Proc. Natl. Acad. Sci. USA*, **72**, 4425–9

17
Animal tests employed to assess the effects of drugs and chemicals on reproduction

T.A. MARKS

Although it has been more than 20 years since the thalidomide tragedy forever laid to rest the idea that a 'placental barrier' existed which served to protect the embryo from prenatal exposure to harmful substances, the phenomenon of chemical ingestion by the father affecting his progeny has only recently received sufficient documentation to be generally recognized (Joffe, 1979; Manson and Simons, 1979). The effects of chemicals and drugs on male as well as female reproductive systems have also been widely studied (Dixon and Hall, 1982).

Public concern about potential human reproductive risks, resulting from exposure to chemicals, drugs, food additives, etc., has led to governmental regulation in this area. In the United States, the National Center for Drugs and Biologics (formerly the Bureau of Drugs) of the Food and Drug Administration (FDA) is responsible for monitoring reproduction studies of drugs, while the FDA's Bureau of Foods regulates direct food additives and colour additives used in food. The United States Environmental Protection Agency (EPA) is responsible for monitoring reproductive testing of chemicals as required under Section 4(a) of the *Toxic Substance Control Act* (TSCA) and the *Federal Insecticide, Fungicide and Rodenticide Act* (FIFRA). Also, reproductive toxicity principles and procedures for evaluating the toxicity of household substances have been developed by the Consumer Products Safety Commission (Tardiff, 1977). In addition, the Occupational Safety and Health Administration (OSHA) of the Department of Labor has been designated to assure that safe and healthful conditions exist in the workplace and to administer the *Occupational Safety and Health Act*.

During the past few years a great deal of attention has been given to the area of reproductive toxicology. The 'Love Canal Incident' in Niagara, New York, as well as other chemical exposure incidents, has led to public concerns about the effects of such exposures to human reproduction. Workers in chemical plants are even more likely to be exposed to reproductive hazards and these potential risks have generated concern in Congress (Committee on Science and Technology, 1982). Much of this activity has resulted in several informative and comprehensive reviews assessing the risks of chemicals and other environmental substances to human reproduction and development by governmental (regulatory and non-regulatory) agencies (Clement Associates, Inc., 1981; EPA, 1982a; NTP/NIEHS, 1980), by academia (Amann, 1982; Thomas, 1981) and by industry (Wilson, 1979).

ASSESSING REPRODUCTIVE RISKS

Teratologists, toxicologists and others responsible for using animal studies to assess the reproductive risks to humans of drugs and chemicals are well aware of the problems in this area (Amann, 1982; Fraser, 1977). In the United States, bioassays for assessing the reproductive risks of drugs have been only slightly updated (Burns, 1983; Kelsey, 1982) since the FDA published *Guidelines for Reproduction and Teratology* in 1966. These guidelines were an outgrowth of the thalidomide tragedy. Since 1979, the FDA has stipulated that non-clinical laboratory studies done to meet FDA requirements must adhere to Good Laboratory Practice (GLP) regulations (FDA, 1978). Other countries have published their own guidelines (Christian, 1983; Health and Welfare Canada, 1975; Palmer, 1981), some of which will be briefly outlined here.

STUDIES TO ASSESS THE REPRODUCTIVE RISKS OF NEW DRUGS

Before a new drug can be marketed, most countries require that it be examined for its potential to affect all aspects of reproduction including spermatogenesis, mating, gestation, parturition and lactation. They generally require a three–segment design similar to that introduced in 1966 FDA Guidelines (Collins, 1978a): 'Study of Fertility and General Reproductive Performance' (Segment I); 'Teratology Study' (Segment II); and 'Perinatal and Postnatal Study' (Segment III).

TERATOLOGY STUDIES

Recent publications (Health and Welfare Canada, 1975; Manson *et al.*, 1982; Schardein, 1976; Tracor Jitco, Inc., 1977) have outlined the techniques employed in teratology testing. One can get some idea of the difficulties involved in performing teratology studies in rodents and rabbits from diagrams (Fig. 17.1) illustrating the embryotoxicity, teratogenicity and lethality dose–response relationships generally seen in such studies. Figure 17.1A represents the findings expected in teratology studies with moderately potent teratogens (Wilson, 1973). Embryotoxicity is often observed at doses lower than those which produce teratogenicity. Frequently such doses also produce maternal toxicity, although the embryo can be expected to be more

246

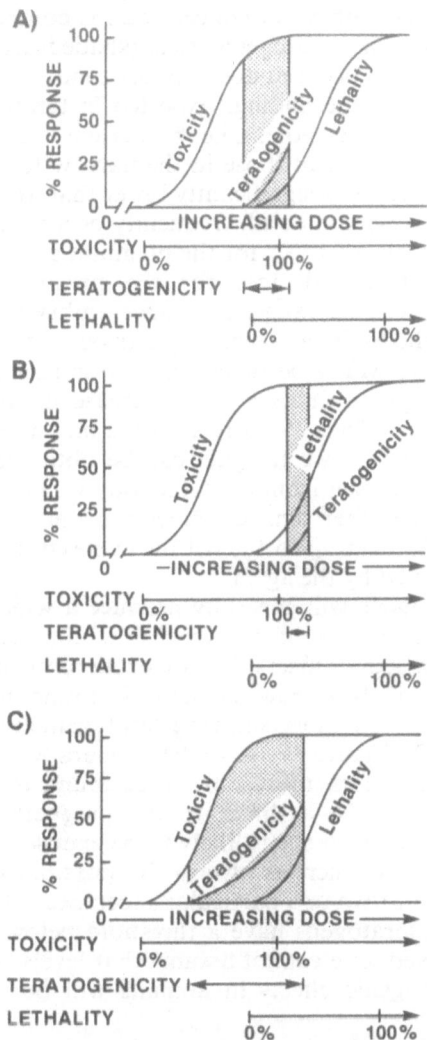

Fig. 17.1 Representative dose-response relationships for embryotoxicity, teratogenicity and lethality in teratology studies. (A) Graphic representation of what is frequently observed with moderately potent teratogens. Note that embryotoxicity has occurred at doses lower than those which produce teratogenicity, the teratogenic zone (shaded area) is narrow, and lethal effects have occurred at doses in this zone. (B) Graphic representation of what is frequently observed with borderline teratogens. Note that embryolethal effects have occurred at doses lower than those which were teratogenic and that embryotoxicity was found at even lower doses. (C) Graphic representation of what should occur if a teratogen is highly potent. Note that the teratogenic zone is wide with a definite dose-response effect; that embryotoxicity was not severe at the lower teratogenic doses and that embryolethal effects did not occur until higher doses were reached

sensitive than the dam to the effects of the agent if the agent or a toxic metabolite(s) reaches the embryo at concentrations comparable to those in the general circulation. The teratogenic zone (shaded area) is usually narrow. Lethal effects also can occur at doses in this zone.

Figure 17.1B represents the findings expected in teratology studies with compounds which are not very potent, i.e. borderline teratogens. Here lethal effects occur at doses lower than those in the narrow teratogenic zone and embryotoxicity occurs at doses significantly lower than those that are lethal. Teratogenic effects, if observed at all, frequently occur only at doses which are one-half to one-eighth the LD_{50} for the pregnant animal (Wilson, 1973). Since the maximum tolerated dose for the pregnant animal (MTD) generally occurs in this same range, and since embryotoxic effects which occur at doses above the MTD are generally attributed to maternal toxicity, it is important that the MTD be determined. For rats the MTD can be defined as the dose that produces a 10% decrease in weight gain during pregnancy, but no lethal effects. A more accurate measurement of the effect of a compound on maternal weight gain can be obtained if the weight of the gravid uterus is subtracted from the final body weight of each dam. The MTD may also produce other signs of toxicity, pronounced pharmacological effects or lethal effects in up to 10% of the exposed dams, if weight gain is not appreciably affected by the agent.

Highly potent teratogens will generally produce a wide teratogenic zone with a definite dose–response effect; toxicity is not severe at the lower teratogenic doses, and lethal effects do not occur until higher doses have been reached (Figure 17.1C). Few substances, found to be teratogenic, follow such a pattern with most showing teratogenicity only at dosages approaching the MTD (Figure 17.1A or B). Generally, similar results can be expected in humans. Thus, most substances found to be teratogenic in animals are not likely to be a threat to the pregnant woman and her offspring at the levels to which she is likely to be exposed. However, as was the case with thalidomide, there is always the possibility that the human embryo will be more sensitive to a particular substance. Therefore, although it is probable that all teratogens have a threshold below which teratogenicity will not be observed, one cannot assume that levels below those necessary to produce teratogenic effects in animals will be absolutely safe in humans.

Two species, one of which often is a nonrodent, are required for teratology studies. Most laboratories use the rat and the rabbit. A vehicle control group and three test groups should be used; each should include at least 20 pregnant rats (or mice) or 10 (IRLG guidelines recommend 12) pregnant does. Figure 17.2 outlines the dosing regimens as recommended by FDA (Collins, 1978a). Although there are exceptions (e.g. Marks *et al.*, 1981), most compounds found to be teratogenic lead to such effects only at doses close to, or higher than, the MTD. Therefore, it is recommended that drugs be tested for teratogenicity at the MTD, one-half the MTD and one-quarter the MTD. Pronounced pharmacological and even toxic effects are frequently observed at the higher doses tested. If the mean body weight gains of the test groups during pregnancy are comparable to that of the vehicle

ANIMAL TESTS TO ASSESS THE EFFECT OF DRUGS

A. RAT or MOUSE

⩾ 20 pregnant dams/group
1 vehicle control and 3 test groups

Examination	% of Pups
Gross	100
Visceral	33-50
Skeletal	50-67

```
                    Cesarean
        Dosing      Section
  •——————|——————————|———————
  0      6          15    20
```

B. RABBIT

⩾ 10 pregnant does/group
1 vehicle control and 3 test groups

Gross	100
Visceral	100
Skeletal	100

```
                         Cesarean
        Dosing           Section
  •——————|———————————————|———————
  0      6               18    28
```

Fig. 17.2 US Food and Drug Administration guidelines for Segment II Teratology Studies. (A) Rat or mouse. Generally the animals are dosed between days 6 and 15 of gestation (day 0 being the day that evidence was obtained that mating had occurred). For rats a caesarean section is performed on day 20 (for mice day 17) and the fetuses examined for gross, visceral and skeletal anomalies. (B) Rabbit. The does are generally dosed between days 6 and 18 of gestation (the dose being mated naturally or artifically on day 0). A cesarean section is performed on day 28 and 100% of the fetuses are examined for gross, visceral and skeletal anomalies

control group, especially between days 6 and 10 of gestation when the weights of the developing embryos are negligible, teratogenic effects occur infrequently. However, other signs of embryotoxicity can be expected at dosages approaching the MTD (Wilson, 1973).

Dosing should be by the most likely route of human exposure; however, for practical reasons the oral or subcutaneous routes are frequently used. The test agent is generally administered once a day during the period of organogenesis—days 6-15 in the rat or mouse and days 6-18 in the rabbit. The test animals are killed on day 20 for the rat or day 28 for the rabbit (Dutch-belted or New Zealand White). The offspring are removed after performing a laparotomy, weighed and examined by established teratological procedures for gross, visceral and skeletal anomalies. Although other *in vivo* methods are used (e.g. Courtney and Chernoff, 1974), most teratology laboratories at present use variations of the Wilson razor blade technique (Barrow and Taylor, 1969; Wilson, 1965) or the Staples technique (Staples, 1974; Stuckhardt and Poppe, 1984), which includes visceral examination of the head as in Wilson's technique, and examination of the skeleton after staining with alizarin red S (Staples and Schnell, 1964).

With minor variations, teratology studies are carried out as just described in all countries except Japan (Japan Ministry of Health and Welfare, 1975) where postpartum behavioural, developmental and fertility tests are also required in the rat study (Fig. 17.3). The Japanese requirements for a rabbit teratology study are essentially the same as those issued by the IRLG (IRLG, 1981). For Japanese studies it is recommended that all lesions and malformations be photographed. At least one photograph of each variation found in a study should also be taken.

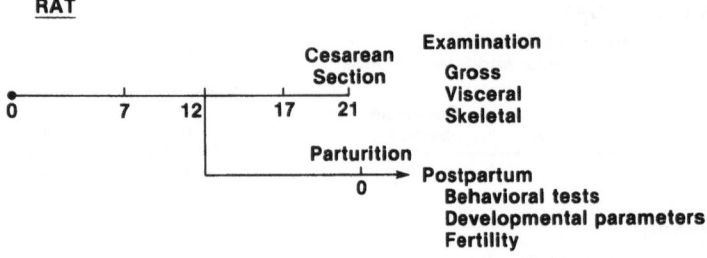

Fig. 17.3 Japanese teratology study in the rat. The dams are dosed between days 7 and 17 (day 0 being the day evidence was obtained that mating had occurred). A caesarean section is performed on about two-thirds of the dams on day 21 with gross, visceral and skeletal examinations carried out. The remaining dams in each group should be allowed to rear their young to weaning, performing behavioural tests and checking developmental parameters with some young reared to maturity and their fertility determined

PERINATAL AND POSTNATAL STUDIES

Testing similar to that used in Japanese teratology studies is required in Japanese perinatal and postnatal studies (Fig. 17.4). The Japanese recommend that pregnant rats be treated from day 17 of gestation until weaning.

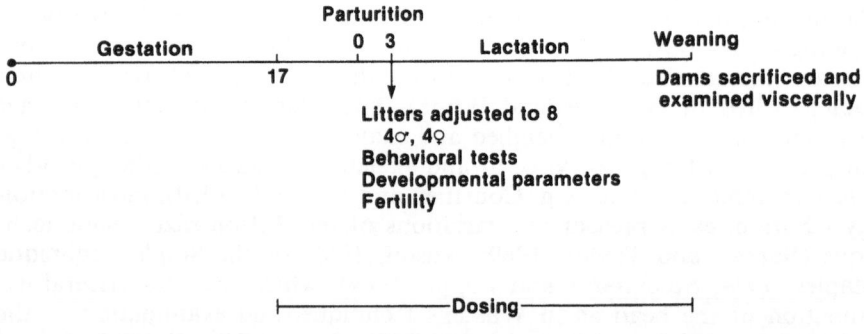

Fig. 17.4 Japanese perinatal and postnatal study. The dams (rats or mice) are dosed from day 17 (day 15 is also acceptable) of gestation, through parturition and lactation, until weaning. The litters are culled to 8 (4 males and 4 females) on postpartum day 3. Behavioural tests should be carried out and developmental parameters monitored with fertility verified at maturity

The litters are culled to 8 on postpartum day 3. The FDA does not require behavioural, developmental or fertility tests for perinatal and postnatal studies (Fig. 17.5). Also, dosing begins on day 15 of gestation.

250

ANIMAL TESTS TO ASSESS THE EFFECT OF DRUGS

≥ 20 pregnant rats/group
1 Vehicle control and
3 test groups

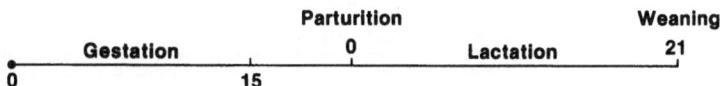

Fig. 17.5 US Food and Drug Administration Segment III perinatal and postnatal study. This study is generally performed in rats. The dams are dosed between day 15 of gestation, through parturition and lactation, until weaning. The weights of the dams and pups are recorded throughout the study, along with pup survival

REPRODUCTION STUDIES

Although Japan's teratology and perinatal and postnatal studies would most likely be acceptable in the rest of the world, their fertility study would not because it does not meet minimum FDA requirements. The basic discrepancy is that in the Japanese study dosing is stopped on day 7 of gestation and an examination similar to a teratology examination is performed after removing the pups on day 21 (Fig. 17.6). In contrast, the FDA recommends that dosing in reproduction studies be continued until weaning of

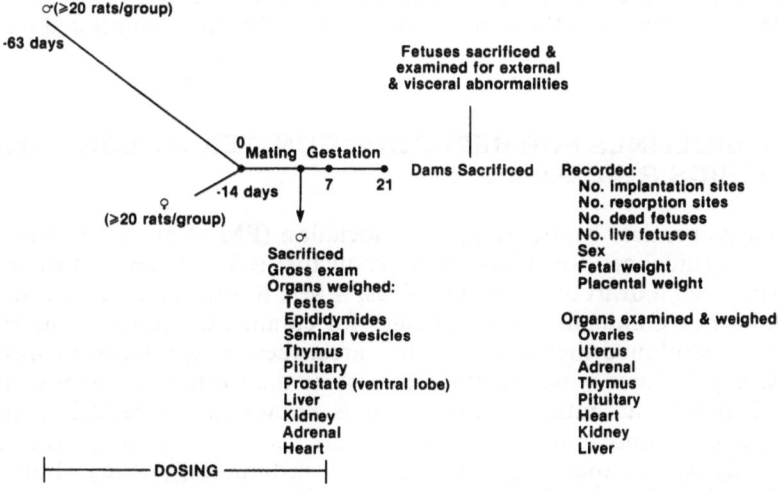

Fig. 17.6 Japanese fertility study. Rats are generally employed in this study. The males are dosed for nine weeks, and the females for two weeks, prior to mating, with dosing continued through the mating period (three weeks), to day 7 of gestation. Note that for both males and females at least the organs listed should be examined and weighed

251

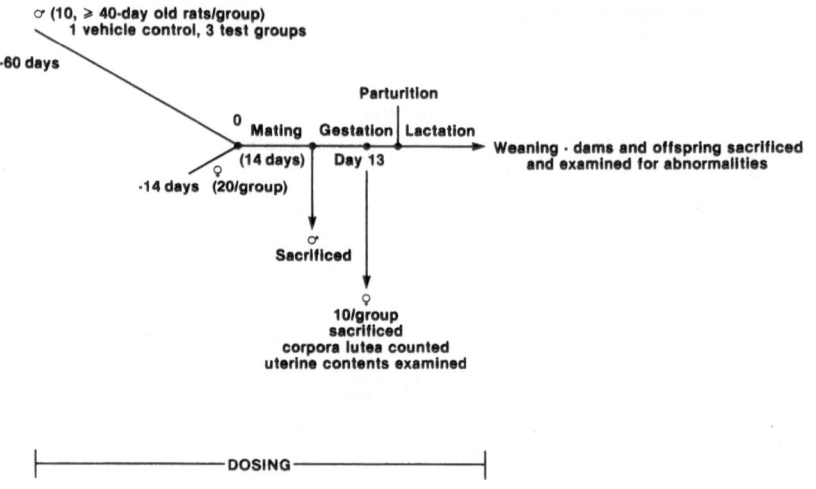

Fig. 17.7 US Food and Drug Administration Segment I study of fertility and reproductive performance. Rats are generally employed in this study. The males should be dosed for 60 days and the females for 14 days, prior to mating. Dosing is continued through the 14-day mating period, gestation, parturition, lactation on to weaning. The males are sacrificed after mating their assigned females or at the end of the 14-day mating period. Half the females, which had shown evidence of having mated, are sacrificed on day 13 of gestation, and their uterine contents examined and their corpora lutea counted. The remaining dams, which had produced litters, and their litters are sacrificed on postpartum day 21

the first generation. On day 13 of gestation half the dams are killed and the corpora lutea are counted and the uterine contents are examined (Fig. 17.7). In both the Japanese and US studies the males are treated for at least 60 days before mating and the females for 14 days. Dosing is continued during the mating period.

PMA GUIDELINES FOR REPRODUCTION, TERATOLOGY AND PEDIATRICS GUIDELINES

The Pharmaceutical Manufacturers Association (PMA) has also shown an interest in guidelines for assessing reproductive risks of new drugs. PMA has distributed a draft of these guidelines, 'PMA Reproduction, Teratology, and Pediatrics Guidelines' to companies for comment. Although the PMA has since abandoned their efforts in this area, there is at least one aspect of the PMA guidelines which is more consistent than other guidelines (international as well as national) with what is known about gestation in the three species (mouse, rat and rabbit) usually used in teratology studies. It is generally agreed that pregnant animals in a teratology study should be treated during the period of organogenesis. However, in spite of evidence that implantation, at least in the rat and rabbit, is still likely on day 6 of gestation, most regulatory agencies recommend that dosing be started on this day. In contrast, the PMA recommended in their draft guidelines that the dosing period for the mouse and rat be days 7–15 of gestation (day 0 being the day spermatozoa are observed in a vaginal smear). In the rabbit, the PMA had recommended that the dosing period be days 8–18 of gestation.

Findings in teratology studies at The Upjohn Company support the PMA's recommendations in this area. Prostaglandins known to produce uterine contractions were found to interfere with implantation when given on days 6–15 of gestation. Other compounds interfered with early postimplantation as early implant sites, not visible on gross inspection of the uteri, were seen with ammonium sulphide staining (Kopf et al., 1964). Since such effects should be detectable in reproduction or perinatal and postnatal studies, there seems to be no need to dose before day 7 in teratology studies.

STUDIES TO ASSESS REPRODUCTIVE RISKS OF FOOD ADDITIVES

New guidelines for reproduction studies in the safety evaluation of direct food additives and colour additives used in foods have recently been released by the FDA's Bureau of Foods (FDA, 1982). The guidelines outlined in this document are more current and comprehensive than those outlined in past publications (Collins, 1978b; FDA, 1970).

The three-generation reproduction study, with optional teratology study, recommended by the Bureau of Foods for the evaluation of additives to food (Fig. 17.8) could take two years or more to complete. The 2–3 litters necessary in each of three generations increases the time and costs for such a study. Also, the suggestion that the highest dose should induce toxicity, but not mortality in parental animals while the lowest dose should not induce any observable effects, is difficult to follow. Predicting such doses is not easy, especially if preliminary toxicity studies were carried out using adult animals while young males are employed in the reproduction study to allow for the 56–day (mouse) or 70–day (rat) dosing period before mating and still have animals of optimum age to sire two or more litters of offspring.

STUDIES TO ASSESS REPRODUCTIVE RISKS OF NEW CHEMICALS

Reproduction and teratology studies have also been used to test chemicals, although the requirements for chemical studies are not as clearly defined as those for drug studies. In the United States, the EPA has the responsibility for monitoring animal toxicology studies of most chemicals. The original EPA guidelines for new chemicals (EPA, 1979b) included a multigeneration study. These guidelines recommended that (1) both males and females should be dosed for 100 days before mating, with dosing continued through mating, gestation and lactation; (2) spermatogenesis must be measured or histopathological examination of the testes must be performed; and (3)

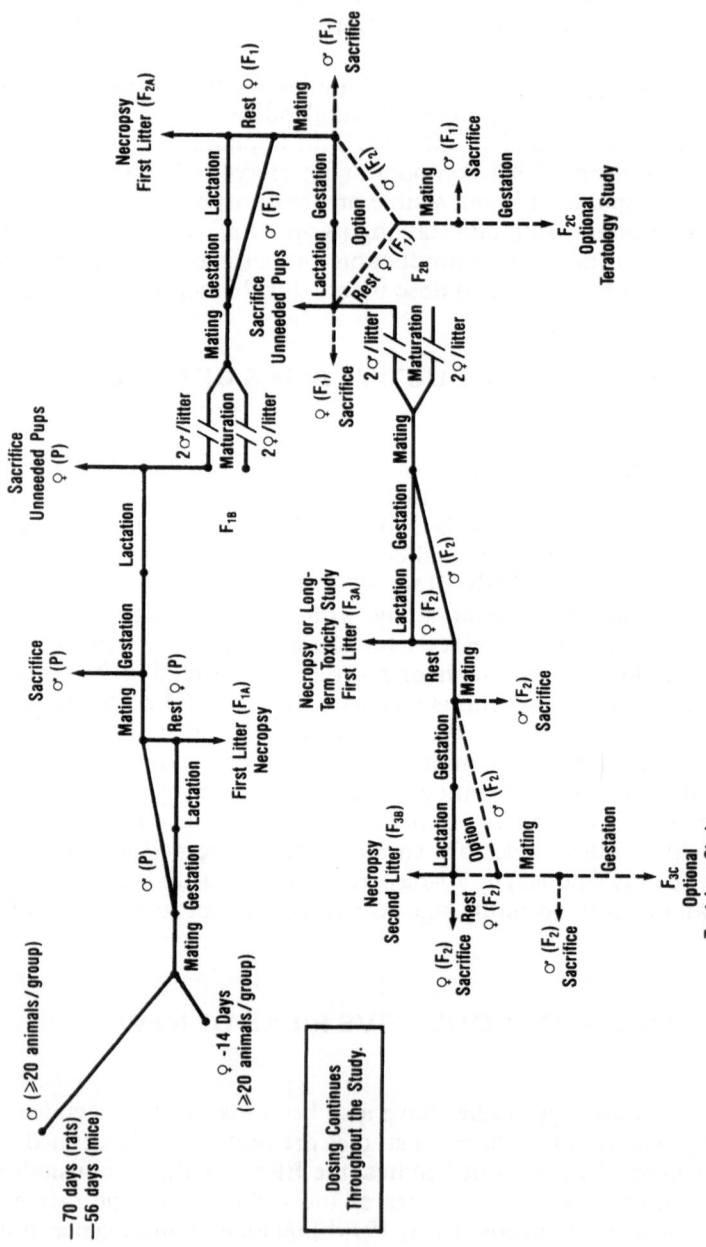

Fig. 17.8 US Food and Drug Administration (Bureau of Foods) three–generation reproduction and teratology study. Rats or mice can be used for this study. Dosing, preferably in the food or water, should be continued throughout the entire study, even during the 10–day rest periods after weaning. Note that it is recommended that the second litter of each of the first two generations be used to produce the subsequent generation with a teratology study run in either the second or the third generation

designated F_1 males and females should be dosed for 120 days before mating with dosing continued through mating, gestation, lactation, weaning and on to postpartum day 60. The EPA also has issued proposed GLP standards (EPA, 1979a).

Health effects test guidelines released by the Office of Toxic Substances of EPA (EPA, 1982b) contain reproduction and fertility, as well as teratogenicity study, test guidelines that may be cited as methodologies to be used in chemical specific test rules promulgated under Section 4(a) of TSCA. The teratology guidelines are very general and are similar to those of the FDA. However, there are several significant changes in these latest EPA guidelines for two-generation reproduction testing as compared with earlier EPA guidelines (EPA, 1979b). One major difference is that the standard for dosing both male and female rats for 100 days before mating has been changed to eight weeks in the first generation. Dosing of the males is to continue through the three-week mating period, after which the males are killed. For the second generation, the 120-day dosing period before mating has also been changed to eight weeks. Again, the males are to continue being dosed until the end of the three-week mating period. Full histopathological examination of the vagina, uterus, ovaries, testes, epididymides, seminal vesicles, prostate, and target organ(s) of all P_1 and F_1 animals selected for mating, at least in control and high dose groups, is recommended. Organs showing pathology in these animals should be examined in animals from other dose groups (thus, these tissues must also be removed and preserved after the animal dies or is killed).

Toxicity data related to an application for registration of a pesticide is administered by the Office of Pesticide Programs of the EPA as required by FIFRA. Unfortunately, pesticide assessment guidelines, released by the office of Pesticide Programs (EPA, 1982c), are inconsistent with the Office of Toxic Substances health effects test guidelines (EPA, 1982b), although they were released at about the same time. For example, the pesticide assessment guidelines indicate that in a two-generation reproduction study the F_1 males and females saved for mating should be dosed from the time they are weaned through the period they are mated (11 weeks for mice and 17 weeks for rats). However, the recommended premating dosing period for parental (P_1) males and females is now eight weeks in both sets of guidelines.

OECD GUIDELINES FOR TERATOLOGY AND REPRODUCTION STUDIES

On the international level, the Organization for Economic Cooperation and Development (OECD) was created to eliminate the non-tariff-related trade restrictions, including those that have resulted from differences in requirements for animal studies to assess reproductive risks (Nichols, 1983). For example, the fact that Japanese guidelines are so different from those in other countries makes it difficult for other countries to enter the Japanese market without performing additional studies. The OECD has prepared teratology and reproduction study guidelines (OECD, 1981), and OECD member nations have agreed that studies carried out according to those guidelines will be mutually acceptable. Unfortunately these guidelines pertain to chemicals but not to drugs. Thus, it is apparent that the costly duplicative procedures for marketing drugs internationally will continue for some time.

In the United States, the chemical industry should benefit from the OECD guidelines since the EPA will probably accept such guidelines for the studies that it regulates. Thus, the need for extensive premating exposure to a chemical for both males and females may no longer be necessary.

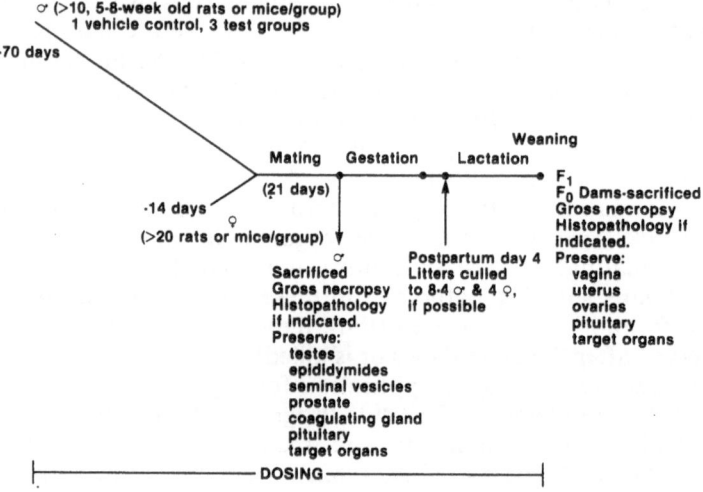

Fig. 17.9 Organization for Economic Cooperation and Development—one generation reproduction toxicity study. If mice are used in this study the males need only be dosed for 56 days prior to mating, not the 70 days noted here for rats. For both species the females are dosed for 14 days prior to being placed with the males. Dosing should be continued during the 21-day mating period, through gestation, parturition, lactation and on to weaning. The litter should be culled to 8 (4 males and 4 females) on postpartum day 4

Recently approved OECD guidelines for a one-generation reproduction study (OECD, 1981) require that males be exposed for 70 days and females for only 14 days (Fig. 17.9). This is in contrast to EPA's former requirement for a 100-day premating exposure for the F_0 animals. Although the EPA has now reduced the premating period to eight weeks, this agency still recommends that both males and females be exposed for this length of time prior to mating.

A two-generation reproduction study is outlined in Fig. 17.10. The procedures through weaning of the F_1 generation is the same as those for a one-generation study. Dosing continues until weaning of the F_2 pups. In both the one- and two-generation studies the designated tissues are preserved for histopathological examination if it is indicated. The coagulating gland and pituitary are included with the organs to be preserved.

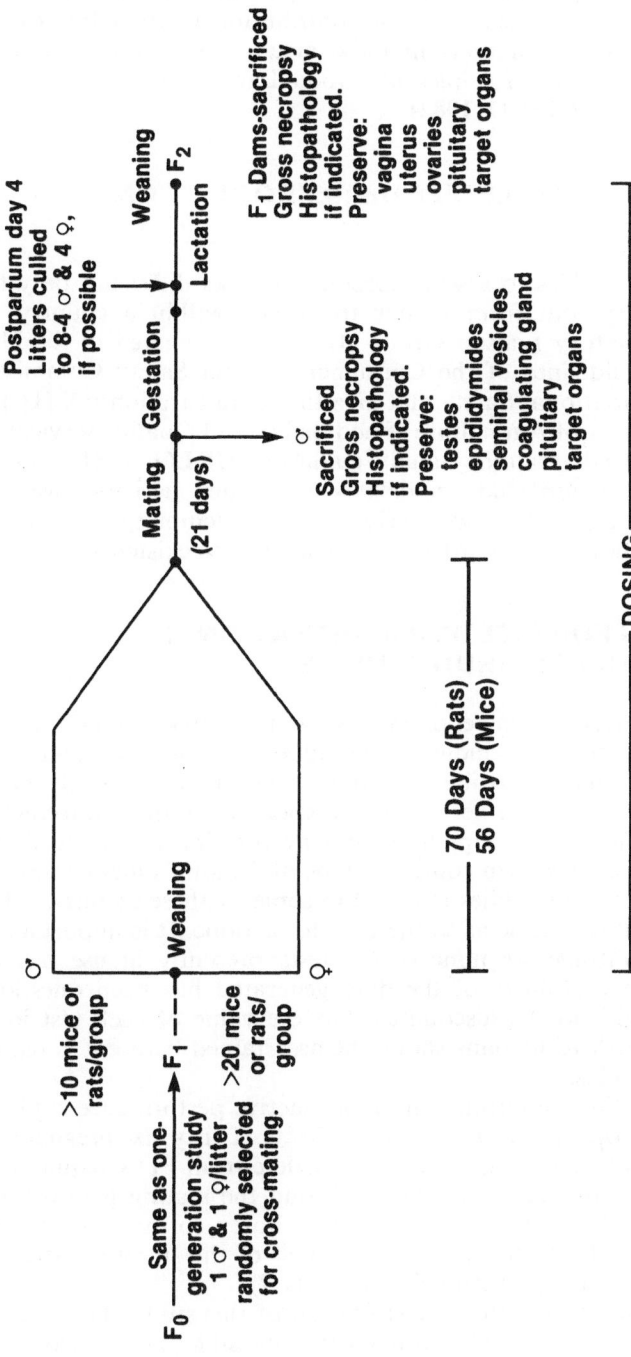

Fig. 17.10 Organization for Economic Cooperation and Development—two generation reproduction toxicity study. The first generation portion of this study is identical to that shown in Fig. 17.9. One male and one female from each litter are randomly selected for cross-mating to produce the second generation (F_1). Dosing of the F_1 animals begins at weaning and ends when they are killed. The remainder of the study is similar to the procedure for the one generation study.

257

Although limited to chemicals, the OECD guidelines for teratology and reproduction studies represent a major contribution to the effort to standardize international regulations in these areas. Also, of interest is the recently released OECD principles of 'Good Laboratory Practice in the Testing of Chemicals' (OECD, 1982).

ATTEMPTS TO STANDARDIZE US REPRODUCTION GUIDELINES

Requirements for studies to assess reproductive risks differ not only from country to country, but from agency to agency within a country. The Interagency Regulatory Liaison Group (IRLG) was created in the US to standardize the guidelines of the Consumer Product Safety Commission, FDA, EPA, Occupational Safety and Health Administration (OSHA) and later the Department of Agriculture (Food Safety and Quality Service). The IRLG had produced teratology study guidelines (IRLG, 1981) and were developing reproduction study guidelines when their activities were curtailed by Congress after they were criticized for attempting to create new guidelines in addition to standardizing those already in existence.

SUGGESTIONS FOR MEETING INTERNATIONAL REQUIREMENTS FOR DRUG STUDIES

Because of the differences in requirements from country to country, scientists in the pharmaceutical industry should try to meet as many international requirements as possible per study. Since Japanese guidelines are so different from those of other countries, scientists doing teratology and reproduction studies at The Upjohn Company concentrate on meeting the requirements of the European countries. One of Upjohn's main concerns is meeting the behavioural studies required in some of these countries. These requirements are not specific as to the tests to be done. It is important that this vagueness continue, as none of the tests presently in use has been validated and the usefulness of the data generated has been questioned. Such testing should not be discounted, but the value of each test in predicting potential risk to humans should be ascertained before it is required by regulatory agencies.

Figure 17.11 outlines a fertility and reproductive performance study modified to meet European and FDA requirements. Thirty six 'pregnant' rats are included in each test group so as not to delete from FDA requirements. Twelve sperm–positive dams are chosen during the mating period for behavioural testing. If possible, these dams are chosen so that no more than four days separate their delivery days. The rest of the study is carried out according to FDA Segment I guidelines (Fig. 17.7).

Figure 17.12 shows the behavioural portion of this study. The litters are culled to eight—four males and four females, if possible. The developmental events and behavioural tests shown are examples of the minimum tests

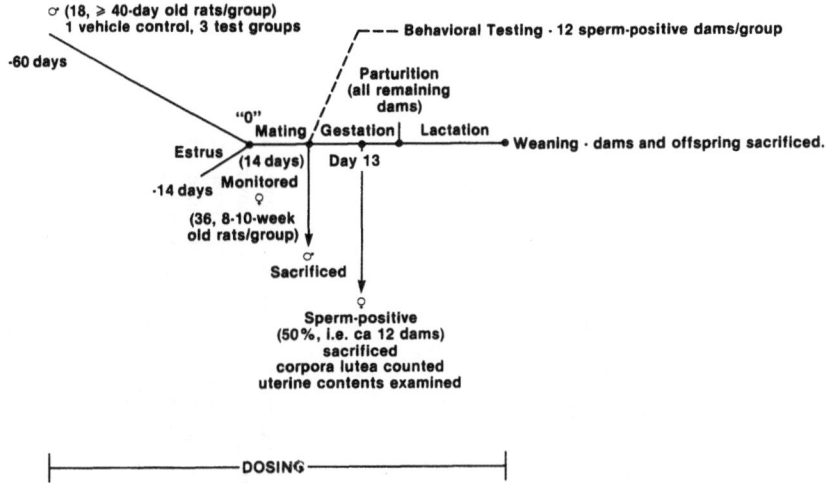

Fig. 17.11 Segment I study of fertility and reproductive performance, modified to meet USA and European requirements. This study is essentially the same as that shown in Fig. 17.7 except that each group contains 18 males and 36 females. After mating, one-third of the dams are removed for behavioural testing, etc., with another third subjected to the '13-day sacrifice' procedure recommended by the FDA. The remaining dams are allowed to give birth and their survival to weaning monitored as in a Segment I study

routinely used in such studies. Several other tests are available for use in place of or in addition to these. No rats are mated within litters. The dams are allowed to deliver their young which are then killed after being checked for abnormalities.

It may be possible to meet both FDA and Japanese requirements for teratology and reproduction studies without repeating studies. FDA guidelines would be used for the reproduction study, and Japanese guidelines would be used for the perinatal and postnatal and the teratology studies. Reportedly both the FDA and Japan have accepted such an approach, which would require a greater effort and be more costly than simply meeting FDA requirements but would make entering both markets easier and more economical.

It seems reasonable that the study requirements for the behavioural portion of the reproduction study in Europe might be met by the behavioural studies required for the prenatal and postnatal and teratology studies in Japan. In fact, it is more practical to perform behavioural tests during the teratology (rat), or perinatal and postnatal studies, since you would only have to dose the dams, and the dosing periods are much shorter than in a reproduction study.

These efforts to meet international teratology and reproduction requirements with one battery of tests are noteworthy, but a better approach would be to establish international guidelines for drugs similar to those which have been finalized by the OECD for chemicals. The Japanese requirements for teratology and perinatal and postnatal studies are not justifiable, considering the present state of the art in these areas. The

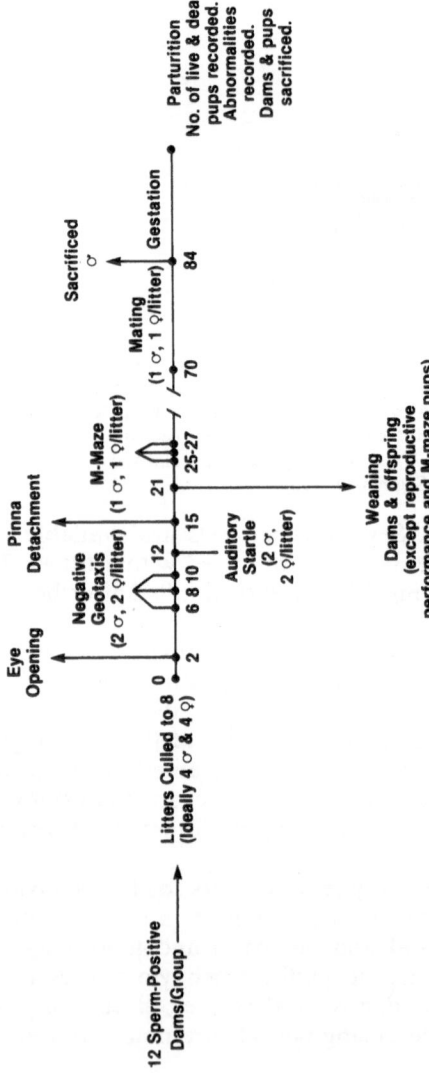

Fig. 17.12 Behavioural and developmental milestones, as well as production of a second generation, in a Segment I study modified to meet USA and European requirements. The litters, from the dams separated from those chosen to meet USA requirements, are culled to 8 (4 males and 4 females, if possible). All 8 pups in each litter are monitored on day 2 for eye opening and day 15 for pinna detachment. Two male and two female pups from each litter are subjected to the negative geotaxis tests on postpartum days 6, 8 and 10, and auditory startle on day 12. Two other pups (one male and one female) from each litter are tested in the water M-maze on days 25–27. The remaining two pups in each litter are designated for reproductive performance and are mated to a pup of the opposite sex from another litter in the same test group

requirement for behavioural studies is premature in light of the poor predictiveness of the results for the human situation and the inconsistent results between, and even within the same, laboratories from the tests generally used in this area. Also, the requirement for weighing fetal organs does not appear to have significant scientific merit.

PROSTAGLANDIN STUDIES AT THE UPJOHN COMPANY

At Upjohn it has been necessary on occasion to deviate from FDA guidelines. Such changes have been discussed with FDA representatives and permission to do so has been obtained. For example, the methyl ester of 15-methylprostaglandin $F_{2\alpha}$ and 9-deoxy-16,16-dimethyl-9-methylene-PGE_2 have pronounced effects on parturition in rats causing induction of labour and/or delayed delivery. After identifying such effects in perinatal and postnatal studies, the decision was made not to administer these prostaglandins during the reproduction study from day 18 of gestation to postpartum day 2.

The validity of using the clinical route (i.v. infusion) in teratology studies was shown in a study in which prostaglandin E_1 (PGE_1) was not teratogenic (Marks *et al.*, 1983), but was teratogenic by the subcutaneous route (Stuckhardt *et al.*, 1983). The teratogenicity possibly resulted from the induction of severe uterine contractions during gestation. PGE_1 also was relatively more toxic to the young male rats (40 days old at the beginning of the dosing period) employed in the reproduction study as compared to the mature females used in this and other studies. These PGE_1-treated males showed reduced mean body weight gains, and significant decreases in the mean weights of the epididymides, seminal vesicles, testes and prostate glands. Pathological changes were also noted, but these changes, like the decreases in tissue weights, might have been the result of general toxic effects. To determine if PGE_1 is specifically toxic for the testes and other reproductive tissues, a second reproduction study using lower doses was carried out. The results confirmed that the effects of PGE_1 on these tissues were most likely the result of general toxicity as there were no toxic effects on reproductive tissues when PGE_1 was administered at doses which did not cause reduced mean body weight gains.

PREDICTIVENESS OF ANIMAL STUDIES FOR HUMAN REPRODUCTIVE RISKS

It is clear that the animal tests now widely used in animal reproduction studies are not as predictive as we'd like them to be (Wilson, 1979). For example, Shepard's '*Catalog of Teratogenic Agents*' (Shepard, 1984) lists over 800 agents which have produced congenital anomalies in experimental animals, and 'only about twenty of these are known to cause defects in the human' (p. xiii) and many of these are highly cytotoxic (Schardein, 1976).

To compensate for the deficiences in the tests used, regulatory agencies have been tempted to require more tests in the hope that the results of such testing will increase the chances that harmful substances can be kept off the market or removed from widespread use. For example, an IRLG workshop was held in September, 1981 to discuss if and how animal and human endpoints (e.g. fetal death, growth retardations, malformation, functional impairment, transient growth retardation, hyperactivity); pharmacokinetic studies; information on mechanisms; and other approaches (statistics, mathematical models, etc.) could be more appropriately used to assess the risks of drugs, chemicals and other substances to human reproduction and development.

Government-sponsored reports (Clement Associates, Inc., 1981; EPA, 1982a; NTP/NIEHS, 1980) have summarized the tests which are currently available to pick from in this area. However, it remains to be proven (i.e. validated) if any of the tests mentioned in these reports is able to assess accurately the risks of drugs and other chemicals to human reproduction. One must realize that the use of tests which have not been validated with non-cytotoxic agents, i.e. have not been shown reliably to predict human health hazards, may only lead to further reductions in the development of new and better (including safer) drugs and chemicals, especially by smaller companies.

TERATOLOGISTS' RESPONSIBILITIES IN ASSESSING REPRODUCTIVE RISKS OF DRUGS AND CHEMICALS

Some have gone so far as to remind teratologists that their responsibility is to develop tests to prevent malformations, not just to study them (Beall, 1980). Others have questioned whether results from animal tests in the near future will be able to predict teratogenicity or guarantee the safety of drugs and chemicals in humans (Brent, 1980) or whether adequate facilities or enough trained personnel are available for such a task (Johnson, 1980). Efforts in this area are underway. Attempts are being made to develop *in vitro* assays (Wilson, 1978). Several of these assays were discussed in a 1981 workshop in Arkadelphia, Arkansas, and were the subject of an entire issue (Vol. 2, No 3/4, 1982) of *Teratogenesis, Carcinogenesis and Mutagenesis*.

Obviously, it is not easy to assess the risk to the unborn human offspring of the thousands of substances in our environment to which we are exposed in our lifetimes. It is frequently difficult even to obtain agreement as to what is a reproductive hazard. For example, if the word teratogenic is assigned to the hundreds of substances which have been shown to produce anomalies in the offspring of any species, then hundreds of teratogens have been identified (Hays, 1981; Shepard, 1980). However, this list places compounds such as aspirin, caffeine and vitamin A in the same category as thalidomide and alcohol. Clearly some discriminatory policy is needed.

In dealing with potential human reproductive hazards, an attempt should be made to avoid the controversies and hysterical connotations presently associated with carcinogens. It must be remembered that available evidence indicates that the general incidence of malformations is not increasing over time (CDC, 1982), in spite of the environmental pollution which has been with us for many years, and that the medical literature indicates that only a small fraction (4-5% at most) of the malformations in humans can be attributed to chemicals or drugs, with the cause of 65-70% unknown (Rao and Schwetz, 1980; Wilson, 1977).

The word 'teratogen' (or reproductive hazard) should not be used alone, as it implies that the substance in question has an established risk to humans. If such is the case, then 'known human teratogen' or some such phrase should be used. In the long run, it is best to establish degrees of teratogenicity by clarifying in which species a substance has been shown to be harmful. Ninety per cent of the teratogens (Shepard, 1983) have not been shown to be a risk to the human and should not be included in the same class as those which have been shown to pose such a risk. The avoidance of the word 'teratogen', without additional information such as 'teratogenic in rats', is especially indicated if test systems other than those recommended by national and/or international guidelines are used in determining teratogenicity. It is also important that unvalidated test systems be identified as such.

The need for inexpensive *in vitro* tests is obvious, but extreme care must be taken in evaluating the merits of such procedures. In all likelihood, no one *in vitro* test will replace any of the teratology and reproduction studies now in widespread use. Although epidemiology studies will play an important role in assessing the risks of a particular agent to the unborn human (Bloom, 1981), such studies will have to be large and well controlled because of the high incidences of reproductive problems.

To improve the information supplied to physicians, the FDA has established five categories (A,B,C, D and X) to indicate a specific drug's potential for causing anomalies at birth (FDA, 1979). These categories range from drugs that fail to demonstrate a risk to the fetus (A) to drugs contraindicated for use during pregnancy because fetal abnormalities have been demonstrated in animal or human studies and potential risks clearly outweigh potential benefits (X). However, Brent (1982) feels that 'package insert statements are confusing, aid negligence lawsuits that are without merit, and lead to unnecessary abortions'.

RECENT ACTIVITIES IN THE AREA OF REPRODUCTIVE HAZARDS

The momentum in the area of assessing reproductive hazards is continuing to build. In April 1983, in Park City, Utah, the University of Utah sponsored a symposium entitled 'Reproduction: The New Frontier in Occupational and Environmental Research'; the proceedings from this symposium will be published. In May 1983, in Arlington, Virginia, the Chemical Manufacturers Association (CMA) Occupational Safety and Health Committee Reproductive Hazards Work Group held a symposium entitled 'Managing

Reproductive Risks in the Workplace'. The objective of this symposium was to provide CMA member companies with information necessary to make reproductive risk assessments within the current legal framework. Attempts to restrict women from hazardous occupations has generated resistance (Chenier, 1982; Lucas–Wallace, 1979) resulting in civil actions and Equal Employment Opportunity Commission guidelines on employment discrimination and reproductive hazards (EEOC, 1980). Thus, in the chemical industry OSHA requirements for providing a safe work place for employees, including women who may be pregnant and their unborn children, Department of Labor (EEOC) antidiscrimination requirements and legal requirements resulting from recent court actions in this area (Bertin, 1982) all must be addressed.

REPRODUCTIVE PROBLEMS WHICH MUST BE ADDRESSED

The long-term effects of any new chemical or drug brought into widespread use is not completely known. Thus the long-term safety levels of most substances cannot be accurately determined. However, better ways of identifying harmful substances must be found so that men and women, as well as their physicians, can better assess the risks to reproduction of the substances to which they frequently come in contact. Also, priorities should be established based on known risks, not the possible risks, of these substances, the cost of assessing the risk and society's willingness to pay the price of reducing that risk.

Clinical surveillance programmes may be the most reliable method of protecting the public from reproductive hazards. Industry can play an important role in such programmes by vigorously maintaining employee surveillance systems. However, the practice of establishing blame must be de-emphasized when harmful substances are identified years after they were introduced into the workplace, or the marketplace, or the environment, or all three. Industry will not readily accept surveillance programmes if the present system (i.e. taking immediate legal action as soon as evidence is found that a substance, or combination of substances, is harmful) continues. We must move toward a mutual goal of identifying reproductive hazards so that exposure to such substances can be eliminated or carefully controlled. Politicians, environmentalists, lawyers, physicians, journalists and the public in general all share with industry and governmental regulatory agencies the responsibility of reaching this goal. Until everyone accepts the fact that our test systems are not foolproof and that the lifestyle to which we are accustomed brings with it a certain degree of risk through exposure to drugs and chemicals, we will not make the effort necessary to minimize such risks.

Acknowledgement

The three diagrams appearing in Fig. 17.1 were prepared by Dr Bernard A. Schwetz of the National Toxicology Program/National Institute of Environmental Health Sciences in Research Triangle Park, NC, for the 1980 'Mid-America Toxicology Course' in Kansas City, MO. I wish to thank Dr Schwetz for generously granting me permission to reproduce these diagrams in this article.

References

Amann, R.P. (1982). Use of animal models for detecting specific alterations in reproduction. *Fund. Appl. Toxicol.*, **2**, 13–26

Barrow, M.V. and Taylor, W.J. (1969). A rapid method for detecting malformations in rat fetuses. *J. Morphol.*, **127**, 291–306

Beall, J.R. (1980). Editorial, A time for change: New activities for the teratology society, to the editor. *Teratology*, **21**, 255–6

Bertin, J.E. (1982). Testimony before the Subcommittee on Investigations and Oversight of the Committee on Science and Technology, US House of Representatives, Ninety-Seventh Congress, First Session, 14, 15 October 1983 (No 53), pp. 173–219 (Washington: US Government Printing Office)

Bloom, A.D. (1981). *Guidelines for Studies of Human Populations Exposed to Mutagenic and Reproductive Hazards.* (White Plains, NY: March of Dimes Birth Defects Foundation) 163 pp.

Brent, R.L. (1980). Expanded activities for the teratology society, editors reply to editorial by James R. Beall, Ph.D. *Teratology*, **21**, 257–8

Brent, R.L. (1982). Drugs and pregnancy: are the insert warnings too dire? *Contempory OB/GYN*, **20**, 42–9

Burns, J. (1983). Overview of safety regulations governing food, drugs and cosmetics in the United States. In Homburger, F. (ed.) *Safety Evaluation and Regulation of Chemicals. 1st International Conference*, Boston, MA, 1982, pp. 9–15 (Basel: Karger)

CDC (1982). *Congenital Malformations Surveillance*, January–December 1980. (Atlanta: Centers for Disease Control) 41 pp

Chenier, N.M. (1982). *Reproductive Hazards at Work. Men, Women and the Fertility Gamble*, (Ottawa: Canadian Advisory Council on the Status of Women) 105 pp

Christian, M.S. (1983). Assessment of reproductivity toxicity—'state of the art'. In Christian, M.S., Galbraith, W.M., Voytek, P. and Mehlman, A. (eds) *Advances in Enviromental Toxicology*, Vol. III. *Assessment of Reproductive and Teratogenic Hazards*, Chapter 8, pp. 65–76 (Princeton: Princeton Scientific Publishers)

Clement Associates, Inc., for the Council on Environmental Quality (1981). *Chemical Hazards to Human Reproduction.* (Washington: US Government Printing Office) 307 pp

Collins, T.F.X. (1978a). Reproduction and teratology guidelines: review of deliberations by the National Toxicology Advisory Committee's Reproduction Panel. *J. Environ. Pathol. Toxicol.*, **2**, 141–7

Collins, T.F.X. (1978b). Multigeneration reproduction studies. In Wilson, J.G. and Fraser, F.C. (eds) *Handbook of Teratology*, Vol. 4, *Research Procedures and Data Analysis*, Chap. 7, pp. 191–214. (New York: Plenum Press)

Committee on Science and Technology (1982). Genetic screening and the handling of high-risk groups in the workplace. Hearings before the Subcommittee on Investigations and Oversight of the Committee on Science and Technology, *US House of Representatives, Ninety-Seventh Congress*, First Session, 14, 15 October 1983 (No 53). (Washington: US Government Printing Office) 319 pp

Courtney, K.D. and Chernoff, N. (1974). *Training Manual for Teratology* (EPA-650/1-73-001) (Research Triangle Park, NC: Environmental Protection Agency), 21 pp.

Dixon, R.L. and Hall, J.L. (1982). Reproductive Toxicology. In Hayes, A.W. (ed.) *Principles and Methods of Toxicology*, pp. 107–40 (New York: Raven Press)

EEOC (1980). Interpretive guidelines on employment discrimination and reproductive hazards, proposed rulemaking. *Federal Register*, **45**, 7514–7

EPA (1979a). Proposed health effects test standards for toxic substances control act test rules, good laboratory practice standards for health effects. *Federal Register*, **44**, 27334–75

EPA (1979b). Proposed rules, subpart F—teratogenic/reproductive health effects. *Federal Register*, **44**, 44087–92

EPA (1982a). Assessment of Risks to Human Reproduction and Development of the Human Conceptus from Exposure to Environmental Substances, *Proceedings of US Environmental Protection Agency Sponsored Conferences;* 1–3 October 1980, Atlanta, GA and 7–10 December 1980, St Louis, MO (ORNL/EIS-197, EPS-600/9-82-001). (Oak Ridge: Oak Ridge National Laboratory)

EPA (1982b). *Health Effects Test Guidelines and Support Documents* (EPA 560/6-82-001, PB 82-232984). (Springfield, VA: National Technical Information Service)

EPA (1982c). *Pesticide Assessment Guidelines Subdivision F, Hazard Evaluation: Human and Domestic Animals by Office of Pesticide Programs* (EPA 540/9-82-025, PB83-153916). (Springfield, VA: National Technical Information Center)

FDA (1970). Food and Drug Administration Advisory Committee on Protocols for Safety Evaluations: Panel on Reproduction Report on Reproduction of Studies in the Safety Evaluation of Food Additives and Pesticide Residues. *Toxicol. Appl. Pharmacol.*, **16**, 264–96

FDA (1978). Nonclinical Laboratory Studies Good Laboratory Practice Regulations. *Federal Register*, **43**, 59986–60025

FDA (1979). Pregnancy labelling. *FDA Drug Bull.*, **9**, 23

FDA (1982). *Toxicological Principles for the Safety Assessment of Direct Food Additives and Color Additives Used in Food.* (Washington: US Food and Drug Administration Bureau of Foods)

Fraser, F.C. (1977). Relation of animal studies to the problem in man. In *Handbook of Teratology*, Vol. 1, *General Principles and Etiology*, Chap. 3

Hays, D.P. (1981). Teratogenesis: a review of the basic principles with a discussion of selected agents: Parts 1, II and III. *Drug Intel. Clin. Pharm.*, **15**, 444–58, 542–66 and 639–50

Health and Welfare Canada (1975). *The Testing of Chemicals for Carcinogenicity, Mutagenicity, and Teratogenicity.* (Ottawa: Health and Welfare Canada) 183 pp.

IRLG (1981). *Recommended Guidelines for Teratogenicity Studies in the Rat, Mouse, or Rabbit.* (Washington, DC: Interagency Regulatory Liaison Group Testing Standards and Guidelines Work Group) 8 pp.

Japan Ministry of Health and Welfare (1975). *Guidelines for Animal Experiments on Reproduction.* (Tokyo: Pharmaceutical Affairs Bureau)

Joffe, J.M. (1979). Influence of drug exposure of the father on perinatal outcome. *Clin. Perinatol.*, **6**, 21–36

Johnson, E.M. (1980). Screening for teratogenic potential: are we asking the proper question? *Teratology*, **21**, 259

Kelsey, F.O. (1982). Regulatory aspects of teratology: role of the Food and Drug Administration. *Teratology*, **25**, 193–9

Kopf, R., Lorenz, D. and Salewski, E. (1964). Der einfluss von thalidomid auf die von ratten in generations ver such über zwei generation. *Naunyn–Schmiedebergs Arch. Exp. Pathol. Pharmacol.*, **247**, 121–35

Lucas–Wallace (1979). Legal considerations bearing on the health and employment of women workers. In Hunt, V.R. (ed.) *Work and the Health of Women*, (Boca Raton, FL: CRC Press)

Manson, J.M. and Simons, R. (1979). Influence of environmental agents on male reproductive failure. In: Hunt, V.R. (ed.), *Work and the Health of Women*, pp. 155–79 (Boca Raton, FL: CRC Press)

Manson, J.M., Zenick, H. and Costlow, R.E. (1982). Teratology test methods for laboratory animals. In Hayes, A.W. (ed.) *Principles and Methods of Toxicology*, pp. 141–84 (New York: Raven Press)

Marks, T.A., Kimmel, G.L. and Staples, R.E. (1981). Influence of symmetrical polychlorinated biphenyl isomers on embryo and fetal development, I. Teratogenicity of 3,3',4,4',5,5'-hexachlorobiphenyl. *Toxicol. Appl. Pharmacol.*, **61**, 269–76

Marks, T.A., Morris, D.F., Weeks, J.R., Stuckhardt, J.L., Poppe, S.M., Moredyk, D.L., Sutter, D.M. and Schaller, P.A. (1983). Teratogen evaluation in rats after continuous i.v. infusion of Prostaglandin E_1. *Teratology*, **27**, 63A

Nichols, J.K. (1983). Chemicals management in the OECD context. In Homburger, F. (ed.)

Safety Evaluation and Regulation of Chemicals. 1st International Conference, Boston, MA, 1982, pp. 31-7 (Basel: Karger)

NTP/NIEHS (1980). Reproductive Toxicology Workshop, 23-25 September 1980, *Workshop Recommendations*, Dixon R.L. (ed.). Research Triangle Park, NC: National Institute of Environmental Health Services) 71 pp.

OECD (1981). *OECD Guidelines for Testing of Chemicals*. (Paris: Organisation for Economic Co-operation and Development)

OECD (1982). *Good Laboratory Practice in the Testing of Chemicals*. (Paris: Organisation for Economic Co-operation and Development) 62 pp.

Palmer, A.K. (1981). Regulatory requirements for reproductive toxicology: theory and practice. In Kimmel, C.A. and Buelke-Sam, J. (eds.) *Developmental Toxicology*, pp. 259-87. (New York: Raven Press)

Rao, K.S. and Schwetz, B.A. (1980). Birth defects in humans and teratogenesis in animals— a perspective. *Down to Earth*, **36**, 26-32

Schardein, J.L. (1976). *Drugs As Teratogens*. (Boca Raton, FL: CRC Press), 291 pp.

Shepard, T.H. (1983). *Catalog of Teratogenic Agents*, 4th Edn. (Baltimore: Johns Hopkins University Press), 410 pp.

Staples, R.E. (1974). Detection of visceral alterations in mammalian fetuses. *Teratology*, **9**, A37-A38

Staples, R.E. and Schnell, V.L. (1964). Refinements in rapid clearing technique in the KOH-Alizarin Red S method for bone. *Stain Technol.*, **39**, 62-3

Stuckhardt, J.L., Marks, T.A., Morris, D.F., Poppe, S.M. and Moerdyk, D.L. (1983). Teratogenicity in rats given subcutaneous doses of prostaglandin E_1. *Teratology*, **27**, in press

Stuckhardt, J.L. and Poppe, S.M. (1984). Fresh visceral examination of rat and rabbit fetuses for teratogenicity screening. *Teratogenesis, Carcinogenesis and Mutagenesis*, **4**, 181-8

Tardiff, R.G. (1977). *Principles and Procedures for Evaluating the Toxicity of Household Substances*. (Washington: National Academy of Sciences, USA)

Thomas, J.A. (1981). Reproductive hazards and environmental chemicals: a review. *Toxic Substances J.* **2**, 318-48

Tracor Jitco, Inc. (1977). Survey and evaluation of techniques used in testing chemical substances for teratogenic effects. Prepared for the Environmental Protection Agency (EPA-560/5-77-007; PB 273195) (Springfield, VA: National Technical Information Service) 95 pp.

Wilson, J.G. (1965). Embryological considerations in teratology. In Wilson, J.G. and Warkany, J. (eds.) *Teratology, Principles and Techniques*, pp. 251-77. (Chicago: University of Chicago Press)

Wilson, J.G. (1973). Principles of teratology. In *Environment and Birth Defects*, Chap. 2., pp. 11-34 (New York: Academic Press)

Wilson, J.G. (1977). Current status of teratology, general principles and mechanisms derived from animal studies. In Wilson, J.G. and Fraser, F.C. (eds.) *Handbook of Teratology*, Vol. 1, *General Principles and Etiology*, Chap. 2, pp. 47-74 (New York: Plenum Press)

Wilson, J.G. (1978). Survey of *in vitro* systems: their potential use in teratogenicity screening. In *Handbook of Teratology*, Vol. 4, *Research Procedures and Data Analysis*, pp. 135-53. (New York: Plenum Press)

Wilson, J.G. (1979). The evaluation of teratological testing. *Teratology*, **20**, 205-12

18
Effects of phenoxy acid herbicides and TCDD on male reproduction

J.C. LAMB, IV and J.A. MOORE

The chlorinated phenoxyacetic acids have been widely used as broad leaf herbicides. The compounds have had both civilian and military applications. The phenoxy acid herbicides 2,4-dichlorophenoxyacetic acid (2,4-D) and 2,4,5-trichlorophenoxyacetic acid (2,4,5-T) are among the most widely used and studied compounds in the class. 2-Methyl-4-chlorophenoxyacetic acid (MCPA), 2-methyl-4-chlorophenoxypropionic acid (MCPP) and Silvex [2-(2,4,5-trichlorophenoxy) propionic acid] are also phenoxy acid herbicides. Human health concerns have centred on inadvertant contaminants of 2,4,5-T which were produced during its manufacture. The contaminant, 2,3,7,8-tetrachlorodibenzo-p-dioxin (TCDD or dioxin), is an extremely toxic compound which has been found at low, but potentially toxic levels in the herbicide mixtures. Other, less toxic, chlorinated dibenzodioxins are also found as contaminants. The original concerns about the potential human reproductive health hazards of the phenoxy acid herbicides were brought to light when studies demonstrated that 2,4,5-T, which was contaminated with 30 parts/10^6 TCDD, caused birth defects in laboratory animals (Courtney et al., 1970). These studies were followed by a number of investigations into the teratogenicity of 2,4,5-T and TCDD. Although a large number of studies have addressed the effects of phenoxy acid and TCDD on development after *in utero* exposure, the number of studies addressing the important question of whether exposure to these same compounds would adversely affect fertility and reproduction in males or in females are still quite limited.

The relevance of the question of potential male reproductive toxicity is enhanced by the knowledge that millions of men may have been exposed to these compounds in military and agricultural applications. The most publicized of the potential exposures is related to the use of the n-butyl esters of 2,4-D and 2,4,5-T in the Vietnam War as a strategic defoliant (Young et al., 1978). The 1:1 mixture of these two herbicides is referred to as Herbicide Orange or Agent Orange. These herbicides were contaminated with as much as 48 parts/10^6 TCDD, although the average contamination level was about 2 parts/10^6 TCDD. A number of other herbicide formulations containing 2,4,5-T and TCDD were also used by the military in Southeast Asia

Table 18.1 Teratogenicity of 2,4-D, 2,4,5-T or TCDD in laboratory animals (listed chronologically)

Compound	Species	Route and Dose level	Gestational days of exposure	Findings	Reference
2,4,5-T (with 30 parts/10⁶ TCDD)	mouse: C57B1/6, AKR, B1/6 × AKR: rat	gavage, also sc for mice; up to 113 mg/kg for rats and mice	6–14 or 9–17 for C57B1/6; 6–15 for AKR; 10–15 for rats	mice: increased % abnormal litters, cystic kidney, cleft palate (sc or oral), fetotoxic rat: fetotoxic, increased cystic kidney, g.i. tract haemorrhagic	Courtney et al. (1970)
2,4,5-T (technical; 0.5 parts/10⁶ TCDD)	mouse: CD-1, C57B1/6J, DBA,/2J rat: CD	sc	6–15	fetocidal at 150 mg/kg mice: cleft palate rat: not teratogenic	Courtney and Moore (1971)
2,4,5-T (analytical; <0.05 parts/10⁶ TCDD)	mouse: CD-1, C57B1/6J, DBA,/2J rat: CD	sc	6–15	mice: cleft palate rat: not teratogenic	Courtney and Moore (1971)
TCDD	mouse: CD-1 C57B1/6J, DBA,/2J rat: CD	sc	6–15	mice: cleft palate, kidney anomalies rat: kidney anomalies	Courtney and Moore (1971)
2,4,5-T (0.5 parts/10⁶ TCDD)	rabbit (NZW)	oral (capsule) 0, 10, 20, 40 mg/kg	6–18	no significant abnormalities, not embryotoxic or teratogenic; occasional dilated renal pelvis not embryotoxic or teratogenic	Emerson et al. (1971)
	rat (S-D)	gavage 0, 1, 3, 6, 12, 24 mg/kg	6–15		
TCDD	rat (S-D)	gavage 0, 0.03, 0.125, 0.5, 2, 8 µg/kg	6–15	decreased maternal weight gain at top 3 doses; no adverse effect at 0.03 µg/kg; fetal mortality, resorptions and intestinal haemorrhage increased at 0.125 µg/kg and above. Attributed early 2,4,5-T teratogenicity findings to TCDD contaminant	Sparschu et al. (1971b)
2,4,5-T (0.5 parts/10⁶ TCDD)	rat (S-D)ʼ	gavage 50 mg/kg 100 mg/kg	6–15 6–10	not teratogenic, delayed ossification fetotoxic, maternally toxic, not teratogenic	Sparschu et al. (1971a)
2,4-D (98.7% 2,4-D)	rat (S-D)	gavage 0, 12.5, 25, 50, 75, 87.5 mg/kg	6–15	pilot showed maternal toxicity at 100 mg/kg; not teratogenic, decreased fetal body weight, sc oedema, delayed ossification; not life threatening; no effect at 25 mg/kg	Schwetz et al. (1971)
2,4-D polyethylene glycol butyl ether ester (61.7%, 2,4-D)	rat (S-D)	gavage (equimolar with above)	6–15	essentially same as above	Schwetz et al. (1971)

270

Compound	Species	Dosage	Days	Effects	Reference
2,4-D isooctyl ester (64.6% 2,4-D)	rat (S-D)	gavage (equimolar with above)	6-15	essentially same as above	Schwetz et al. (1971)
2,4-D (three commercial sources)	hamster	gavage 0, 20, 40, 60, 100 mg/kg	6-10	no significant or clearly dose-related increase in malformations	Collins and Williams (1971)
2,4,5-T (N.D., 0.1, 0.5, 2.9 or 4.5 parts/10^6 TCDD controlled mixtures)	hamster	gavage 0, 20, 40, 80, 100 mg/kg 2,4,5-T	6-10	no abnormalities, but fetotoxicity at high levels of 2,4,5-T with low or N.D. TCDD levels. Abnormalities increased with increased TCDD concentrations	Collins and Williams (1971)
2,4-D and 2,4-D butyl, butoxyethanol or isooctyl ester or diethylamine salt	rat (Wistar)	gavage 25, 50, 100, 150 or 300 mg/kg	6-15	increased skeletal malformations and fetotoxicity	Khera and McKinley (1972)
2,4,5-T and 2,4,5-T butyl ester (<0.5 mg/kg TCDD)	rat (Wistar)	gavage 25, 50, 100, 150 mg/kg	6-15	increased skeletal malformations and fetotoxicity	Khera and McKinley (1972)
2,4,5-T and 2,4,5-T butyl ester, (TCDD as low as <0.02 parts/10^6) and TCDD and 2,4,5-T plus TCDD	mice (NMRI)	gavage 0-120 mg/kg 2,4,5-T, 0.3-9 µg/kg TCDD	6-15; also TCDD on 7, 8, 9, 10, 11, 12 or 13	purest 2,4,5-T caused cleft palate at 20 mg/kg; TCDD caused cleft palate at 1 µg/kg or single dose of 20-50 µg/kg; peak day of sensitivity was day 11; 2,4,5-T plus TCDD resulted in a potentiated response	Neubert and Dillman (1972)
2,4,5-T TCDD and 2,4,5-T plus TCDD	mice	gavage	6-15; 13	reviewed studies on the teratogenicity of TCDD in combination with 2,4,5-T; demonstrated potentiation	Neubert et al. (1973)
TCDD	mice (C57B1/6J)	gavage 0, 1, 3, 10 µg/kg	10; 10-13 (cross-fostered animals to control postnatal exposure)	showed that postnatal (nursing) exposure to TCDD caused significant kidney lesions; hydronephrosis was dose- and length of exposure-related	Moore et al. (1973)
2,7-DCDD Hexa-CDD (mixed isomers) OCDD	rat (S-D)	DCDD: 100 mg/kg HCDD: 0.1-100 µg/kg OCDD: 100, 500 mg/kg	6-15	DCDD: no fetotoxicity or anomalies HCDD: 10 or 100 µg/kg fetoxic; increased visceral and skeletal anomalies at 100 µg/kg OCDD: no significant anomalies	Schwetz et al. (1973)
TCDD	mice (CF-1)	0, 0.001, 0.01, 0.1, 1, 3 µg/kg	6-15	cleft palate at 1 and 3 µg/kg; dilated renal pelvis at 3 µg/kg. No increase in malformations at ≤0.1 µg/kg	Smith et al. (1976)

Table 18.1 cont. Teratogenicity of 2,4-D, 2,4,5-T or TCDD in laboratory animals (listed chronologically)

Compound	Species	Route and Dose level	Gestational days of exposure	Findings	Reference
TCDD	rat (S–D)	0.2–0.6 µg/kg	17	increased aryl hydrocarbon hydroxylase activity 14-fold in maternal liver and 100-fold in fetal liver	Berry et al. (1976)
TCDD	rat (F344) mouse (C57B1/6)	gavage 0, 1, 5 µg/kg	11 and 18 and/or 0, 7, 14 d postnatal	depletion of lymphocytes in thymic cortex; allograft rejection time prolonged	Vos and Moore (1974)
2,4,5-T (0.05 parts/ 10^6 TCDD)	monkey (Macaca mulatta)	oral (capsule) 0.05, 1, 10 mg/kg	22–38	no evidence of teratogenesis	Dougherty et al. (1976)
2,4,5-T (0.01 parts/ 10^6 TCDD) or TCDD-free; <0.001 parts/10^6 2,4,5-Trichlorophenol; phenoxy acetic	mice (CD-1)	gavage 800–900 mg/kg	either 8, 9, 10, 11, 12, 13, 14 or 15	2,4,5-T teratogenic in single or multiple dosages	Hood et al. (1979)
		200–300 mg/kg	7–10, 10–12 or 13–15	2,4,5-Trichlorophenol and phenoxyacetic acid were not strongly teratogenic or fetotoxic	
2,4,5-T (<0.5 parts/ 10^6 TCDD)	mice (CD-1)	gavage 20, 100 mg/kg	6–15	increase in skeletal variations after maternal exposure to 2,4,5-T	Beck (1981)
2,4,5-T (<0.5 parts/ 10^6 TCDD)	mice (CD-1)	100 mg/kg	6–17	changes in heart and serum creatine kinase and lactic dehydrogenase activity	Courtney and Ebron (1981)
TCDD	mice (NMRI)	oral, sc, ip 5, 12.5, 25 µg/kg	16; 7–10; 7–11; 9–15	low levels of TCDD do cross the placenta and accumulate in fetal tissue, especially liver. Levels greatest at gestational days 9 and 10	Nau and Bass (1981)
2,4-D as propylene glycol butyl ether (PGBE) and isooctyl ester (10)	rat (CD)	gavage molar equivalents to 0, 6.25, 12.5, 25 or 87.5 mg/kg of 2,4-D	6–15	PGBE and IO minor embryotoxicity but not deleterious to growth or survival; not teratogenic; no maternal toxicity	Unger et al. (1981)

(Young *et al.*, 1978). Accurate measures of herbicide exposures were not taken. Estimates of the exposure to TCDD by soldiers have been based on various assumptions of chemical concentration and intake of the chemical. These estimates indicated that a soldier directly sprayed would receive 1/1750 of the minimum toxic dose, the toxic dose was also estimated by the author (Stevens, 1981). However, these estimates did not consider that the group which worked in the spray units may have received a higher dosage of the herbicides.

The purpose of this paper is to review the limited published research available on the effects of the phenoxy acid herbicides and the contaminant TCDD on male fertility and reproduction. There are a number of other potential health effects of these compounds which have been reviewed by others which will not be described in this paper (for reviews see: Bovey and Young, 1988; Hay, 1982; Hutzinger *et al.*, 1982; Tucker *et al.*, 1983). Selected findings on the influence of these compounds on development as a result of *in utero* exposure will be described only to help put the data on the toxicity to the male reproductive system into perspective. Also the genetic toxicity of these chemicals will not be addressed in detail, but will only be described as it may be related to the potential male reproductive toxicity of the chemicals. The teratogenicity and mutagenicity of 2,4-D, 2,4,5-T and TCDD have been recently reviewed in some detail (Friedman, 1984).

TERATOGENICITY OF PHENOXY HERBICIDES AND TCDD

The ability of 2,4-D, 2,4,5-T and TCDD to cause birth defects seems to be highly dose and species dependent (Gehring and Betso, 1978). A number of the original papers on the teratogenicity of these compounds are summarized in Table 18.1. The original studies demonstrating the teratogenicity of 2,4,5-T were confounded by the contamination of the herbicide with 30 parts/10^6 TCDD (Courtney *et al.*, 1978). Those investigators showed that 2,4,5-T with TCDD caused cleft palate and dilated renal pelvis in mice and cystic kidney and gastrointestinal haemorrhages in rats. Subsequent studies indicated that TCDD was teratogenic in both species, whereas 2,4,5-T (0.05 parts/10^6 TCDD or less) was teratogenic only in mice (Courtney and Moore, 1971). TCDD is teratogenic in rats at maternal doses of 0.125 μg/kg and above (Sparschu *et al.*, 1971a) and mice at 1 or 3 μg/kg (Smith *et al.*, 1976). The teratogenicity of 2,4,5-T in mice seems to be potentiated by TCDD (or TCDD potentiated by 2,4,5-T) (Neubert and Dillmann, 1972; Neubert *et al.*, 1973). 2,4,5-T was not demonstrated teratogenic in rabbits (Emerson *et al.*, 1971) or monkeys (Dougherty *et al.*, 1976). High levels of 2,4-D acid and esters were fetotoxic and embryotoxic, but not clearly teratogenic in rats and hamsters (Collins and Williams, 1971; Khera and McKinley, 1972; Schwetz *et al.*, 1971).

The effects of phenoxy acid herbicides and TCDD on human development have been studied, but the results to date are inconclusive. The risk of exposure to phenoxy herbicides is considerably greater for applicators of the spray than for residents of areas sprayed with the herbicides (Newton and Norris, 1981). The potential toxicity is dependent upon the dose level and the duration of exposure to the chemical. Calculations based on the general toxicity of 2,4,5-T and TCDD together with estimates of exposure potential indicate that applicators are unlikely to receive exposures which would lead to a safety factor lower than 300:1 for 2,4,5-T or 600:1 for TCDD (Newton and Norris, 1981). These calculations rely upon very speculative dose and toxicity estimations. Two significant studies on the incidence of miscarriages in women living in Oregon were subjected to a panel review concerned with the epidemiology of 2,4,5-T, the panel concluded that the studies (Alsea I and II) were insufficient in design and implementation (Coulston and Olajos, 1980). Those studies failed to document 2,4,5-T exposure and did not demonstrate an increase in spontaneous abortions above background levels for the general population.

Studies on the relationship of TCDD to a variety of human health effects and reproductive toxicity in 79 workers showed no correlation between exposure and birth defects (May, 1982). Also, exposure to TCDD after accidental environmental contamination in Seveso, Italy was not associated with an increase in the incidence of birth defects, despite levels sufficient to kill livestock and cause severe chloracne in people in the contaminated area (Reggiani, 1978; Fanelli et al., 1980). The TCDD was dispersed over the Italian countryside after the explosion of a chemical plant which produced trichlorophenol, the precursor to hexachlorophene and 2,4,5-T.

MALE REPRODUCTIVE TOXICITY OF PHENOXY ACIDS AND TCDD

There are a number of mechanisms by which chemical exposures might interfere with normal reproductive function in males. Chemicals acting on the male reproductive system can act: by inhibiting libido and preventing normal mating; by decreasing spermatogenesis and sperm concentrations; by increasing the proportion of abnormal or mutated sperm; and by altering accessory sex organ function which controls the constitution of the seminal plasma. Male chemical exposures may also lead to exposure of females either through direct contact with contaminated persons or clothing or by exposure to the chemical concentrated in the seminal plasma or the sperm and possibly altering fertility of the sperm or development of the fertilized ovum. Although the consideration of these various mechanisms seems to complicate the study of this area, the critical endpoints to consider are first, was there a fertile mating, and second, did the offspring develop normally?

In the specific case of the phenoxy acid herbicides and TCDD, the data on human exposures must be considered in two groups. The first group would be men who were exposed during commercial or agricultural use or in accidental exposures and the adverse effects on reproduction are described recently after the exposure. The second group would be the military men exposed to the chemicals and who, years after the potential exposure, have expressed concern over reproductive dysfunction or siring malformed children. The reason for the distinction is that in the first group the wives of the exposed men might receive a direct exposure to the chemicals, but in the second group direct maternal exposure to the chemical is highly unlikely. The exposure via sperm or seminal plasma would seem unlikely for the second group because of the long periods of time between the male exposure and female contact, compared to the biological half-lives of the phenoxy acids and TCDD. However, neither human nor animal studies have attempted to measure the concentrations of these chemicals in the sperm or semen. Also, there is no information on the definitive half-life of 2,4,5-T or TCDD in humans. The potential for various chemicals to pass into the semen has been reviewed by Mann and Mann (1981). The influence of chemical exposures to males on the development of their offspring has been reviewed by Soyka and Joffe (1980).

Despite intense public interest in this area, there still are few studies on the effects of phenoxy acid and TCCD exposure to men and the effects on fertility and offspring development. A review of 79 workers exposed to TCDD who developed chloracne (clinical evidence of TCDD toxicity) demonstrated no association between the chemical exposure and altered reproduction or offspring development (May, 1980). This study considered data collected over a ten year period after documented TCDD exposure; half of the subjects still had mild chloracne and in isolated cases wives and children of the workers had developed chloracne as well. The review of the pregnancies from those exposed men revealed no chemical related problems. In a study from New Zealand comparing agricultural sprayers using 2,4,5-T to agricultural contractors not using 2,4,5-T during a two year period there was no significant effect on the incidence of miscarriages or congenital defects (Smith A.H. et al., 1981; Smith et al., 1982). An earlier study from New Zealand had shown a significant increase in the incidence in talipes (club foot) and hypospadias in children from areas where 2,4,5-T was used for aerial spraying compared to non-spray areas (Hanify et al., 1981). These effects were not confirmed in the subsequent study (Smith et al., 1982). A survey of wives of Dow Chemical employees found no overall significant associations between TCDD exposures and pregnancy outcome (Townsend et al., 1982). A review of existing data by the American Medical Association also found no evidence of a link between human Agent Orange exposure and sterility, spontaneous abortions or birth defects (Beljan et al., 1982).

Very few animal studies have directly addressed the question of whether the phenoxyacetic acids and/or TCDD can directly affect male reproductive function. Table 18.2 summarizes the majority of the animal studies which have considered the male reproductive system as an endpoint of toxicity. There are no studies which indicate that the phenoxy acid herbicides or TCDD affect male reproductive function at levels below those causing systemic toxicity or mortality.

Several general toxicity studies on the effects of TCDD have identified the testis as a potential target organ. The species studied include the monkey and chicken (Allen and Carstens, 1967; Norback and Allen, 1973), guinea pig and mouse (McConnell et al., 1978) and rat (Kociba et al., 1976). All of these studies indicate that the testicular effects were noted in animals

Table 18.2 Studies considering the effects of phenoxy acids or TCDD on male reproductive function in laboratory animals (listed chromologically)

Compound	Species	Route and Dose level	Type of Study	Findings	Reference
'Toxic fat' (contained chemical, TCDD, not identified at that time)	monkey (Macaca mulatta)	diet containing 0.125 to 10% toxic fat	chronic toxicity (until death of animals)	testes, grossly normal but tubules contained only spermagonia and Sertoli cells (dosage levels not specified, all animals were killed by dosing)	Allen and Carstens (1967)
2,4,-D	rat	diet 0, 5, 25, 125, 625, 1250 parts /10^6 0, 100, 500, 1500 parts/10^6	chronic toxicity 6-litter reproduction	no effects on testes no effect on fertility or reproduction in males, decrease in offspring survival to weaning at 1500 parts/10^6 (due to maternal exposure)	Hansen et al. (1971)
	dog	0, 10, 50, 100, 500 parts/10^6	chronic toxicity	no effects on testes	
TCCD	monkey	not specified	toxicity not specified	decreased spermatogenesis at lethal dosages	Norback and Allen (1973)
	chicken	not specified	toxicity not specified	decreased spermatogenesis at lethal dosages	
TCDD	rat (Wistar)	oral, 0, 4, 8, 12 µg/ kg^{-1} day^{-1} for 7 days	dominant lethal	12 µg/kg lethal to 20/20; 8 µg/kg lethal to 11/20; 4 µg/kg lethal to 2/20; no dominant lethal mutations for 7 week post-treatment; testes histologically normal; sperm granulomas in epididymis; mating incidence reduced	Khera and Ruddick (1973)
2,4,5-T	mouse	gavage 6.25, 12.5, 25 mg/kg daily 10 days	hormone binding	2,4,5-T inhibited uptake and metabolism of [3H]testosterone in prostate	Lloyd et al. (1973)
MCPA	rat	diet 0, 50, 40, 3200 parts/10^6, dermal 0, 0.5, 1, 2 g/kg	short-term toxicity	slight non-significant decreased in prostate weight at 3200, parts/10^6 in diet only	Verschuuren et al. (1975)
MCPA	rat	drinking water 0, 100, 500, 1000, 2000, 3000 parts / 10^6	60-day, testicular toxicity	no change in testis weight; high concentrations were related to slight morphological changes in testis	Elo and Parvinen (1976)

Compound	Species	Study	Dosage	Effect	Reference
TCDD	rat (Sprague–Dawley)	13-week subchronic toxicity	gavage 0, 0.001, 0.01, 0.1, 1 µg/kg (5 days/week)	decrease testis size and spermatogenesis in 1/5 rats at 1 µg/kg; decrease accessory sex gland size in 2/5 at 1µg/kg; mortality = 2/12	Kociba et al. (1978)
TCDD	rat (Sprague–Dawley)	two-year chronic toxicity	diet 0, 0.001, 0.01, 0.1 µg/kg^{-1} day^{-1} dosage	no adverse effect	McConnell et al. (1978)
TCDD	guinea pig			decreased spermatogenesis and testis weight at lethal dosages	McConnell et al. (1978)
	mice (C57B1/6)			decreased spermatogenesis and testis weight at lethal dosages	
MCPA; 2,4-D	rat (Sprague–Dawley)	chemical disposition	intravenous injection of [^{14}C]MCPA and [^{14}C]2, 4-D and competed with water intake of cold MCPA unlabelled	low levels of MCPA and 2,4-D were found in testis. Maximal concentrations at 4 h after injection. By 24 h levels in all tissues were 1/2 the 4 h levels	Elo and Ylitalo (1979)
TCDD	rat (Sprague–Dawley)	3-generation reproduction	diet 0, 0.001, 0.01, 0.1 µg/kg^{-1} day^{-1}	adverse effects on pairs given 0.01 and 0.1 µg/kg^{-1} day^{-1}; no apparent adverse effects in males (0.1 µg/kg) mated to untreated females	Murray et al. (1979)
TCDD	rat (Wistar)	metabolism of testosterone	gavage, 20 µg/kg single dose	significant decrease in testosterone catabolism by the liver	Nienstedt et al. (1979)
2,4-D; 2,4,5-T isooctyl ester of 2,4,5-T, MCPA; MCPP (2-methyl-4-chlorophenoxy-propionic acid); and 2,4-DP (2,4-dichlorophenoxy-propionic acid)	mice	DNA synthesis	oral, 200 mg/kg for all except 2,4,5-T ester which included 50, 100, 200, 400 mg/kg	2,4-D, 2,4,5-T, 2,4,5-T-isooctyl ester, MCPA and MCPP (but not 2,4-DP) inhibited testicular thymidine putake at dosages of 200 mg/kg (animals received 1 µCi [^{3}H]thymidine 1 h before dosing and were given 10 µCi [^{3}H]thymidine 3 h later and killed in 30 min). No effect at 50 or 100 mg/kg 2,4,5-T isooctyl ester	Seiler (1979)

Table 18.2 cont. Studies considering the effects of phenoxy acids or TCDD on male reproductive function in laboratory animals (listed chromologically)

Compound	Species	Route and Dose level	Type of Study	Findings	Reference
2,4,5-T (propylene glycol butyl ether ester)	rat (Long–Evans)	gavage, 0, 25, 50, 100 mg/kg	spermatotoxicity	no apparent effect on testicular weight, epididymal weight or sperm morphology; increase DNA synthesis 1 wk after dosing, no effect at 4, 7 or 10 wk	Koller–Goldsmith *et al.* (1980)
2,4-D and 2,4,5-T plus TCDD (2 or 30 parts/10⁶)	mouse (C57B1/6)	diet 0; 40 mg kg^{-1} day^{-1} 2,4-D, 40 mg kg^{-1} day^{-1} 2,4,5-T and 2.4 μg kg^{-1} day^{-1} TCDD; 20/20/1.2; or 40/40/0.6	male reproductive toxicity	simulated phenoxy acid mixture with controlled levels of TCDD did not adversely affect reproduction, fertility, offspring development or, spermagenesis	Lamb *et al.* (1980)
TCDD	rat (Sprague–Dawley)	gavage 2.5, 5 or 10 mg/kg	TCDD induced benzo(a)pyrene metabolism	TCDD significantly increased testicular and prostatic metabolism of benzo(a)pyrene and increased AHH and cytochrome P-450 activity (maximal at 48 h)	Lee and Suzuki (1980); Lee and Nagayama (1980); Lee *et al.* (1981); Nagayama and Lee (1982)
TCDD	guinea pig (Hartley)	gavage 1 μg/kg	TCDD and microsomal activity	TCDD decreased cytochrome P-450 activity (52% at one day) which persisted for at least 9 days; haem, SDH and ALA synthetase were not affected	Tofilon *et al.* (1980)
2,4,5-T	rat (Sprague–Dawley)	diet 0, 3, 10, 30 mg/kg^{-1} day^{-1}	3-generation reproduction	2,4,5-T reduced neonatal survival, but did not alter reproduction	Smith *et al.* (1981)

severely affected by the chemical exposure, with the exception of the exposure of young chickens to TCDD where a decrease in testis size occurred without other signs of toxicity (Norback and Allen, 1973). Unfortunately the experimental design and exposure conditions were not included in the description of those findings. Reproductive toxicity studies on TCDD, in the form of either multigeneration studies (Murray et al., 1979) or dominant lethal studies (Khera and Ruddick, 1973) have demonstrated that the male rat reproductive system is not especially sensitive to TCDD exposure and adverse effects were not seen without significant toxicity or mortality. Rat testicular and prostatic metabolism of the carcinogen benzo(a)pyrene are elevated by exposure to 2.5–18 µg/kg TCDD; aryl hydrocarbon hydroxylase (AHH) and cytochrome P–450 activity are increased by TCDD (Lee and Suzuki, 1980; Lee and Nagayama, 1980; Lee et al., 1981; Nagayama and Lee, 1982). These effects are not observed in the guinea pig (Tofilon et al., 1980).

Data on the effects of the phenoxyacetic acids on male reproduction are also quite limited. A six-generation reproduction study of 2,4,-D (Hansen et al., 1971) and a three-generation reproduction study of 2,4,5-T (Smith F.A. et al., 1981) did not show any association between the chemical exposure and compromised reproductive function in male rats. Significant exposures to various phenoxy acids, such as 2-methyl-4-chlorophenoxy-acetic acid (MCPA), 2,4-D and 2,4,5-T have been related to decreased testicular weight, decreased accessory sex organ weight, altered hormone binding, decreased metabolism of testosterone and altered DNA synthesis in the testis (see Table 18.2). None of these target organ effects has been associated with functional alterations in fertility and no adverse effects have been noted at levels which do not also adversely affect other organ systems or increase mortality.

In a study designed specifically to model potential reproductive toxicity in males after exposure to phenoxy acid mixtures containing TCDD, C57B1/6 male mice were given 2,4-D plus 2,4,5-T adulterated with controlled levels of TCDD (Lamb et al., 1980, 1981a, b, c). The mice were treated with the chemical mixtures in the diet continuously for eight weeks. The treated diet contained equal amounts of 2,4-D and 2,4,5-T and TCDD in concentrations of either 2 or 30 parts/10^6 in the phenoxy acid mixtures. The four treatment groups included controls (Group I) and three treated groups. Approximate daily dosage levels were 40 mg/kg 2,4-D, 40 mg/kg 2,4,5-T and 2.4 µg/kg TCDD (Group II), or 40 mg/kg 2,4-D, 40 mg/kg 2,4,5-T and 0.16 µg/kg TCDD (Group III), or 20 mg/kg 2,4-D, 20 mg/kg 2,4,5-T and 1.2 µg/kg TCDD (Group IV).

Chemical toxicity was evaluated in males killed at various times during the eight week dosing period and in the eight weeks following dosing. A parallel set of male mice were treated (25 males per dose group) and at the end of the eight week dosing period the males in the second set were tested for fertility and reproductive performance. Over the following eight weeks those males were each cohabited with three untreated female mice for five days a week each week.

The exposure levels were high enough to cause decreased body weight

Table 18.3 Fertility and mating efficiency in C57BL/6N mice treated with phenoxy acid and TCDD and in control mice (8 wk total)

Treatment group[a]	Mating frequency[b] (%)	Fertility index[c] (%)	Total fertility[d] (%)
I (control	74.6 ± 1.6	56.2 ± 2.2	42.0 ± 1.9
II (80/2.4)	70.3 ± 2.4	58.3 ± 2.9	41.0 ± 2.6
III (80/0.16)	67.8 ± 2.4[e]	55.3 ± 2.3	37.7 ± 2.2
IV (40/1.2)	73.0 ± 2.0	60.8 ± 2.9	44.2 ± 2.3

[a]Calculated daily exposure is given in parentheses as phenoxy acid (mg/kg) over TCDD (μg/kg)
[b]Plugs observed divided by total females housed with males
[c]Fertile matings divided by females with plugs
[d]Fertile matings divided by total females housed with males
[e]$p < 0.05$ relative to controls. Values are means ± SE; $n = 25$ males per group
Reprinted by permission of *J. Toxicol. Environ. Health* (Lamb et al., 1981b)

gain, thymic involution and increased hepatic weight, but there were no clinical signs of toxicity. Body weight and thymus weight returned to control levels four weeks after dosing was suspended. Liver weight returned to normal more slowly. No significant treatment-related effects were observed in testis–epidodymis, spleen, kidney or brain weights. Sperm counts per mg of epididymis, sperm motility and sperm morphology were not affected by treatment.

Despite the evidence of chemical toxicity (decreased weight gain, thymic involution, liver enlargement), the mating frequency and fertility index (Table 18.3) were not affected by the chemical exposure. There was a significant decrease in the mating frequency in group III, but no such effect was noted in group II which received equal exposure to the phenoxy acids and fifteen times the exposure to TCDD. The fertility index and total fertility were not significantly affected by treatment. All of the reproductive

Table 18.4 Effect of 2,4-D, 2,4,5-T, and TCDD on fetal development[a]

Measurement	Treatment group			
	I	II	III	IV
Number of females examined	171	148	145	164
Maternal weight gain (g)	11.8 ± 0.3	12.0 ± .03	11.6 ± 0.3	11.5 ± 0.3
Number of implants per litter	7.1 ± 0.2	7.4 ± 0.2	7.2 ± 0.2	7.0 ± 0.2
Number of resorptions per litter	2.18 ± 0.11	2.37 ± 0.14	2.26 ± 0.1	2.11 ± 0.14
Number of live fetuses per litter	4.9 ± 0.2	5.0 ± 0.2	4.9 ± 0.2	5.0 ± 0.2
Average fetal weight per litter (g)	1.03 ± 0.01	1.08 ± 0.01	1.08 ± 0.01	1.10 ± 0.01
Males/females	404/419	356/376	356/349	376/420
Visceral malformations:				
Number of fetuses examined	455	393	394	443
Number with visceral malformations	2	2	5	5
Skeletal and external malformations:				
Number of fetuses examined	830	744	711	805
Number of malformed fetuses	26	26	20	25

[a]Values are means ± SE
Reprinted by permission of *J. Toxicol. Environ. Health* (Lamb et al., 1981c)

Table 18.5 Summary of malformations observed in fetuses sired by males treated with 2,4-D, 2,4,5-T, and TCDD

Observation	Treatment group			
	I	II	III	IV
Visceral malformations[a]				
Heart/vessel anomalies	0.2(1/455)	0.5(2/393)	1.0(4/394)	0.7(3/443)
Kidney agenesis	0.2(1/455)	0.0(0/393)	0.3(1/394)	0.0(0/443)
Liver, two lobes only	0.0(0/455)	0.0(0/393)	0.0(0/394)	0.2(1/443)
Lung, lobes two-thirds normal size	0.2(1/455)	0.0(0/393)	0.0(0/394)	0.0(0/443)
Right kidney, half normal size	0.0(0/455)	0.0(0/393)	0.0(0/394)	0.2(1/443)
Skeletal and external malformations[a]				
Anophthalmia/microphthalmia	1.4(12/830)	1.9(14/744)	2.0(14/711)	2.4(19/805)
Agnathia/micrognathia	1.3(11/830)	1.2(9/744)	1.4(10/711)	1.6(13/805)
Cleft palate	0.6(5/830)	0.7(5/744)	0.7(5/711)	0.7(6/805)
Cleft lip/nose	0.0(/830)	0.0(0/744)	0.3(2/711)	0.0(0/805)
Open eye	0.5(4/830)	0.0(0/744)	0.0(0/711)	0.0(0/805)
Exencephaly/hydrocephaly	0.2(2/830)	0.4(3/744)	0.1(1/711)	0.2(2/850)
No tongue	0.0(0/830)	0.0(0/744)	0.1(1/711)	0.0(0/805)
Umbilical hernia	0.1(1/830)	0.3(2/744)	0.1(1/711)	0.1(1/805)
Ribs fused/missing	0.1(1/830)	0.3(2/744)	0.3(2/711)	0.1(1/805)
Spinal centra doubled/misaligned	0.1(1/830)	0.0(0/744)	0.0(0/711)	0.0(0/805)
Spinal arches fused	0.0(0/830)	0.0(0/744)	0.1(1/711)	0.0(0/805)
Mandibles fused	0.0(0/830)	0.0(0/744)	0.1(1/711)	0.0(0/805)
Skull bones missing	0.0(0/830)	0.1(1/744)	0.1(1/711)	0.0(0/805)
Eye bones missing	0.0(0/830)	0.1(1/744)	0.0(0/711)	0.0(0/805)
Facial bones fused	0.2(2/830)	0.5(4/744)	0.4(3/711)	0.0(0/805)
Kinked tail	0.1(1/830)	0.0(0/744)	0.0(0/711)	0.0(0/805)
Total malformations[b]	5.2(43/830)	5.8(43/744)	6.6(47/711)	5.7(46/805)
Total malformed fetuses[b]	3.1(26/830)	3.6(27/744)	3.2(23/711)	3.6(29/805)

[a] Percentage incidence of specific anomalies; number of specific malformations per number of observations is given in parentheses
[b] Percentage incidence of malformations or malformed fetuses; number of malformations or malformed fetuses per number of observations is given in parentheses
Reprinted by permission of *J. Toxicol. Environ. Health* (Lamb et al., 1981c)

Table 18.6 Effect of 2,4-D, 2,4,5-T, and TCDD on postnatal development of offspring of treated males[a]

Measurement	Treatment group			
	I	II	III	IV
Day 0:				
Number of litters	80	94	81	107
Number of live pups per litter	4.40 ± 0.32	4.19 ± 0.29	4.44 ± 0.32	4.41 ± 0.29
Number of dead pups per litter	0.92 ± 0.16	0.92 ± 0.14	0.67 ± 0.13	0.84 ± 0.11
Average pup weight (g)	1.37 ± 0.01	1.39 ± 0.01	1.36 ± 0.01	1.39 ± 0.01
Day 4:				
Number of litters	44	60	48	56
Number of live pups per litter	5.30 ± 0.33	4.79 ± 0.25	4.91 ± 0.25	5.13 ± 0.27
Average pup weight (g)	2.22 ± 0.07	2.33 ± 0.05	2.37 ± 0.06	2.41 ± 0.08
Day 7:				
Number of litters	42	60	48	56
Number of live pups per litter	5.32 ± 0.31	4.58 ± 0.25	4.92 ± 0.24	5.04 ± 0.26
Average pup weight (g)	3.83 ± 0.12	3.79 ± 0.09	3.82 ± 0.12	3.94 ± 0.10
Day 21:				
Number of litters	41	56	46	56
Number of live pups per litter	5.15 ± 0.32	4.59 ± 0.25	4.87 ± 0.23	4.96 ± 0.25
Average pup weight (g)	7.48 ± 0.21	7.60 ± 0.16	7.67 ± 0.15	7.80 ± 0.18

[a]Values are means $\pm$ SE
Reprinted by permission of *J. Toxicol. Environ. Health* (Lamb *et al.*, 1981c)

toxicity data are expressed as the summation of all the eight week breeding trials; however, no treatment-related effects were observed in any single week (see Lamb *et al.*, 1980).

In addition to monitoring fertility, fetal development and postnatal survival and growth were evaluated. Pregnant females were selected either for sacrifice near the end of gestation (fetal development) or were allowed to deliver their litters (postnatal studies). No significant changes were observed in the number of implants per litter, live fetuses per litter or resportions per litter (Table 18.4). Fetal weight and sex ratios were not significantly affected by paternal exposure to the compounds. Gross examination, fresh tissue dissection and skeletal examination of the fetuses did not demonstrate any treatment-related anomalies (Table 18.5).

Table 18.7 Summary of specific malformations in the postnatal study

Observation	Treatment group			
	I	II	III	IV
Anophthalmia/microphthalmia	1.9(8/429)	2.6(12/468)	2.5(11/432)	1.7(10/579)
Agnathia/micrognathia	1.4(6/429)	1.3(6/468)	1.9(8/432)	1.4(8/579)
Cleft lip/palate	0.2(1/429)	0.4(2/468)	0.0(0/432)	0.0(0/579)
All else	0.0(0/429)	0.0(0/468)	0.5(2/432)[a]	0.0(0/579)
Total	3.0(13/429)	3.8(18/468)	4.4(19/432)	2.9(17/579)

[a]One exencephaly; one clubbed right hind limb. All fetuses (live or dead) were assumed to be at risk
Reprinted by permission of *J. Toxicol. Environ. Health* (Lamb *et al.*, 1981c)

In the postnatal study, the number of live pups and mean pup weight at 0, 4, 7 or 14 days of age were not significantly affected by the treatment (Table 18.6). External malformations were not significantly increased in the postnatal study (Table 18.7).

CONCLUDING REMARKS

The chlorinated phenoxy acids are broad leaf herbicides which have been used in agriculture, landscaping and commercial and military deforestation. Compounds in this class include the phenoxyacetic acids, 2,4-dichlorophenoxyacetic acid (2,4-D) and 2,4,5-trichlorophenoxyacetic acid (2,4,5-T), and the phenoxypropionic acids, Silvex and 2-methyl-4-chlorophenoxypropionic acid (MCPP). 2,4,5-T has been identified as a teratogen in animal models, as is the contaminant 2,3,7,8-tetrachlorodibenzo-p-dioxin (TCDD) which is found in 2,4,5-T. Data on the effects of these compounds in humans are not conclusive. The influence of the phenoxy acids and the contaminant TCDD on male reproductive function in males has been studied in very few toxicological investigations. Studies on 2,4-D, 2,4,5-T and TCDD have failed to demonstrate male reproductive toxicity, or adverse effects on the offspring of exposed males at dose levels which are not lethal to the test animals. Human studies, to date, have not demonstrated a link between exposure to these compounds and adverse effects on reproductive function. The existing metabolism data support the use of the rodent as a model for TCDD toxicity. Studies on additional species and with new experimental designs have been slow in coming. Evaluations of human data should include verification of exposure levels, to the extent possible, and proper selection of control population if they are intended to address the question of whether these chemicals can affect human male reproductive function.

References

Allen, J.R. and Carstens, L.A. (1967). Light and electron microscopic observations in *Macaca mulatta* monkeys fed toxic fat. *Am. J. Vet. Res.*, **28**, 1513

Beck, S.L. (1981). Assessment of adult skeletons to detect prenatal exposure to 2,4,5-T or trifuluralin in mice. *Teratology*, **23**, 33

Beljan, J.R., Irey, N.S., Kilgore, W.W., Kimura, K., Suskind, R.R., Vostal, J.J. and Wheater, R.H. (1982). Health effects of agent orange and dioxin contaminants. *J. Am. Med. Assoc.*, **248**, 1895

Berry, D.L., Zachariah, P.K., Namkung, M.J. and Juchau, M.R. (1976). Transplacental induction of carcinogen-hydroxylating systems with 2,3,7,8-tetrachlorodibenzo-p-dioxin. *Toxicol. Appl. Pharmacol.*, **36**, 569

Bovey, R.W. and Young, A.L. (1980). *The Science of 2,4,5-T and Associated Phenoxy Herbicides.* (New York: Wiley)

Collins, T.F.X. and Williams, C.H. (1971). Teratogenic studies with 2,4,5-T and 2,4-D in the hamster. *Bull. Environ. Contam. Toxicol.*, **6**, 559

Coulston, F. and Olajos, E.J. (1980). Panel report: panel to discuss the epidemiology of 2,4,5-T. *Ecotoxicol. Environ. Safety*, **4**, 96

Courtney, K.D. and Ebron, M.T. (1981). 2,4,5-T effects on cardiac and serum lactic dehydrogenase (LDH) and creatine kinase (CK) isozymes II. Neonatal enzyme activities and isozyme profiles. *Arch. Environ. Contam. Toxicol.*, **10**, 583

Courtney, K.D., Gaylor, D.W., Hogan, M.D. and Falk, H.L. (1970). Teratogenic evaluation of 2,4,5-T. *Science*, **168**, 864

Courtney, K.D. and Moore, J.A. (1971). Teratology studies with 2,4,5-trichlorophenoxyacetic acid and 2,3,7,8-tetrachlorodibenzo-*p*-dioxin. *Toxicol. Appl. Pharmacol.*, **20**, 396

Dougherty, W.J., Coulston, F. and Golberg, L. (1976). The evaluation of the teratogenic effects of 2,4,5-trichlorophenoxyacetic acid in the rhesus monkey. *Environ. Qual. Saf.*, **5**, 89

Elo, H.A. and Ylitalo, P. (1979). Distribution of 2-methyl-4-chlorophenoxyacetic acid and 2,4-dichlorophenoxyacetic acid in male rats: Evidence for the involvement of the central nervous system in their toxicity. *Toxicol. Appl. Pharmacol.*, **51**, 439

Elo, H. and Parvinen, M. (1976). Effect of sodium 2-methyl-4-chlorophenoxyacetate on spermatogenesis in the rat. *J. Reprod. Fert.*, **48**, 243

Emerson, J.L., Thompson, D.J., Strebing, R.J., Gerbig, C.G. and Robinson, V.B. (1971). Teratogenic studies on, 2,4,5-trichlorophenoxyacetic acid in the rat and rabbit. *Food Cosmet. Toxicol.*, **9**, 395

Fanelli, R., Bertoni, M.P., Castelli, M.G., Chiabrando, C., Martelli, G.P., Noseda, A., Garattini, S., Binaghi, C., Marazza, V. and Pezza, F. (1980). 2,3,7,8-Tetrachlorodibenzo-*p*-dioxin toxic effects and tissue levels in animals from the contaminated area of Seveso, Italy. *Arch. Environ. Contam. Toxicol.*, **9**, 569

Friedman, J.M. (1984). Does agent orange cause birth defects? *Teratology*, **29**, 193

Gehring, P.J. and Betso, J.E. (1978). Phenoxy acids: Effects and fate in mammals. *Ecol. Bull.* (Stockholm), **27**, 122

Hanify, J.A., Metcalf, P., Nobbs, C.L. and Worsley, K.J. (1981). Aerial spraying of 2,4,5-T and human birth malformations: An epidemiological investigation. *Science*, **212**, 349

Hansen, W.H., Quaife, M.L., Habermann, R.T. and Fitzhugh, O.G. (1971). Chronic toxicity of 2,4-dichlorophenoxyacetic acid in rats and dogs. *Toxicol. Appl. Pharmacol.*, **20**, 122

Hay, A. (1982). *The Chemical Scythe, Lessons of 2,4,5-T and Dioxin*. (New York: Plenum)

Hood, R.D., Patterson, B.L., Thacker, G.T., Sloan, G.L. and Szczech, G.M. (1979). Prenatal effects of 2,4,5-T, 2,4,5-trichlorophenol, and phenoxyacetic acid in mice. *J. Environ. Sci. Health*, **C13**, 189

Hutzinger, O., Frei, R.W., Merian, E. and Pocchiari, F. (eds.) (1982). *Chlorinated Dioxins and Related Compounds: Impact on the Environment*. (New York: Pergamon)

Khera, K.S. and Ruddick, J.A. (1973). Polychlorodibenzo-*p*-dioxins: Perinatal effects and the dominant lethal test in Wistar rats. In Blair, E.H. (ed.), *Chlorodioxins—Origin and Fate*, pp. 70–84. (American Chemical Society)

Khera, K.S. and McKinley, W.P. (1972). Pre- and postnatal studies on 2,4,5-trichlorophenoxyacetic acid, 2,4-dichlorophenoxyacetic acid and their derivatives in rats. *Toxicol. Appl. Pharmacol.*, **22**, 14

Kociba, R.J., Keeler, P.A., Park, C.N. and Gehring, P.J. (1976). 2,3,7,8-tetrachlorodibenzo-*p*-dioxin (TCDD): Results of a 13-week oral toxicity study in rats. *Toxicol. Appl. Pharmacol.*, **35**, 553

Kociba, R.J., Keyes, D.G., Beyer, J.E., Carreon, R.M., Wade, C.E., Dittenber, D.A., Kalnins, R.P., Frauson, L.E., Park, C.N., Barnard, S.D., Hummel, R.A. and Humiston, C.G. (1978). Results of a two-year chronic toxicity and oncogenicity study of 2,3,7,8-tetrachlorodibenzo-*p*-dioxin in rats. *Toxicol. Appl. Pharmacol.*, **46**, 279

Koller-Goldsmith, R.M., Zenick, H. and Manson, J. (1980). Evaluation of the spermatotoxicity of 2,4,5-trichlorophenoxyacetic acid (2,4,5-T) in rats. *Annual Report*, Center for the Study of the Human Environment, USPHS ES00159, 31 March

Lamb, J.C. IV, Marks, T.A., Gladen, B.C., Allen, J.W. and Moore, J.A. (1981b). Male fertility, sister chromatid exchange, and germ cell toxicity following exposure to mixtures of chlorinated phenoxy acids containing 2,3,7,8-tetrachlorodibenzo-*p*-dioxin. *J. Toxicol. Environ. Health*, **8**, 825

Lamb, J.C. IV, Marks, T.A. and McConnell, E.E. (1981a). Toxicity of chlorinated phenoxy acids in combination with 2,3,7,8-tetrachlorodibenzo-*p*-dioxin in C57BL/6 male mice. *J. Toxicol. Environ. Health*, **8**, 815

Lamb, J.C. IV, Moore, J.A. and Marks, T.A. (1980). Evaluation of 2,4-dichlorophenoxyacetic acid (2,4-D), 2,4,5-trichlorophenoxyacetic acid (2,4,5-T), and 2,3,7,8-tetrachlorodibenzo-*p*-dioxin (TCDD) toxicity in C57BL/6 mice: Reproduction and fertility in treated male mice and evaluation of congenital malformations in their offspring. *National Toxicology Program Technical Report*, No NTP-80-44

Lamb, J.C. IV, Moore, J.A., Marks, T.A. and Haseman, J.K. (1981c). Development and viability of offspring of male mice treated with chlorinated phenoxy acids and 2,3,7,8-tetrachlorodibenzo-*p*-dioxin. *J. Toxicol. Environ. Health*, **8**, 835

Lee, I.P. and Nagayama, J. (1980). Metabolism of benzo(a)pyrene by the isolated perfused rat testis. *Cancer Res.*, **40**, 3297

Lee, I.P. and Suzuki, K. (1980). Induction of aryl hydrocarbon hydroxylase activity in the rat prostate glands by 2,3,7,8-tetrachlorodibenzo-*p*-dioxin. *J. Pharmacol. Exp. Ther.*, **215**, 601

Lee, I.P., Suzuki, K. and Nagayama, J. (1981). Metabolism of benzo(a)pyrene in rat prostate glands following 2,3,7,8-tetrachlorodibenzo-*p*-dioxin exposure. *Carcinogenesis*, **2**, 823

Lloyd, J.W., Thomas, J.A. and Mawhinney, M.G. (1973). 2,4,5-T and the metabolism of testosterone-1,2-^{3}H$_2$ by mouse prostate glands. *Environ. Health*, **26**, 217

Mann, T. and Mann, C.L. (1981). Passage of chemicals into human and animal semen: Mechanisms and significance. *CRC Crit. Rev. Toxicol.*, **11**, 1

May, G. (1982). Tetrachlorodibenzodioxin: a survey of subjects ten years after exposure. *Br. J. Ind. Med.*, **39**, 128

McConnell, E.E. (1980). Acute and chronic toxicity, carcinogenesis, reproduction, teratogenesis and mutagenesis in animals. In Kimbrough, R.(ed.), *Halogenated Biphenyls, Terphenyls, Naphthalenes, Dibenzodioxins and Related Products*, pp. 109-50. (Amsterdam; Elsevier/North-Holland Biomedical)

McConnell, E.E., Moore, J.A., Haseman, and Harris, M.W. (1978). The comparative toxicity of chlorinated dibenzo-*p*-dioxins in mice and guinea pigs. *Toxicol. Appl. Pharmacol.*, **44**, 335

Moore, J.A., Gupta, B.N., Zinkl, J.G. and Vos, J.G. (1973). Postnatal effects of maternal exposure to 2,3,7,8-tetrachlorodibenzo-*p*-dioxin (TCDD). *Environ Health, Perspec.*, **5**, 81

Murray, F.J., Smith, F.A., Nitschke, K.D., Humiston, C.G., Kociba, R.J. and Schwetz, B.A. (1979). Three-generation reproduction study of rats given 2,3,7,8-tetrachlorodibenzo-*p*-dioxin (TCDD) in the diet. *Toxicol. Appl. Pharmacol.*, **50**, 241

Nagayama, J. and Lee, I.P. (1982). Comparison of benzo(a)pyrene metabolism by testicular homogenate and the isolated perfused testis of rat following 2,3,7,8-tetrachlorodibenzo-*p*-dioxin treatment. *Arch. Toxicol.*, **51**, 121

Nau, H. and Bass, R. (1981). Transfer of 2,3,7,8-tetrachlorodibenzo-*p*-dioxin (TCDD) to the mouse embryo and fetus. *Toxicology*, **20**, 299

Neubert, D. and Dillmann, I. (1972). Embryotoxic effects in mice treated with 2,4,5-trichlorophenoxyacetic acid and 2,3,7,8-tetrachlorodibenzo-*p*-dioxin. *Naunyn–Schmiedeberg's Arch. Pharmacol.*, **272**, 243

Neubert, D., Zens, P., Rothenwallner, A. and Merker, H.-J. (1973). A survey of the embryotoxic effects of TCDD in mammalian species. *Environ. Health Perspec.*, **5**, 67

Newton, M. and Norris, L.A. (1981). Potential exposure of humans to 2,4,5-T and TCDD in the Oregon coast ranges. *Fund. Appl. Toxicol.*, **1**, 339

Nienstedt, W., Parkki, M., Uotila, P. and Aitio, A. (1979). Effect of 2,3,7,8-tetrachlorodibenzo-*p*-dioxin on the hepatic metabolism of testosterone in the rat. *Toxicology*, **13**, 233

Norback, D.H. and Allen, J.R. (1973). Biological responses of the nonhuman primate, chicken and rat to chlorinated dibenzo-*p*-dioxin ingestion. *Environ. Health Perspec.*, **5**, 233

Reggiani, G. (1978). Medical problems raised by the TCDD contamination in Seveso, Italy. *Arch. Toxicol.*, **40**, 161

Schwetz, B.A., Sparschu, G.L. and Gehring, P.J. (1971). The effect of 2,4-dichlorophenoxyacetic acid (2,4-D) and esters of 2,4-D on rat embryonal, foetal and neonatal growth and development. *Food Cosmet. Toxicol.*, **9**, 801

Seiler, J.P. (1979). Phenoxyacids as inhibitors of testicular DNA synthesis in male mice. *Bull. Environ. Contam. Toxicol.*, **21**, 89

Smith, A.H., Fisher, D.O., Pearce, N. and Chapman, C.J. (1982). Congenital defects and miscarriages among New Zealand 2,4,5-T sprayers. *Arch. Environ. Health*, **37**, 197

Smith, A.H., Matheson, D.P., Fisher, D.O. and Chapman, C.J. (1981). Preliminary report of reproductive outcomes among pesticide applicators using 2,4,5-T. *N. Zealand Med. J.*, **93**, 178

Smith, F.A., Murray, F.J., John, J.A., Nitschke, K.D., Kociba, R.J. and Schwetz, B.A. (1981). Three-generation reproduction study of rats ingesting 2,4,5-trichlorophenoxyacetic acid in the diet. *Food Cosmet. Toxicol.*, **19**, 41

Smith, F.A., Schwetz, B.A. and Nitschke, K.D. (1976). Teratogenicity of 2,3,7,8-tetrachlorodibenzo-*p*-dioxin in CF-1 mice. *Toxicol. Appl. Pharmacol.*, **38**, 517

Soyka, L.F. and Joffe, J.M. (1980). Male mediated drug effects on offspring. In Schwarz, R.H. and Yaffe, S.J. (eds.), *Drug and Chemical Risks to the Fetus and Newborn*, pp. 49–66. (New York: Alan R. Liss

Sparschu, G.L., Dunn, F.L., Lisowe, R.W. and Rowe, V.K. (1971a). Study of the effects of high levels of 2,4,5-trichlorophenoxyacetic acid on foetal development in the rat. *Food Cosmet. Toxicol.*, **9**, 527

Sparschu, G.L., Dunn, F.L. and Rowe, V.K. (1971b). Study of the teratogenicity of 2,3,7,8-tetrachlorodibenzo-*p*-dioxin in the rat. *Food Cosmet. Toxicol.*, **9**, 405

Stevens, K.M. (1981). Agent Orange toxicity: A quantitative perspective. *Human Toxicol.*, **1**, 31

Tofilon, P.J., Peters, P.G., Clement, R.P., Hardwicke, D.M. and Piper, W.N. (1980). Depressed guinea-pig testicular microsomal cytochrome P-450 content by 2,3,7,8-tetrachlorodibenzo-*p*-dioxin. *Life Sci.*, **27**, 871.

Townsend, J.C., Bodner, K.M., Van. Peenen, P.F.D., Olson, R.D. and Cook, R.R. (1982). Survey of reproductive events of wives of employees exposed to chlorinated dioxins. *Am J. Epidemiol.*, **115**, 695

Tucker, R.E., Young, A.L. and Gray, A.P. (eds.) (1983). *Human and Environmental Risks of Chlorinated Dioxins and Related Compounds*. (New York: Plenum)

Unger, T.M., Kliethermes, J., Van Goethem, D. and Short, R.D. (1981). Teratology and postnatal studies in rats of the propylene glycol butyl ether and isooctyl esters of 2,4-dichlorophenoxyacetic acid. EPA-600/S1-81-035

Verschuuren, H.G., Kores, R. and Den Tonkelaar, E.M. (1975). Short-term oral and dermal toxicity of MCPA and MCPP. *Toxicology*, **3**, 349

Vos, J.G. and Moore, J.A. (1974). Suppression of cellular immunity in rats and mice by maternal treatment with 2,3,7,8-tetrachlorodibenzo-*p*-dioxin. *Int. Arch. Allergy Appl. Immunol.*, **47**, 777

Young, A.L., Calcagni, J.A., Thalken, C.E. and Tremblay, J.W. (1978). *The Toxicology, Environmental Fate, and Human Risk of Herbicide Orange and Its Associated Dioxin*. US Air Force OEHL Technical Report No TR-78-92.

19
Human spermatogenesis and fertility following exposure to dibromochloropropane (DBCP)

G. POTASHNIK

1,2-Dibromo-3-chloropropane (DBCP) is a highly effective nematocide and soil fumigant which was widely used in agriculture between 1955 and 1977. The first report of its gonadotoxic effect in animals appeared in 1961 (Torkelson, *et al.*, 1961), but it was only during the summer of 1977 that epidemiological studies conducted at chemical plants manufacturing this compound indicated that employees who had been exposed to it showed oligospermia or azoospermia and infertility (Potashnik *et al.*, 1978; Whorton *et al.*, 1977). A thorough investigation was initiated and the suppressive effect of DBCP on human testicular function was confirmed. It was not clear at that time whether this compound selectively affects the seminiferous tubules or whether it also exerts some toxic effect on the interstitial (Leydig) cells, leading to peripheral testosterone depletion and sexual disturbances, as initially claimed by some of the affected individuals. In addition, the questions relating to the mechanism of this gonadal effect and its possible reversibility could not be answered at that time.

Periodic follow-up of the affected workers for more than five years and intensive clinical and experimental research has improved our understanding of these questions. This chapter presents the latest information and data accumulated on this subject.

CHEMICAL CHARACTERIZATION AND COMMERCIAL USE

Until 1977 DBCP was available on the market under the trade names, Fumazone, Nemazone and Nemaset. The compound is a dark yellow or amber liquid with a pungent odour. The molecular structure of DBCP is presented in Fig. 19.1. The compound has a specific gravity of 2.08 (at 25°C), a boiling point of 195°C and a vapour pressure of 0.8 mm Hg (at 20°C). DBCP is slightly soluble in water and miscible in methanol, acetone, carbon tetrachloride and dimethylsulphoxide (DMSO).

DBCP was used on a variety of crops, including cotton, soybeans, fruits,

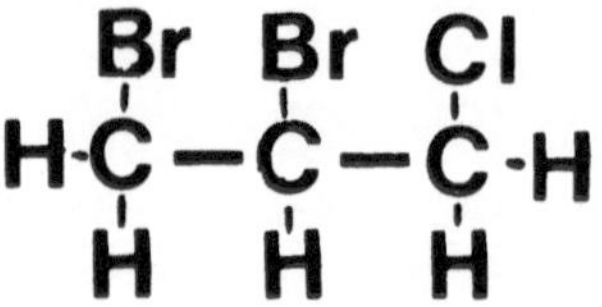

$$\underset{\underset{\textstyle H}{|}}{\overset{\overset{\textstyle Br}{|}}{H\text{-}C}} - \underset{\underset{\textstyle H}{|}}{\overset{\overset{\textstyle Br}{|}}{C}} - \underset{\underset{\textstyle H}{|}}{\overset{\overset{\textstyle Cl}{|}}{C}}\text{-}H$$

Fig. 19.1   Molecular structure of 1,2-dibromo-3-chloropropane (DBCP)

nuts, vegetables and ornamentals. DBCP is not phytotoxic and can be applied directly to the soil. It was applied to the soil by injection, granular deposition, or sprinkler irrigation. The combination of its relatively low vapour pressure and high density ensured a long residence time of the compound in soil. Its fumigation action in the soil was attributed to its slow rate of volatilization.

EXPERIMENTAL STUDIES

Effect on the reproductive system

In 1961 DBCP was found to exert acute and chronic toxicological effects on the rat, guinea pig, rabbit and monkey. Respiratory exposure to DBCP vapour at a concentration of 10 or more parts/10^6 over a period of more than 7 weeks resulted in a significant decrease in sperm count, degeneration of the seminiferous tubules and severe atrophy of the testes (Torkelson *et al.*, 1961). Oral ingestion of DBCP similarly reduced sperm count and motility, increased the rate of formation of morphologically abnormal sperm cells and caused testicular atrophy (Faydysh *et al.*, 1970).

The suppressive effect of DBCP on rat testes is reversible. In a recent study fertile male rats were injected subcutaneously with DBCP, dissolved in DMSO, at a dosage of 20 mg DBCP per kg body weight, once a week for three consecutive weeks. One testis of each rat was removed 3–7 weeks after the last injection. The second testis was removed 27 weeks later. About 70% of the animals with atrophy of the seminiferous tubules in the first testis showed reversibility of the suppressive effect. Active spermatogenesis was observed on histological sections of the second testis (Shemi *et al.*, 1981).

Other toxicological effects of DBCP

A bioassay for the possible carcinogenicity of DBCP was conducted on rats and mice of both sexes (Olson *et al.*, 1973; Powers *et al.*, 1975). DBCP dissolved in corn oil was administered by gavage five days a week for a total of 78 weeks. As early as 10 weeks after the study was initiated, squamous cell carcinomas of the stomach were detected in both male and female rats and mice. The incidence of adrenocarcinoma of the mammary gland was statistically significant only in female rats. Based on these data, under certain bioassay conditions, DBCP is a stomach carcinogen in rats and mice of both sexes, and is carcinogenic to the mammary gland in female rats. However, no cases of cancer have been reported in men exposed to the compound during its production or in men fumigating fields with DBCP. In Israel, this is true for the 12-year period for which severely affected patients who became azoospermic have been followed up (Potashnik, 1983).

DBCP exerts significant genetic activity. It induced dominant lethal mutations in rats, but not in mice, in the postmeiotic stage of spermatogenesis (Teramoto et al., 1980). In addition, its mutagenicity on certain strains of *Salmonella typhimurium* has also been demonstrated (Biles et al., 1978).

HUMAN EXPOSURE TO DBCP

Diagnostic approach

The following predetermined protocol is applied to all male workers presenting with occupationally related testicular dysfunction: Detailed exposure histories include specific occupation, mode of exposure to the chemical, cumulated exposure time and time lapse since last exposure. The latter factor is of value since it bears a relationship to the possible reversibility of the effect. Genital examination includes location and measurement of testes, its consistency and examination for the presence of a variocele. Three analyses of seminal fluid, obtained by masturbation following five days of sexual abstinence, are recommended. Plasma levels of FSH, LH and testosterone (measured by the radioimmunoassay) reflect the integrity of the function of the hypophyseal testicular axis. Elevated concentrations of gonadotrophins combined with a moderate decrease in testosterone indicate late effects associated with severe damage to the seminiferous tubules; and thus has limited value in serving as an early indicator of gonadotoxic effect. In cases in which sperm count depression is associated with normal basal levels of FSH and LH, the use of the LHRH challenge test might be helpful in establishing a cause–effect relationship between exposure to the toxic agent and testicular dysfunction. Exaggerated plasma concentrations of gonadotrophins in response to LHRH injection is suggestive of testicular failure.

Testicular biopsy is indicated in cases presenting with azoospermia and normal levels of FSH and LH in order to rule out the possibility of epididymal or vas obstruction. This procedure is also indicated in cases with azoospermia whose histories do not include any records of fertile semen or pregnancy of the spouse. In such cases, karyotyping of the affected individuals is also recommended to exclude a genetic basis for the testicular failure.

List 1   Investigation protocol for possible occupationally related, chemically induced testicular dysfunction

1. Explanation of the protocol to each patient.

2. Exposure history: cumulated exposure time, mode of contact with the chemical, history of poisoning.
3. Medical history with emphasis on marital status and previous reproductive history.
4. Physical examination including genitalia and prostate.
5. Seminal fluid analysis.
6. Laboratory tests: complete blood count and urine analysis; plasma hormones—FSH, LH, testosterone, prolactin, T_4, TSH; dynamic tests—LHRH test.
7. Testicular biopsy when indicated.
8. Karyotype in selected cases.

The above-described evaluation of all employees at risk is followed by annual evaluations of sperm count which have proved to be a sensitive indicator of possible adverse environmental effects on testicular function.

Effect of DBCP on human spermatogenesis

Today DBCP is known to exert a suppressive effect on human testicular function. It damages selectively the seminiferous tubules thus leading to oligospermia or azoospermia.

In 1977 a study at a local factory revealed severe impairment of spermatogensis in workers exposed to DBCP during production (Potashnik *et al.*, 1979). Azoospermia was diagnosed in 13 workers with estimated cumulated exposure times of 100–6726 hours (Table 19.1). All 13 were operators directly involved in the production process. Eight of the men were previously fertile (on the basis of pregnancies in their wives). The other five had normal karyotypes, thus excluding a genetic basis for the testicular failure. With a value of 20 million sperm cells/ml being taken as the lower limit of normal, oligospermia was diagnosed in seven employees whose exposure time varied from 34–310 hours (Table 19.2). Four men in this group were operators and the other three were packers of DBCP. Normal sperm counts were found in five employees, all packers (Table 19.3). Duration of exposure to DBCP ranged from 10 to 30 hours in four men, and was 60 hours in the fifth. Thus, a close correlation between exposure time to DBCP and severity of damage was established. Azoospermia was diagnosed in men with exposure times of more than 100 hours, whereas exposure time in the oligospermic men ranged from 34 to 310 hours. DBCP is a potent testicular toxin even after a relatively short exposure. Sperm density provides a reliable and sensitive early indicator of the gonadotoxic effect of the compound.

Testicular morphology of individuals exposed to DBCP

DBCP exerts a direct effect on the seminiferous epithelium, selectively damaging the spermatogenic cells. Evaluation of biopsies obtained from azoospermic patients revealed no evidence of active spermatogenesis. The seminiferous tubules were lined only by Sertoli cells (Fig. 19.2a). Small groups

Table 19.1 Comparison of sperm counts and hormone profiles in 1977 and 1981 in 13 workers with 1,2-dibromo-3-chloropropane (DBCP)-induced azoospermia (Potashnik, 1983)

Patient no.	Age (years)	Exposure time (hs)	October 1977				October 1981			
			Sperm count (millions/ml)	FSH (miu/ml)	LH (miu/ml)	T (ng/ml)	Sperm count (millions/ml)	FSH (miu/ml)	LH (miu/ml)	T (ng/ml)
A. Recovered with pregnancy										
1	1	390	0	27.0	6.7	6.0	7.0	46.0	26.0	4.5
2	22	120	0	5.4	3.4	8.5	48.0	6.0	6.2	7.6
B. Recovered without pregnancy										
3	20	114	0	10.0	5.0	7.8	8.0	15.0	8.0	6.6
4	35	115	0	12.5	10.5	4.8	1.5[a]	14.0[a]	13.0[a]	4.5[a]
C. Not recovered										
5	39	6726	0	13.4	4.0	7.8	0	35.0	15.0	4.8
6	29	488	0	21.5	6.2	5.4	0[a]	40.0[a]	19.0[a]	5.6[a]
7	24	1426	0	15.7	6.8	6.3	0	35.0	19.0	5.9
8	48	243	0	27.0	4.3	6.7	0	40.0	23.0	4.6
9	47	1504	0	18.1	4.3	4.2	0	23.0	11.0	4.0
10	50	618	0	16.4	3.7	10.4	0	40.0	16.0	4.8
11	30	901	0	30.0	12.5	3.8	0	66.0	34.0	7.0
12	35	120	0	20.0	9.0	8.0	0	48.0	20.0	5.0
13	33	100	0	25.4	5.3	4.8	0[a]	36.0[a]	N.A.	N.A.

a = Updated to July 1980
T = Testosterone
N.A. = Data not available

Table 19.2 Sperm counts and hormone profiles in 1977 and 1981 in 7 workers with 1,2-dibromo-3-chloropropane (DBCP)-induced oligospermia (Potashnik, 1983)

Patient no.	Age (years)	Exposure time (h)	October 1977				October 1981			
			Sperm count (millions/ml)	FSH (miu/ml)	LH (miu/ml)	T (ng/ml)	Sperm count (millions/ml)	FSH (miu/ml)	LH (miu/ml)	T (ng/ml)
A. Recovered with pregnancy										
14	20	70	0.5	3.5	6.2	5.8	1.7[a]	3.0[a]	3.3[a]	4.2[a]
15	37	79	0.5	6.0	5.6	6.2	37.0	12.0	7.6	6.5
16	26	70	1.5	9.4	3.9	6.7	5.0	13.0	11.0	5.0
17	23	38	10.0	3.2	6.0	9.0	17.0	6.0	11.0	5.8
18	22	34	2.7	11.0	4.0	10.0	121.0	10.0	13.0	8.7
B. Not recovered										
19	36	220	6.3	9.8	10.0	5.0	2.0	18.0	18.0	7.0
20	37	310	8.3	6.6	12.0	4.4	4.0	11.0	20.0	4.1

[a] = Updated to July 1979
T = Testosterone

Table 19.3 Clinical and laboratory data in five normospermic men exposed to 1,2-dibromo-3-chloropropane (DBCP)

Patient no.	Age (years)	No. of previous pregnancies of spouse	Exposure time (h)	Sperm count (millions/ml)	FSH (miu/ml)	LH (miu/ml)	T (ng/ml)
21	22	0[a]	30	20.5	2.8	3.7	4.7
22	26	3	30	21.5	6.4	4.2	7.8
23	25	2	30	24.0	3.5	3.5	8.2
24	23	0[a]	60	60.0	3.5	3.1	4.5
25	24	2	10	65.0	6.0	6.4	5.7

[a] = Unmarried

of tubules were completely hyalinized and clusters of normal Leydig cells were present in the interstitial tissues of all cases examined (Fig. 19.2b). A similar histological picture in the biopsies taken from the oligospermic patients, although evidence of partial spermatogenesis could be detected. The loss of spermatogenic cells in these cases was found at all stages of differentiation, from stem cells to mature forms (Fig. 19.2c). Electron microscopy of biopsies obtained from severely affected individuals following exposure to DBCP revealed no ultrastructural alterations in the cytoplasmic organelles and nuclear components of the spermatocytes, spermatozoa or spermatides. Sertoli cells and their intercellular junctions were found to be well preserved (Biava *et al.*, 1978).

Sertoli and Leydig cell integrity described has recently been questioned.

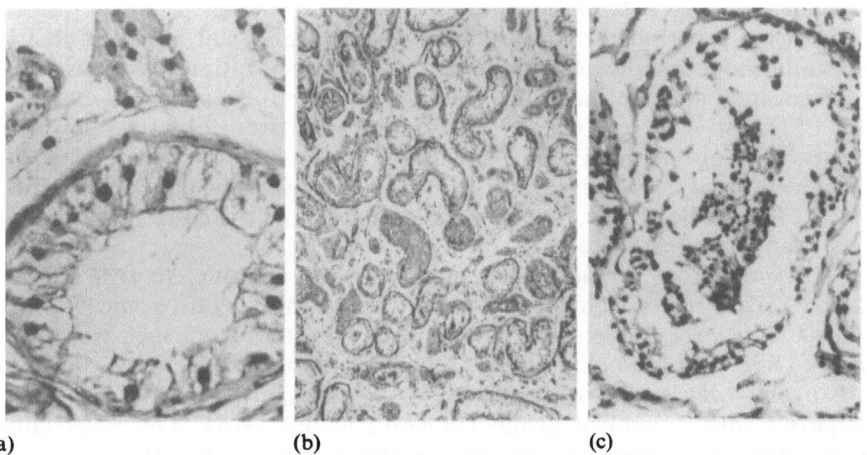

(a) (b) (c)

Fig. 19.2 Seminiferous tubule lined only by Sertoli cells. There is slight thickening of the tubule basement membrane. Intact Leydig cells are present in the interstitial tissue (Haematoxylin and eosin × 165) (b) Testicular biopsy showing atrophy of the germinal epithelium and hyalinization of occasional tubules. Groups of normal appearing Leydig cells are seen in the interstitial tissue (Haematoxylin and eosin × 34). (c) Seminiferous tubule lined mainly by Sertoli cells but showing minimal spermatogenic activity and desquamation of the spermatogenic cells (Haematoxylin and eosin × 165)

Despite lack of histological evidence, DBCP does have an adverse effect on the integrity and function of these cells. In a four-year reassessment study of workers with DBCP-induced azoospermia and oligospermia, further significant increases in basally elevated FSH levels were observed in workers who had been exposed to the compound and did not present with any improvement of sperm count (Tables 19.1 and 19.2). Similarly, significant increases in LH to levels above the upper limit of normal combined with decreases in testosterone concentrations were detected in these patients (Potashnik, 1983). These dynamic hormonal changes suggest that DBCP might exert a delayed gonadotoxic effect leading to Sertoli and Leydig cell dysfunction.

The gonadotoxic effect of DBCP is directly correlated with cumulated exposure time and sperm density. The toxin acts first on the seminiferous tubules, causing a selective decrease or loss of the spermatogenic cells only. Following heavy exposure, dysfunction of the Leydig and Sertoli cells is likely to occur as a delayed toxic effect of DBCP, thus explaining the lack of spermatogenic recovery over a prolonged period of time.

Hormonal changes associated with DBCP-induced testicular dysfunction

Prolonged exposure to DBCP in workers presenting with azoospermia is usually associated with a significant increase in plasma FSH to levels higher than the upper limit of normal. In moderately affected individuals, most of whom present with oligospermia, slight plasma FSH elevations falling within the normal limits were observed. Significantly elevated FSH levels is an indicator for severity of damage.

Following a period of more than four years, significant increases in LH levels and moderate decreases in testosterone concentrations were observed in the severely affected individuals (Potashnik, 1983). In addition, exaggerated FSH and LH response to LHRH injection were observed in these patients (LeRoith et al., 1981). These observations, combined with a report of elevated basal LH levels in DBCP-induced azoospermic patients (Egantz, et al., 1980) indicate the involvement of Leydig cells in the pathological process affecting the testes.

The dynamics of prolactin secretion following exposure to DBCP, was studied in severely affected individuals who became azoospermic. Twelve such patients were challenged intravenously with thyrotropin-releasing hormone (TRH) and metoclopramide. The peak plasma prolactin response to both agents was significantly increased in the azoospermic group, when compared with a control group (LeRoith et al., 1981). The underlying mechanism responsible for this hyper-responsiveness was attributed to a state of oestrogen excess in those patients. However, the role of the gonadotoxic effect of DBCP in modulating these hormonal changes, is still to be clarified.

RECOVERY FROM DBCP-INDUCED TESTICULAR DYSFUNCTION

Improvement of spermatogenesis

Annual follow-up for more than four years of workers exposed to DBCP has shown clearly that the suppressive effect of DBCP on human spermatogenesis is reversible (Potashnik, 1983). In a recent study, sperm count improvement was observed in 5 of 7 oligospermic men after 14–36 months from their last exposure, and in 4 of 13 azoospermic workers after 20–45 months from their last exposure (Table 19.4). In all but one of these patients, recorded exposure time to DBCP did not exceed 120 hours and plasma FSH and LH levels were within the normal range on the initial evaluation (Tables 19.1 and 19.2). In the case with a recorded exposure time of 390 hours, spermatogenic recovery was associated with persistently high FSH levels. Improvement of fertility was further confirmed in these men by the occurrence of nine pregnancies (Table 19.4). Eight of the pregnancies have so far been followed to term. They culminated uneventfully in the spontaneous delivery of healthy infants with no detectable congenital abnormalities. After more than 60 months from the last exposure, no signs of sperm count improvement were detected in the azoospermic and oligospermic men with exposure times of more than 120 hours.

Normal basal plasma FSH levels were found on initial evaluation of oligospermic and azoospermic patients who showed various degrees of sperm count improvement. In contrast, basally high FSH levels and further significant increases during a four-year follow-up characterized the severely affected workers who became azoospermic and did not show evidence of sperm count recovery

The gonadotoxic effect of DBCP on human testicular function is reversible, being inversely related to previous exposure time, although time lapse since last exposure does also play a role in favour of this reversibility. This was confirmed by recent experimental studies in rats, in which complete spermatogenic recovery was detected, depending on the dose of DBCP, exposure period and time-interval between last exposure and testicular evaluation (Shemi *et al.*, 1981). The combination of spermatogenesis on testicular biopsy and normal plasma FSH levels is a reliable indicator of the recovery. Significantly high FSH levels maintained for a prolonged period of time are indicative of an extensive and probably irreversible toxic effect of DBCP, explaining the lack of recovery over a prolonged period of time.

Reproductive outcome

A recent epidemiological study based on medical records of 68 children whose fathers were production workers potentially exposed to DBCP at the time of conception, did not reveal any significant increase in the prevalence of congenital malformations (Potashnik, 1983). Similarly, physical examinations of all eight children conceived during the spermatogenic recovery process were unremarkable and no malformations were observed (Table 19.4).

Table 19.4 Reproductive outcome in relation to sperm count improvement in 9 workers with 1,2-dibromo-3-chloropropane (DBCP)-induced oligospermia (Potashnik, 1983)

Patient no.	Sperm count (millions/ml)		Recovery time[a] (months)	Pregnancy time[b] (months)	Outcome of pregnancy in spouse
	Initial Evaluation	First improvement			
1	0	0.4	20	26	Full-term normal female weighing 3150 g
2	0	3.0	45	42	Full-term normal female weighing 2750 g
3		1.0	42	—	No pregnancy occurred
4	0	N.A.	N.A.	—	Wife had hysterectomy in 1974
14 I	0.5	1.4	17	22[c]	Full-term normal female weighing 3400 g
II		—	—	—	Full-term normal female weighing 3580 g
15	0.5	13.0	34	66	Still pregnant
16	1.5	5.0	20	20	Full-term normal male weighing 3080 g
17	10.0	20.0	14	24	Full-term normal female weighing 3470 g
18 I	2.7	64.0	36	30[c]	Full-term normal female weighing 4010 g
II	—	—	—	—	Full-term normal male weighing 3860 g

a = From last exposure to first improved count
b = From last exposure to first missed period in spouse
c = Referred to first pregnancy only
N.A. = Data not available

Paternal exposure to DBCP might be asociated with a significant decrease in the sex ratio among offspring conceived during the exposure period. In a recent retrospective study, a population consisting of 30 families of which 13 fathers had become azoospermic, 8 oligospermic and 9 had remained normospermic after exposure to DBCP, were evaluated. Of the 89 pregnancies recorded, 68 culminated in the birth of live infants. The prevalence of male infants conceived during the pre-exposure period was 52.9%, a value close to that of 52% observed in the normal population. In contrast, the male rate for all the exposed groups (azoospermic, oligospermic and normospermic) was found to be as low as 35.2%. Furthermore, when the data from only the exposed azoospermic and oligospermic groups were combined and compared with the pre-exposure figure of 52.9%, a highly sigificant low male rate of 16.6% was found ($p < 0.025$) (Table 19.5). Similarly,

Table 19.5 Relationship between first paternal exposure and fetal sex ratio in 1,2-dibromo-3-chloropropane (DBCP) - exposed production workers

Group	Total no. of births	Sex ratio in offsprings		
		No. of males	No. of females	Males (%)
Pre-exposure and non-exposed	51	27	24	52.9
All exposed groups[a]	17	6	11	35.2
Exposed azoospermic and oligospermia	12	2	10	16.6

[a] = Including the DBCP-exposed azoospermic, oligospermic and normospermic workers

fetal sex distribution of two males and six females was observed among pregnancies during the recovery process from the azoospermic and oligospermic states (Table 19.4). The adverse effect of DBCP is initially reflected by some damage to the Y-bearing sperm cells, without a significant decrease in the male fertility. Conceptions occuring during the early stage of such an exposure result in a significantly low sex ratio. When exposure to such a noxious factor is continued, it may result in further damage to the testes, expressing itself as oligospermia or azoospermia and infertility. In subjects showing recovery, the same chain of events seems to take place in the reverse order. During the early stage of recovery, there is an increase in sperm density and recovery of fertility potential, as indicated by conceptions occurring during this period. The low sex ratio observed during the first stage of recovery supports the assumption that fertility potential of the Y-bearing sperm cells is restored only later on. Semen obtained from workers exposed to DBCP might have a higher incidence of sperm cells containing 2 Y chromosomes as compared with non-exposed workers, thus suggesting a disjunctional error in the maturing process of the Y-bearing sperm cells (Kapp et al., 1979).

Chronic paternal exposure to DBCP among production workers does not seem to increase the spontaneous abortion rate. In the above-described study, a spontaneous abortion rate of 13.6% (3 of 22 conceptions) was observed among the wives of all exposed groups. This figure is similar to the spontaneous abortion rate of 13.4% (9 of 67) recorded in the pre-exposure and non-exposed groups.

EFFECT OF DBCP ON SPERMATOGENESIS IN AGRICULTURAL WORKERS

Until 1977 DBCP was widely used in agriculture as a nematocide; it was applied mainly by means of injection, drench application, granular deposition or via sprinkler irrigation. The largest group of people potentially exposed to DBCP was thus agricultural workers who had been exposed to the compound intermittently by cutaneous contact or by inhalation while applying it in the fields. Results of the study carried on such field applications indicated that while infertility was not a problem, cumulated exposure time to DBCP of two months or more over a one-year period was associated with statistically significant but clinically unimportant sperm count depression and plasma basal FSH elevation (Glass et al., 1979). Similarly, significant differences in median sperm counts have been found among various occupational groups, with the lowest counts being detected among formulators, applicators and farmers. Intermediate counts were found in sales personnel, and the highest sperm counts, in researchers (Sandifer et al., 1979). Reports of these studies did not include any information regarding the outcome of pregnancies.

In a recent epidemiological study the effect of exposure to DBCP on reproductive outcome was evaluated among families of field applications (Kharrazi et al., 1980). Of 197 pregnancies reported for the total study group, 76 occurred before any contact with DBCP had been made and 121 after initial exposure. Of the 76 pregnancies before DBCP contact, 71 resulted in live births and 5 (6.6% of pregnancies) in spontaneous abortion; of the 121 pregnancies occurring after initial DBCP exposure, 97 resulted in live births and 24 (19.8% of pregnancies), in spontaneous abortion (Table 19.6). A subsample consisting of workers whose wives conceived both be-

Table 19.6 Outcomes of pregnancies in families of agricultural workers exposed to 1,2-dibromo-3-chloropropane (DBCP) (Kharrazi et al., 1980)

	Total population (n = 62)		Subsample (n = 16)[a]	
	Before exposure	After exposure	Before exposure	After exposure
No. of pregnancies	76	121	34	40
No. of live births	71	97	32	29
No. of spontaneous abortions	5	24	2	11
% of pregnancies	6.6	19.8*	5.9	27.5**

[a] = Consists of workers whose wives conceived both before and after the exposure to DBCP

The differences in rates of spontaneous abortion before and after exposure were significant at *0.01 $< p <$ 0.025 ($\chi^2 = 5.52$); **$p < 0.05$ ($\chi^2 = 4.60$)

fore and after exposure to DBCP was also evaluated. Of 74 pregnancies reported for the subsample, 2 of 34 (5.9%) pre-exposure pregnancies and 11 of 40 (27.5%) postexposure pregnancies ended in spontaneous abortion (Table 19.6). This high abortion rate represents a type of increased pregnancy wastage. This increased wastage can be related to mild irregular chronic paternal exposure to DBCP resulting in transient low sperm counts with or without a high frequency of morphological changes in the sperm cells. All pregnancies ending in live births conceived before the father had contact with DBCP were compared with those conceived after such contact for birth weight, type of delivery, prevalence of congenital malformations, disease at birth, premature birth, postmature birth and infant death. No differences were found between the two groups.

CONCLUDING REMARKS

DBCP is widely used in agriculture as a highly effective nematocide. People exposed to this compound developed a dose/exposure related oligospermia or azoospermia which appears to be a reliable and sensitive indicator of tubular changes. DBCP causes selective damage to the seminiferous tubules in the presence of normal appearing Sertoli cells and intact functioning Leydig cells. Significant elevation of plasma FSH was observed in severely affected individuals presenting with azoospermia, whereas in midly affected oligospermic men, normal basal FSH values were found. Plasma LH and testosterone concentrations fell within the normal range. The gonadotoxic effect of DBCP is reversible, the reversibility being inversely related to previous exposure time and occurs in the presence of normal basal FSH levels.

Children conceived during the time of paternal exposure to DBCP did not reveal any significant increase in rate of congenital malformations. Recovery observed among the azoospermic and oligospermic men was associated with uncomplicated pregnancies and uneventful spontaneous deliveries of eight physically normal infants. A significantly low prevalence of male infants among pregnancies conceived during paternal exposure to DBCP was detected.

Acknowledgments

Previous and ongoing experimental studies described in this chapter are kindly supported by a grant from Bromine Compounds Ltd, Beer-Sheva, Israel. The professional assistance of nurse Sabina Harush in proper handling of the patients is greatly appreciated.

References

Biava, C.G., Smuckler, E.D. and Whorton, D. (1978). The testicular morphology of individuals exposed to dibromochloropropane. *Exp. Mol. Pathol.*, **29**, 448–58
Biles, R.W., Connor, T.H., Trieff, N.M. and Legator, M.S. (1978). The influence of contaminants on the mutagenic activity of dibromochloropropane (DBCP). *J. Environ. Pathol. Toxicol.*, **2**, 301–21

Egnatz, D.B. Ott, M.G., Townsend, J.C., Olson, R.D. and Jons, D.D. (1980). DBCP and testicular effects in chemical workers: An epidemiological survey in Midland, Michigan. *J. Occup. Med.*, **22**, 727–32.

Faydysh, E.V., Rakmatullayev, N.N. and Varshavskii, V.A. (1970). The cytotoxic action of nemagon in a subacute experiment. *Med. Zh. Uzbetistana*, **1**, 64–5

Glass, R.I., Lyness, R.N., Megle, D.C., Powell, K.E. and Kahn, E. (1979). Sperm count depression in pesticide applicators exposed to dibromochloropropane. *Am. J. Epidemiol.*, **109**, 346–51

Kapp, R.W., Picciano, D.J. and Jacobson, C.B. (1979). Y-chromosomal non-disjunction in dibromochloropropane exposed workmen. *Mutat. Res.*, **64**, 47–51

Kharrazi, M., Potashnik, G. and Goldsmith, J.R. (1980). Reproductive effects of dibromo-chloropropane. *Isr. J. Med. Sci.*, **16**, 403–6

LeRoith, D., Potashnik, G., Dunn, J. and Spitz, I.M. (1981). The exaggerated prolactin response to thyrotropin-releasing hormone and metoclopramide in 1,2-dibromo-3-chloropropane-induced azoospermia. *J. Clin. Endocrinol. Metab.*, **52**, 38–42

Olson, W.A., Habermann, R.T., Weisburger, E.K., Ward, J.M. and Weisburger, J.H. (1973). Induction of stomach cancer in rats and mice by halogenated aliphatic fumigants. *J. Natl. Cancer Inst.*, **51**, 1993–5

Potashnik, G. (1983). A four-year reassessment of workers with dibromochloropropane-induced testicular dysfunction. *Andrologia*, 15, 164–70

Potashnik, G., Ben-Aderet, N., Israeli, R., Yanai-Inbar, I. and Sober, I. (1978). Suppressive effect of 1,2-dibromo-3-chloropropane on human spermatogenesis. *Fertil. Steril.*, **30**, 444–7

Potashnik, G., Yanai-Inbar, I., Sacks, M.U. and Israeli, R. (1979). Effect of dibromochloropropane-induced testicular dysfunction. *Isr. J. Med. Sci.*, **25**, 438–42

Powers, M.B., Woelker, R.W., Page, N.P. Weisburger, E.R. and Kraybill, J.F. (1975). Car-cinogenicity of ethylene dibromide (EDB) and 1,2-dibromo-3-chloropropane (DBCP) after oral administration in rats and mice. *Toxicol. Appl. Pharmacol.*, **33**, 171–2

Sandifer, S.H., Wilkins, R.T., Loadholt, B., Lane, L.G. and Eldridge, J.C. (1979). Sperma-togenesis in agricultural workers exposed to dibromochloropropane (DBCP). *Bull. Environ. Contam. Toxicol.*, **23**, 703–10

Shemi, D., Sod-Moriah, U.A., Kaplanski, J., Potashnik, G. and Yanai-Inbar, I. (1981). Suppression and recovery of spermatogenesis in dibromochloropropane-treated rats. *An-drologia*, **14**, 191–9

Teramoto, S., Saito, R., Aoyama, H. and Sirasu, Y. (1980). Dominant lethal mutation induced in male rats by 1,2-dibromo-3-chloropropane (DBCP). *Mutat. Res.*, **77**, 71–8

Torkelson, T.R., Sadek, S.E. and Rowe, V.K. (1961). Toxicologic investigations of 1,2-dibromo-3-chloropropane. *Toxicol. Appl. Pharmacol.*, **3**, 545–59

Whorton, D., Krauss, R.M., Marshall, S. and Milby, T.H. (1977). Infertility in male pesticide workers. *Lancet*, **2**, 1259–61

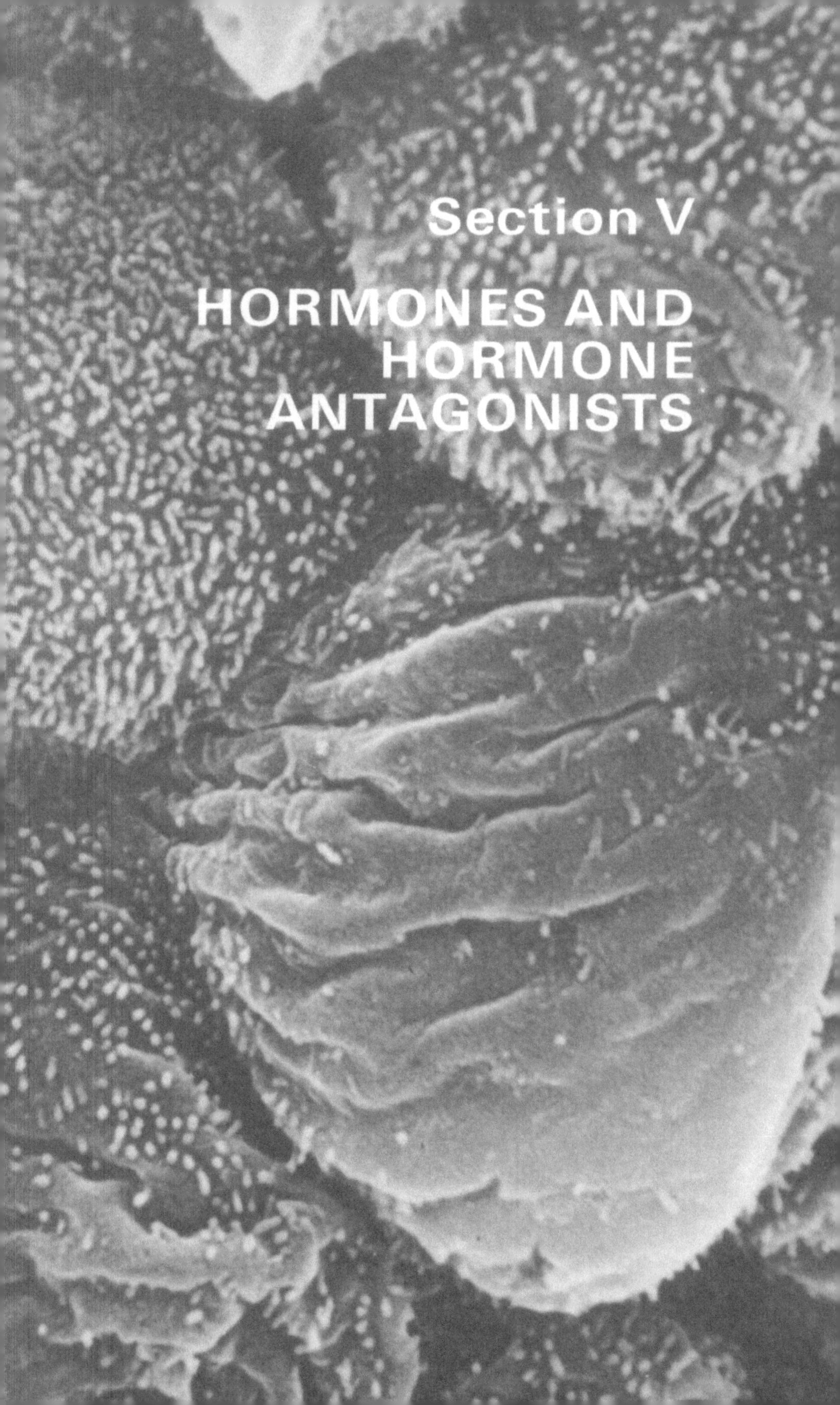

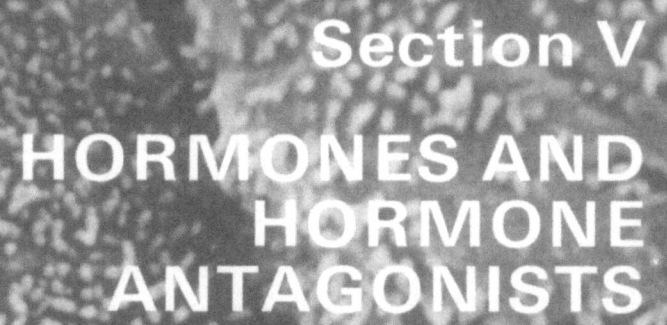

Section V
HORMONES AND
HORMONE
ANTAGONISTS

20

LHRH and its analogues: potential for male contraception and for therapy of androgen-dependent syndromes

B.H. VICKERY

It is more than a decade since the isolation, sequencing and synthesis of LHRH was reported. Initially it was forseeen that LHRH (Fig. 20.1) would be of use in correcting infertility of hypthalamic origin. Early hopes were also expressed that structural modification of the molecule would result in analogues which would retain binding activity to the LHRH receptors but be without intrinsic gonadotropin-releasing activity and thus antagonize the releasing activity of endogenous LHRH. These LHRH antagonists were foreseen as potential contraceptive agents.

Treatment of infertility with LHRH in either men or women, however, gave disappointingly poor results. LHRH agonist potency is particularly responsive to minor modifications of the molecule, i.e. substitution of D-amino acids for the 6-position glycine, and replacement of the 10-position glycine by alkylamide (Table 20.1). Such modified analogues, by virtue of

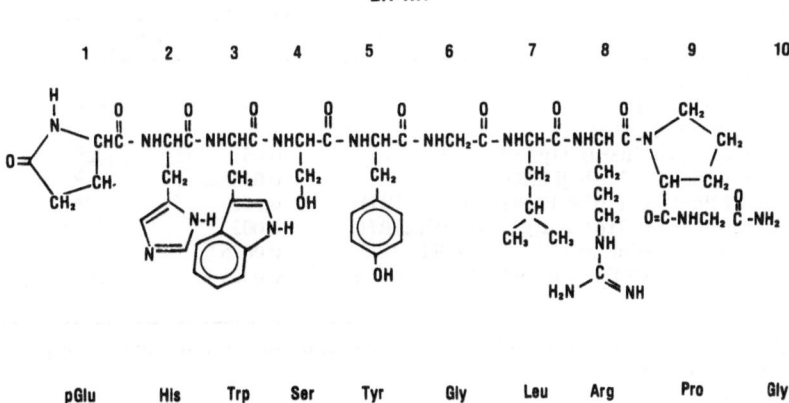

Fig. 20.1 Structure of luteinizing hormone–releasing hormone

Table 20.1 Representative highly potent agonist analogues of LHRH

Structure	Name	Potency
LHRH		1
[D-Leu⁶]LHRH EA	(Leuprolide)	15[a]
[D-Ser(tBu⁶)]LHRH EA	(Buserelin)	15[b]
[D-His(Bzl)⁶]LHRH EA		21[a]
[D-Ser(tBu⁶)]LHRH AzaGly ICI-118630		100[b]
[D-Trp⁶]LHRH		100[c]
[D-Trp⁶]LHRH EA		100[c]
[D-Nal(2)⁶]LHRH	(Nafarelin acetate)	200[c]
[D-Nal(2)⁶]LHRH EA		90[c]
[D-Nal(2)⁶]LHRH AzaGly		225[c]

[a] LH release (Rivier et al., 1975)
[b] Ovulation induction (Dutta et al., 1978)
[c] Oestrus suppression (Nestor et al., 1982)

increased receptor binding and protection from enzymatic degradation, achieved potency increases versus the native LHRH of more than 200-fold and have been referred to as 'superagonists.' Clinical evaluation of these more potent agents, however, demonstrated that, far from improving infertility therapy, the situation was worsened. Studies in animals and man revealed that, to exert profertility actions, LHRH is required in short duration bursts at intervals of 1 hour or longer. Thus, because of their resistance to inactivation and, therefore, their long biological and receptor life, the highly potent agonist analogues of LHRH will not be useful for stimulation of fertility. However, due to their ability to down regulate pituitary gonadotropin secretion, and possibly actions at other sites including the gonads, they exert 'paradoxical' gonadal suppressive effects. These effects have made the agonists prime candidates for contraceptive use and,

Table 20.2 Representative antagonistic analogues of LHRH

Structure	Dose (mg)	Blockade of ovulation (%)
[Des-His²]LHRH	—*	—*
[D-Phe²,D-Ala⁶]LHRH	6 × 0.5	95[a]
[D-Phe²,D-Trp³,D-Phe⁶]LHRH	1	90[b]
[N-Ac-D-Phe¹,D-pCl-Phe²,D-Trp³,⁶]LHRH	0.06	100[b]
[N-Ac-D-pCl-Phe¹,²,D-Trp³,⁶]LHRH	0.015	70[b]
[N-Ac-D-pCl-Phe¹,²,D-Trp³,D-Phe⁶,D-Ala¹⁰]LHRH	0.010	100[b]
[N-Ac-D-pCl-Phe¹,²,D-Trp³,D-Arg⁶,D-Ala¹⁰]LHRH	0.003	78[b]
[N-Ac-Δ³-Pro¹,D-pF-Phe²,D-Nal(2)³,⁶]LHRH	0.0025	100[c]
[N-Ac-D-Nal(2)¹,D-pCl-Phe²,D-Trp³,D-hArg(Et₂)⁶,D-Ala¹⁰]LHRH	0.0005	50[d]

*Compound antagonistic in vitro but of insufficient potency to block ovulation in vivo
[a] Yardley et al., (1975)
[b] Schally (1983)
[c] Rivier et al. (1981b)
[d] Nestor et al. (1983)

more recently, for therapy of a variety of gonadal hormone-dependent syndromes and neoplasms.

The paradoxical suppressive effects of agonist analogues, of LHRH were first noted in animals in 1975 and, since that time, have been increasingly pursued in animals and man. In the meantime, synthetic structure–activity studies of the LHRH molecule have been rewarded with antagonistic structures (Table 20.2). Beginning with the discovery that deletion or substitution of postition 2 (His), followed by substitution of positions 3, 6, 1 and 10, four and five-substituted analogues are now available which are several orders of magnitude more potent than the first reported antagonists, and have binding affinities equal to those of the most potent agonists. The antagonists now have sufficient potency to make it feasible to evaluate their properties *in vivo*.

LABORATORY ANIMAL STUDIES

Rats

As little as $0.5\,\mu$g per day of LHRH is able to delay puberty and affect testicular steroidogenisis in male rats (Oshima *et al.*, 1975). Demonstration of inhibition of spermatogenesis and steroidogenesis in mature rats by daily dosing with LHRH agonist analogues followed (Bex and Corbin, 1978; Labrie *et al.*, 1978). Daily administration is not necessary to produce the effect: administration on alternate days, twice weekly or even as infrequently as once every four days, without increased dosage requirements, is still suppressive (Rivier and Vale, 1979; Rivier *et al.*, 1979). The decreases in testicular steroidogenesis are associated with decreases in accessory organ weight but not to the extent observed in castrate animals. Greater suppression of accessory organ weight results from combination treatment with LHRH agonist and antiandrogens (Labrie *et al.*, 1982; Auclair and Givner, 1982). It is possible selectively to suppress accessory organ weight without effect on spermatogenesis (Tcholakian *et al.*, 1978) and spermatogenesis without effect on accessory organ weight (Vickery *et al.*, 1983a). However, it is not possible in the rat totally to abolish spermatogenesis with agonist analogues of LHRH, as revealed by long-term fertility trials (Vickery *et al.*, 1983a) and by the fact that testosterone supplementation, far from reversing the effects, synergistically further suppresses spermatogenesis (Heber and Swerdloff, 1981). A testicular calcification is routinely observed following even acute administration of these agents to rats but not any other species (Vickery, 1981; L. Penumarthy, personal communication, 1981). The calcification may be a reflection of testosterone withdrawal, however, as it appears to be prevented by testosterone supplementation (L. Shott, personal communication, 1981). Some doubt is cast upon this explanation by the fact that testicular calcifications do not result from administration of LHRH antagonists.

Injection of an adequate dose of an LHRH antagonist (which is still greater than normal for agonists, even with the most potent antagonists available) causes abrupt falls in LH and testosterone levels (Rivier *et al.*, 1980) which may persist for up to 72 hours (McRae *et al.*, 1983). Effects on FSH levels are slower to appear and are of lesser magnitude than effects on LH levels. Daily treatment is associated with inhibition of spermatogenesis (Vickery *et al.*, 1983d) and of fertility (Rivier *et al.*, 1981a). Testosterone supplementation has restored both mating activity and fertility (Rivier *et al.*, 1981). Accessory organ weights in animals treated with antagonists are equivalent to those in castrated animals and much more severely suppressed than can be achieved with agonist analogues (McRae *et al.*, 1983).

Monkeys

Male macaques appear, from early studies, to be particularly insensitive to the down-regulatory effects of LHRH agonists (Arimura *et al.*, 1973; Levitan *et al.*, 1977), although increased levels of gonadotropins and steroids result from *in vivo* administration. For example, daily long-term dosing of cynomolgus monkeys causes repetitive daily testosterone rises (Fig. 20.2) but no sign of lowering of basal levels of testosterone or interference with spermatogenesis. Similar findings are reported even following twice-daily dosing of rhesus monkeys (Wickings *et al.*, 1981; Akhtar *et al.*, 1982). If dosing continues long enough (4-6 months), a degree of testicular suppression may result in a certain percentage of monkeys of either species (Sundaram *et al.*, 1981; L. Shott, personal communication, 1981); however interpretation of this observation is clouded by the known seasonality of testicular function in macaques (Wickings and Nieschlag, 1980).

Continuous administration by Alzet® minipump of [D-Ser(tBu)⁶,Pro⁹-NHEt]LHRH (Buserelin, Hoe 766) at the comparatively low dose of 2 µg/h to rhesus monkeys will result in marked suppression of both testicular steroidogenesis and spermatogenesis within 3 weeks (Akhtar *et al.*,

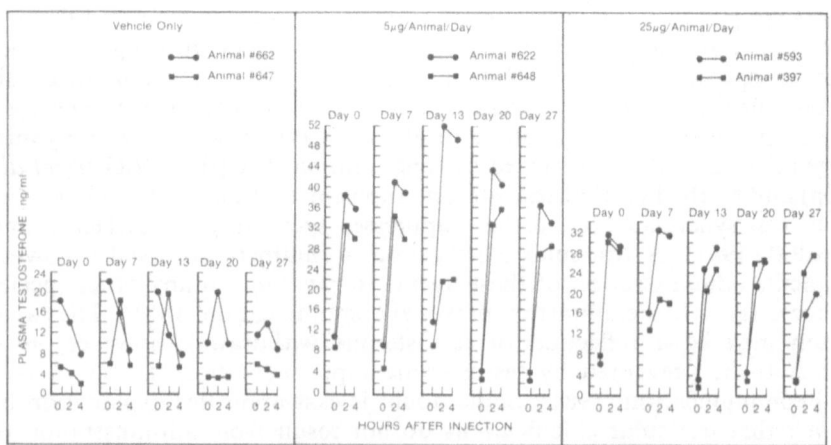

Fig. 20.2 Effect of chronic daily intramuscular injection of vehicle or 5 µg or 25 µg per animal per day of naferelin acetate to male cynomolgus monkeys on circulating levels of testosterone ●, ■ indicate individual animals.

1983). Supplementation in these animals with testosterone restored potentia and resulted in azoospermic ejaculates (by electroejaculation). Subcutaneous implantation of pellets of [D-Trp⁶,Pro⁹-NHEt]LHRH in rhesus monkeys also shows effects of continuous administration (Vickery et al., 1980). The pattern of circulating levels of testosterone during and after treatment in the two studies is remarkably similar (Fig. 20.3). It is not known whether the marked suppression of circulating levels of testosterone noted for baboons treated with [D-Trp⁶,Pro⁹-NHEt]LHRH was a reflection of the continuous mode of administration from pellets (Vickery and McRae, 1980), as no daily injection studies have been reported for male baboons.

Long-term treatment possibilities are opened up by recent studies in male

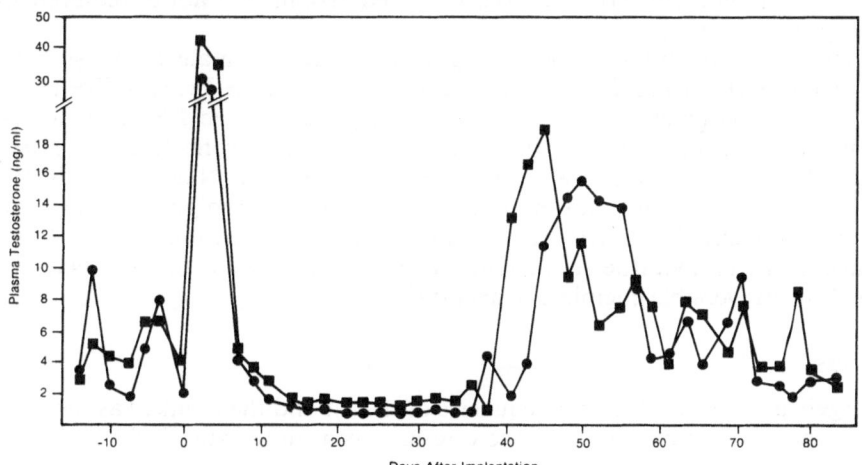

Fig. 20.3 Circulating levels of testosterone in two male rhesus monkeys before and after subcutaneous implantation of cholesterol pellets containing 2.5 mg of [D-Trp⁶,Pro⁹-NHEt]LHRH.

rhesus monkeys using a subcutaneously implanted silastic matrix formulation of nafarelin acetate (E. Nieschlag and B. Vickery, unpublished work). The formulation, which has a duration of release in excess of one year, suppressed testosterone levels, ejaculation and testicular volumes by six weeks after implantation.

The suppressive effects on testicular function in rhesus monkeys, which result from continuous administration of LHRH agonist, are associated with a fall in circulating levels of LH, which are then maintained at or below the limits of detection of the assay (Akhtar et al., 1983). This does not happen in animals receiving once- or twice-daily treatment. Similar discrepancies are noted in female macaques receiving continuous versus daily administration of these analogues (Vickery et al., 1983e). These qualitative differences in response if verified in man have important implications for male contraception and, particularly, for therapy of androgen-dependent neoplasms. The recently described 'mega-dose' therapy with leuprolide ([D-Leu⁶,Pro⁹-NHEt]LHRH), by loading up the circulation and compensating for the short intrinsic biological half-life of this analogue may be an alternative although less cost-effective approach (Santen *et al.*, 1983).

The effects of testosterone replacement in macaques, under continuous therapy with buserelin, have been mentioned. If start of testosterone supplementation (from subcutaneously implanted silastic capsules) is delayed until after ejaculation has been abolished, then ejaculation can be restored and be compatible with azoospermia (Akhtar *et al.*, 1983). If, however, testosterone supplementation is begun at the onset of buserelin treatment then azoospermia is not achieved, at least over the length of two spermatogenic cycles (E. Nieschlag, personal communication, 1983). Perhaps the supplemented levels of testosterone are capable of maintaining spermatogenesis in the presence of low levels of gonadotropins but not of reestablishing spermatogenesis.

The effects of antagonistic analogues of LHRH in male monkeys have been less well explored. A dose of 2 mg/kg of [Ac-Δ^3-Pro^1,D-*p*F-Phe^2,D-Trp^{3,6}]LHRH given to castrate male monkeys suppressed LH levels for 24 hours but the same dose had no effect upon testosterone levels in intact animals (Spiliotis *et al.*, 1983). [*N*-Ac-Pro^1,D-*p*F-Phe^2,D-Nal(2)^{3,6}]LHRH is capable, after a single injection of 5 mg/kg in cynomolgus monkeys, of suppressing circulating testosterone levels within 1 h, and suppression is still marked at 24 h (McRae *et al.*, 1983). Daily administration should therefore result in a reversible chemical castration.

Dogs

Largely as a result of the inadequacies of the rat and the monkey as sensitive or responsive animal models, the dog has been quite extensively evaluated

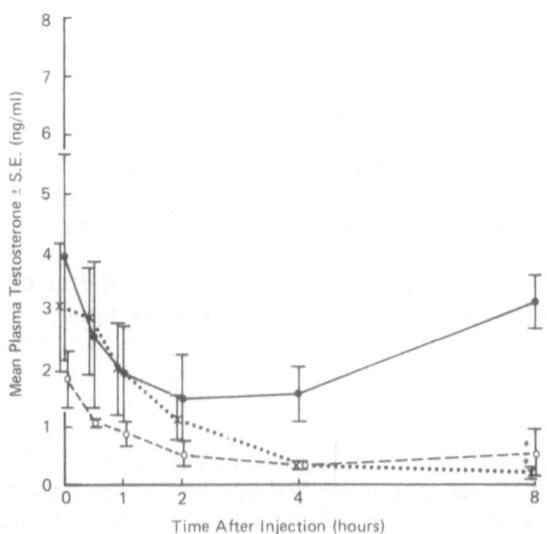

Fig. 20.4 Effect of a single intramuscular injection of 100 µg/kg or 1000 µg/kg of [*N*-Ac-Pro^1,D-*p*F-Phe^2,D-Nal(2)^{3,6}]LHRH on circulating levels of testosterone in male beagle dogs

for suppressive effect of LHRH agonists. Initial studies using pelleted [D-Trp^6,Pro^9-NHEt]LHRH established the ability, after a transitory stimulation, to reduce circulating levels of testosterone to 5% of normal (Vickery *et al.*, 1980). These lowered levels resulted in progressive diminution in size of hyperplastic prostates in geriatric dogs (Vickery *et al.*, 1983b). Reversibility and effects of testosterone supplementation (Vickery *et al.*, 1984a) have been well-characterized for daily administration of nafarelin acetate, ([D-Nal(2)^6]LHRH; RS-94991) and, depending on the final correlation of data from dogs and men, could auger well for the contraceptive and therapeutic utilities.

The degree and duration of effect of single doses of [*N*-Ac-Pro^1,D-*p*F-Phe^2,D-Nal(2)^{3,6}]LHRH in the dog (McRae *et al.*, 1983) suggests that once-daily administration will be adequate to suppress pituitary and testicular function (Fig. 20.4).

CONTRACEPTION IN MEN

LHRH agonists alone

Following upon the observation of paradoxical suppression of gonadotropin responsivity in men (Hashimoto *et al.*, 1975; Davies *et al.*, 1977) and the reports of suppression of sexual function in adult male rats (Bex and Corbin, 1978; Labrie *et al.*, 1978), the first studies evaluated the effect of chronic administration of buserelin in normal men (Bergquist *et al.*, 1979). The effects were disappointing, largely due to the fact that the study preceded the realization that suppressive effects in males generally require higher doses than in females. Thus, this first study used 5 μg per day, the dose of the LHRH agonist which suppressed ovulation in women (Nillius *et al.*, 1978). A later study evaluated 100 μg per day of another agonist, [D-Trp^6,Pro^9-NHEt]LHRH, and documented clear-cut effects on output of testicular steroids (Linde *et al.*, 1981), so clear in fact that treatment was terminated early, in 5 of 9 men, due to occurrence of impotence and hot flushes. Effects on sperm output were obscured by the fact that treatment was stopped when the men became impotent. However all subjects had a fall in sperm density. In the three subjects who completed 10 weeks of treatment, sperm densities of $0-5 \times 10^6$/ml were noted (Doelle *et al.*, 1983).

Intermittent treatment with LHRH agonists

In an effort to avoid the unacceptable side-effects of testosterone withdrawal, a study was performed in men based upon the observation that daily administration of LHRH agonist was not necessary to depress spermatogenesis in rats (Rivier and Vale, 1979). Unfortunately, in men, treatment every fourth day with 50 μg s.c. of [D-Trp^6,Pro^9-NHEt]LHRH had no consistent effect on sperm output, libido or potency (Doelle *et al.*, 1982). In men, therefore, under this treatment regimen, pituitary responsiveness is maintained and receptor down-regulation does not take place.

Continuous treatment with LHRH agonists

Building upon studies performed in male macaques, Nieschlag and colleagues report consistent induction of oligospermia in men with buserelin administered chronically by subcutaneous infusion (E. Nieschlag, personal communication, 1983). Whereas this study demonstrates feasibility but not practicality, the recent demonstration of efficacy of nafarelin acetate administered from a subcutaneous silastic matrix implant to rhesus monkeys (E. Nieschlag and B. Vickery, unpublished) suggests a practical approach is possible.

Testosterone replacement

Testosterone supplementation has been routinely included in longer-term studies of administration of LHRH analogues to men. For this purpose testosterone enanthate injection every two weeks has been the method of choice. It may be recalled that testosterone enanthate as a single agent is capable of producing severe oligospermia in man (Steinberger and Smith, 1977). In addition, testosterone and LHRH agonist combination treatment in rats synergistically suppressed spermatogenesis (Heber and Swerdloff, 1981).

Two long-term studies have been conducted in men. In the first, $50\,\mu g$ per day of [D-Trp⁶,Pro⁹-NHEt]LHRH was administered for 10 weeks together with 100 mg testosterone enanthate every 2 weeks. Libido and potency were maintained under this regimen. Although mean sperm density was significantly lower after 10 weeks of treatment than in pretreatment, the actual values ($25 \pm 3 \times 10^6$/ml) were disappointingly high. The testosterone enanthate treatment alone, as assessed in other men, had no effect on sperm density (Doelle et al., 1983).

The more potent agonist, nafarelin acetate, has been administered daily at a higher dose ($200\,\mu g$/day) for a longer period of time (116 days) in combination with 200 mg testosterone enanthate every 2 weeks (R. Swerdloff, personal communication, 1983). Again, consistent oligozoospermia was not induced. Of course, biopsy material from these normal volunteers is not available. Biopsy material from prostatic cancer patients who had received high dose therapy with leuprolide reveals total shutdown of spermatogenesis (Rajfer et al., 1983). This, together with the apparently greater effect of LHRH agonist alone in normal volunteers, suggests a protective action of testosterone. Such a protective action has been noted in male macaques even under sustained treatment (E. Nieschlag, personal communication, 1983). It may be worthwhile to evaluate the effect of sustained administration of LHRH agonists in men, while delaying onset of testosterone supplementation for the first few weeks of treatment, before abandoning hope for utility of LHRH agonists for contraception in men.

MECHANISMS OF ACTION

Hypophysial effects

LHRH and its analogues bind with high affinity to specific LHRH receptors on the gonadotropes in the anterior pituitary to stimulate release and synthesis of LH and FSH. Continued presence of LHRH or long-lived agonist analogues can cause a down regulation of the receptors leading to a cessation of release of the gonadotropins. These findings have been graphically illustrated in the studies by Knobil and colleagues on the circhoral requirement of LHRH for normal reproductive function (Pohl *et al.*, 1983).

Down regulation of LHRH receptors has not been reported to occur following administration of LHRH antagonists. Indeed, the dosage requirements are in keeping with a mechanism of competitive inhibition of endogenous LHRH binding.

Qualitative differences in response to low versus high or continuous levels of both agonist and antagonist are noted. Thus, the disappearance of pituitary response to LHRH challenge can be dissociated from the lowering of circulating levels of gonadotropins by LHRH agonists. Similarly with the LHRH antagonists, it is possible to abolish circhoral pulses of LH release at lower doses than are required to lower basal levels of gonadotropins (Spiliotis *et al.*, 1983).

Gonadal effects

In certain species, notably the rat, a similar phenomenon occurs at the gonad in response to gonadotropins. Thus LH binds to specific high-affinity receptors to trigger gametogenesis and particularly steroidogenesis. High maintained gonadotropin levels can then down regulate homologous gonadal receptors leading to depressed gonadal function (Labrie *et al.*, 1981). In the rat this can be mimicked with exogenous chorionic gonadotropin (Chasalow *et al.*, 1979).

Further, in the rat, specific gonadal LHRH receptors, of equal affinity to those in the pituitary, have been demonstrated (Clayton *et al.*, 1980). LHRH agonists have been shown *in vitro* and *in vivo* in hypophysectomized animals to suppress directly testicular 17α-hydroxylase and 17,20-desmolase activity by action at a site distal to cAMP (Hsueh *et al.*, 1981; Hsueh and Jones, 1981). LHRH antagonists, while apparently not exerting any direct effects of their own, can antagonize the direct gonadal effects of the agonists (Jones and Hsueh, 1984). The demonstration of LHRH-like materials in rat and rhesus monkey testes with biological activity argues for the existence of a paracrine role of LHRH-like materials in the testes (Sharpe *et al.*, 1981). The material may act as messenger between Sertoli and Leydig cells with short-term stimulatory and longer-term inhibitory actions (Sharpe *et al.*, 1982; Fraser *et al.*, 1984).

Comparative aspects

The early consequence of LHRH agonist treatment in men is loss of pituitary responsiveness to LHRH. Daily injection of highly potent LHRH agonists in male rats results in high gonadotropin levels, equivalent to those in castrate animals, and it is only after a period of some weeks that pituitary responsiveness declines.

High levels of gonadotropin in rats can suppress testicular steroidogenesis. There is no evidence that this phenomenon occurs in man: repetitive injection of hCG in men is not associated with lowered gonadal responsivity.

High affinity LHRH receptors have not been found in testicular tissue from cadavers although present in pituitary tissue from the same cadavers. LHRH receptors are present in testicular tissue from rats.

In sum, there is no evidence for other than a hypophyseal site of action for LHRH analogues in man. Results of studies in other species, particularly in the rat, should be regarded with caution, and may not be extrapolable to man. With that caveat, however, the qualitatively greater effect exerted by continuous infusion of LHRH agonists relative to daily administration could involve interaction with low-affinity LHRH receptors which have been found in human testicular tissue (R. Sharpe, personal communication, 1983).

THERAPEUTIC APPLICATIONS

The pronounced suppressive effects on testicular steroidogenesis achieved with LHRH agonists alone is receiving increasing attention for dyscrasias in which the effects of testosterone withdrawal are acceptable or even desirable.

Prostate cancer

Studies such as those in male transexuals (Tolis *et al.*, 1981), in addition to the studies reported above, support the safety and consistently effective suppression of testicular steroidogenesis by long-term LHRH agonist treatment. The LHRH agonists were therefore evaluated for alleviation of prostate cancer, a disease which is in 80% of cases testosterone dependent, but for which established hormonal manipulation, i.e. orchiectomy or oestrogen treatment, is either poorly accepted or poorly tolerated.

Studies with leuprolide megadose therapy by injection have been reported and are ongoing (Santen *et al.*, 1983). In Stage D carcinoma, early amelioration of bone pain and stabilization or remission of metastases can be achieved, at least over the short term. The very high doses (1–10 mg/day) and the need for daily injection with leuprolide are however inconvenient.

Studies with the more potent analogue, buserelin, have utilized nasal administration of 200–500 µg twice daily (Faure *et al.*, 1983). Testosterone levels decreased progressively after a lag of 2–5 weeks. The time course and maximal degree of suppression however was highly variable between subjects. The effect of 50 µg s.c. daily was therefore assessed. Castration levels of testosterone were rapidly reached. A hybrid regimen with buserelin is under consideration, in which the material is administered over the first 3–7 days by injection and followed thereafter by 1–3 times daily intranasal administration (Wenderoth et al., 1982).

Interest in this area is intensifying and new clinical trials are being conducted with other LHRH agonists such as [D-Ser(tBu⁶)Azagly¹⁰]LHRH (ICI 118,630, Allen et al., 1983) and nafarelin acetate (M. Henzl, personal communication, 1983).

Benign prostatic hypertrophy

Whereas the studies in prostatic carcinoma are concentrating on stage D patients and remission of metastases, it would also be logical to use LHRH analogues for their primary effect of regression of the prostate *in situ*, for example for treatment of benign prostatic hypertrophy (BPH). Striking responses were obtained in the geriatric dog, the only other species in which massive hyperplasia develops spontaneously (Vickery et al., 1982). The side-effects of testosterone withdrawal, impotence and hot flushes, may be deemed unacceptable for BPH therapy. However, the alternative of transurethral prostatectomy is not without its sequelae of impotence and retrograde ejaculation. Clinical trials are required to assess acceptability of side-effects and might even pursue the possibility that low level testosterone supplementation of LHRH analogue therapy can restore libido without affecting prostate size (Vickery et al., 1983c).

Precocious puberty

LHRH agonists are also being used in the treatment of true, idiopathic or hamartoma-induced precocious puberty. The studies with daily injections of 4 µg/kg of [D-Trp⁶,Pro⁹-NHEt]LHRH document disappearance of pubic hair and regression of testicular volumes after only a few months of treatment (Comite et al., 1983). These successes have now led to investigations of blockade of growth hormone-induced puberty and of therapy in short stature, normal age puberty (F. Comite, personal communication, 1983).

Other possibilities

Should the inhibition of spermatogenesis be achievable in men with either LHRH agonists or antagonists, then they may prove useful to protect against the sterilizing effects of certain cancer chemotherapeutic agents. There is a high remission rate being achieved with chemotherapy in certain lymphomas such as Hodgkin's disease (Sutcliffe et al., 1978). However, the high remission is associated with a high degree of poor to irreversible infertility due to induction of azoospermia (Whitehead et al., 1982). These young patients are presently advised to avail themselves of sperm cryopreservation before treatment but would no doubt prefer the method to preserve reproductive function.

The rationale and early studies were based on studies performed in mice (Glode *et al.*, 1981). As the chemotherapeutic agents used, particularly the alkylating agents, exert their effects on post spermatogonial elements (Jackson, 1970, 1972), regression of the germinal elements to spermatogonia was hoped to eliminate the gonadotoxicity. Although these studies have not been replicated (M. Meistrich, personal communication, 1983) and in fact it is difficult to understand how they could be in mice because of this species' insensitivity to LHRH agonists (Bex *et al.*, 1982), they did spark a great deal of interest. Perhaps the 'protection' noted results from a stimulation of spermatogenesis, such as noted for cobolamine derivatives (Kimura *et al.*, 1983). Modelling studies in the dog (a species in which spermatogenesis can be totally abolished with LHRH analogues) have been reported (Goodpasture *et al.*, 1983; Link *et al.*, 1983) and both nafarelin acetate (Vickery *et al.*, unpublished observations) and buserelin (Nyose and Pontes, personal communication, 1983) are under intensive study for this indication.

CONCLUDING REMARKS

It now seems clear that the LHRH analogues will be an addition to our pharmacopoeia. These agents, with remarkable lack of toxicity, are providing very encouraging results in therapeutic areas and will probably be the drugs of choice for precocious puberty and related syndromes. It is too soon to tell whether the beneficial effects in prostatic carcinoma will affect the life expectancy of the patients but they appear to provide a viable alternative to orchidectomy and/or oestrogen treatment.

Utility for male contraception is less clear. Perhaps if the studies on continuous administration of LHRH agonists are extended to men or if the antagonists are of greater efficacy, then the early promise of these agents may be fulfilled. However, the need for testosterone supplementation as well as adjunctive contraception during the early oligospermia of several weeks to months duration will have to be considered.

Further developments with LHRH analogues will, because of their unavailability by the oral route, involve research into alternative delivery systems and routes. Absorptiion through mucous membranes is being studied and there is promising research into sustained release bioerodable, injectable and implantable systems (Vickery *et al.*, 1984b). These systems will enable the assessment of the relative worth of LHRH analogues in large-scale trials.

References

Ahmed, S.R., Shalet, S.M., Brooman, P.J.C., Howell, A. and Blacklock, N.J. (1983). Treatment of metastatic carcinoma of the prostate with LHRH-analogue, ICI 118630 (abstr.). *2nd Joint Meeting, British Endocrine Society*, University of York

Akhtar, B.F., Marshall, G.R., Wickings, E.J. and Nieschlag, E. (1983). Reversible induction of azoospermia in rhesus monkeys by constant infusion of a GnRH agonist using osmotic minipumps. *J. Clin. Endocrinol. Metab.*, **56**, 534-40

Akhtar, B.F., Wickings, E.J., Zaidi, P. and Nieschlag, E. (1982). Pituitary and testicular functions in sexually mature rhesus monkeys under high dose LRH agonist treatment. *Acta Endocrinol.*, *(Copenh.)*, **101**, 113-8

Allen, J.M., O'Shea, J.P., Ghanadian, R., Mashiter, K., Williams, G and Bloom, S.R. (1983). LHRH analogues in treatment of advanced prostatic cancer: preliminary data. *Clin. Sci.*, **64**, 59p

Arimura, A., Spies, H.G. and Schally, A.V. (1973). Relative insensitivity of rhesus monkeys to the LH releasing hormone (LHRH). *J. Clin. Endocrinol. Metab.*, **36**, 372-4

Auclair, C. and Givner, M.L. (1982). Medrogestrone and an LHRH analogue as potential combination therapy for hormone-dependent cancers. *Arch, Androl.*, **86**, 21-4

Belanger, A., Labrie, F., Lemay, A., Caron, S. and Raynaud, J.P. (1980). Inhibitory effects of a single intranasal administration of [D-Ser-(tBu)^6,des-Gly-NH$_2$^{10}]LHRH agonist, on serum steroid levels in normal men. *J. Steroid Biochem.*, **13**, 123-6

Bergquist, C., Nillius, S.J., Berg, T., Skarin, G. and Wide, L. (1979). Inhibitory effects on gonadotropin secretion and gonadal function in men during chronic treatment with a potent stimulatory luteinizing hormone-releasing hormone analogue. *Acta Endocrinol.*, *(Copenh.)*, **91**, 601-8

Bex, F.J. and Corbin, A. (1978). Inhibition of reproductive processes in the immature and mature male rat with an LHRH agonist (abstr. no. 6). *Third Annual Meeting of the American Society for Andrology* Nashville, TN

Bex, F.J., Corbin, A. and France, E. (1982). Resistance of the mouse to the antifertility effects of LHRH agonists. *Life Sci.*, **30**, 1263-9

Chasalow, F., Marr, H., Haour, F. and Saez, J.M. (1979). Testicular steroidogenesis after human chorionic gonadotropin. Desensitization in rats. *J. Biol. Chem.*, **254**, 5613-7

Clayton, R.N., Katikineni, M. Chan, V., Dufau, M.L. and Catt, K.J. (1980). Direct inhibition of testicular function by gonadotropin-releasing hormones: mediation by specific gonadotropin-releasing hormone receptors in interstitial cells. *Proc. Natl. Acad. Sci. USA*, **77**, 4459-63

Comite, F., Cutler, G.B. Jr. and Loriaux, D.L. (1983). LHRH analog therapy of precocious puberty. In Vickery, B.H., Nestor, J.J. Jr. and Hafez, E.S.E. (eds.) *LHRH and its Analogs: Contraceptive and Therapeutic Applications* pp. 315-28. (Lancaster: MTP)

Davies, T.F., Gomez-Pan, A., Watson, M.J., Mountjoy, C.A., Hanker, J.P., Besser, G.M. and Hall, R. (1977). Reduced 'gonadotropin response to releasing hormone'. after chronic administration to impotent men. *Clin. Endocrinol. (Oxf.)*, **6**, 213-18

Doelle, G.C., Evans, R.M., Alexander, A.N. and Rabin, D. (1983). Antifertility effects of an LHRH agonist in men. In Vickery, B.H., Nestor, J.J. Jr and Hafez, E.S.E. (eds.) *LHRH and its Analogs: Contraceptive and Therapeutic Applications*, pp. 271-82. (Lancaster: MTP)

Doelle, G., Linde, R., Alexander, N., Kirchner, F., Vale, W., Rivier, J. and Rabin, D. (1982). Intermittent long-term administration of a potent gonadotropin-releasing hormone agonist in normal men. *Int. J. Fertil.*, **27**, 234-7

Dutta, A.S., Furr, B.J.A., Giles, M.B., Valcaccia, B. and Walpole, A.L. (1978). Potent agonist and antagonist analogues of luliberin containing an azaglycine residue in position 10. *Biochem. Biophys. Res. Commun.*, **81**, 382-90

Faure, N., Lemay, A., Tolis, G., Labrie, F., Belanger, A. and Fazekas, A.T.A. (1983). Buserelin therapy for prostatic carcinoma. In Vickery, B.H., Nestor, J.J. Jr and Hafez, E.S.E. (eds.) *LHRH and its Analogs: Contraceptive and Therapeutic Applications*, pp. 337-50. (Lancaster: MTP)

Fraser, H.M., Sharpe, R.M. and Popkin, R.M. (1984). Direct gonadal stimulation with LHRH. In Vickery, B.H., Nestor, J.J. Jr. and Hafez, E.S.E. (eds.) *LHRH and its Analogs: Contraceptive and Therapeutic Applications*, pp. 181-96. (Lancaster: MTP)

Glode, L.M., Robinson, J. and Gould, S.F. (1981). Protection from cyclophosphamide-induced testicular damage with an analogue of gonadotropin releasing hormone. *Lancet*, **1**, 1132-4

Goodpasture, J.C., Vickery, B.H., Zaneveld, L.J.D. and Waller, D.P. (1983). Antireproductive effects in dogs of chronic cyclophosphamide administration. *Program*, *ASPET*, Philadelphia

Happ, J., Scholz, P., Weber, T., Cordes, U., Schramm, P., Neubauer, M. and Beyer, J. (1978).

Gonadotropin secretion in eugonadotropic human males and post-menopausal females under long-term application of a potent analogue of gonadotropin-releasing hormone. *Fertil. Steril.*, **30**, 674-8

Hashimoto, T., Miyar, K., Vozumi, T., Mori, S., Watanabe, M. and Kumahara, Y. (1975). Effect of prolonged LH-releasing hormone administration on gonadotropin response in patients with hypothalamic and pituitary tumors. *J. Clin. Endorcinol. Metab.*, **41**, 712-16

Heber, D. and Swerdloff, R.S. (1981). Gonadotropin-releasing hormone analog and testosterone synergistically inhibit spermatogenesis. *Endocrinology*, **108**, 2019-21

Hsueh, A.J.W. and Jones, P.B.C. (1981). Extrapituitary actions of gonadotropin-releasing hormone. *Endocr. Rev.*, **2**, 437-61

Hsueh, A.J.W., Schreiber, J.R. and Erickson, G.F. (1981). Inhibitory effects of gonadotropin releasing hormone upon cultured testicular cells. *Mol. Cell. Endocrinol.*, **21**, 43-9

Jackson, H. (1970). Antispermatogenic agents. *Br. Med. Bull.*, **26**, 79-86

Jackson, H. (1972). Chemical methods of male contraception In Austin, C.R. and Short, R.V. (eds.) *Reproduction in Mammals*, Vol. 5, pp. 67-86, (Cambridge: Cambridge University Press)

Jones, P.B.C. and Hsueh, A.J.W. (1984). Direct antigonadal actions of LHRH. In Vickery, B.H., Nestor, J.J. Jr. and Hafez, E.S.E. (eds.) *LHRH and its Analogs: Contraceptive and Therapeutic Applications*, pp. 163-80. (Lancaster: MTP)

Kimura, M., Ishikawa, H., Mitsukawa, S., Orikasa, S. and Kumamoto, Y. (1983). Effect of mecobolamin on spermatogenesis in rats treated with cancer chemotherapeutic drugs. *J. Androl.*, **4**, 36

Labrie, F., Auclair, C., Cusan, L., Kelly, P.A., Pelletier, G. and Ferland, L. (1978). Inhibitory effects of LHRH and its agonists on testicular gonadotropin receptors and spermatogenesis in the rat. *Int. J. Androl. Suppl. 2*, 303-18

Labrie, F. Dupont, A., Belanger, A., Cusan, L., Lacourciere, Y., Monfette, G., Laberge, J.G., Emond, J.P., Fazekas, A.T.A., Raynaud, J.P. and Husson, J.M. (1982). New hormonal therapy in prostatic carcinoma: combined treatment with an LHRH agonist and an antiandrogen. *Clin. Invest. Med.*, **5**, 267-75

Labrie, F., Godbout, M., Belanger, A., Seguin, C., Pelletier, G., Cusan, L., Kelly, P.A. and Reeves, J.J. (1981). Mechanisms of the antifertility effects of LHRH agonists in the male rat. In Zatuchni, G.I., Shelton, J.D. and Sciarra, J.J. (eds.) *LHRH Peptides as Female and Male Contraceptives.* pp. 246-60. (Philadelphia: Harper & Row)

Levitan, D., Beitins, I.Z., Milton, G., Barnes, A. and McArthur, J.W. (1977). Insensitivity of bonnet monkeys to (D-Ala^6,DesGly^{10})LHRH ethylamide, a potent new luteinizing hormone releasing hormone analogue in rats and mice. *Endocrinology*, **100**, 918-22

Linde, R., Doelle, G.C., Alexander, A.N., Kirchner, F., Vale, W., Rivier, J. and Rabin, D. (1981). Reversible inhibition of testicular steroidogenesis and spermatogenesis by a potent GnRH agonist in normal men. *N. Engl. J. Med.*, **305**, 663-7

Link, D.V., Waller, D.P., Goodpasture, J.C., Zaneveld, L.J.D. and Vickery, B.H. (1983). Effects of combined cyclophosphamide-doxorubicin on male reproductive function in dogs. *Program, ASPET*, Philadelphia

McRae, G.I., Vickery, B.H., Nestor, J.J. Jr., Bremner, W.J. and Badger, T.M. (1983). Biological activity of a highly potent LHRH antagonist. In Vickery, B.H., Nestor, J.J., Jr. and Hafez, E.S.E. (eds.) *LHRH and its Analogs: Contraceptive and Therapeutic Applications*, pp. 137-52. (Lancaster: MTP)

Nestor, J.J., Jr., Ho, T.L., Simpson, R.A., Horner, B.L., Jones, G.H., McRae, G.I. and Vickery, B.H. (1982). Synthesis and biological activity of some very hydrophobic superagonist analogues of luteinizing hormone-releasing hormone. *J. Med. Chem.*, **25**, 795-801

Nestor, J.J., Jr., Tahilramani, R., Ho, T.L., McRae, G.I. and Vickery, B.H. (1983). New luteinizing hormone-releasing factor antagonists. In Hruby, V.J. and Rick, D.H. (eds.) *Peptides: Structure, Function. Proceedings 8th Peptide Symposium*, pp. 861-4. Pierce Chem. Co., Rockford, Illinois

Nillius, S.J., Bergquist, C. and Wide, L. (1978). Inhibition of ovulation in women by chronic treatment with a stimulatory LRH analogue: a new approach to birth control? *Contraception*, **17**, 537-45

Oshima, H., Nankin, H.R., Fan, D.F., Troen, P., Yanaihara, T., Niizato, N., Yoshida, K.I.,

Ochiai, K.-I. (1975). Delay in sexual maturation of rats caused by synthetic LH-releasing hormone: enhancement of steroid $\Delta^{4-5}\alpha$-hydrogenase in testes. *Biol. Reprod.*, **12**, 491-7

Pohl, C.R., Richardson, D.W., Hutchinson, J.S., Germak, J.A. and Knobil, E. (1983). Hypophysiotropic signal frequency and the functioning of the pituitary-ovarian system in the rhesus monkey. *Endocrinology*, **112**, 2076-80

Rajfer, J., Swerdroff, R.S. and Heber, D. (1983). Human testicular morphologic characteristics after chronic GnRH analog therapy. *Fertil. Steril.*, **39**, 440

Rivier, C. and Vale, W. (1979). Hormonal secretion in male rats chronically treated with D-Trp⁶,Pro⁹NEt-LRF. *Life Sci.*, **25**, 1065-74

Rivier, C., Rivier, J. and Vale, W.(1979). Chronic effects of [D-Trp⁶,Pro⁹-NHEt] luteinizing hormone-releasing factor on reproductive processes in the male rat. *Endocrinology*, **105**, 1191-201

Rivier, C., Rivier, J. and Vale, W. (1980). Antireproductive effects of a potent gonadotropin-releasing hormone antagonist in the male rat. *Science*, **210**, 93-4

Rivier, C., Rivier, J. and Vale, W. (1981a). Effect of a potent GnRH antagonist and testosterone propionate on mating behavior and fertility in the male rat. *Endocrinology*, **108**, 1988-2001

Rivier, J., Ling, N., Monahan, M., Rivier, C., Brown, M. and Vale, W. (1975). Luteinizing hormone releasing factor and somatostatin analogs. In Walter, R. and Meienhofer (eds.) *Peptides: Chemistry, Structure and Biology-Proceedings of the Fourth American Peptide Symposium*, pp. 863-70. (Ann Arbor: Ann Arbor Science Publishers)

Rivier, J., Rivier, C., Perrin, M., Porter, J. and Vale, W. (1981b). GnRH analogs: structure-activity relationships. In Zatuchni, G.I., Shelton, J.D. and Sciarra, J.J. (eds.) *LHRH Peptides as Female and Male Contraceptives*. pp. 13-23. (Philadelphia: Harper & Row)

Santen, R.J., Smith, J.A., Dufau, M., Warner, B. (1983). Leuprolide therapy for prostatic carcinoma. In Vickery, B.H., Nestor, J.J. Jr. and Hafez, E.S.E. (eds.) *LHRH and its Analogs: Contraceptive and Therapeutic Applications*. 351-64. (Lancaster: MTP Press)

Schally, A.V. (1983). Current status of antagonistic analogs of LHRH as a contraceptive method in the female. In Zatuchni, G.I. (ed.) *Research Frontiers in Fertility Regulation*, PARFR, Vol. 2

Sharpe, R.M., Fraser, H.M., Cooper, I. and Rommerts, F.F.G. (1981). Sertoli-Leydig cell communication via an LHRH-like factor. *Nature*, **290**, 785-7

Sharpe, R.M., Fraser, H.M., Cooper, I. and Rommerts, F.F.G. (1982). The secretion, measurement and function of a testicular LHRH-like factor. In Bardin, C.W. and Sherins, R.J. (eds.) *Cell Biology of the Testis. Ann. N.Y. Acad. Sci.*, **383**, 272-94

Smith, R., Donald, R.A., Espiner, E.A., Stromach, S.G., Edwards, R.A. (1979). Normal adults and subjects with hypogonadotropic hypogonadism respond differently to [D-Ser(tBu)⁶,des-Gly-NH₂¹⁰]LHRH-EA. *J. Clin. Endocrinol. Metab.*, **48**, 167-70

Spiliotis, B.E., Lee, B.C., Brown, T.J., Pineda, J.L., Vale, W., Rivier, J., Nixon, W., Reid, R. and Bercu, B.B. (1983). Effect of a potent GnRH antagonist on pulsatile secretion in the male subhuman primate (macaque). *J. Androl.*, **4**, 46

Steinberger, E. and Smith, R.D. (1977). Effect of chronic administration of testosterone enanthate on sperm production and plasma testosterone, follicle stimulating hormone, and luteinizing hormone levels: A preliminary evaluation of a possible male contraceptive. *Fertil. Steril.*, **28**, 1320-8

Sundaram, K., Wang, N.-G., Bardin, C.W. (1981). Antigonadal, antisteroidal and antifertility effects of LHRH agonist in male animals. In Zatuchni, G.I., Shelton, J.D. and Sciarra, J.J. (eds.) *LHRH Peptides as Female and Male Contraceptives*, pp. 261-74. (Philadelphia: Harper & Row)

Sutcliffe, S.B., Wrigley, P.F.M. and Peto, J. (1978). MVPP chemotherapy regimen for advanced Hodgkin's disease. *Br. Med. J.*, **1**, 679-83

Tcholakian, R.K., De la Cruz, A., Chowdhury, M., Steinberger, A., Coy, D.H. and Schally, A.V. (1978). Unusual anti-reproductive properties of the analog [D-leu desgly-NH₂¹⁰] luteinizing hormone-releasing hormone ethylamide in male rats. *Fertil. Steril.*, **30**, 600-3

Tolis, G., Mehta, A., Comaru-Schally, A.M., Schally, A.V. (1981). Suppression of androgen production by D-tryptophan-6-luteinizing hormone-releasing hormone in man. *J. Clin. Invest.*, **68**, 819

Vickery, B.H. (1981). Physiology and antifertility effects of LHRH and agonistic analogs in male animals. In Zatuchni, G.I., Shelton, J.D. and Sciarra, J.J. (eds.) *LHRH Peptides as Female and Male Contraceptives*, pp. 275-90. (Philadelphia: Harper & Row)

Vickery, B.H. and McRae, G.I. (1980). Effects of continuous treatment of male baboons with superagonists of LHRH. *Int. J. Fertil.*, **25**, 179-84

Vickery, B.H., McRae, G.I. and Briones, W. (1980). Responses of the males of different laboratory species to continuous administration of an LHRH agonist. *J. Androl.*, **1**, 62

Vickery, B.H., McRae, G.I. and Bonasch, H. (1982). Effect of chronic administration of a highly potent LHRH agonist on prostate size and secretory function in geriatric dogs. *The Prostate*, **3**, 123-30

Vickery, B.H., McRae, G.I., Bergstrom, K., Briones, W., Worden, A. and Seidenberg, R. (1983a). Inability of twice weekly administration of an agonist analog of LHRH to abolish fertility in male rats. *J. Androl.*, (in press)

Vickery, B.H., McRae, G.I., Schanbacher, B.D. and Falvo, R.E. (1983b). Dose-response studies on male reproductive parameters in dogs with a highly potent LHRH agonist. *J. Androl.*, **4**, 56

Vickery, B.H., McRae, G.I., Nestor, J.J. Jr. and Bremner, W. (1983c). Effects of a highly potent LHRH antagonist in rats, dogs and cynomolgus monkeys. *J. Androl.*, **4**, 35

Vickery, B., McRae, G. and Tallentire, D. (1983e). Disparate effects of daily versus continuous administration of a potent LHRH agonist on plasma LH levels in female rhesus monkeys. *Fertil. Steril.*, **39**, 417

Vickery, B.H., McRae, G.I., Briones, W., Worden, A., Seidenberg, R., Schanbacher, B.D. and Falvo, R.E. (1984a). Effect of an LHRH agonist analog upon sexual function in male dogs: suppression, reversibility and effect of testosterone replacement. *J. Androl.*, **5**, 28-42

Vickery, B.H., McRae, G.I., Nestor, J.J. Jr., Sanders, L.M. and Kent, J. (1984b). *In vivo* assessment of long acting formulations of LHRH analogs. In Zatuchni, G.I., Shelton, J.D. and Sciarra, J.J. (eds.) *Long acting Contraceptive Delivery Systems*, pp. 180-9. (Philadelphia: Harper & Row)

Wenderoth, U.K., Happ. J., Krause, U., Adenauer, H. and Jacobi, G.H. (1982). Endocrine studies with a gonadotropin-releasing hormone analogue to achieve withdrawal of testosterone in prostate cancer patients. *Eur. J. Urol.*, **8**, 343-7

Whitehead, E., Shalet, S.M., Blackledge, G., Todd, I., Crowther, D. and Beardwell, C.G. (1982). The effects of Hodgkin's disease and combination chemotherapy on gonad function in the adult male. *Cancer*, **49**, 418-22

Wickings, E.J. and Nieschlag, E. (1980). Seasonability in endocrine and exocrine testicular function of the adult rhesus monkey (*Macaca mulatta*) maintained in a controlled laboratory environment. *Int. J. Androl.*, **3**, 87-104

Wickings, E.J., Zaidi, P. and Nieschlag, E. (1981). Effect of chronic high-dose LHRH-agonist treatment on pituitary and testicular functions in rhesus monkeys. *J. Androl.*, **2**, 72-9

Yardley, J.P., Foell, T.J., Beattie, C.W. and Grant, N.H. (1975). Antagonism of luteinizing hormone release and of ovulation by an analog of the luteinizing hormone releasing hormone. *J. Med. Chem.*, **18**, 1244-7

21
Direct regulation of Leydig cell functions by neuropeptides

E.Y. ADASHI and A.J.W. HSUEH

REGULATION OF LEYDIG CELL FUNCTIONS BY GnRH

Since pituitary gonadotropins are essential for normal gonadal functions and since hypothalamic GnRH was believed to act solely on the pituitary gland, treatment with high doses of GnRH or its agonists had been predicted to be a potential means for enhancing fertility. However, early studies using GnRH as an ovulation-inducing agent in anovulatory women have been only partially successful. Similarly, the early use of GnRH and GnRH agonists in the therapy of hypogonadotropic hypogonadism in men resulted in only limited success, and actual decreases in testicular steroidogenesis were reported.

The paradoxical inhibitory actions of GnRH and agonists have been well-documented in animal models (Hsueh and Jones, 1981). In female rats, the long-term administration of pharmacological doses of GnRH or potent GnRH agonists inhibits ovarian steroidogenesis, ovulation, ovum transport, ovum implantation, pregnancy, uterine growth, and ovarian-dependent mammary tumourigenesis. Similarly, in male rats, long-term administration of high doses of GnRH or GnRH agonists has been shown to inhibit

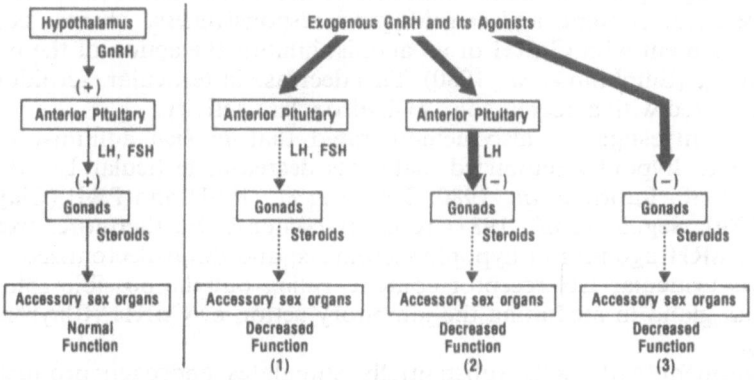

Fig. 21.1 Mechanisms of action

319

testicular steroidogenesis, spermatogenesis, and growth of male accessory sex organs and some prostate tumours.

At least three possible mechanisms can be proposed to explain the paradoxical, inhibitory actions of GnRH and its agonists (Fig. 21.1): (1) chronic stimulation of the anterior pituitary by high doses of GnRH or its agonists may desensitize the gonadotrophs to hypothalamic GnRH, resulting in decreased circulating gonadotropins and subsequent atrophy of reproductive organs; (2) treatment with pharmacological doses of GnRH or its agonists may stimulate the release of high levels of LH which, in turn, results in LH-induced desensitization of gonadal cells to subsequent LH action; and (3) GnRH and its agonists may exert an extrapituitary, direct inhibitory action upon gonadal cells.

We have used an ovarian primary cell culture to provide conclusive evidence of the direct inhibitory effect of GnRH and its agonists on ovarian granulosa cell functions *in vitro*. Ovarian granulosa cells, obtained from preantral follicles of immature hypophysectomized rats, respond *in vitro* to follicle-stimulating hormone (FSH) with the production of oestrogens and progestins. Concomitant treatment with GnRH or a GnRH agonist results in the inhibition of FSH-stimulated oestrogen and progestin production (Hsueh and Erickson, 1979a; Hsueh and Ling, 1979). These results demonstrate the extrapituitary, direct inhibitory effect of GnRH on ovarian functions and provide the basis for further studies in male animals.

DIRECT INHIBITORY EFFECTS OF GnRH ON TESTICULAR FUNCTIONS

An extrapituitary inhibitory effect of GnRH on testicular functions has been observed in male hypophysectomized rats. Treatment with high doses of GnRH or a GnRH agonist for 5 days in immature, hypophysectomized male rats decreases the FSH maintenance of testis weight, LH receptor content (Fig. 21.2) and Leydig cell androgen biosynthesis (Hsueh and Erickson, 1979b). Moreover, treatment with FSH or PRL and growth hormone in hypophysectomized immature or adult rats maintains testis weight, LH receptor content, and steroidogenic responsiveness, whereas concomitant treatment with GnRH or an agonist inhibits the action of the pituitary hormones (Bambino *et al.*, 1980). This decrease in testicular steroidogenesis is associated with a decrease in 17α-hydroxylase activity.

Other investigators also demonstrated that *in vivo* administration of GnRH to hypophysectomized male rats decreases testicular LH (Clayton *et al.*, 1980; Labrie *et al.*, 1980; Seguin *et al.*, 1981) and PRL (Clayton *et al.*, 1980; Seguin *et al.*, 1981) receptor contents. Furthermore, treatment with GnRH agonists in hypophysectomized and adrenalectomized rats decreases testicular LH receptor content, ruling out the possible role of the adrenal gland in mediating the inhibitory action of GnRH (Clayton *et al.*, 1980).

Treatment with hCG substantially stimulates androgen production in cultured testicular cells obtained from hypophysectomized, immature or

DIRECT REGULATION OF LEYDIG CELL FUNCTIONS

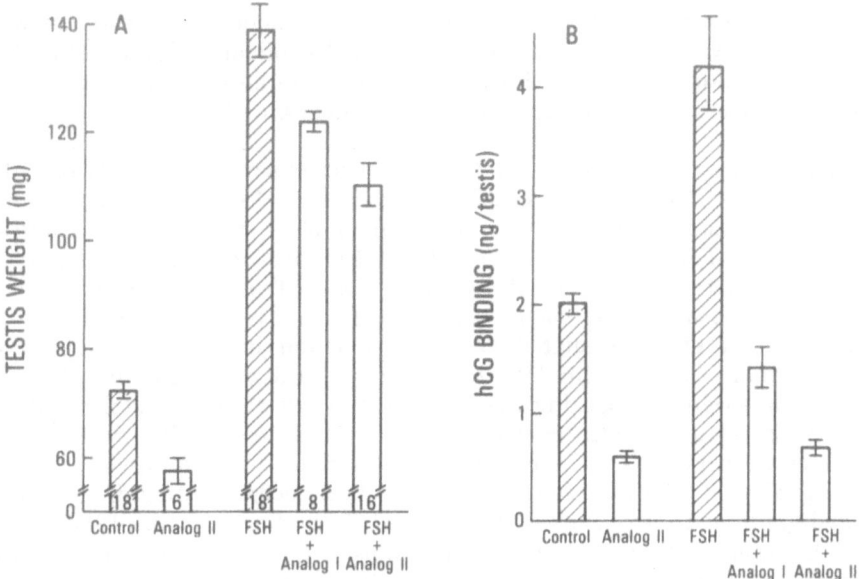

Fig. 21.2   Effects on testis weight and hCG binding

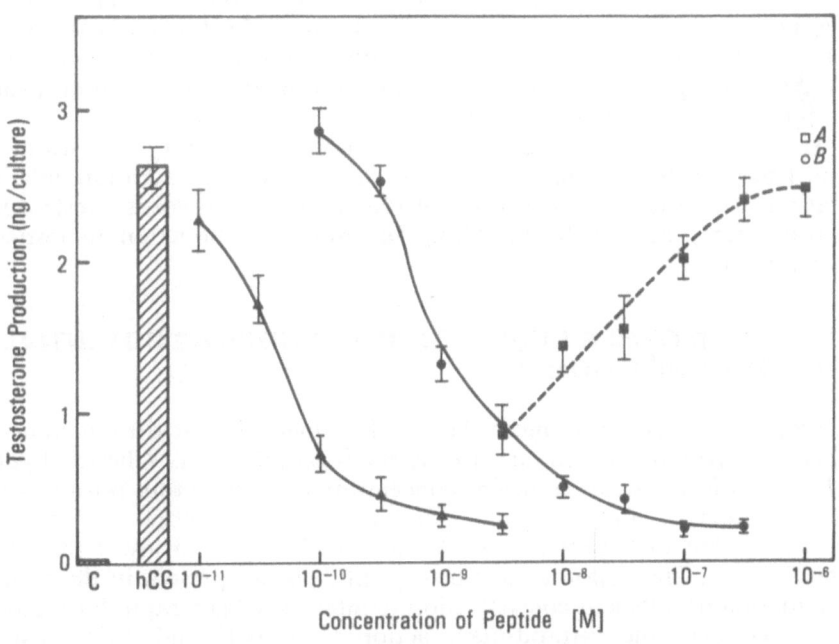

Fig. 21.3   Testosterone production and concentration of peptides

adult rats (Hsueh *et al.*, 1981; Hsueh, 1982). Concomitant treatment with GnRH or a GnRH agonist results in a dose-dependent inhibition of androgen production (Fig. 21.3). Furthermore, the inhibitory effect of GnRH is blocked by concomitant treatment with a potent GnRH antagonist (Hsueh, 1982).

The mechanism of action of GnRH on testicular Leydig cells has also been studied. Primary cultures of adult testicular cells were used to examine the mechanism of the GnRH inhibition of hCG-stimulated testosterone production. The inhibitory effect of GnRH on testicular androgen production appears to be the result of decreases in the activities of 17α-hydroxylase and 17,20-desmolase (Hsueh *et al.*, 1983). This is not accompanied by decreases in hCG-stimulated cAMP production in GnRH-treated cells. Furthermore, GnRH inhibits testosterone production stimulated by a cAMP analogue, suggesting that GnRH may act at steps distal to cAMP synthesis (Hsueh, 1982, Hsueh *et al.*, 1983). These inhibitory effects of GnRH are believed to be mediated by the specific, high affinity ($Kd \sim 10^{-10}$ mol/l) GnRH binding sites which have been demonstrated in testicular Leydig, but not Sertoli, cells (Clayton *et al.*, 1980; Bourne *et al.*, 1980).

The adult testis culture system contains both Leydig and Sertoli cells, which are known to contain LH and FSH receptors, respectively. Since GnRH or its agonists inhibit testosterone production maintained by hCG (Hsueh, 1982), the most likely site of action of GnRH in these cultures is at the Leydig cell (Hunter, *et al.*, 1982). Primary cultures of purified Sertoli cells have also been used to study GnRH action. Treatment with high doses of GnRH or an agonist does not interfere with aromatase activity or the synthesis of plasminogen activator stimulated by FSH, cholera toxin, or a cAMP analogue (Gore-Langton *et al.*, 1981). In contrast, treatment with a GnRH agonist inhibits the FSH stimulation of androgen binding protein secretion (Rich and Bardin, 1981).

In summary, GnRH and its agonists stimulate pituitary releases of LH and FSH which, in turn, enhance gonadal functions. In addition, administration of pharmacological doses of GnRH and its agonists exerts direct, extrapituitary actions by inhibiting testosterone production in testicular Leydig cells.

GnRH AND OTHER REGULATORY PEPTIDES AS POTENTIAL GONADAL HORMONES

GnRH is different from most classical hormones in that the circulation of this neuropeptide is restricted to the brain portal vessel. Whereas hypothalamic GnRH reaches sufficient concentrations in the brain portal circulation to interact effectively with pituitary GnRH receptors, the peripheral concentration of hypothalamic GnRH is believed to be lower than 10^{-11} mol/l. Thus, The hypothalamic neuropeptide is not present in the systemic circulation in sufficient concentration to interact with extrapituitary binding sites. Whereas the extrapituitary actions of GnRH and its agonists on gonadal functions may represent an evolutionary vestigial phenomenon, recent evidence indicates that GnRH-like peptides are secreted by extrahypothalamic tissues.

The presence of GnRH-like peptides has been demonstrated in testicular, placental, mammary, and pancreatic tissues (Hsueh and Jones, 1981). GnRH-like peptides have also been found in rat testicular tissue (Sharpe and Fraser, 1980; Dutlow and Millar, 1981; Paull et al., 1981) and placental tissues from women (Gibbons et al., 1975; Khodr and Siler-Khodr, 1980; Lee et al., 1981), rats (Gautron et al., 1981) and rabbits (Nowak and Wiseman, 1982). Thus, GnRH or GnRH-like peptides may play an important paracrine role in the regulation of various extrapituitary organs.

The direct inhibitory actions of GnRH and its agonists on gonadal functions may explain, at least partially, the paradoxical inhibitory effect of these peptides on various male and female reproductive functions. Subsequent demonstration of GnRH receptors and GnRH-like peptides in the gonads further raises questions regarding a paracrine control role of this and other regulatory peptides in the gonads. Future studies on the intragonadal role of various regulatory peptides on gonadal development should afford important information regarding the maturation of ovarian follicles and testicular seminiferous tubules.

REGULATION OF LEYDIG CELL FUNCTIONS BY NEUROHYPOPHYSEAL HORMONES

The neurohypophyseal hormones of the vertebrates are best known for their antidiuretic, oxytocic and pressor properties (Sawyer, 1961; Acher et al., 1969). However, arginine vasotocin (AVT), found throughout vertebrate phylogeny (Sawyer, 1961), has also been shown to exert profound pharmacological inhibitory effects on male reproductive functions in vivo (Vaughan et al., 1974a,b; Yamashita et al., 1979, 1980), Specifically, treatment with pharmacological doses of AVT has been shown to retard the growth of testes and accessory sex organs of intact prepubertal male rodents (Vaughan et al., 1974a,b) and to inhibit the testicular steroidogenic response to gonadotropic stimulation in intact adult (Yamashita et al., 1979) and immature (Yamashita et al., 1980) male dogs. Although AVT may exert its inhibitory effect in vivo by reducing the release of pituitary gonadotropins (Vaughan et al., 1979; Pavel et al., 1979), the possibility of a direct antigonadal effect could not be ruled out.

Addressing this latter possibility, Adashi and Hsueh have recently shown that AVT can act independently of the hypothalamic–pituitary unit to exert a direct inhibitory effect on the hCG-stimulated accumulation of testosterone by cultured rat testicular cells in vitro (Fig. 21.4) (Adashi and Hsueh, 1981a). Eight other naturally occurring neurohypophyseal hormones have been shown to have a similar effect (Adashi and Hsueh, 1981a). Ranked in order of relative 'antigonadal' (i.e. the ability to inhibit the hCG-stimulated accumulation of testosterone) potency, arginine vasopressin (AVP), AVT and lysine vasopressin (LVP) proved most potent with a projected minimal effective concentration of about 10^{-10}mol/l. These peptides were about

100-fold more potent than oxytocin, mesotocin and valitocin, whereas iso-tocin, glumitocin and aspartocin were virtually without effect (Adashi and Hsueh, 1981a).

The possibility that the 'antigonadal' activity of the neurohypophyseal hormones is mediated by testicular receptors for gonadotropin releasing hormone (GnRH) has also been investigated (Hsueh and Jones, 1981). However, a synthetic antagonistic analogue of GnRH capable of antagon-izing the 'antigonadal' activity of GnRH, was without effect on the AVT-induced inhibition of androgen biosynthesis (Adashi and Hsueh, 1981a).

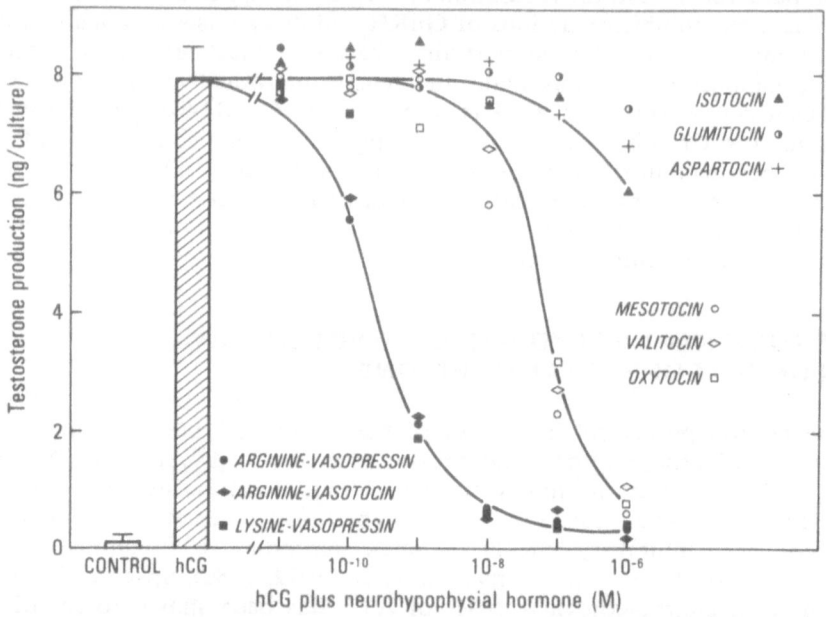

Fig. 21.4 Potency of various peptides

Moreover, a synthetic, pressor-selective antagonistic analogue of the neu-rohypophyseal hormones [d(CH$_2$)$_5$Tyr(Me)-AVP] (Kruszynski *et al.*, 1980) capable of antagonizing the 'antigonadal' activity of AVP (Adashi and Hsueh, 1981b), was without effect on the GnRH-induced inhibition of an-drogen biosynthesis (unpublished).

To elucidate further the specificity of the putative testicular recognition sites mediating the 'antigonadal' activity of the neurohypophyseal hor-mones, Adashi and Hsueh (1981b) have demonstrated that pressor ([Phe^{2}Orn^8] oxytocin) but not antidiuretic (dVDAVP) or oxytocic ([Thr^{4}Gly^7] oxytocin)-selective agonistic peptide analogues of the neuro-hypophyseal hormones exerted dose–dependent inhibition of the hCG-stimulated accumulation of testosterone by cultured rat testicular cells *in vitro* (Fig. 21.5a).

In addition, pressor [d(CH$_2$)$_5$Tyr (Me)AVP and dPVDAVP] but not oxytocic [d(CH$_2$)$_5$TOT]-selective antagonistic peptide analogues of the

DIRECT REGULATION OF LEYDIG CELL FUNCTIONS

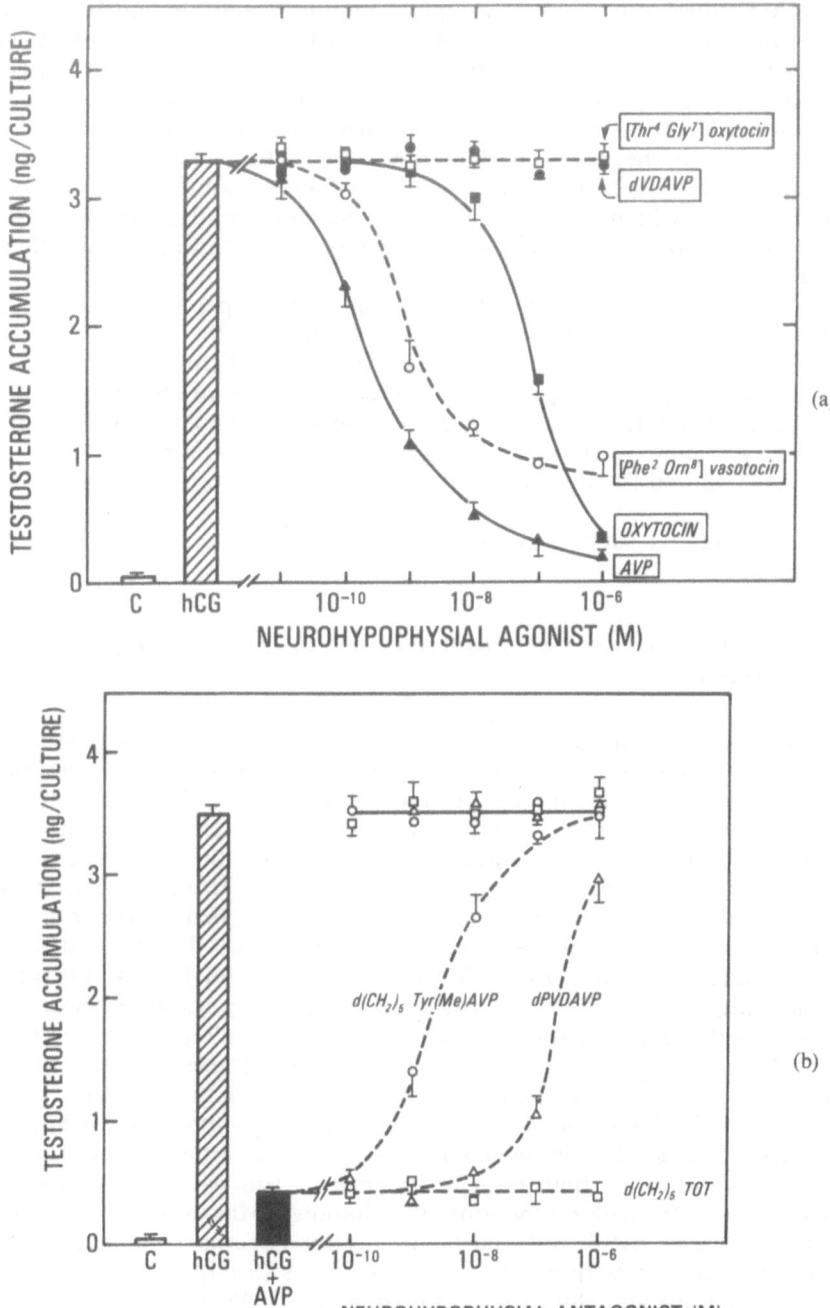

Fig. 21.5 Testosterone Production: (a) neurohypophyseal agonists (b) neurohypophyseal antagonists

neurohypophyseal hormones brought about a dose-dependent blockade of the 'antigonadal' activity of AVP (Fig. 21.5b) (Adashi and Hsueh, 1981b).

Taken together, these and previous findings indicate that the 'antigonadal' activity of the neurohypophyseal hormones is mediated by putative pressor-selective testicular recognition sites which differ in specificity from those mediating the 'antigonadal' activity of GnRH.

Adashi and Hsueh (1982) have also characterized some aspects related to the cellular mechanism(s) and site(s) of the 'antigonadal' action of AVT. Using a primary culture of rat testicular cells, the 'antigonadal' effect of AVT was found to be:

(1) Specific, i.e. not stimulated by 16 other unrelated peptides tested.
(2) Time-dependent with onset of action of approx. 12h.
(3) Partially reversible 5 days after discontinuation of treatment.
(4) Exerted, in part, at a point distal to the generation of cAMP.
(5) Accounted for, in part, by selective suppression of the activity of the steroidogenic enzymes 17α-hydroxylase and 17,20-desmolase.
(6) Unaccounted for by simple interference with the binding of hCG to its receptors.
(7) Unaccounted for by alterations in the total testicular cell number or viability.

NEUROHYPOPHYSEAL PEPTIDES AS POTENTIAL GONADAL HORMONES

These studies of the 'antigonadal' activity of the neurohypophyseal hormones provided an alternative explanation for their recognized pharmacological antireproductive activity *in vivo* (Vaughan *et al.*, 1974a,b; Yamashita *et al.*, 1979, 1980). The finding of specific, pressor-selecting putative testicular recognition sites is intriguing. However, since the reported circulating concentrations of the neurohypophyseal hormones in various adult mammals including man are of the order of 10^{-12}mol/l (Robertson *et al.*, 1973; Chard *et al.*, 1970; Keil and Severs, 1977), and since the minimal effective 'antigonadal' dose *in vitro* is 10^{-10}mol/l (Adashi and Hsueh, 1981a), systemic 'antigonadal' effects of exogenous neurohypophyseal hormones must be regarded as pharmacological. It is unlikely that endogenous, blood-borne neurohypophyseal principles are of physiological relevance to testicular function. It is therefore tempting to speculate that the putative, pressor-selective testicular recognition sites subserve neurohypophyseal hormones or closely related peptides which may be produced within the testis, yielding local concentrations high enough to exert *in situ* paracrine or autocrine regulation of testicular functions. In addition to the possible existence of intratesticular GnRH and neurohypophyseal hormones, testicular immunoreactive propiomelanocortin-related peptides (Sharp *et al.*, 1980; Tsong *et al.*, 1982a, b) and thyrotropin-releasing factor (Pekary *et al.*, 1980) have also been recently described.

More recently, the pertinence of the neurohypophyseal hormones to ovarian functions has also been vigorously pursued. Bovine (Heap, 1983) corpus luteum tissues have been shown to contain high concentrations of oxytocin-like immuno and bioactivity and to secrete it under $PGF_{2\alpha}$ stimulation (Flint and Sheldrick, 1982). Human ovarian tissues of non-pregnant women were also found to contain high concentrations of oxytocin and arginine vasopressin-like immunoreactivity (Wathes *et al.*, 1982). Although the role of the neurohypophyseal hormones in the regulation of ovarian function remains uncertain, mounting evidence suggests a luteolytic role (Neely, *et al.*, 1979; Sheldrick *et al.*, 1980; Tan *et al.*, 1982a,b). These observations lend additional credence to the postulate that the neurohypophyseal hormones may play a paracrine or autocrine role at the gonadal level, subserving different functions in the ovary and testis.

NEUROPEPTIDES AS POSSIBLE CONTRACEPTIVE AGENTS

Although the possible direct action of GnRH on testis function in men has not been tested, GnRH and its agonists have been shown to inhibit steroidogenesis by cultured human granulosa cells (Tureck *et al.*, 1982). Combined with its potent pituitary 'desensitizing' action, GnRH may act at both pituitary and testicular sites to achieve 'chemical castration' of males. Recent studies have indicated the potential of decreasing male reproductive functions using potent GnRH agonists (Heber and Swerdloff, 1980). Furthermore, GnRH may also be used in the treatment of prostatic cancer.

Studies of the 'antigonadal' activity of the neurohypophyseal hormones may also offer the potential for the development of a new group of highly potent and selective contraceptive peptides capable of interfering directly with Leydig cell androgen biosynthesis. Although extratesticular pressor-related side-effects may preclude the systemic use of pressor-selective 'antigonadal' peptides *in vivo*, the putative testicular recognition sites may represent a unique subset of pressor-selective receptors distinct from those in extratesticular sites. It has been suggested that receptors mediating uterine responses to oxytocin differ in their specificity from those mediating milk ejection at the breast level. The possible existence of a unique subset of testis-specific, pressor-selective receptor sites should allow the design and synthesis of 'testis-selective' analogues of the neurohypophyseal hormones with 'antigonadal' contraceptive potential, but devoid of extratesticular pressor-related side-effects.

Acknowledgements

Supported by National Institutes of Health Research Grant HD-14084 and Program Project Grant HD-12303. AJWH is the recipient of Research Career Development Award HD-00375.

References

Acher, R., Chauvet, J. and Chauvet, M.T. (1969). Evolution of the neurohypophysial hormones with reference to amphibian. *Nature*, **221**, 759-60

Adashi, E.Y. and Hsueh, A.J.W. (1981a). Direct inhibition of testicular androgen biosynthesis revealing antigonadal activity of neurohypophysial hormones. *Nature*, **293**, 650-2.

Adashi, E.Y. and Hsueh, A.J.W. (1981b). Direct inhibition of testicular androgen biosynthesis by arginine-vasopressin: Mediation through pressor-selective testicular recognition sites. *Endocrinology*, **109**, 1793-5

Adashi, E.Y. and Hsueh, A.J.W. (1982). Direct inhibition of rat testicular androgen biosynthesis by arginine vasotocin: Studies on mechanisms of action. *J. Biol. Chem.*, **257**, 1301-8

Bambino, T.H., Schreiber, J.R. and Hsueh, A.J.W. (1980). Gonadotropin-releasing hormone and its agonist inhibit testicular luteinizing hormone receptor and steroidogenesis in immature and adult hypophysectomized rats. *Endocrinology*, **107**, 908-17

Bourne, G.A., Regiani, S., Payne, A.H. and Marshall, J.C. (1980). Testicular GnRH receptors—characterization and localization on interstitial tissue. *J. Clin. Endocrinol. Metab.*, **51**, 407-9

Chard, T., Boyd, N.R.H., Forsling, M.L., McNeilly, A.S. and Landon, J. (1970). The development of a radioimmunoassay for oxytocin: The extraction of oxytocin from plasma, and its measurement during parturition in human and goat blood. *J. Endocrinol.*, **48**, 223-34

Clayton, R.N., Katikeneni, M., Chan, V., Dufau, M.L. and Catt, K.J. (1980). Direct inhibition of testicular function by gonadotropin-releasing hormone: mediation by specific gonadotropin-releasing hormone receptors in interstitial cells. *Proc. Natl. Acad. Sci. USA*, **77**, 4459-63

Dutlow, C.M. and Millar, R.P. (1981). Rat testis immunoreactive LH-RH differs structurally from hypothalamic LH-RH. *Biochem. Biophys. Res. Commun.*, **101**, 486-94

Fields, P.A., Elridge, R.K., Fuchs, A.R., Roberts, R.F. and Fields, M.J. (1983). Human placental and bovine corpora luteal oxytocin. *Endocrinology*, **112**, 1544-6

Flint, A.P.E. and Sheldrick, E.L. (1982). Ovarian secretion of oxytocin is stimulated by prostaglandin. *Nature*, **297**, 587-8

Gautron, J.P., Pattou, E. and Kordon, C. (1981). Occurrence of higher molecular forms of LHRH in fractionated extracts from rat hypothalamus, cortex and placenta. *Mol. Cell. Endocrinol.*, **24**, 1-15

Gibbons, J.M., Mitnick, M. and Chieffo, V. (1975). *In vitro* biosynthesis of TSH- and LH-releasing factors by the human placenta. *Am. J. Obstet, Gynecol.*, **121**, 127-31

Gore-Langton, R.E., Lacroix, M. and Dorrington, J.H. (1981). Differential effects of luteinizing hormone-releasing hormone on follicle-stimulating hormone-dependent responses in rat granulosa cells and Sertoli cells *in vitro*. *Endocrinology*, **108**, 812-9

Heap, R.B. (1983). New functions for oxytocin? *Nature*, **301**, 115

Heber, D. and Swerdloff, R.S. (1980). Male contraception: Synergism of gonadotropin-releasing hormone analog and testosterone in suppressing gonadotropins. *Science*, **209**, 936-8

Hsueh, A.J.W. (1982). Direct effects of gonadotropin-releasing hormone on testicular Leydig cell functions. *Ann. NY Acad. Sci. USA*, **383**, 249-71

Hsueh, A.J.W., Bambino, T.H., Zhuang, L.Z., Welsh, T.H. Jr. and Ling, N.C. (1983). Mechanism of the direct action of gonadotropin-releasing hormone and its antagonist on androgen biosynthesis by cultured rat testicular cells. *Endocrinology*, **112**, 1653-61

Hsueh, A.J.W. and Erickson, G.F. (1979a). Extrapituitary action of gonadotropin releasing hormone: Direct inhibition of ovarian steroidogenesis. *Science*, **204**, 854-5

Hsueh, A.J.W. and Erickson, G.F. (1979b). Extrapituitary inhibition of testicular function by luteinizing hormone releasing hormone. *Nature*, **281**, 66-7

Hsueh, A.J.W. and Jones, P.B.C. (1981). Extrapituitary actions of gonadotropin-releasing hormone. *Endocrinol. Rev.*, **2**, 437-61

Hsueh, A.J.W. and Ling, N.C. (1979). Effect of an antagonistic analog of gonadotropin-releasing hormone upon ovarian granulosa cell function. *Life Sci.*, **25**, 1223-30

Hsueh, A.J.W., Schreiber, J.R. and Erickson, G.F. (1981). Inhibitory effect of gonadotropin-releasing hormone upon cultured testicular cells. *Mol. Cell. Endocrinol.*, **21**, 43-9

Hunter, M.G., Sullivan, M.H.F., Dix, C.J., Aldred, L.F. and Cooke, B.A. (1982). Stimulation and inhibition by LHRH analogues of cultured rat Leydig cell function and lack of effect on mouse Leydig cells. *Mol. Cell Endocrinology.*, **21**, 31-44

Keil, L.C. and Severs, W.B. (1977). Reduction in plasma vasopressin levels of dehydrated rats following acute stress. *Endocrinology*, **100**, 30-8

Khodr, G.S. and Siler-Khodr, T.M. (1980). Placental luteinizing hormone-releasing factor and its synthesis. *Science*, **207**, 315-7

Kruszynski, M., Lammek, B., Manning, M., Seto, J., Haldar, J. and Sawyer, W.H. (1980). [1-(β-Mercapto-β, β-cyclopentamethylenepropionic acid), a-(O-methyl)tyrosine] arginine vasopressin and [1-(β-mercapto-β, β-cyclopentamethylenepropionic acid)] arginine vasopressin, two highly potent antagonists of the vasopressor response to arginine vasopressin. *J. Med. Chem.*, **23**, 364-8

Labrie, F., Belanger, A., Cusan, L., Seguin, C., Pelletier, G., Kelly, P.A., Reeves, J.J., Lefebvre, F.-A., Lemay, A., Groudeau, Y. and Raynaud, J.-P. (1980). Antifertility effects of LHRH agonists in the male. *J. Androl.*, **1**, 209-28

Lee, J-N., Seppala, M. and Chard, T. (1981). Characterization of placental luteinizing hormone-releasing factor-like material. *Acta Endocrinol. (Copenh.)*, **96**, 394-7

Michell, R.H., Kirk, C.J. and Billah, M.M. (1979). Hormonal stimulation of phosphatidylinositol breakdown, with particular reference to the hepatic effects of vasopressin. *Biochem. Soc. Trans.*, **7**, 861-5

Neely, D.P., Stabenfedt, G.H., and Sauter, C.L. (1979). The effect of exogenous oxytocin on luteal function in mares. *J. Reprod. Fertil.*, **55**, 303-8

Nowak, R. and Wiseman, B. (1982). Secretion of a GnRH-like factor by the rabbit fetal placenta. *Biol. Reprod.*, **26** (Suppl.), 76A

Paull, W.K., Turkelson, C.M., Thomas, C.R. and Arimura, A. (1981). Immunohistochemical demonstration of a testicular substance related to luteinizing hormone-releasing hormone. *Science*, **213**, 1263-4

Pavel, S., Luca, N., Calb, M. and Goldstein, R. (1979). Inhibition of release of luteinizing hormone in the male rat by extremely small amounts of arginine vasotocin: Further evidence for the involvement of 5-hydroxytryptamine-containing neurons in the mechanism of action of arginine vasotocin. *Endocrinology*, **104**, 517-23

Pekary, A.E., Meyer, N.V., Vaillant, C. and Hershman, J.M. (1980). Thyrotropin releasing hormone and a homologous peptide in the male reproductive system. *Biochem. Biophys. Res. Commun.*, **95**, 618-23

Rich, K.A. and Bardin, C.W. (1981). Direct inhibitory effect of a GnRH agonist on secretion of androgen binding protein (ABP) from Sertoli cells in primary culture. *Biol. Reprod.*, **24** (Suppl.), 133A

Robertson, G.L., Mahr, E.A., Athar, S. and Sinha, T. (1973). Development and clinical application of a new method for the radioimmunoassay of arginine vasopressin in human plasma. *J. Clin. Invest.*, **52**, 2340-52

Sawyer, W.H. (1961). Hormones and electrolyte metabolism, comparative physiology and pharmacology of the neurohypophysis. *Recent Prog. Horm. Res.*, **17**, 437-65

Seguin, C., Cusan, L., Belanger, A., Kelly, P.A., Labrie, F. and Raynaud, J.P. (1981). Additive inhibitory effects of treatment with an LHRH agonist and an antiandrogen on androgen-dependent tissues in the rat. *Mol. Cell Endocrinol.*, **21**, 37-41

Sharp, B., Pekary, A.E., Meyer, N.V. and Hersham, J.M. (1980). β-Endorphin in male rat reproductive organs. *Biochem. Biophys. Res. Commun.*, **95**, 618-23

Sharpe, R.M. and Fraser, H.M. (1980). HCG stimulation of testicular LHRH-like activity. *Nature*, **287**, 642-3

Sheldrick, E.L., Mitchell, M.D. and Flint, A.P.E. (1980). Delayed luteal regression in ewes immunized against oxytocin. *J. Reprod. Fertil.*, **59**, 37-42

Tan, G.J.S., Tweedale, R.T. and Biggs, J.S.G. (1982a). Effects of oxytocin on the bovine corpus luteum of early pregnancy. *J. Reprod. Fertil.*, **66**, 75-8

Tan, G.J.S., Tweedale, R.T. and Biggs, J.S.G. (1982b). Oxytocin may play a role in the control of the human corpus luteum. *J. Endocrinol.*, **95**, 65-70

Tsong, S.D., Phillips, O.M., Bardin, C.W., Halmi, N., Liotta, A.S., Margioris, A. and Krieger, D.T. (1982a). ACTH and β-endorphin-related peptides are present in multiple sites in the reproductive tract of the rat. *Endocrinology*, **110**, 2204-6

Tsong, S.D., Phillips, D.M., Halmi, N., Krieger, D.T. and Bardin, C.W. (1982b). β-endorphin is present in the male reproductive tract of five species. *Biol. Reprod.*, **27**, 755-64

Tureck, R.W., Mastroianni, L., Blasco, L. and Strauss, III, J.F. (1982). Inhibition of human granulosa cell progesterone secretion by a gonadotropin-releasing hormone agonist. *J. Clin. Endocrinol. Metab.*, **54**, 1078-80

Vaughan, M.K., Black, D.E., Johnson, L.Y. and Reiter, R.J. (1979). The effect of subcutaneous injections of melatonin, arginine vasotocin and related peptides on pituitary and plasma levels of luteinizing hormone, follicle-stimulating hormone, and prolactin in castrated adult male rats. *Endocrinology*, **104**, 212-7

Vaughan, M.K., Reiter, R.J., McKinney, T. and Vaughan, G.M. (1974b). Inhibition of growth of gonadal dependent structures by arginine vasotocin and purified bovine pineal fractions in immature mice and hamsters. *Int. J. Fertil.*, **19**, 103-6

Vaughan, M.K., Vaughan, G.M. and Klein, D.C. (1974a). Arginine vasotocin: Effects on development of reproductive organs. *Science*, **186**, 938-9

Wathes, D.C., Pickering, B.T., Swann, R.W., Porter, D.G., Hull, M.G.R. and Drife, J.O. (1982). Neurohypophysial hormones in the human ovary. *Lancet*, **2**, 410-2

Wathes, D.C. and Swann, R.W. (1982). Is oxytocin an ovarian hormone? *Nature*, **297**, 225-7

Yamashita, K., Mieno, M. and Yamashita E.R. (1979). Suppression of the luteinizing hormone releasing effect of luteinizing hormone releasing hormone by arginine vasotocin. *J. Endocrinol.*, **81**, 103-8

Yamashita, K., Mieno, M. and Yamashita, E.R. (1980). Suppression of the luteinizing hormone releasing effect of luteinizing hormone releasing hormone by arginine vasotocin in immature male dogs. *J. Endocrinol.*, **84**, 449-52

22
Non-steroidal inhibitors of androgen transport and metabolism

G.G. ROUSSEAU, J.I. QUIVY, C.F. ROLIN JACQUEMYNS, D.A.N.
SIRETT, M.T. de REVIERS, M.C. VIGUIER-MARTINEZ, S. DELPECH
and G. COLAS

The testicular and epididymal androgen-binding protein (ABP) appears to have an essential role in the processes of spermatogenesis and sperm maturation in the rat. The appearance of ABP coincides with the onset of fertility in normal rats (Hansson *et al.*, 1973), and its disappearance in mature H^{re} rats coincides with the onset of sterility characteristic of this mutant (Musto and Bardin, 1976). In addition to its presumed role as a transport protein for testicular androgens, both within the Sertoli cell, where it is synthesized, and through the tubular system towards the epididymis, ABP could be an 'androgen-concentrating factor' maintaining a concentration of androgen at the caput epididymis sufficient for the maturation of the spermatozoa (Hansson *et al.*, 1973; Purvis and Hansson, 1978). Finally, a transmembrane carrier function, facilitating the uptake of androgens by the epididymis, is possible (Bardin *et al.*, 1981).

It may be possible to modify or interrupt sperm maturation by inhibiting the formation of the androgen–ABP complex. We have studied ligands which bind specifically and reversibly to rat ABP, but which are unlikely to demonstrate undesirable androgen agonist or antagonist activity, in view of their inability to bind to the androgen receptor. To date very few steroids possess any degree of specificity for each of these two proteins (Kirchhoff *et al.*, 1979). For this reason we chose the dicyclohexane structure as a basis for investigation. We hoped it was less likely to show crossreactivity at the level of mechanisms implicating steroid-binding proteins (carrier, receptor, enzyme) than steroids themselves. The following chapter reviews the work with these novel structures.

EFFECTS OF DICYCLOHEXANE DERIVATIVES *IN VITRO*

Binding to rat epididymal ABP

Five dicyclohexane derivatives have been tested for their ability to inhibit the binding of dihydrotestosterone (DHT) to rat epididymal ABP. Typical results are given in Table 22.1. These binding studies were carried out using the dextran-coated charcoal method for separating bound and free ligand, and the equilibrium dissociation constants for the inhibitors (K_i) were calculated from double-reciprocal plots (details are given in Table 22.1). The inhibition was competitive in nature. The racemic diastereoisomers of the dicyclohexane derivatives (with both ethyl groups on the same side of the plane of the molecule given by the two rings) showed, in general, a higher affinity for ABP than their meso analogues (the two ethyl groups on opposite sides of the plane of the rings). The compound PRDX showed a high affinity for rat ABP (K_i of the order of 100 nmol/l). This contrasts with the affinities observed for steroids including two ketone functions in their rings A or D, such as 5α-androstane-3,17-dione and 4-androstene-3,17-dione, which have K_i values greater than 500 nmol/l. The synthetic oestrogen diethylstilboestrol (DES) has the same carbon skeleton as the dicyclohexane compounds (which are chemically derived from DES) but has a very low affinity for ABP ($K_i = 2630$ nmol/l).

Binding to rat prostate androgen receptor

The binding of the dicyclohexane compounds to the rat prostatic androgen receptor (AR), measured by competition with the synthetic ligand [³H]methyltrienolone (17β-hydroxy-17α-methylestra-4,9,11-trien-3-one), was weak or undetectable. Therefore their specificity for ABP is considerable. The ratio of the inhibition constants (K_i for AR divided by K_i for ABP) was high for PRDX, PRXL and PRCL (Table 22.1). It was lower for the meso derivative PMDX, which bound relatively more strongly to the receptor than the other non-steroidal compounds. It was also established that PRDX does not bind to the rat uterine oestrogen receptor (Quivy, unpublished observations), and that PRDX, PMDX, PRCL and PRTL do not compete with dexamethasone (9α-fluoro-16α-methyl-11β,17α,21-hydroxy-1,4-pregnadiene-3,20-dione) for the glucocorticoid receptor in cultured rat hepatoma cells (Rousseau, unpublished observations).

Binding to human testosterone-estradiol binding protein (TeBG) in plasma and TeBG-like protein (hABP) in epididymis and testis

A protein (hABP) capable of binding androgens is known to be present in the epididymis and testis of the human (Vigersky *et al.*, 1976; Lipshultz *et al.*, 1977; Hsu and Troen, 1978). The physiochemical characteristics of hABP are very similar to those of another protein, testosterone–oestradiol binding globulin (TeBG), which binds androgens in human plasma and is

Table 22.1 Inhibition by dicyclohexane derivatives of androgen binding to rat ABP and androgen receptor (AR) *in vitro*

Structure[a]	Name[b,c]	Inhibition[d] constant (K_i)		Inhibition ratio[e]
		ABP (nmol/l)	AR (nmol/l)	(ABP vs AR)
	PRDX	160	14 000	87
	PRXL	240	6 900	29
	PMDX	390	2 660	7
	PRCL	600	12 010	20
	PRTL	3100	∞	—

[a] Only one enantiomer is represented for the racemic derivatives (d, l)
[b] Nomenclature: PRDX, d,1-3,4-bis(4-oxocyclohexyl)-hexane; PRXL, d,1-3-(4-oxocyclohexyl)-4(cis-4-hydroxycyclohexyl)-hexane; PMDX, meso-3,4-bis(4-hydroxycyclohexyl)-hexane; PRCL, d,1-3-(cis-4-hydroxycyclohexyl)-4-(trans-4-hydroxycyclohexyl)-hexane
[c] Synthesis see Devis *et al* (1979) and Verhoeven *et al* (1983)
[d] K_i values are obtained after linear regression analysis of Lineweaver–Burk plots, using at least four binding determinations in duplicate (Kirchhoff *et al.*, 1979). Estimates given are mean values from at least three experiments
[e] Inhibition ratio is K_i for AR divided by K_i for ABP

secreted by the liver. The binding affinity of the three racemic dicyclohexane derivatives, PRDX, PRCL and PRTL, with relatively high affinities for rat ABP, was studied in both hABP and TeBG preparations. These two proteins were partially purified by ammonium sulphate precipitation (45–60% saturation) in order to minimize the effects of non-specific binding of the inhibitors, and to prepare hABP and TeBG for use in similar experimental conditions. The affinity of the test compounds for each protein was determined in two types of experiment (Table 22.2). In one method, various concentrations of [³H]DHT were incubated in the presence and absence of a single, constant concentration of inhibitor; the inhibition constant K_i was derived from Lineweaver–Burk plots. The second method involved the in-

Table 22.2 Inhibition by dicyclohexane derivatives of androgen binding to human ABP and TeBG

| Name | $K_i\ hABP$ (nmol/l) | | $K_i\ hTeBG$ (nmol/l) | |
	a	b	a	b
PRDX	1950	5400	1920	3700
PRCL	215	365	245	1955
PRXL	395	580	230	305

a and b refer to the two methods described in the text
hABP was prepared from testicular or epididymal cytosol by precipitation with ammonium sulphate (45–60% saturation), after treatment with charcoal for 30 min at 30°C to remove endogenous androgenic steroids and androgen receptor. TeBG was obtained by the same method, from dilute normal male plasma

cubation of constant concentrations of [³H]testosterone alone or in the presence of increasing concentrations of inhibitor; K_i was calculated using Dixon plots.

The two methods showed the same trend: compounds possessing at least one hydroxyl group (PRCL, PRXL) bound more strongly to both proteins than PRDX, which has no hydroxyl substituents. In a study of the structural requirements for binding to TeBG, the presence of a hydroxyl group at one of the extremities of the steroid (for example, position 17β in androstanes and oestrenes) was shown to be a necessary condition for binding with high affinity to this protein (Cunningham et al., 1981). However, our work has not demonstrated any fundamental differences between the structural requirements for binding to hABP and TeBG in our preparations. We cannot exclude the possibility that the androgen binding activity in our 'hABP' preparation resulted from contamination of the testicular or epididymal cytosol with plasma TeBG.

Inhibition of aromatase activity in cultured rat Sertoli cells and in human placental microsome preparations

So far the dicyclohexane compounds have been discussed in the context of their selective inhibition of androgen binding to ABP. Our aim was to identify compounds which could interfere with androgen transport in the seminiferous tubule and epididymis, without provoking side-effects mediated by the androgen receptor. The observations of a reduction in sperm motility when rats were treated *in vivo* with the most potent inhibitor of binding to ABP (p. 337) were encouraging. However, it cannot be assumed that the effect was obtained by way of the mechanism outlined above. Since all steps in spermatogenesis subsequent to the leptotene stage of the meiotic prophase take place in a milieu regulated by the Sertoli cells (Kerr and de Kretser, 1981; Ritzen *et al.*, 1981), we examined the influence of the dicyclohexane compounds on cell function in Sertoli cell enriched cultures from prepubertal rats. One indicator of normal Sertoli cell function is the increased aromatization of testosterone to oestradiol-17β in response to treatment of the cells with FSH (Armstrong and Dorrington, 1977); indeed, this property has been used to develop a specific *in vitro* bioassay for FSH (van Damme *et al.*, 1979). In our experiments aromatase activity was monitored by following the conversion of exogenous testosterone to oestradiol-17β. The product was measured in the culture medium by radioimmunossay (Verhoeven *et al.*, 1979), following incubation of the cells with ovine FSH or pregnant mare serum gonadotrophin (Verhoeven *et al.*, 1983). The presence of PRDX in the culture medium during the incubation reduced the gonadotrophin-induced increase in Sertoli cell oestradiol-17β production in a reversible, dose-dependent manner (Fig. 22.1a). This inhibition did not seem to involve the early stages of the hormone response, since the gonadotrophin-induced rise in the concentration of cyclic AMP was still observed in the presence of PRDX. Furthermore, stimulation of aromatase activity by treatment of the cultures with $N^6,O^{2'}$-dibutyryl-adenosine-3′,5′-cyclic monophosphate ((Bu)$_2$cAMP), an analogue of cyclic AMP, was sensitive to inhibition by the dicyclohexane. The derivatives PMDX and PRXL (Table 22.1) could also inhibit the aromatase activity induced in Sertoli cell cultures by gonadotrophins and (Bu)$_2$cAMP, without affecting the concentration of cyclic AMP. The compound PRTL, however, had no effect on cellular aromatase activity.

The suggestion in the Sertoli cell culture system that dicyclohexane compounds acted to reduce oestradiol production without affecting the integrity of the early gonadotrophin response mechanism prompted an examination of their interaction with the aromatase enzyme complex itself. Accordingly, a cell-free system was set up using microsomes prepared from human term placenta, a convenient source of aromatase activity (Ryan, 1959). A preliminary assay used a single concentration of substrate (testosterone) and showed that the production of oestradiol-17β, measured by radioimmunoassay as in the Sertoli cell studies, was substantially reduced in the presence of PRDX (Verhoeven *et al.*, 1983). The degree of inhibition decreased through the dicyclohexane series PMDX, PRXL and PRTL. For a more extensive investigation the placental microsome preparation was retained, but the assay procedure was changed to measure the production of [^{3}H]oestradiol-17β and [^{3}H]oestrone from [^{3}H]testosterone as substrate. Oestrone is formed from oestradiol-17β by 17β-hydroxysteroid dehydrogenase activity present in the microsome preparation as a contaminant. Several concentrations of substrate were used to give a range of partial saturations of the enzyme activity, and the results were analysed on double-reciprocal

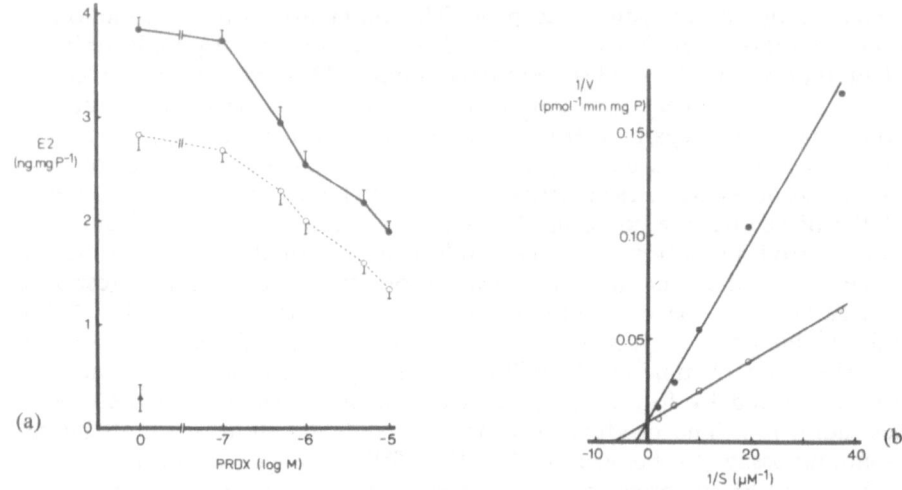

Fig. 22.1 (a) Dose–response relationship of the inhibitory effects of PRDX on aromatase in Sertoli cells. Sertoli cell-enriched monolayers were incubated in the presence of PMSG (●—●, 1 U/ml; ○—○, 10 U/ml), testosterone (0.5 µmol/l), MIX (3-isobutyl-1-methyl-xanthine, 0.1 mmol/l) and concentrations of PRDX between 0 and 10 µmol/l. The concentration of oestradiol-17β (E2) in the medium was determined after a 24 h incubation period. The triangle corresponds to determinations in absence of PMSG stimulation. Values given are mean ±SD of incubations in triplicate. (Taken from Verhoeven *et al.*. (1983) with permission from author and publisher.) (b) Inhibition of human placental microsome aromatase activity by PRDX. Microsomes (15 µg protein) were incubated with [^{3}H]testosterone (0.1 µCi) and testosterone (25–500 nmol/l) at 37°C for 7.5 min., in the presence (●—●) or absence (○—○) of PRDX (1.6 µmol/l). The amount of oestradiol-17β and oestrone formed was measured after extraction and separation of the products by TLC. Points are mean values of duplicate incubations. The lines are the result of simple linear regression using the individual data points. In this experiment, K_m (testosterone) = 0.15 µmol/l, K_i (PRDX) = 0.89 µmol/l.

plots. These graphs were linear in the presence and absence of PRDX, and showed that the inhibition of aromatase activity was competitive (Fig. 22.1b). The other dicyclohexane compounds tested so far have given the same type of results; values for the inhibition constants K_i obtained from double-reciprocal plots for each compound are presented in Table 22.3. The K_m value for testosterone, the substrate, was 0.1 ± 0.01 µmol/l in our system.

Table 22.3 Inhibition of human placental microsome aromatase activity by dicyclohexane compounds

Compounds	K_i (µmol/l)
PRDX	0.60 ± 0.12 (6)
PMDX	0.99 ± 0.26 (4)
PRXL	1.08 ± 0.29 (4)
PRCL	6.07 ± 2.60 (5)
PRTL	9.12 ± 2.10 (3)

Results are given as mean ±SEM (number of experiments). For method, see legend to Fig. 22.1b

PRDX was the most potent aromatase inhibitor in this group of compounds, reflected in the relatively low value of K_i observed.

EFFECTS OF DICYCLOHEXANE DERIVATIVES IN THE RAT *IN VIVO*

Sperm motility

Among the dicyclohexane derivatives examined, PRDX showed the best affinity for rat ABP, and the best specificity in that it did not interact significantly with steroid receptors. Therefore the effect of the administration of PRDX to adult rats on different physiological parameters related to reproductive function was studied. A decrease in the percentage of motile epididymal sperm was observed following subcutaneous injection of PRDX at different doses ($0.1-2$ mg kg^{-1} day^{-1}) for various periods (14-29 days) (Table 22.4). Each rat was mated with three proven fertile females. The

Table 22.4 Effect of PRDX administration on motility of cauda epididymal sperm and on fertility in the rat

Treatment		Motile sperm (%)		Pregnant females (%)*	
Daily dose (mg/kg)	Length (days)	Control	Treated	Control	Treated
0.1	18	41	16	58	33[a]
0.3	18	35	17	60	53[b]
0.5	18	60	42	—	—
0.3	29	39	34[b]	41	22[b]
2.0	14	39	17	43	40[b]

Control and treated groups were compared using Student's t-test
Differences were significant ($p < 0.05$), except [a], $0.1 > p > 0.05$ and [b], not significant ($p > 0.1$). ($n = 5-10$/group)
* Each male was mated with three females during the last three to five days of treatment

results of these experiments were not conclusive, due to lack of reproducibility and an overall poor performance amongst the control, vehicle-injected rats. A treatment-associated diminution in fertility was noted but the effect was not highly significant.

There was no clear dose–response curve for PRDX. The largest reductions in sperm motility (60%) were observed at widely different doses of PRDX (0.1 mg kg^{-1} day^{-1} and 2 mg kg^{-1} day^{-1} for periods of 18 and 14 days, respectively). It appeared that there was a saturation effect, perhaps inherent in the mode of administration of PRDX (a lipophilic compound), or in the processes of transport to the testis or excretion.

Organ weights and histology

None of the treatments affected the weight of either the whole animal or of the organs of the reproductive tract, except in one case where testis weight

Table 22.5 Effect of PRDX administration on organ and body weight in adult rats

Treatment		Weights				
Daily dose (mg/kg)	Length (days)	Body (g)	Left testis (g)	Epididymis (g)	Seminal vesicles (g)	Ventral prostate (g)
—	18	359	1.60	0.49	1.00	0.29
0.3	18	356	1.51*	0.47	0.93	0.28
—	18	467	1.72	0.52	1.03	0.36
0.5	18	469	1.73	0.51	0.95	0.45
—	14	482	1.55	0.49	0.93	0.38
2.0	14	476	1.55	0.49	0.96	0.39

* Significantly different from control (*t*-test: $p < 0.05$)

was slightly decreased (Table 22.5). The lack of modification in the weights of the ventral prostate and the seminal vesicles suggested that PRDX does not possess significant androgenic or anti-androgenic activity; this corroborated the lack of binding to the androgen receptor observed *in vitro*.

By histological criteria there was no major change in spermatogenesis. However, in some cases there was a decrease in the number of type I zygotene spermatocytes and in the nuclear area of Sertoli cells (Table 22.6). In one experiment, in which rats were treated with PRDX at $0.3 \, \mathrm{mg \, kg^{-1}}$ $\mathrm{day^{-1}}$ for 18 days, more extensive histological investigations showed no change in the area of intertubular material or of Leydig cells; the length of the seminiferous tubules was unchanged, while the diameter of the tubules was slightly but significantly reduced (to $264 \, \mu m$ from $277 \, \mu m$).

Table 22.6 Effect of PRDX administration on the number of type I zygotene spermatocytes per orthogonal section of seminiferous tubules and the nuclear area of Sertoli cells in the adult rat (mean).

Treatment		Zygotene spermatocytes		Nuclear area of Sertoli cells (μm^2)	
Daily dose (mg/kg)	Length (days)	Treated	Controls	Treated	Controls
0.1	18	44.9	49.9	59.3	64.3
0.3	18	44.8*	49.3	61.0*	68.6
0.3	29	43.2	50.8	55.3	63.6
0.5	29	46.4*	50.8	65.3	63.6

* Significantly different from controls (*t*-test: $p < 0.05$)
Quantitative histological procedures have been described elsewhere (Hochereau-de Reviers *et al.*, 1976, 1979)

Plasma hormone concentrations

Rats which had received 0.1, 0.3 or $0.5 \, \mathrm{mg \, kg^{-1} \, day^{-1}}$ of PRDX for 18 days showed no significant changes in their plasma concentrations of LH,

FSH, PRL and testosterone. Levels of pituitary hormones in plasma were also unchanged by treatment at the higher dose of $2\,mg\,kg^{-1}\,day^{-1}$ for 14 days. Hormone assay methodology has been summarized, with further references, elsewhere (Viguier-Martinez et al., 1983).

Studies in immature rats

In prepubertal rats PRDX had no effect on statural growth or on the weight of reproductive organs, except for one group (group 1 in Table 22.7), in which epididymal and ventral prostate weights were decreased. By histological criteria there was no effect, in this group, on the first stages of spermatogenesis. Plasma levels of LH and FSH remained unchanged. However, there was a decrease in prolactin levels in group 2 (from 8.8 ± 2.0 to $3.5 \pm 0.4\,ng/ml$).

Table 22.7 Effect of PRDX administration for 14 days to prepubertal rats

Treatment	Weights				
Daily dose (mg/kg)	Body (g)	Testis (mg)	Epididymis (mg)	Ventral prostate (mg)	Seminal vesicle (mg)
Group 1					
—	140	763	91	51	55
0.3	140	716	72*	43*	49
Group 2					
—	120	527	117	44	25
2.0	121	527	113	41	26

* Significantly different from controls (t-test: $p < 0.05$)

DISCUSSION AND CONCLUDING REMARKS

It has been demonstrated that, in the rat, the non-steroidal molecule PRDX, which can inhibit the binding of androgens to ABP without binding to the androgen receptor *in vitro*, does not interfere with the development of androgen target tissues or with the secretion of pituitary hormones and testosterone itself. This dicyclohexane derivative, therefore, probably does not possess significant androgenic or anti-androgenic activity at the doses used; in contrast, a synthetic steroid (17β-methoxy-2α-methyl-5α-androstan-3-one) with a similar binding specificity showed some androgenic activity (Lobl, 1982). An appreciable reduction in the motility of epididymal sperm was observed even at relatively low doses of PRDX ($0.1\,mg\,kg^{-1}\,day^{-1}$). We believe that a modification of the maturation of the spermatozoa is implied, rather than an effect on an earlier stage of sperm development. The process of spermatogenesis in the rat requires at least six weeks, and is followed by a period of about eight days during which the sperm move through the epididymis (Hammerstedt, 1981). The fact that 14 days of treatment is sufficient to produce an effect on sperm motility is difficult to reconcile with a perturbation of any stage in sperm development prior to the final week of spermatogenesis. After their transit of the epididymis, mature sperm are retained in the caudal region for 2–13 days; samples of caudal fluid obtained after 14 days of treatment for motility studies could contain a mixture of sperm which had completed maturation before the start of treatment, sperm which had been in the process of epididymal transit and maturation during treatment, and sperm which had completed the final stages of spermatogenesis and the process of maturation during treatment.

With certain treatments slight histological modifications in the seminiferous tubules were observed, but in view of the time factor it is unlikely that such changes could be linked with the altered state of the mature spermatozoa recovered from the cauda epididymis. In some experiments there was a reduction in the size of Sertoli cell nuclei, a parameter which can reflect changes in the synthetic activity of the cells and in their sensitivity to hormones (Hochereau-de Reviers *et al.*, 1976); this is unlikely to be associated with the inhibition of aromatase activity demonstrated *in vitro* by several of the dicyclohexane derivatives, including PRDX. Our studies suggest that the reduction in aromatase activity is the result of direct competition at the enzyme complex, rather than an alteration in the amount of enzyme available mediated at the level of the nucleus. The possibility cannot be excluded that a perturbation of Sertoli cell function in such a manner by PRDX could influence the subsequent motility of epididymal sperm, whether by altering a late step in spermatogenesis or by decreasing the production of a Sertoli cell factor required for sperm maturation in the epididymis. This type of mechanism is purely speculative, and must remain so until we have tested more specific aromatase inhibitors for their ability to reduce sperm motility *in vivo*, or the full extent of the supportive role of the Sertoli cell and its products in spermatogenesis and sperm maturation has been elucidated. We continue to favour a mechanism directed at ABP function to explain the action of PRDX on sperm properties *in vivo*.

The lack of effect of PRDX on plasma concentrations of pituitary hormones and testosterone in adult rats suggests that the dicyclohexane derivative does not act on the hypothalamo-pituitary axis. The reduction in plasma levels of prolactin in immature rats following treatment with a relatively high dose of PRDX ($2\,\text{mg}\,\text{kg}^{-1}\,\text{day}^{-1}$) is interesting in view both of the dependence of this parameter on plasma oestradiol in the male rat (Kalra *et al.*, 1973), and of the higher levels of Sertoli cell aromatase activity in younger rats (Armstrong and Dorrington, 1977). However, the attribution of this effect to the ability of PRDX to inhibit aromatase activity must await further experiments.

Finally we reviewed the data showing that two dicyclohexanes, PRCL and PRXL, have a satisfactory affinity for human TeBG, a protein similar if not identical to hABP, but species differences in structural requirements for binding to ABP or equivalent proteins were indicated. In the human as in the rat, these non-steroidal molecules, or derivatives with an improved affinity for TeBG/hABP, constitute an interesting tool for the investigation of the different stages of sperm development.

Acknowledgements

The assistance of M. Place, K. Wauters and T. Lambert (at Brussels) and of C. Perreau and the staff of the rodent animal house (at Nouzilly) is gratefully acknowledged. Some of the studies presented in this paper were supported by Grant No. 820-0444 of the Ford, Mellon, and Rockefeller Foundations, and by a grant 'ATP Internationale' of the CNRS (France).

References

Armstrong, D.T. and Dorrington, J.H. (1977). Estrogen biosynthesis in the ovaries and testes. In Thomas, J.H. and Singhal, R.L. (eds.), *Advances in Sex Hormone Research, Regulatory Mechanisms Affecting Gonadal Hormone Action*, pp 217-58. (Baltimore: University Park Press)

Bardin, C.W., Musto, N., Gunsalus, G., Kotite, N., Cheng, S.-L., Larrea, F. and Becker, R. (1981). Extracellular androgen binding proteins. *Ann. Rev. Physiol.*, **43**, 189-98

Cunningham, G.R., Tindall, D.J., Lobl, T.J., Campbell, J.A. and Means, A.R. (1981). Steroid structural requirements for high affinity binding to human sex steroid binding protein (SBP). *Steroids*, **38**, 243-62

van Damme, M.-P., Robertson, D.M., Marana, R., Ritzén, E.M. and Diczfalusy, E. (1979). A sensitive and specific *in vitro* bioassay method for the measurement of follicle-stimulating hormone activity. *Acta Endocrinol.* **91**, 224-37

Devis, R. and Bui, X.-H. (1979). Contribution à l'étude des androgènes synthétiques non stéroïdes. Partie I. Perhydrohexestrols et dicétones correspondantes. *Bull. Soc. Chim. France*, **2**, 1-8

Hammerstedt, R.H. (1981). Monitoring the metabolic rate of germ cells and sperm. In McKerns, K.W. (ed.) *Reproductive Processes and Contraception*, pp. 353-91 (New York: Plenum)

Hansson, V., Ritzen, E.M., French, F.S. and Nayfeh, S.N. (1973). Androgen transport and receptor mechanisms in testis and epididymis. In Hamilton, D.W. and Greep, R.O. (eds.) *Handbook of Physiology, Section 7: Endocrinology*, Vol. 5 pp. 173-201 (Baltimore: Williams and Wilkins)

Hochereau-de Reviers, M.T., Blanc, M.R., Cahoreau, C., Courot, M., Dacheux, J.L. and Pisselet, C. (1979). Histological parameters in bilateral cryptorchid adult rams. *Ann. Biol. Anim. Biochim. Biophys.* **19**, 1141-6

Hochereau-de Reviers, M.T., Loir, M. and Pelletier, J. (1976). Seasonal variations in the response of the testis and LH levels to hemicastration in adult rams. *J. Reprod. Fertil.*, **46**, 203-9

Hsu, A.-F. and Troen, P. (1978). An androgen binding protein in the testicular cytosol of human testis. Comparison with human plasma testosterone-estrogen binding globulin. *J. Clin. Invest.*, **61**, 1611-9

Kalra, P.S., Fawcett, C.P., Krulich, L. and McCann, S.M. (1973). The effect of gonadal steroids on plasma gonadotrophins and prolactin in the rat. *Endocrinology*, **92**, 1256-68

Kerr, J.B. and de Kretser, D.M. (1981). The cytology of the human testis. In Burger, H. and de Kretser, D.M. (eds.) *The Testis* pp. 141-69 (New York: Raven)

Kirchhoff, J., Soffié, M. and Rousseau, G.G. (1979). Differences in the steroid-binding site specificities of rat prostate androgen receptor and epididymal androgen-binding protein (ABP). *J. Steroid Biochem.* **10**, 487-97

Lipshultz, L.I., Tsai, Y.-H., Sanborn, B.M. and Steinberger, E. (1977). Androgen-binding activity in the human testis and epididymis. *Fertil. Steril.*, **28**, 947-51

Lobl, T.J. (1982). Steroid binding proteins: receptors and transporters. (Abstract). *Arch. Androl.*, **9**, 55

Musto, N.A. and Bardin, C.W. (1976). Decreased levels of androgen binding protein in the reproductive tract of the restricted (H^re) rat. *Steroids*, **28**, 1-11

Purvis, K. and Hansson, V. (1978). Androgens and androgen-binding protein in the rat epididymis. *J. Reprod. Fertil.*, **52**, 59-63

Ritzén, E.M., Hansson, V. and French, F.S. (1981). The Sertoli cell. In Burger, H. and de Krester, D.M. (eds.) *The Testis* pp. 171–94. (New York: Raven)

Ryan, K.J. (1959). Biological aromatization of steroids. *J. Biol. Chem.*, **234**, 268–72

Verhoeven, G., Cailleau, J., Quivy, J.I. and Rousseau, G.G. (1983). Dicyclohexane derivatives that bind to androgen-binding protein (ABP) also inhibit hormone stimulated aromatase activity in rat Sertoli cells. *J. Steroid Biochem.*, **18**, 127–33

Verhoeven, G., Dierickx, P. and De Moor, P. (1979). Stimulation effect of neurotransmitters on the aromatization of testosterone by Sertoli cell-enriched cultures. *Mol. Cell Endocrinol.*, **13**, 241–53

Vigersky, R.A., Loriaux, D.L., Howards, S.S., Hodgen, G.B., Lipsett, M.B. and Chrambach, A.C. (1976). Androgen binding proteins of testis, epididymis and plasma in man and monkey. *J. Clin. Invest.*, **58**, 1061–8

Viguier-Martinez, M.C., Hochereau-de Reviers, M.T., Barenton, B. and Perreau, C. (1983). Effect of a non-steroidal antiandrogen, flutamide, on the hypothalamo-pituitary axis, genital tract and testis in growing male rats: endocrinological and histological data. *Acta Endocrinol.*, **102**, 299–306

23
Danazol plus testosterone enanthate in male langur monkey

N.K. LOHIYA and O.P. SHARMA

Danazol (100 mg/day; oral) in combination with testosterone enanthate (50 mg/15 days; i.m.) was tested for reversible sterilization of male langur monkey. Seminal characteristics, hormone assay, blood serum biochemical and haematological studies were performed for efficacy and side-effects. Oligospermia or azoospermia was noted after 60 days of treatment. Semen weight, volume and percentage of sperm vitality, motility and morphology were impaired progressively. pH of semen and libido remained unimpaired. The azoospermic state continued during maintenance phase. Serum testosterone levels decreased non-significantly. Changes in seminal characteristics reversed to normal range following 60–120 days recovery. No severe side-effects were noticed.

Attempts at pharmacological fertility control in laboratory animals and human males have mainly made use of steroids (Neumann *et al.*, 1976; Frick and Bartsch, 1976). Suppression or complete inhibition of spermatogenesis may be achieved in this way (Nieschlag *et al.*, 1978; Lotz and Krause, 1981; Faundes *et al.*, 1981).

Danazol, a heterocyclic steroid (17α-pregna-2,4-diene-20-yno(2,3-d) isoxazol-17β-ol), suppresses fertility in a variety of animal species including human, either through the suppression of pituitary gonadotropin secretion (Dmowski, 1979) or by inhibiting gonadal steroidogenesis (Victor and Lauersen, 1982). Reduced sperm concentration following danazol administration was associated with impaired libido (Sherins *et al.*, 1971). Testosterone, in combination with danazol was administered exogenously to maintain libido and extratesticular androgen actions (Skoglund and Paulsen, 1973; Ulstein *et al.*, 1975; Paulsen and Leonard, 1976) but consistent azoospermia could be achieved in a small percentage of subjects (Paulsen and Leonard, 1976). The present chapter deals with contraceptive efficacy and side-effects of danazol plus testosterone enanthate in langur monkey (*Presbytis entellus entellus* Dufresne).

EXPERIMENTATION

Animals

Five adult male langurs, weighing between 15 and 18 kg, trapped around Jaipur, India, were subjected to quarantine for 2 months. Animals were housed individually in metallic cages (measuring $3.5 \times 2.5 \times 2.5$ ft) ($1.07 \times 0.76 \times 0.76$ m) under semi-natural laboratory conditions. Animals were provided with green leaves, roasted-soaked grains, wheat chapaties, seasonal fruits and unrestricted access to water.

Experimental protocol

The study period was divided into four phases, i.e. (1) control phase, 30 days; (2) treatment phase, 60 days; (3) maintenance phase, 60 days; and (4) post-treatment recovery phase, 120 days. Danazol (100 mg/day; oral) suspended in olive oil was administered with testosterone enanthate (TE) (50 mg/15 days; i.m.) followed by maintenance doses of danazol (50 mg/day; oral) plus TE (50 mg/15 days; i.m.) for another 60 days.

Semen analysis

Semen samples were collected fortnightly by electro-ejaculation (Mastroianni and Manson, 1963) and were assessed for seminal characteristics, i.e. semen weight, volume, pH, sperm density, sperm morphology and percentage of vital and motile spermatozoa, as outlined in the WHO Laboratory Manual (Belsey et al., 1980). The sperm counts were made only in seminal fluid exuded from coagulum.

Toxicological studies

Blood samples were collected every month for haematology (Lynch et al., 1969), serum electrolytes (Na$^+$ and K$^+$), serum glutamic oxaloacetic transaminase (SGOT), serum glutamic pyruvic transaminase (SGPT) (Reitman and Frankel, 1957), alkaline phosphatase (Fiske and Subbarow, 1925), LDH (Cabaud and Wroblewski, 1958) and bilirubin (King and Coxon, 1950) determination throughout the study.

Radioimmunoassay

Three blood samples were collected at 15 min intervals (08.00, 08.15 and 08.30h) during different phases of the study. Samples were clotted at 37°C and centrifuged at 3000 r.p.m. for 20 min. Serum was drawn off and stored at -20°C for subsequent analysis. Serum levels of testosterone were assayed in triplicates using a specific radioimmunoassay (RIA) method (WHO, 1981). Antisera was raised against T-3-carboxymethyloxime-BSA in sheep. Binding of antisera ranged from 45 to 60%. Serum pools gave a within-assay coefficient of variation of 3.98% and interassay coefficient of variation of 9.32% with 10 pg sensitivity. About 8000–10000 counts min⁻¹ tube⁻¹ of [1,2,6,7-³H]testosterone was used as tracer.

Data analysis

Testosterone values were determined from the best-fit straight line of standard curve linearized on logit-log co-ordinates by Hewlett–Packard programmable calculator model 9831 A. The data were compared by Student's '*t*' test.

EFFICACY

Seminological studies

A gradual but non-significant decrease in semen weight, volume and seminal fluid volume was observed up to 60 days of treatment (Fig. 23.1a). Seminal fluid sperm density, vitality and motility decreased gradually to severe oligospermia or azoospermia (Figs 23.1b,c). Animals remained azoospermic throughout the maintenance dose regimen. Sperm abnormalities increased with the duration of treatment (Fig. 23.1c). Semen pH did not change. Semen parameters were within the pretreatment range following 120 days of recovery.

The results revealed reversible inhibition of spermatogenesis following danazol plus TE in langur monkeys. Danazol might exert its effects by (1) inhibition of multiple enzymes of steroidogenesis; (2) inhibition of gonadotropin synthesis and/or release; (3) interaction with androgen and glucocorticoid receptors in target tissues; and (4) alteration of endogenous steroid metabolism (Barbieri et al., 1979). Administration of danazol plus TE exerts a variable but definite inhibitory effect on the pituitary–testicular system, resulting in decreased spermatogenesis (Paulsen and Leonard, 1976). The severe oligospermia or azoospermia which developed within 60 days of treatment and continued during the maintenance phase may be due to either diminished steroidogenesis in the testis or antigonadotropic action of the combination.

Impaired sperm motility is related to inadequate Leydig cell activity resulting in an insufficient androgen supply (MacLeod et al., 1964). A combination drug might affect the process of spermiogenesis and possibly sperm maturation within the epididymis resulting in increased sperm abnormalities along with reduced sperm vitality and motility (MacLeod, 1965; Ulstein et al., 1975; Paulsen and Leonard, 1976). The altered proportion of seminal plasma constituents may also impair functional properties of the spermatozoa (Eliasson et al., 1974; Eliasson, 1982).

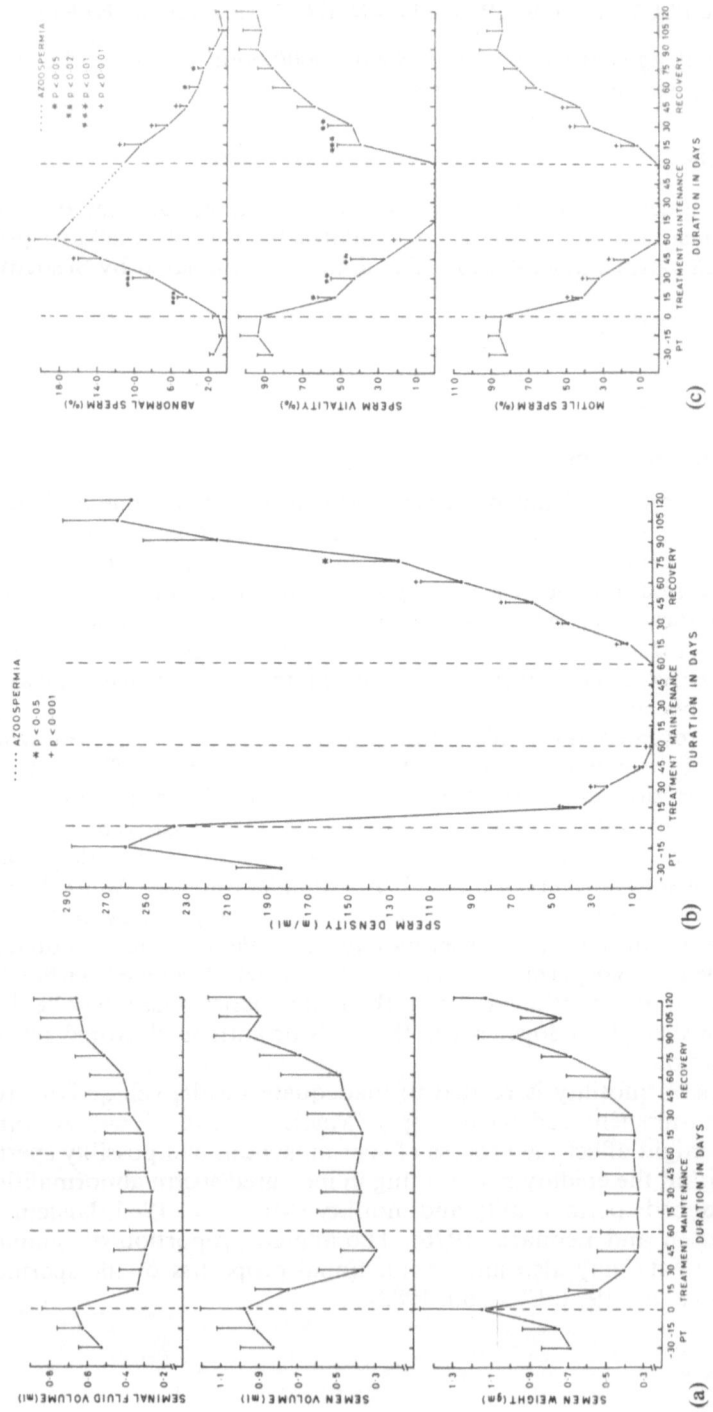

Fig. 23.1 Changes in different seminological variables of langur monkey prior to, during treatment (danazol, 100 mg/day; oral plus TE, 50 mg/15 days; i.m.), maintenance (danazol, 50 mg/day; oral plus TE, 50 mg/15 days; i.m.) and recovery. Each value represents the mean ± SEM (vertical bars). (a) Semen weight, volume and seminal fluid volume during different phases of the study. Changes are non-significant. (b) Changes in the sperm density during different phases of the study. Sperm density reduced progressively to azoospermia on day 15 of maintenance phase. (c) Percentage of motile, vital and abnormal spermatozoa during different phases of the study. Changes are dose dependent.

346

TOXICOLOGY AND SIDE-EFFECTS

Clinical chemistry

No significant alterations were noticed in serum transaminases, alkaline phosphatase, LDH and bilirubin. Haematological variables and serum electrolytes remained normal. These results indicate that there were no drug-related changes in general body metabolism, liver and kidney function. Reversible slight weight gain was expected owing to anabolic properties of both danazol and TE (Paulsen and Leonard, 1976).

Androgenicity

Serum testosterone levels were decreased slightly on days 15, 30 and 60 of treatment (Fig. 23.2). All animals exhibited normal mounting and copulatory behaviour throughout the study. It is evident that circulating levels of testosterone are required for the maintenance of extra-testicular androgen actions, i.e. accessory sex organ function, libido and potency. Slightly decreased weight and volume of semen and seminal fluid might be due to lowered peripheral testosterone level.

Normal mounting and copulatory behaviour and normal response to electrostimulation by all animals throughout the study suggested that the achieved sterility was not due to impaired libido and potency (Skoglund

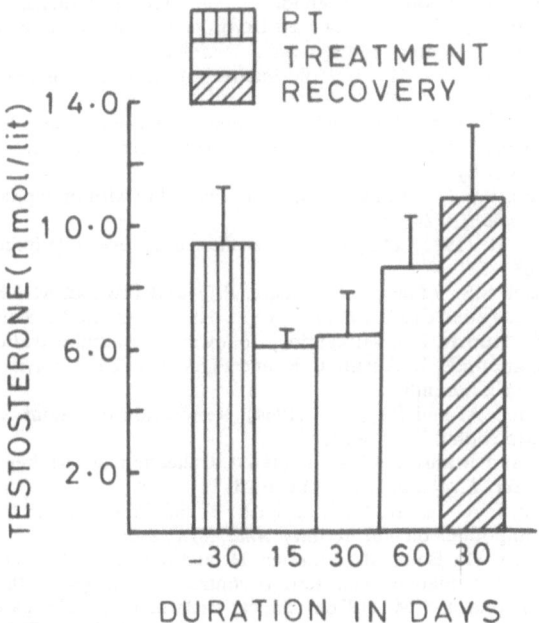

Fig. 23.2 Circulating levels of testosterone during different phases of the study. A non-significant reduction during treatment phase is reversible

and Paulsen, 1973). It is further suggested that the present testosterone level in peripheral blood was adequate to maintain normal androgenicity.

Acknowledgements

This investigation was supported by a grant from the University Grants Commission, New Delhi under Career Award Scheme. Thanks are due to Prof. A.S. Kapoor for his interest in this study and Sterling Winthrop Research Institute, Rensselaer, New York, for the generous gift of danazol.

References

Barbieri, R.L., Lee, H. and Ryan, K.J. (1979). Danazol binding to rat androgen, glucocorticoid, progesterone, and estrogen receptors; Correlation with biologic activity. *Fertil. Steril.*, **31**, 182–6

Belsey, M.A., Eliasson, R., Gallegos, A.J., Moghissi, K.S., Paulsen, C.A. and Prasad, M.R.N. (1980). *Laboratory Manual for the Examination of Human Semen and Semen. Cervical Mucus Interaction*, pp. 1–43 (Singapore: Press Concern)

Cabaud, P.G. and Wroblewski, F. (1958). Colorimetric measurement of lactic dehydrogenase activity of body fluids. *Am. J. Clin. Pathol.*, **30**, 234–6

Dmowski, W.P. (1979). Endocrine properties and clinical application of danazol. *Fertil. Steril.*, **31**, 237–51

Eliasson, R. (1982). Biochemical analysis of human semen. *Int. J. Androl. (Suppl.)*, **5**, 109–19

Eliasson, R., Johnsen, O. and Lindholmer, C. (1974). Effects of seminal plasma on some functional properties of human spermatozoa. In Mancini, R.E. and Martini, L. (eds.) *Male Fertility and Sterility*, pp. 107–22 (New York: Academic Press)

Faundes, A., Brache, V., Leon, P., Schmidt, F. and Alvarez-Sanchez, F. (1981). Sperm suppression with monthly injections of medroxyprogesterone acetate combined with testosterone enanthate at a high dose (500 mg). *Int. J. Androl.*, **4**, 235–45

Fiske, C.H. and Subbarow, Y. (1925). Colorimetric determination of phosphorous. *J. Biol. Chem.*, **66**, 375–400

Frick, J. and Bartsch, G. (1976). Reversible inhibition of spermatogenesis by various steroidal compounds. In Hafez, E.S.E. (ed.) *Human Semen and Fertility Regulation in Men*, pp. 533–42 (St Louis: C.V. Mosby)

King, E.J. and Coxon, V.J. (1950). Determination of bilirubin with precipitation of the plasma proteins. *J. Clin. Pathol.*, **3**, 248–59

Lotz, W. and Krause, R. (1981). Dihydrotestosterone causes reversible infertility in male rats. *Fertil. Steril.*, **35**, 691–5

Lynch, M.J., Raphael, S.S., Mellor, L.D., Spare, P.D. and Inwood, M.J.H. (1969). *Medical Laboratory Technology and Clinical Pathology*, pp. 619–753. (London: Saunders)

MacLeod, J. (1965). Human seminal cytology following the administration of certain antispermatogenic compounds. In Austin, C.R. and Perry, J.S. (eds.) *Agents Affecting Fertility*, pp. 93–123 (London: Churchill)

MacLeod, J., Pazianos, A. and Ray, B.S. (1964). Restoration of human spermatogenesis by menopausal gonadotrophins. *Lancet*, **1**, 1196–7

Mastroianni, L. Jr. and Manson, W.A. Jr. (1963). Collection of monkey semen by electroejaculation. *Proc. Soc. Exp. Biol. Med.*, **112**, 1025–7

Neumann, F., Diallo, F.A., Hasan, S.H., Schenck, B. and Traore, I. (1976). The influence of pharmaceutical compounds on male fertility. *Andrologia*, **8**, 203–35

Nieschlag, E., Hoogen, H., Bolk, M., Schuster, H. and Wickings, E.J. (1978). Clinical trial with testosterone undecanoate for male fertility control. *Contraception*, **18**, 607–14

Paulsen, C.A. and Leonard, J.M. (1976). Clinical trials in reversible male contraception. I. Combination of danazol plus testosterone. In Spilman, C.H., Lobl, T.J. and Kirton, K.T. (eds.) *Regulatory Mechanisms of Male Reproductive Physiology*, pp. 197–211 (Amsterdam: Excerpta Medica)

Reitman, S. and Frankel, S. (1957). A colorimetric method for the determination of serum glutamic oxalacetic and glutamic pyruvic transaminases. *Am. J. Clin. Pathol.*, **28**, 56-63

Sherins, R.J., Gandy, H.M., Thorslund, T.W. and Paulsen, C.A. (1971). Pituitary and testicular function studies. I. Experience with a new gonadal inhibitor, 17α-pregn-4-en-20-yno-(2,3-d)isoxazol-17-ol (Danazol). *J. Clin. Endocrinol. Metab.*, **32**, 522-31

Skoglund, R.D. and Paulsen, C.A. (1973). Danazol-testosterone combination: a potentially effective means for reversible male contraception. A preliminary report. *Contraception*, **7**, 357-65

Ulstein, M., Netto, N., Leonard, J. and Paulsen, C.A. (1975). Changes in sperm morphology in normal men treated with danazol and testosterone. *Contraception*, **12**, 437-44

Victor, R.J. and Lauersen, N.H. (1982). Danazol—a versatile pharmacologic agent. *Fertil. Steril.*, **37**, 475-7

WHO (1981). Programme for the provision of matched assay reagents for the radioimmunoassay of hormones in reproductive physiology. *WHO Method Manual*, 5th Edn, pp. 1-66

24
Inhibin and male contraception

A.R. SHETH, B.S. SARVAMANGALA, K.A. KRISHNAN and G.R. VANAGE

The development of a safe and effective new male contraceptive is a major goal of current reproductive research. The increased interest in a hormonal male contraceptive is due to the widely publicized side-effects of regular female hormonal contraceptives which make them less attractive. A male contraceptive agent should cause azoospermia without impairment of libido and potency although administration of low doses of androgens completely arrests spermatogenesis, high dosages must be carefully considered because of some severe side-effects. An approach to male contraception would be the use of 'inhibin' a gonadal peptide, that selectively inhibits the secretion of FSH by the pituitary. This chapter describes our efforts to purify and characterize this peptide.

GONADOTROPINS AND TESTICULAR FUNCTION

Endocrine control of spermatogenesis is a complex process requiring the presence of follicle stimulating hormone (FSH) and high intratesticular levels of testosterone. The relative contribution of FSH and testosterone to the spermatogenic process is still not clear. Leydig cells are the target cells for luteinizing hormone (LH) and Sertoli cells for FSH (Steinberger et al., 1979). The action of LH on Leydig cells results in the secretion of testosterone which is required for normal spermatogenesis (Steinberger, 1981; Steinberger et al., 1973). The action of FSH on Sertoli cells triggers a series of events to protein synthesis (Means, 1971; Steinberger, 1975). One of the proteins secreted by Sertoli cells is androgen binding protein (ABP) which helps maintain high androgen concentration in the tubule and promote cytological differentiation of the epithelium of the epididymis (Hansson et al., 1975; Rosenberg, 1981).

FSH is required for the initiation of spermatogenesis during the first wave and may not be required for its maintenance (Raj et al., 1978, Nandedkar et al., 1982). High intratesticular testosterone concentration is required for the completion of meiosis in the rat (Steinberger and Duckett, 1967). In adult rats, FSH supports spermatogenesis, multiplication and

351

differentiation (Courot *et al.*, 1971; Vernon *et al.*, 1975). Dual pathways may operate here (Clermont and Harvey, 1967; Dym *et al.*, 1979), since testosterone was able to maintain or restore spermatogenesis (Harries *et al.*, 1977). Quantitative analysis revealed that undifferentiated type A (A_0-A_2) spermatogenesis is sustained by testosterone, but it only partially restores A_3 to intermediate spermatogonial multiplication (Chowdhary, 1979). Qualitative spermatogenesis can be maintained in the rat despite low levels of intratesticular testosterone (Cunning and Huckins, 1979).

In the human there is no conclusive evidence that any stage of spermatogenesis may be independent of gonadotropins, and both FSH and testosterone are required for the maintenance of spermatogenesis in adult male.

INHIBIN

The secretion of FSH is partially regulated by the negative feedback effect of gonadal steroids. Steroids not only suppress FSH secretion, but also LH secretion. A testicular factor implicated in the negative feedback control of FSH secretion has been named inhibin by McCullagh (1932). Experimental evidence for the existence of inhibin has been provided only in the past few years.

Sources

Inhibin is found in several different sources, including seminal plasma, rete testis fluid, spermatozoa and follicular fluid of various species (Franchimont *et al.*, 1979).

Purification and characterization

Substances with inhibin like activity have been isolated from the gonads and their secretions of several species (Hafez, 1980; de Jong, 1979a). Inhibin has been isolated additionally from human seminal plasma (Thakur *et al.*, 1981), sheep testes (Moodbidri *et al.*, 1976), ovaries (Vijayalakshmi *et al.*, 1980a) and human placenta (Bandivdekar *et al.*, 1981). No homology has been established between the various preparations. It is generally accepted that inhibin is a non-steroidal, water-soluble, trypsin sensitive peptidic or proteinaceous substance. The molecular size of this peptide has not yet been determined with certainty. The apparent disparity in the molecular size may be due to the existence of multiple forms of inhibin, polymer formation, association with the carrier protein or differences in the purification procedures employed (Krishnan *et al.*, 1982). The variability could be due to proteolysis of inhibin occurring during purification with conventional materials (Channing and Franchimont, 1981).

Inhibin obtained from human seminal plasma and placenta is of high molecular weight, whereas that from sheep testes and ovaries are low-molecular-weight peptides, this typical purification procedure is depicted in Fig 24.1.

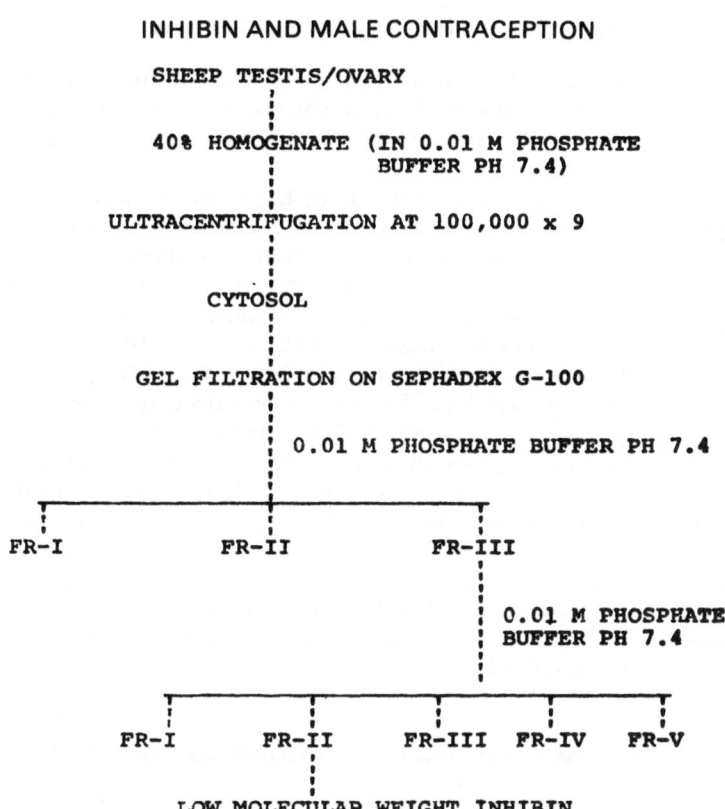

Fig. 24.1   Flow chart for the purification procedure employed for sheep testis and ovary

Bioassay and radioimmunoassay for inhibin

In the purification of any hormone, a suitable assay is required to check the biological activity at various steps. Suppression of FSH secretion is the common end point in the systems described for the detection of inhibin activity. Most of the *in vivo* systems used, detect rather than measure inhibin activity. The various *in vivo* assays are: (a) FSH suppression in intact rats and short and long-term castrated rats or in large animal models such as sheep and monkey; (b) inhibition of FSH augmentation (Hudson *et al.*, 1979). *In vivo* assays are laborious, time consuming and lack precision because elicitation of response is largely dependent on dose, route of administration of test material, and age and physiological status of animal. *In vitro* bioassays for inhibin have also been developed using pituitary halves or culture of dispersed pituitary cells, either in the presence or absence of GnRH (de Jong *et al.*, 1976). Scott *et al.* (1980) reported a simple and rapid *in vitro* bioassay for inhibin based on inhibition of a cellular FSH content using ovine testicular lymph protein preparation as a standard. Specificity, reproducibility, precision, simplicity and large capacity of the assay system makes it more advantageous over other bioassay systems. Recently, Ramasharma *et al.* (1981) developed an *in vitro* bioassay using the mouse whole pituitary in short-term incubation at 37°C. The inhibition of FSH and/or LH release was measured by a specific radioreceptor assay. An estimation of inhibition of bioactive (binding activity) FSH release can be obtained within 24 h.

A sensitive and specific radioimmunoassay has been developed for human seminal plasma inhibin (Vaze et al., 1979). The antibody to inhibin, raised in rabbit by active immunization, had an affinity constant (K_a) of 2.379×10^9 M^{-1}. The assay sensitivity was 1-2 ng/tube and the intra and interassay coefficients of variation were 5-7% and 15% respectively. The recovery for inhibin added to the serum of a castrated man was 95-110%. The antisera raised against inhibin was capable of neutralizing the endogenous inhibin activity resulting in increased FSH levels. It has been demonstrated that antiserum to bovine seminal plasma inhibin provokes a significant increase in FSH levels in serum of intact adult male rats (Franchimont et al., 1977). The antisera against inhibin (high molecular weight) could neutralize the biological activity of low-molecular-weight inhibin from ram testis (Vijay-alakshmi et al., 1981). This suggests that there can be more than one molecular species having an immunologically similar site. The development of an RIA has served as a powerful tool for monitoring purification, measurement of inhibin in other body fluids and tissues, and for under-standing its physiological role.

Cell types involved in synthesis or biotransformation of inhibin

Several investigators consider late spermatids or Sertoli cell/spermatid associations as the source of inhibin (Davies et al., 1978; Dematrova, 1978). Others have attributed Sertoli cell and/or spermatogonia as the likely source of inhibin secretion (Krueger et al., 1974). Although there is direct evidence for the production of inhibin by Sertoli cells in culture (Steinberger and Steinberger, 1976), this does not rule out the possibility of the involvement of the other cell types in inhibin production. Using enriched fractions of various testicular types, Sheth et al. (1981a) have shown that the spermatid-enriched fraction exhibits high inhibin activity as assessed by bioassay and RIA methods. Subsequently, receptors for inhibin have been identified in spermatids (Dandekar et al., 1983), suggesting that inhibin may be concentrated in spermatids rather than being synthesized.

Receptors for inhibin

Inhibin acts directly on pituitary cells to control FSH secretion, and re-ceptors for inhibin have been identified in the pituitary tissue (Sairam et al., 1981; Vanage and Sheth, 1982). The receptors are specific since, other hor-mones like FSH, LH, PRL and LHRH failed to displace the labelled inhibin from the membranes.

The occurrence of immunoreactive inhibin in human prostate has been reported, which is similar to inhibin isolated from human seminal plasma

(Sheth *et al.*, 1981b). Recently, specific receptors to inhibin have been demonstrated in human prostate (Phadke *et al.*, 1982). These observations indicate that inhibin may be concentrated in the prostate, but it is not known whether the prostate synthesizes it. Inhibin also binds specifically to rat ventral prostate. Accordingly a sensitive and specific radioreceptor assay has been developed. The binding of inhibin was a saturable process with an association constant of 2.3×10^{11} M^{-1}. Other hormones such as LH, FSH, PRL and TSH from rat and human origin failed to inhibit the binding of inhibin to rat ventral prostate. The assay sensitivity was 5 ng/tube. The

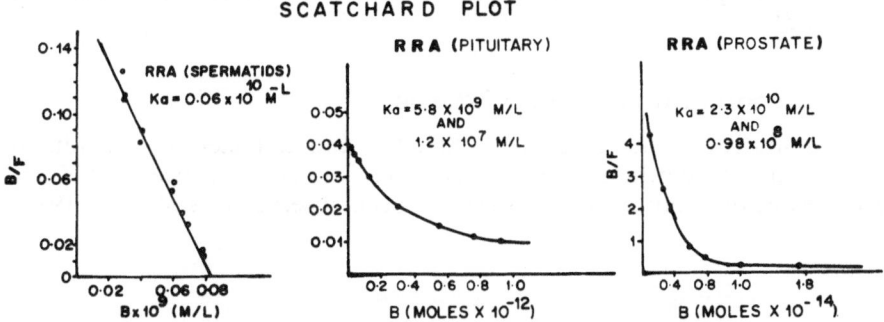

Fig. 24.2 Scatchard analysis of the inhibin radioreceptor assay data. The ordinate represents bound/free ration of inhibin and the abscissa indicates the total bound inhibin

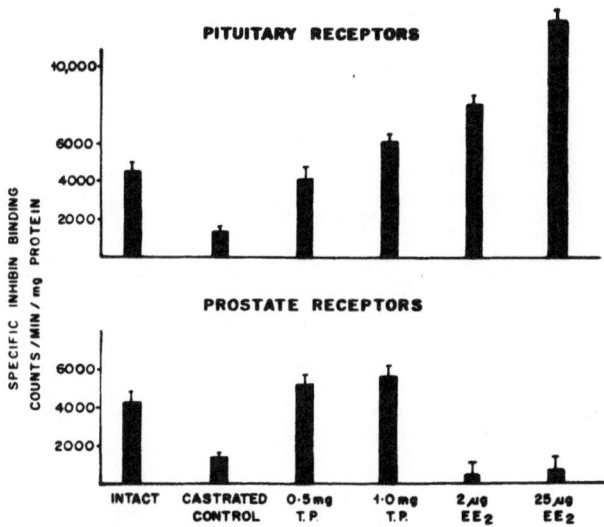

Fig. 24.3 Effect of testosterone propionate and oestradiol on the binding of inhibin to rat prostate and pituitary membrane preparation. Adult male rats were castrated for 24 h and injected subcutaneously with testosterone or oestradiol for 10 days. Control rats received olive oil. 24 h after the last injection animals were killed and prostate and pituitary glands were removed

specific binding of inhibin to rat prostate obtained from animals of different age groups revealed that the maximum binding was observed using prostate of 75 day old rats. Only those fractions in the purification scheme which had inhibin activity as detected in *in vivo* bioassay, also competed for the binding. This sensitivity, specificity and precision ($p < 0.002$) as well as quickness will make possible its use as a suitable assay for detection as well as quantitation of inhibin activity. Inhibin has greater affinity for prostate than pituitary and spermatids (Fig. 24.2). The preliminary experiments indicated that testosterone was involved in controlling inhibin receptors at the prostatic level whereas, oestradiol had no effect. However, oestradiol increased the pituitary sensitivity for inhibin as compared to testosterone (Fig. 24.3).

Factors regulating inhibin synthesis

In vitro studies in rat reveal that FSH, LH and testosterone individually regulate inhibin synthesis/secretion. A synergistic action between FSH and testosterone on inhibin secretion has also been observed (Steinberger, 1980).

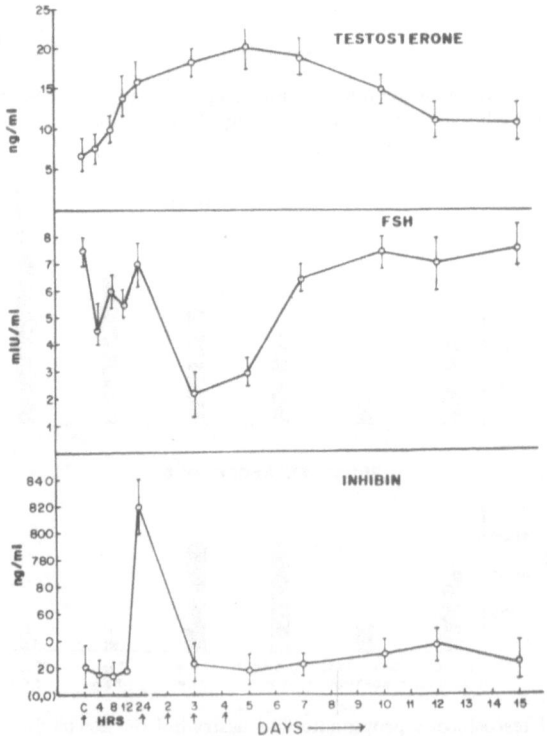

Fig. 24.4 Effect of hCG on serum FSH, testosterone and inhibin levels. hCG (1000 IU per day for 5 days) was injected intramuscularly into male volunteers and blood samples were collected 4 h after the last injection. (n = 6)

In females FSH, LH and DHT seem to regulate inhibin secretion (Channing *et al.*, 1981). An increase in serum and ovarian inhibin levels induced by PMSG has been observed in immature female rats (Lee and Findley, 1982). Administration of hCG to male volunteers increased inhibin levels 24 h later, followed by a suppression in FSH levels at 72 h (Fig. 24.4). When testosterone was injected a sharp increase in serum and seminal plasma inhibin levels were observed on days 8 and 12 respectively (Fig. 24.5). Injection of Sertoli cell medium treated with DHT showed no inhibin activity (Nagendranath *et al.*, 1982).

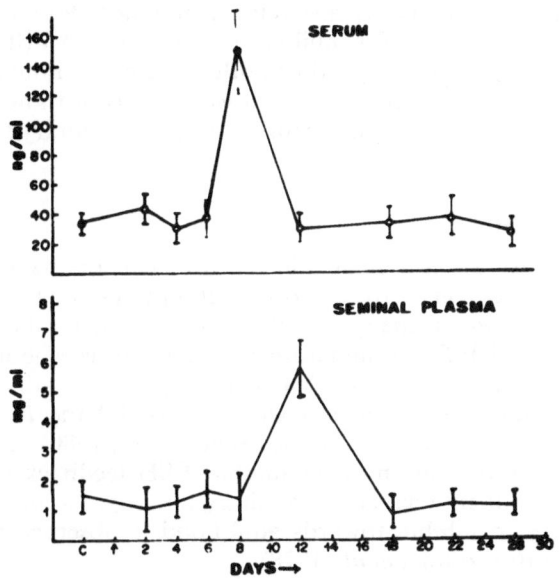

Fig. 24.5 Effect of single injection of testosterone enanthate (250 mg) on serum and seminal plasma inhibin levels in male volunteers. Blood and seminal plasma samples were collected on alternate days for the first 15 days and once a week for two weeks. (n = 6)

PHYSIOLOGY OF INHIBIN

Localization

Although FSH is required for the initiation of spermatogenesis at puberty and for the reinitiation of spermatogenesis in the adult, it is not clear whether the secretion of inhibin is stage of spermatogenesis dependent. Using immunofluorescent localization of inhibin it has been shown that a shift in the distribution of inhibin from extratubular to intratubular occurs during maturation. In the adult testis, inhibin is distributed in the basal compartment in tubules devoid of spermatozoa and spermatids but in adluminal compartment in tubules with spermatozoa. Such a relationship is suggestive of an inhibin feedback effect (Johnson *et al.*, 1981).

357

Metabolic half life

The duration of hormonal effect is dependent on the hormone metabolism rate. Studies of the half life ($T_{\frac{1}{2}}$) and metabolic clearance rate (MCR) for inhibin show that $T_{\frac{1}{2}}$ is shorter in adult rats than in immature rats. The MCR of inhibin is faster in adult rats than in immature rats. The specific uptake of labelled inhibin by the pituitary is higher in immature rats than adult rats. *In vitro* studies have shown that inhibin binding to pituitary plasma membrane obtained from immature rats was greater than from adult rats (Vanage *et al.*, 1980). The uptake of inhibin by the pituitary of adult and immature animals is age related and not dose related. These results suggest a critical role for inhibin in the control of FSH secretion in immature animals. The pineal gland of both mature and immature rats has also been observed to take up inhibin. However, it is not known if inhibin plays an active role in extra-hypothalamic control of pituitary function.

Age and sex difference

During sexual maturation a change in sensitivity of the feedback between gonadal steroids and gonadotropins occurs (Gupta *et al.*, 1975). Studies of FSH and inhibin levels in the serum of developing male rats revealed high levels of inhibin and FSH in immature rats. The levels of both substances decline with maturity. The FSH released in response to administration of antiserum to inhibin also decreased with age as did the *in vitro* binding capacity of pituitary plasma membrane (Sheth *et al.*, 1980). These observations show that the regulation of the inhibin–FSH feedback relationship is related to age-dependent changes in pituitary binding. An increase in sensitivity of pituitary to inhibin towards adulthood is observed in the female but not in male rats (de Jong *et al.*, 1978).

Accessory reproductive organ function

Using a sensitive and specific RIA, immunoreactive inhibin has been detected in rat seminal vesicles and epididymis and human prostate (Table 24.1). Prostate exhibited a very much higher content of inhibin than testis. Inhibin is absorbed by the epididymis which passes through it and enters

Table 24.1 Inhibin activity in human reproductive tissues by RIA

Source	Inhibin (ng/mg *protein* mean ± SE)
Testis	36.2 ± 12.6
Epididymis	28.1 ± 4.77
Seminal vesicles	72.0 ± 12.0
Prostate (normal)	158 ± 34
Benign prostatic hypertrophy	1366 ± 560
Prostate (after castration)	38 ± 15

circulation. The significance of high concentration of inhibin in the prostate is not understood.

Higher levels of inhibin have been observed in patients with benign prostatic hyperplasia and in prostatic cancer than in normal controls. Determination of inhibin levels may therefore, serve as a therapeutic tool to monitor prostate disease.

BIOLOGICAL ACTION

Pituitary

It has now been established that inhibin affects the pituitary synthesis and release of FSH. Much of the data has come from *in vitro* studies using dispersed pituitary cells (Steinberger and Steinberger, 1976; de Jong *et al.*, 1979). Inhibin suppresses FSH secretion both in the presence and absence of LHRH. There is a significant decrease in the LHRH–induced FSH release in animals pretreated with low-molecular-weight ovarian or testicular inhibin (Vijayalakshmi *et al.*, 1980). *In vitro* pituitary response to LHRH indicated a significant increase in both FSH and LH in LHRH-treated groups as compared to controls. At both 50 μg and 100 μg dose levels of ovarian inhibin, there is a significant suppression of FSH (Table 24.2).

Table 24.2   Effect of inhibin on LHRH induced release of FSH and LH *in vitro*

Dose	FSH (ng/ml medium $\pm$ SEM)	LH (ng/ml medium $\pm$ SEM)
Control	1.59 $\pm$ 0.18	1.46 $\pm$ 0.27
LHRH	5.73 $\pm$ 0.43	11.2 $\pm$ 1.3
Ovarian inhibin		
50 μg	4.1 $\pm$ 0.22*	11.0 $\pm$ 0.9
100 μg	3.23 $\pm$ 0.24**	12.18 $\pm$ 1.55

(n = 4); *$p < 0.05$; **$p < 0.1$

However, LH levels remained unaffected, whereas other investigators have reported that bovine testicular extracts or ram rete testis fluid preferentially suppresses FSH but may equally reduce LH secretion when administered in doses higher than those inducing significant decreases in FSH (Franchimont *et al.*, 1975, 1977). Purified ram ovarian inhibin produces a selective suppression of LHRH–induced FSH levels at both the 50 μg and 100 μg dose levels.

Both *in vivo* and *in vitro* studies reveal that either ovarian or testicular inhibin acts at the pituitary level by interfering with the action of LHRH. The interaction of LHRH and inhibin is reversible at the pituitary level (Rush and Lipner, 1979). Inhibin suppresses the binding of labelled LHRH to pituitary receptors both *in vivo* and *in vitro* (Sheth *et al.*, 1981).

The studies of inhibin and TRH at the pituitary level showed that TRH blocks the effect of inhibin on FSH release while inhibin delays the pituitary

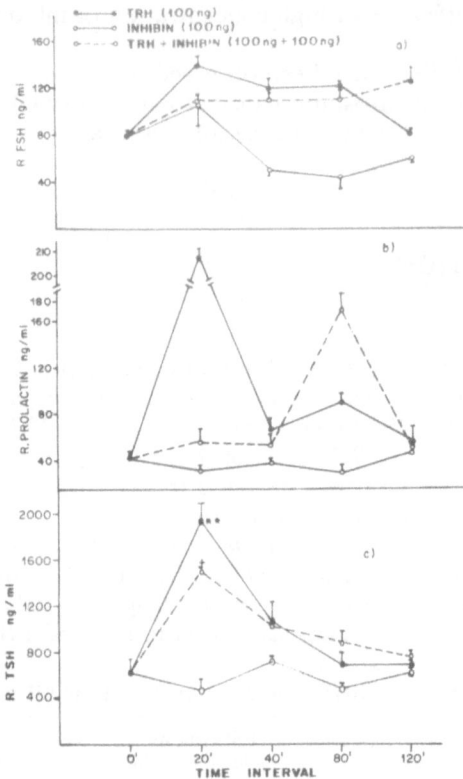

Fig. 24.6 *In vivo* responsiveness of pituitary to TRH, inhibin and inhibin + TRH in terms of circulating FSH (a), PRL (b), and TSH (c) levels. Values are expressed as means ± SD (n = 5)

responsiveness to TRH (Fig. 24.6). Human seminal plasma inhibin (100 ng) administered along with TRH (100 ng) to adult male rats delayed *in vivo* pituitary release of PRl into the serum (Fig. 24.6b). It also lowered the induced TSH levels in serum, thereby decreasing the sensitivity of the pituitary gland to TRH (Fig. 24.6c). Inhibin alone did not alter either the serum PRL and TSH levels although it suppressed serum FSH levels. Inhibin's effect on FSH release was blocked by TRH (Fig. 24.6a), indicating that inhibin may influence the responsiveness of the pituitary to TRH.

Inhibin reverses completely the stimulatory effect of oestrogen on LHRH-induced LH and FSH secretion. The control of gonadotropin secretion in the intact animal may be dependent on the modulatory role of sex steroid and inhibin and their interaction with LHRH (Lagace *et al.*, 1979).

Hypothalamus

Inhibin may act at the hypothalamic level. Interference of inhibin with the

Table 24.3 Effect of ovarian inhibin on hypothalamic LHRH content

Dose	LHRH (ng/*hypothalamus* ± *SEM*	FSH (ng/ml ± *SEM*)	LH (ng/ml ± *SEM*)
Control	2.58 ± 0.06 (4)	2.83 ± 0.05 (4)	1.28 ± 0.06 (4)
Ovarian inhibin 300 μg	1.72 ± 0.08* (5)	2.22 ± 0.05** (5)	1.24 ± 0.05 (5)

*$p < 0.001$; **$p < 0.05$; numbers in parentheses are the number of observations

production of hypothetical FSH-RH has been suggested (Lugaro *et al.*, 1974; LeLannou and Chambon, 1977). Compared to controls ovarian inhibin treated rats have decreased hypothalamic LHRH content (Table 24.3). More recently, Lumpkin *et al.* (1981) described the evidence for a hypothalamic site of action of inhibin from rete testis fluid to suppress FSH release.

Gonads

A variety of relatively low as well as high-molecular-weight inhibin preparations have been reported from gonads. None of these inhibitors however, have been tested for their *in vivo* effect at the gonadal level. Simultaneous administration of labelled FSH (10 ng) along with inhibin (50 μg) inhibits the *in vivo* uptake of labelled FSH by immature rat testis (Vanage *et al.*, 1980). Inhibin preparations from human seminal plasma, ram testis and ovaries have been found to inhibit the ^{125}I-labelled hFSH binding to testicular receptors (Moodbidri *et al.*, 1980; Vijayalakshmi *et al.*, 1981). Further, a dose-dependent inhibition of cAMP accumulation parallels the reduction in FSH binding (Vijayalakshmi *et al.*, 1980b).

An inhibition kinetic study by Lineweaver–Burk analysis revealed that the low-molecular-weight inhibin acts as a competitive binder, thus preventing the interaction of FSH to testicular receptors. The K_d value for FSH binding in the absence of inhibin was 1.34×10^{-9} M. Inhibin enhances the cAMP-PDE activity in testicular tissue from immature rat testis. However, PDE activity in adult rat testis was not affected by FSH over various concentrations studied. Inhibin may have a function during gonadal development and differentiation, but once maturity is attained, it may play only a limited role.

Franchimont *et al.* (1981) observed inhibin inhibition of testicular DNA synthesis both *in vivo* and *in vitro*. Inhibin may also interfere with protein synthesis. Preliminary studies indicate that ram testicular inhibin affects the transcriptional process in a cell-free system using a calf thymus DNA template.

INHIBIN LEVELS IN INFERTILE CASES

The cause of infertility cannot be easily identified in many men. This may be due to the wide spectrum of abnormalities of semen and seminiferous tubules as well as involvement of more than one pathogenic process. Abnormal spermatogenesis, abnormal Leydig cell function and abnormal pituitary function occur in varying degrees in most types of infertility. In patients with oligospermia, FSH levels are either elevated or normal (Setchell *et al.*, 1977). Both groups show supranormal FSH response to LHRH, which has been interpreted as decreased secretion of a tubular factor that inhibits FSH secretion. In several species seminal plasma exhibits inhibin like activity. Hence patients with severe tubular damage and raised FSH levels should show reduced inhibin activity in seminal plasma. With the availability of sensitive and specific RIA for inhibin (Vaze *et al.*, 1979) semen samples of infertile patients have been screened for inhibin levels. The results indicate higher inhibin levels in serum and semen of normospermic men than in oligospermic, vasectomized and Klinefelter's syndrome subjects (Ash *et al.*, 1980). No direct correlation was observed between inhibin levels in serum or semen with number of sperm in the ejaculate (Vaze *et al.*, 1979).

Using a bioassay, Scott and Burger (1980) have demonstrated the absence of inhibin in azoospermic men, which is consistent with a relationship between tubular damage and decreased production of inhibin.

CORRELATION BETWEEN TESTICULAR BIOPSY, INHIBIN AND FSH CONCENTRATIONS

Testicular biopsy provides important information about the integrity of the seminiferous tubule. Serum FSH levels are elevated in patients with severely damaged seminiferous tubules when spermatids are absent (Franchimont *et al.*, 1972). An inverse relationship exists between serum FSH concentrations and the mean number of spermatogonia (de Kretser *et al.*, 1974). This has been supported by the finding that the Vitamin A-deficient rat has normal FSH levels despite loss of cell types other than spermatogonia (Krueger *et al.*, 1974).

Our studies indicate an inverse relationship between serum FSH and inhibin levels in patients with germinal arrest at the primary spermatocytes and spermatid stages (Fig. 24.7). Hence, measurement of inhibin levels could be used as an important tool in the diagnosis of infertility.

CONTRACEPTIVE EFFECT

Interest in the inhibin hypothesis has been generated by the need to develop a suitable male contraceptive which will not affect libido and potency. Since inhibin preferentially inhibits FSH secretion without affecting LH, it may fulfill the basic requirements of a contraceptive agent.

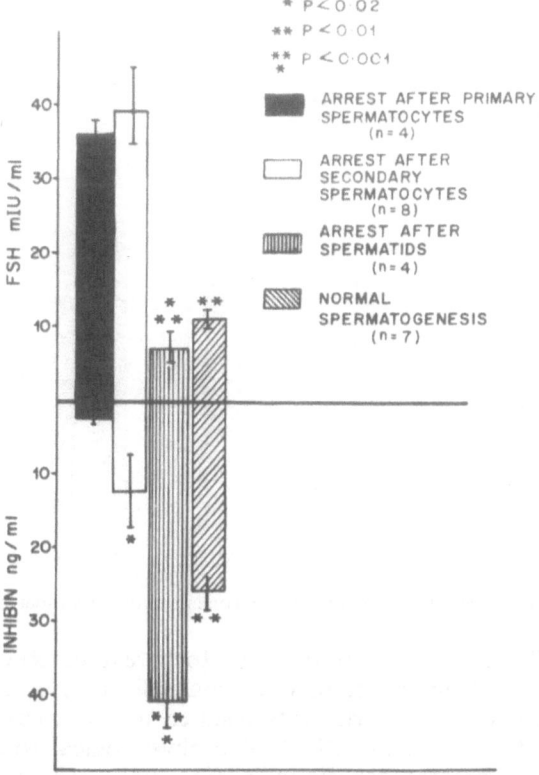

Fig. 24.7 Comparison between the levels of inhibin and FSH in serum obtained from infertile patients

Inhibin alone

Studies of the long-term effect of inhibin on testicular function has been limited. Davies *et al.* (1979) did not find any change in testicular sperm count in adult male rats after treatment with a crude preparation of inhibin from rete testis fluid for 90 days. In contrast to their report, our study has revealed a decrease in both testicular and epididymal sperm count, when a low-molecular-weight inhibin preparation from ram testes was injected for 30 days (Fig. 24.8). This could be due to a direct action of inhibin at the testicular level in addition to its effect on FSH secretion.

Inhibin + testosterone

In order to evaluate the effect of inhibin enhancement in combination with testosterone, inhibin was administered along with a 2.5 cm testosterone implant or 50 µg/day of testosterone propionate (Fig. 24.8). With both the combinations, greater suppression of sperm count was observed.

A decrease in preleptotene and pachytene spermatocytes in adult rats

MALE FERTILITY AND ITS REGULATION

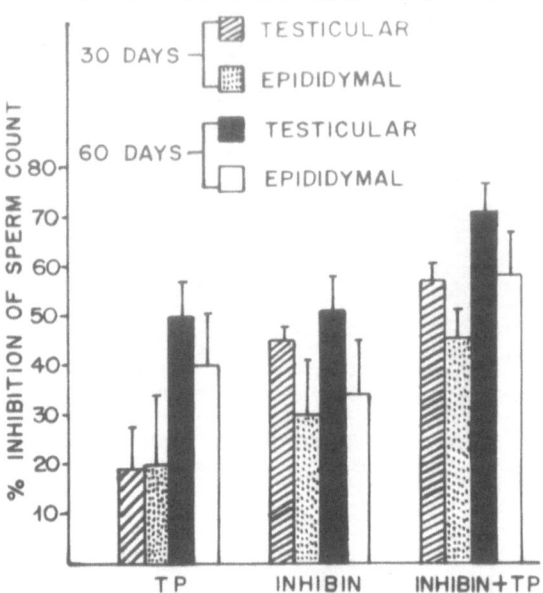

Fig. 24.8   Effect of inhibin and testosterone propionate on sperm count

treated with RTF has been reported by Hochereau-de Reviers (1981). In addition, RTF acted on spermatogonial multiplication in adult rat testes. Inhibin treatment of prepubertal rats resulted in a decrease in pachytene spermatocytes (de Jong *et al.*, 1978). The physiological role of inhibin in the regulation of spermatogenesis in mature males will be clarified once pure preparations of inhibin become available.

CONCLUDING REMARKS

Inhibin, a peptidic factor that lowers the rate of follicle stimulating hormone (FSH) secretion, has been purified from gonads of different species and human placenta. A sensitive and specific radioimmunoassay for inhibin has been developed, by which the amount of inhibin in various biological fluids and tissues was measured. The seminal and serum inhibin concentrations in normospermic subjects were significantly higher than those of oligospermic, vasectomized, Klinefelter's syndrome, Sertoli cell-only syndrome subjects. An inverse relationship exists between serum FSH and inhibin concentrations in patients with germinal arrest at primary spermatocytes and spermatid stage. Prostate exhibited a very high content of inhibin which was greater than in testis. Greater than normal inhibin levels were observed in patients with benign prostatic hyperplasia and in prostatic cancer. The half-life of inhibin was much shorter in adult rats than in immature rats. The metabolic clearance rate of inhibin was much faster in adult rats than in immature rats. Specific receptors for inhibin were observed in pituitary, prostate and spermatids. However, inhibin receptor affinity was greater in prostate than pituitary or spermatids.

Testosterone as well as hCG is involved in the regulation of circulating inhibin levels in male volunteers. Inhibin reduces the LHRH synthesis at the hypothalamic level. Inhibin reduced LHRH-induced FSH secretion at the pituitary level. The interaction of TRH and inhibin at the pituitary level revealed that TRH blocks the effect of inhibin on FSH release and inhibin in turn, delayed pituitary responsiveness to TRH. Inhibin inhibits the binding of FSH to testicular receptor at the gonadal level and acts as a competitive binder. Further, it affects the transcriptional process in the cell free system. Apart from Sertoli cells, the germ cells may also secrete inhibin as high amounts of bioactive and immunoreactive inhibin were found in spermatid-enriched fractions of rat testis extract. There was a decrease in both testicular and epididymal sperm count with the injection of inhibin for a longer period in adult male rats. The effect was more pronounced with combination of inhibin and testosterone. Apart from its possible contraceptive application in the male, inhibin shows the role of FSH in reproductive disorders.

References

Ash, R.H., Vaze, A.Y., Thakur, A.N. and Sheth, A.R. (1980). Concentration of immunoreactive inhibin in seminal plasma and serum from normospermic, oligospermic, vasectomized, Klinefelter's syndrome and Sertoli-cell-only syndrome subject. *J. Androl.* **1**, 252-4

Bandivdekar, A., Vijayalakshmi, S., Jaswaney, V. and Sheth, A.R. (1981). Inhibin in human placenta. *Ind. J. Exp. Biol.*, **19**, 744-5

Channing, C.P., Anderson, L.D. and Hoover, D.J. (1981). Hormonal control of granulosa cell secretion of oocyte maturation inhibitor and inhibin-F activity. In Rolland, R., van Hall, E.V., Hillier, S.G., McNatty, K.P. and Schoemarker, J. (eds.) *Proceedings of IV Renier D. Graaf Symposium on Follicular Maturation and Ovulation*, pp. 219-23 (Amsterdam-Oxford-Princeton: Excerpta Medica)

Channing, C.P. and Franchimont, P. (1981). Some concluding remarks on the subject of intragonadal regulation of reproduction. In Franchimont, P. and Channing, E.P. (eds.) *Intragonadal Regulation of Reproduction*, pp. 419-23 (London, New York, Toronto, Sydney, San Franisco)

Chowdhary, A.K. (1979). Dependence of testicular germ cell hormone: A quantitative study in hypophysectomized testosterone-treated rats. *J. Endocrinol.*, **82**, 331-40

Clermont, Y. and Harvey, S.C. (1967). Effect of hormones on spermatogenesis of immature rats. *Biol. Reprod.*, **14**, 332-8

Courot, M., Ortavant, R., de-Reviers, M.M. (1971). Variations due controle gonadotrope du testicule selon. *L'age des animaxo Exp. Anim.*, **4**, 201-11

Cunning, G.R. and Huckins, C. (1979). Persistence of complete spermatogenesis in the presence of low intratesticular concentrations of testosterone. *Endocrinology*, **105**, 177-86

Dandekar, S.P., Sheth, A.R. and Ghosh, D. (1983). Presence of specific receptor binding sites for inhibin in rat spermatids. *Andrologia*, **14**, 274-8

Davies, R.V., Main, S.J., Laurie, M.S. and Setchell, B.P. (1979). The effect of long-term administration of either a crude inhibin preparation or an antiserum to FSH on serum hormone levels, testicular function and fertility of adult male rats. *J. Reprod. Fertil. Suppl.*, **26**, 183-91

Davies, R.V., Main, S.J. and Setchell, B.P. (1978). Inhibin: evidence for its existence, methods of bioassay and nature of active material. *Int. J. Androl. Suppl.*, **2**, 102-14

de Jong, F.H. (1979). Inhibin—Fact or Artifact. *Mol. Cell. Endocrinol.*, **13**, 1-10 de Jong, F.H., Smith, S.D. and Van der Molen (1979). Bioassay of inhibin like activity using pituitary cells *in vitro*. *J. Endocrinol.*, **80**, 91–102

de Jong, F.H., Welschen, R., Hermans, W.R., Smith, S.D. and Van der Molen, H.J. (1978). Effect of testicular and ovarian inhibin like activity in using *in-vitro* and *in-vivo* systems. *Int. J. Androl. Suppl.*, **2**, 125–38

de Kretser, D.M., Burger, H.G. and Hudson, B. (1974). The relationship between germinal cells and serum FSH levels in males with infertility. *J. Clin. Endocrinol. Metab.*, **38**, 787–93

Dematrova, M. (1978). Localization of inhibin. In *Proceedings of the IV International Symposium on Immunology of Reproduction*. Varna

Dym, M., Raj, H.G.M., Lin, Y.C., Chemes, H.E., Kotite, N.J., Nayfeh, S.N. and French, F.S. (1979). Is FSH required for maintenance of spermatogenesis in adult rats? *J. Reprod. Fertil. Suppl.*, **26**, 175–81

Franchimont, P., Chari, S., Hagelstein, M.T. and Duraiswami, S. (1975). Existence of a follicle stimulating hormone inhibiting factor 'Inhibin' in bull seminal plasma. *Nature (London)*, **157**, 402–4

Franchimont, P., Chari, S., Hazee-Hagelstein, M.T., Debruche, M.L. and Duraiswami, S. (1977). Evidence for the existence of inhibin. In Troen, P. and Nankin, H.R. (eds.) *The Testis in Normal and Infertile Men*, pp. 253–69 (New York: Raven Press)

Franchimont, P., Croze, F., Demoulin, A., Bologne, R. and Hustin, J. (1981). Effect of inhibin on rat testicular desoxyribonucleic acid (DNA) synthesis *in-vivo* and *in-vitro*. *Acta Endocrinologica*, **98**, 312–20

Franchimont, P. Millet, D., Vendrely, E., Letawe, J., Legros, J.J. and Netter, A. (1972). Relationship between spermatogenesis and serum gonadotropin levels in azoospermia and oligospermia. *J. Clin. Endocrinol. Metab.*, **34**, 1003–8

Franchimont, P., Verstraclen-Proyard, J., Hazee-Hagelstein, M.T., Renard, C.H., Demoulin, A., Bourguignon, J.P. and Hustin, J. (1979). *Vitam. Horm.*, **37**, 243–302

Gupta, D., Rager, K., Zaryki, J. and Eichner, M. (1975). Levels of luteinizing hormone, follicle stimulating hormone, testosterone, and dihydrotestosterone in circulation of sexually maturing intact male rats and after orchidectomy and experimental bilateral cryptorchidism. *J. Endocrinol.*, **66**, 183–93

Hafez, E.S.E. (1980). Male and female inhibin. *Arch. Androl.*, **5**, 131–58

Hansson, V., French, F.S., Weddington, S., Nayfeh, S.N. and Ritsen, E.M. (1974). Stimulation of testicular androgen binding protein (ABP). In Dufau, M.L. and Means, A.R. (eds.) *Hormone Binding and Target Cell Activation in the Testis, Current Topics in Molecular and Cellular Endocrinology*, Vol. 1, pp. 287–91 (New York: Plenum Press)

Hansson, V., Ritzen, E.M., French, F.S. and Nayfeh, S.N. (1975). Androgen transport and receptor mechanism in testis and epididymis. In Hamilton, D.W. and Greep, R.O. (eds.) *Handbook of Physiology*, vol. 5, pp. 173–202 (Washington: American Physiological Society)

Harries, M.E., Bartke, A., Weisz, J. and Waston, D. (1977). Effects of testosterone and dihydrotestosterone on spermatogenesis, rete testis fluid and peripheral androgen levels in hypophysectomized rats. *Fertil. Steril.*, **28**, 1113–7

Hochereau-de-Reviers, M.T. (1981). Control of spermatogonial multiplication. In Kenneth, W. and McKern, S. (eds.) *Reproductive Processes and Contraception*, pp. 307–31 (New York: Plenum Press)

Hudson, B., Baker, H.W.G., Eddie, L.W., Higginson, R.E., Burger, H.G., deKretser, D.M., Dobos, M. and Lee, V.W.K. (1979). Bioassays for inhibin, a critical review. *J. Reprod. Fertil. Suppl.*, **26**, 17–29

Johnson, M.H., Thakur, A.N. and Sheth, A.R. (1981). Distribution of inhibin in testis of neonatal, pubertal and adult rats. *Arch. Androl.*, **7**, 127–31

Krishnan, K.A., Panse, G.T. and Sheth, A.R. (1982). Comparative study of inhibin from human testis, prostate and seminal plasma. *Andrologia*, **14**, 409–15

Krueger, P.M., Hodgen, G.D. and Sherins, R.J. (1974). New evidence for the role of the Sertoli cell and spermatogonia in feedback control of FSH secretion in male rats. *Endocrinology*, **95**, 355–62

Lagace, L., Massicotte, J., Drouin, J., Giguer, V., Dupont, A. and Labrie, F. (1979). Interaction between LHRH, steroids and inhibin at the pituitary level in the control of LH and FSH secretion in the rat. In Talwar, G.P. (ed.) *Recent Advances in Reproduction and Regulation of Fertility*, pp. 73–85

LeLannou, D. and Chambon, Y. (1977). Presence dans l'epididyme d'un facteur abaissant fortement le taux sanguin de FSH chez'le rat. *C.R. Seances, Soc. Biol.*, **171**, 636-9

Lee, V.W.K. and Findly, J.K. (1982). Changes in ovarian and peripheral blood inhibin levels in immature female rats after PMSG treatment. In Rolland, R., Van Hall, E.V., Hillier, S.G., McNatty, K.P. and Schoemaker, J. (eds.) *Follicular Maturation and Ovulation*, (Amsterdam-Oxford-Princeton: Excerpta Medica)

Lugaro, G., Cassellato, M.M., Mazzola, G., Fachini, G. and Carrea, G. (1974). Evidence for the existence in spermatozoa of a factor inhibiting hormone synthesis. *Neuroendocrinology*, **15**, 62-8

Lumpkin, M., Negro-vilar, A., Franchimont, P. and McCann, S. (1981). Evidence for a hypothalamic site of action of inhibin to suppress FSH release. *Endocrinology*, **108**, 1101

McCullagh, D.R. (1932). Dual endocrine activity of the testis. *Science NY*, **76**, 19-20

Means, A.R. (1971). Concerning the mechanism of FSH action: Rapid stimulation of testicular synthesis of nuclear RNA. *Endocrinology*, **89**, 981-9

Moodbidri, S.B., Joshi, L.R. and Sheth, A.R. (1976). Isolation of an inhibin-like substance from ram testis. *IRCS Med. Sci.*, **4**, 217-9

Moodbidri, S.B., Joshi, L.R. and Sheth, A.R. (1980). On the mechanism of action of low molecular weight inhibin from ram testis. *Ind. J. Exp. Biol.*, **18**, 100-1

Nagendranath, N., Jose, T.M., Sheth, A.R. and Juneja, H.S. (1982). Effect of testosterone, estradiol-17-beta and 5-alpha-dihydrotestosterone on inhibin production by Sertoli cells in culture. *Arch. Androl.*, **9**, 217-22

Nandedkar, T.D., Sarvamangala, B.S., Raghavan, V.P. and Sheth, A.R. (1982). Effect of FSH deprivation on spermatogenesis in prepubertal mice. *Arch. Androl.*, **8**, 257-60

Phadke, M., Vijayalakshmi, S. and Sheth, A.R. (1982). Evidence for the presence of specific receptors for inhibin in human prostate. *Ind. J. Exp. Biol.*, **20**, 419-20

Raj, H.G.M., Dym, M., Chemes, H.E., Kotite, N.J., Nayfeh, S.N. and French, F.S. (1978). Effect of passive immunity to FSH on male reproduction in immature and adult rat. *Proceedings of the Third Annual Meeting, Am. Soc. Androl.* (Abstr.)

Ramasharma, K., Sairam, M.R. and Ranganathan, M.R. (1981). Effect of inhibin-like factors on gonadotropin release by mouse pituitary *in-vitro*. *Acta Endocrinologica*, **98**, 496-505

Rosenberg, E. (1981). Advances in male reproductive research. In Corte's-Prieto, J., Campos, da-Paz-A. and Neves-e-castro, M. (eds.) *Research on Fertility and Sterility*, pp. 75-81. (Lancaster: MTP)

Rush, M.E. and Lipner, H. (1979). Blockade of gonadotrophin releasing hormone induced secretion preparation. *Endocrinology*, **105**, 187-93

Sairam, M.R., Ranganathan, M.R. and Ramasharma, K. (1981). Binding of inhibin-like protein from bull seminal plasma to ovine pituitary membranes. *Mol. Cell. Endocrinol.*, **22**, 251-64

Scott, R.S. and Burger, H.G. (1980). Inhibin is absent from azoospermic semen of infertile men. *Nature*, **285**, 246-7

Scott, R.S., Burger, H.G. and Quigg, H. (1980). A simple and rapid *in-vitro* bioassay for inhibin. *Endocrinology*, **107**, 1536-42

Setchell, B.P., Davies, R.V. and Mains, J. (1977). Inhibin. In Johnson, A.D. and Gommes, W.R. (eds.) *The Testis*, vol. IV pp. 189-238 (New York: Academic Press)

Sheth, P.R., Dandekar, S.P., Seethalakshmi, N. and Sheth, A.R. (1982). Inhibin interaction with LHRH receptors at the pituitary level. *Arch. Androl.*, **8**, 185-8

Sheth, A.R., Koregaokar, S.U. and Seethalakshmi, N. (1981a). Occurrence of bioimmuno-reactive inhibin in rat spermatids. *Andrologia*, **13**, 232-5

Sheth, A.R., Panse, G.T., Vaze, A.Y., Geller, J. and Albert, J. (1981b). Inhibin in human prostate. *Arch. Androl.*, **6**, 317-21

Sheth, A.R., Vanage, G.R., Vaze, A.Y. and Thakur, A.N. (1980). Negative feedback of secretion of follicle stimulating hormone by pituitary gland of developing male rats. *J. Endocrinol.*, **87**, 401-7

Steinberger, A. (1980). Factors affecting *in-vitro* secretion of inhibin by isolated Sertoli cells. In Cunning, I.A., Funder, J.W. and Mendelsohn, F.A. (eds.) *Proceedings of the VI International Congress of Endocrinology*, pp. 259-62 (Amsterdam: Elsevier-North Holland)

Steinberger, A. and Steinberger, E. (1976). Secretion of a FSH inhibiting factor by cultured Sertoli cells. *Endocrinology*, **99**, 918-21

Steinberger, E. (1975). Hormonal regulation of the seminiferous tubule function. In French, F.S., Hansson, V., Ritzen, E.M. and Nayfeh, S.N. (eds.) *Hormonal Regulation of Spermatogenesis*, pp. 337–54 (New York: Plenum)

Steinberger, E. (1981). Spermatogenesis, its control and its evaluation. In Prieto, C. and Campos, da-Paz, A. (eds.) *Research on Fertility and Sterility*, pp. 91–101. (Lancaster: MTP)

Steinberger, E. and Duckett, G.E. (1967). Hormonal control of spermatogenesis. *J. Reprod. Fertil.*, **2** (Suppl.), 75–87

Steinberger, E., Sanborn, B. and Steinberger, A. (1979). Sertoli cell function. In Talwar, G.P. (ed.) *Recent Advances in the Reproduction and Regulation of Fertility*, pp. 219–31 (Amsterdam: Elsevier–North Holland)

Steinberger, E., Smith, K.D., Tcholakian, R.K., Chowdhary, M., Steinberger, A., Fischer, M. and Paulsen, C.A. (1973). Steroidogenesis in human testes. In Mancini, R.E. and Martin, L. (eds.) *Male Fertility and Sterility*, pp. 149–151 (New York, Academic Press)

Thakur, A.N., Vaze, A.Y., Dattatreyamurthy, B. and Sheth, A.R. (1981). Isolation and characterization of inhibin from human seminal plasma. *Ind. J. Exp. Biol.*, **19**, 307–13

Vanage, G.R., Sheth, A.R. and Kadam, M.S. (1981). *In-vivo* effect of inhibin on FSH uptake by rat testis. *Experientia*, **37**, 433–4

Vanage, G.R. and Sheth, A.R. (1982). Binding characteristics of inhibin to rat pituitary plasma membrane. *Ind. J. Exp. Biol.*, **20**, 445–57

Vanage, G.R., Thakur, A.N., Kadam, M.S. and Sheth, A.R. (1980). Metabolic clearance rate of inhibin in mature and immature male rats. *Biol. Reprod.*, **23**, 606–10

Vaze, A.Y., Thakur, A.N. and Sheth, A.R. (1979). Development of a radioimmunoassay for human seminal plasma inhibin. *J. Reprod. Fertil. Suppl.*, **26**, 135–46

Vaze, A.Y., Thakur, A.N. and Sheth, A.R. (1980). Levels of inhibin in human semen and accessory reproductive organs. *Andrologia*, **12**, 66–71

Vernon, R.G., Go, V.L.W. and Fritz, I.B. (1975). Hormonal requirements of the different cycles of the seminiferous epithelium during reinitiation of spermatogenesis in long term hypophysectomized rats. *J. Reprod. Fertil.*, **47**, 77–94

Vijayalakshmi, S., Bandivdekar, A.H., Joshi, L.R., Moodbidri, S.B. and Sheth, A.R. (1980a). Isolation and characterization of ovine testicular and ovarian inhibin. *Arch. Androl.*, **5**, 179–88

Vijayalakshmi, S., Moodbidri, S.B., Bandivdekar, A.H. and Sheth, A.R. (1980b). Modulation of FSH action by inhibin. *Arch. Androl.*, **5**, 231–5

Vijayalakshmi, S., Sheth, P.R., Dandekar, S.P., Vaze, A.Y., Moodbidri, S.B. and Sheth, A.R. (1981). Biological studies with low and high molecular weight inhibin preparations. *Int. J. Androl.*, **4**, 691–702

Section VI

BLOOD-TESTICULAR AND EPIDIDYMAL BARRIERS

25
The blood–epididymis barrier

B.T. HINTON

For several years, evidence has accumulated to suggest that, as in the testis, there is a barrier between blood and the epididymal lumen. This finding is perhaps not surprising in view of the known functions of the blood–testis barrier. Spermatozoa, once shed from the germinal epithelium, need continuous protection and an environment favourable for maturation and survival as they progress along the epididymal duct. With the introduction of micropuncture, microperfusion and microanalytical techniques to study male reproductive physiology, it has been possible to obtain new, additional information on several aspects of epididymal physiology. The luminal fluid or microenvironment that surrounds the maturing spermatozoa can be studied in considerable detail. Such studies provide clues as to the importance of this microenvironment towards sperm maturation. Furthermore, we now have a better idea of how the epididymal epithelium contributes to the formation of the microenvironment. Many molecules do not simply traverse the epididymal epithelium but do seem to be regulated.

Due to space limitation, this chapter will not attempt to give an exhaustive overview of all the physiological aspects of the blood–epididymis barrier, but will use examples to highlight the various properties of the epididymis. For more detailed references, the reader should consult the reviews cited within this chapter. Thus many of the excellent pieces of work published within the field of epididymal physiology have been omitted.

MORPHOLOGICAL EVIDENCE

Although this chapter will deal with the physiological aspects of the blood–epididymis barrier, a brief word will be said with respect to the morphological characteristics. Friend and Gilula (1972) wrote, 'Among the various epithelial cell contacts examined, the zonula occludens of the epididymis is the most highly developed'. Through some rather elegant freeze-fracture studies by Suzuki and Nagano (1978a), an extensive tight junctional meshwork can be seen between the cells along the entire length of the epididymal duct. Several other types of cell contacts such as desmosomes and gap junctions are also abundant in this epithelium (Friend and Gilula, 1972;

Suzuki and Nagano, 1978a,b). However, it is the tight junctions which ultimately separate the epididymal luminal compartment from the blood compartment (Hoffer and Hinton, 1984).

COMPOSITION OF EPIDIDYMAL LUMINAL FLUID

One major piece of evidence for the existence of a blood–epididymis barrier is that the composition of epididymal luminal fluid is distinctly different from that of blood plasma (see reviews by Jones, 1978; Turner, 1979; Howards *et al.*, 1979; Brooks, 1979a; Hinton, 1980; Setchell and Hinton, 1981). Each of the ions (sodium, potassium, calcium, magnesium, chloride, bicarbonate, sulphate, phosphate) and the organic compounds (glucose, lactate, amino acids, androgens, *myo*-inositol, L-carnitine, glycerylphosphocholine, sialic acids) are found in different concentrations in the luminal fluid at different regions along the epididymal duct. The concentration of many of

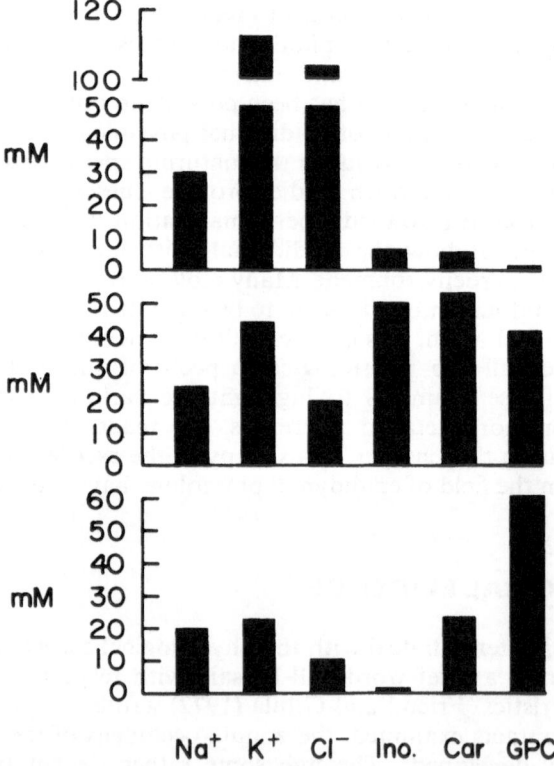

Fig. 25.1 Concentration of sodium (Na$^+$), potassium (K$^+$), chloride (Cl$^-$), inositol (Ino), L-carnitine (Car) and glycerylphosphocholine (GPC) in the luminal fluid of the ductus deferens from the human (top), rat (middle) and rabbit (lower). Note that in the rat and rabbit the organic solutes are in greater concentration compared to the ions, whereas in the human male it is the reverse (data from Levine and Marsh, 1971; Hinton *et al.*, 1979, 1980, 1981)

the organic solutes within the epididymal luminal fluid can reach very high values. For example, 90 mmol/l and 50 mmol/l *myo*-inositol in cauda fluid for the hamster and rat respectively, and a 2000-fold concentration gradient of L-carnitine across the rat cauda epithelium. There is also considerable species differences in the composition of epididymal luminal fluid (Fig. 25.1). Even luminal fluid collected from the human ductus deferens is considerably different in composition compared to other species (Hinton *et al.*, 1981; Fig. 25.1). Therefore, it is not clear which animal model to choose for the study of epididymal physiology in man. This is an important point for investigators searching for a male contraceptive agent acting on the epididymis.

Changes in the composition of luminal fluid along the epididymis are due to several factors: (1) water resorption, (ii) secretion, (iii) absorption or (iv) metabolism of a particular solute by the spermatozoa. Water resorption in the proximal regions of the epididymis (Levine and Marsh, 1971; Crabo, 1965) increase both the concentration of various ions and solutes, and spermatozoa (from 10^6 per ml to 10^8–10^9 per ml). The mechanism by which the epididymis can move water so effectively from its lumen is probably linked to the active outward movement of ions (e.g. Na^+, see Levine and Marsh, 1971; Wong *et al.*, 1978). Secretion of a solute may be via (i) direct transfer from blood to lumen (e.g. L-carnitine transport) or (ii) synthesis by the epididymal epithelium from a precursor which is blood derived (e.g. inositol from glucose; proteins from amino acids). Absorption of solutes from the lumen can occur by the epididymal cells. Utilization of various solutes by the spermatozoa will also affect the composition of epididymal luminal fluid (e.g. L-carnitine uptake into spermatozoa).

Recently, there has been considerable emphasis from investigators on the study of protein secretion into the epididymal luminal fluid. Many proteins are secreted in the luminal fluid at different areas along the epididymal duct (Barker and Amann, 1971; Amann *et al.*, 1973; Koskimies and Kormano, 1975; Turner *et al.*, 1979; Olson and Hinton, 1984). Studies have continued to identify several proteins in the hope of finding a role for these proteins. Several proteins secreted into the epididymal luminal fluid that have a known function include Forward Motility Protein (Brandt *et al.*, 1978), Acrosome Stabilizing Factor (Thomas *et al.*, 1984; see Fig. 25.2), 'Immobilin' (Usselman and Cone, 1983) and sperm motility inhibiting factor (Turner and Giles, 1982). Angiotensin converting enzyme (Holburger *et al.*, 1982) and alpha lactalbumin (Hamilton, 1981; Jones and Brown, 1982) are two proteins known to be present in epididymal luminal fluid, but their precise function awaits further elucidation. Many proteins secreted by the epididymal cells are for sperm utilization, especially as sperm surface components. This seems to be the case for many species, e.g. rat (Brown *et al.*, 1983), rabbit (Oliphant and Singhas, 1979; Nicolson *et al.*, 1979) and human (Young and Goodman, 1980). The precise role of many of the sperm surface components is not known, although many are responsible for the antigenic properties of the spermatozoa.

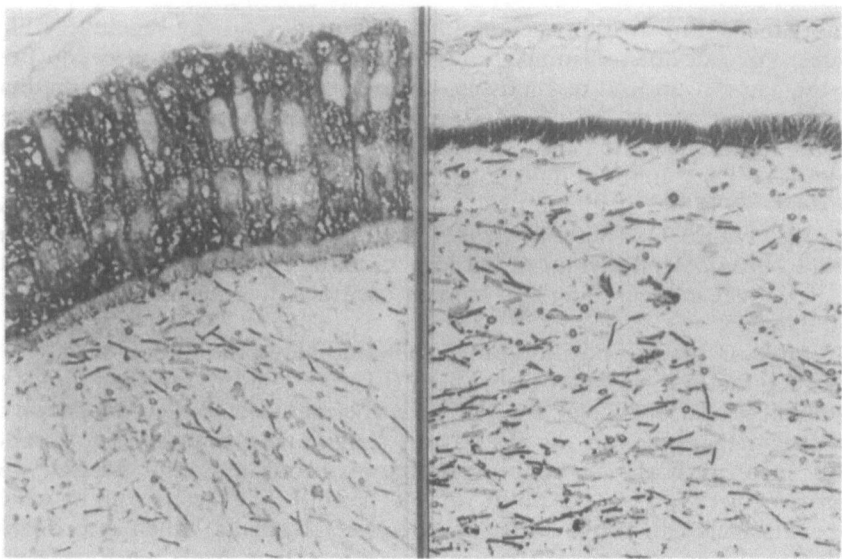

Fig. 25.2 Immunohistochemical localization of Acrosome Stabilizing Factor (ASF) in the rabbit epididymis. Left: corpus; right: cauda. Note staining localized within cytoplasm of principal cells in corpus region and some staining asssociated with the spermatozoa. Localization of ASF in cauda region is confined to the luminal surface membrane and microvilli. Spermatozoa are more intensely stained in this region. Localization of ASF was not demonstrated within the epithelial cells or spermatozoa of the caput epididymidis. Magnification × 700. (Photograph kindly supplied by Drs T.S. Thomas and G. Oliphant)

PERMEABILITY OF THE EPIDIDYMAL EPITHELIUM TO MOLECULES

The epididymis does not readily allow molecules to traverse its epithelia. The fact that compounds of different molecular weight enter the epididymal lumen from blood at different rates is further evidence for a blood–epididymis barrier (Howards *et al.*, 1976; Cooper and Waites, 1979a; Turner *et al.*, 1979; Hinton and Howards, 1981). In general, small molecular weight compounds such as water or urea readily enter the epididymal lumen whereas the larger molecular weight compounds such as inulin, dextran or proteins do not; even L-glucose (MW 180) is considerably restricted. The passive diffusion rates of these molecules across the epididymal epithelium do not appear to be very different between epididymal region or between species. However, there is considerable species and epididymal regional differences in the uptake of organic solutes such as sugars, amino acids and steroids (see Figs 25.3 and 25.4). The epididymis is able to utilize various transporting mechanisms, situated on the basolateral membranes, selectively to move different solutes either down or against their concentration gradient. For example, there is a saturable, stereospecific carrier mediated mechanism (presumably facilitated diffusion) which transports D-glucose down a concentration gradient from blood to cells and lumen (Brooks,

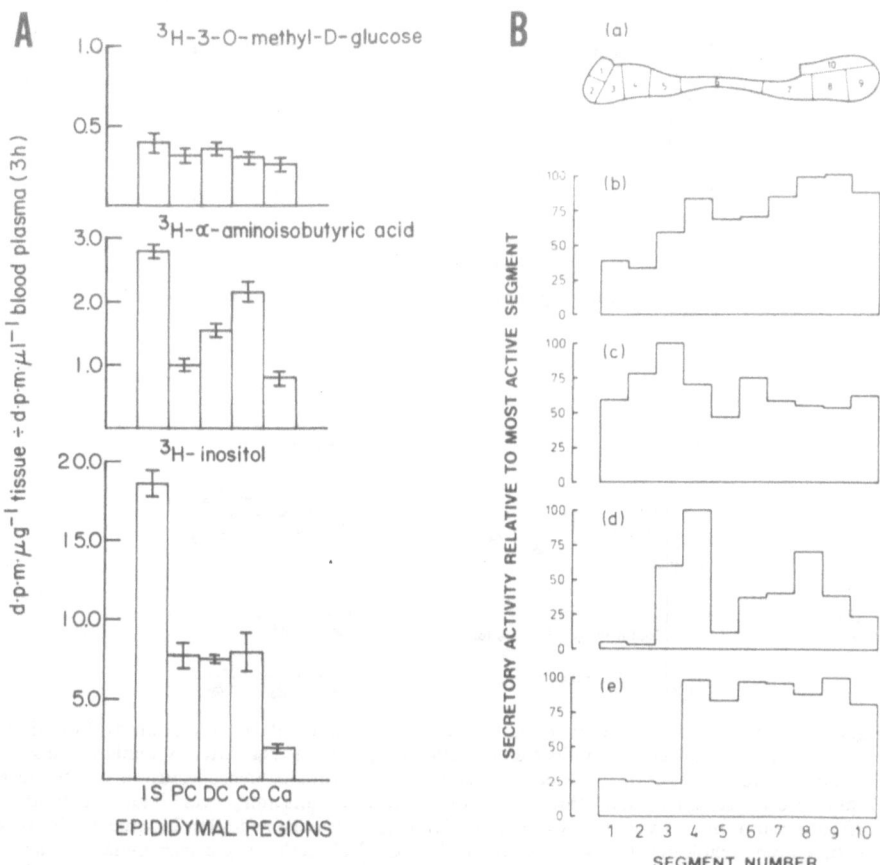

Fig. 25.3 (A) Appearance of 3-*O*-[³H]methyl-D-glucose, α-[³H]aminoisobutyric acid and [³H]-inositol into the different regions of the rat epididymis 3 h after systemic infusion of isotope. Results are expressed as a ratio of d min⁻¹ μg⁻¹ tissue ÷ d min⁻¹ μl⁻¹ blood plasma for each epididymal region: IS, initial segment; PC, proximal caput; DC, distal caput; Co, corpus; Ca, cauda. Data redrawn from Hinton and Howards (1982). (B) Incorporation of U-¹⁴C-labelled amino acids (b), [³H]-galactose (c), [³H]mannose (d) and [³H]fucose (e) into secreted proteins by epididymal tissue *in vitro*. Reproduced with permission of Dr D.E. Brooks and *Biology of Reproduction* (1981). Both figures demonstrate that uptake of different organic solutes is not necessarily similar for each epididymal region

1979b; Hinton and Howards, 1982). The reverse transport process is illustrated by inositol and L-carnitine which are transported against a concentration gradient (presumably via an active transport process, Brooks *et al.*, 1973; Johansen and Bohmer, 1979; Hinton and Setchell, 1980). Both of these compounds are accumulated by the epididymis in a region-dependent manner (see Fig. 25.4); for example, the distal caput and corpus regions are extremely active in transporting L-carnitine from blood into cell, whereas the initial segment is particularly active in inositol transport (Brooks *et al.*, 1973; Johansen and Bohmer, 1979; Hinton and Setchell, 1980; Hinton and

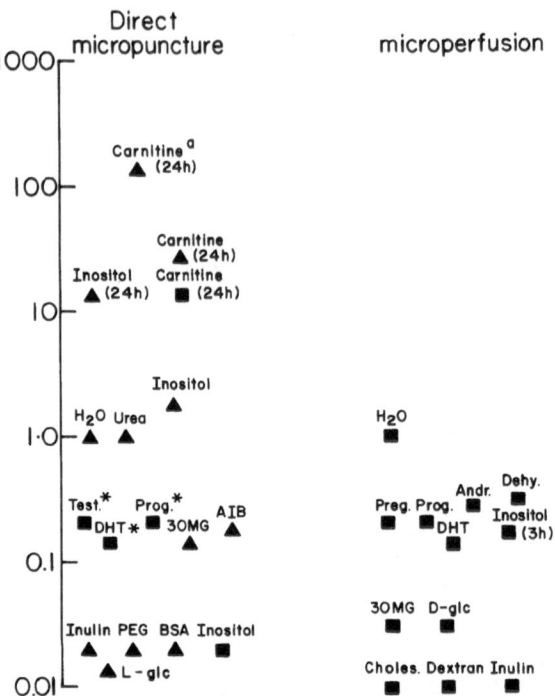

Fig. 25.4 Appearance of different organic solutes in the lumen of the rat (*, hamster) proximal caput (a, distal caput) epididymidis (▲) or cauda epididymidis (■) after systemic infusion of the radioactive compound, followed by direct micropunture of microperfusion of the duct. Results are expressed in logarithmic form of the ratio counts min^{-1} vol^{-1} luminal fluid or perfusate/counts min^{-1} vol^{-1} blood plasma. Samples were collected after 2 h unless otherwise stated. Choles, cholesterol; D-glc, D-glucose; 30MG, 3-O-methyl-D-glucose; L-glc, L-glucose; PEG, polyethylene glycol; AIB, α-aminoisobutyric acid; BSA, bovine serum albumin; H_2O, water; Test, testosterone; DHT, 5-α-dihydrotestosterone; Prog, progesterone; Preg, pregnenalone; Andr, androstenedione; Dehy, dehydroepiandrosterone. Each compound was isotopically labelled with either ^3H, ^{14}C or ^{125}I. Data from Cooper (1982), Cooper and Waites (1979a,b), Turner et al., (1981); Hinton and Howards (1981, 1982)

Howards, 1982). There appears to be another transporting step for L-carnitine situated on the luminal membrane which transports this compound against a concentration gradient from cell into lumen; it has been suggested that this transporting step is androgen-dependent (Bohmer et al., 1979). The non-metabolizable neutral amino acid, α-aminoisobutyric acid, has been shown to be accumulated by a saturable transport system (Hinton and Howards, 1982).

There has been considerable interest in the literature with respect to the origin of glycerylphosphocholine (GPC) in epididymal lumen. There is now evidence (Hammerstedt and Rowan, 1982) to suggest that the epididymal basolateral membrane can transfer lipoproteins, a source of GPC for secretion, from blood into cell. The lipoproteins would then presumably be degraded by the epididymal cells to GPC (and other related compounds, e.g. phosphocholine). This type of movement into the epididymal cells is highly suggestive of a receptor-mediated endocytotic event. It would therefore be of considerable interest to determine if the epididymis can transfer large molecular weight compounds, like proteins, into its cell from the blood. Presumably, via a similar mechanism, some immunoglobulins are able to enter the cauda epididymal fluid (Weininger et al., 1982).

Since many of the transporting systems are saturable, then the epididymis is able to regulate the flow of important organic solutes into its cells and lumen. Interestingly, the composition of the epididymal luminal fluid can

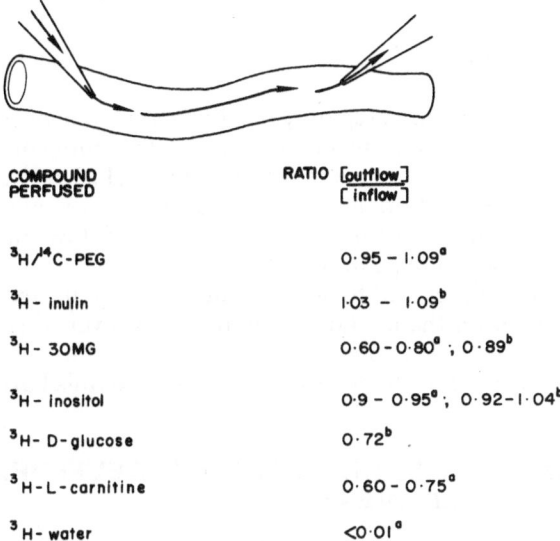

COMPOUND PERFUSED	RATIO $\left[\dfrac{outflow}{inflow}\right]$
$^3H/^{14}C$-PEG	0·95 – 1·09[a]
^3H – inulin	1·03 – 1·09[b]
^3H – 30MG	0·60 – 0·80[a]; 0·89[b]
^3H – inositol	0·9 – 0·95[a]; 0·92–1·04[b]
^3H – D–glucose	0·72[b]
^3H–L–carnitine	0·60 – 0·75[a]
^3H– water	<0·01[a]

Fig. 25.5 The movement of various radioactive compounds out of the lumen of the rat caput epididymidis (a) or the cauda epididymidis (b). Each compound was microperfused into the epididymal lumen at rates from 8 to 13.5 μl h^{-1} for the caput and 1.2 to 15.4 μl min^{-1} for the cauda. Results are shown as a ratio of counts min^{-1}. vol^{-1} collected fluid (outflow) counts min^{-1} vol^{-1} perfused fluid (inflow). Data for cauda epididymidis was taken from Cooper (1982), and data for caput epididymidis from Hinton et al., 1984)

also influence the transfer of various molecules across the epithelium from blood to lumen. The presence of proteins within the cauda luminal fluid is known to increase androgen transfer (Cooper and Waites, 1979b), and high intraluminal glucose within the caput luminal fluid decreases transfer of glucose (Hinton et al., 1984). These findings probably demonstrate a close interaction between luminal fluid and epithelium in such a way as to regulate further the movement of various compounds into the epididymis. Another factor contributing to differences in transfer of substances across the epithelium along different regions of the epididymis will be blood flow.

The epididymis regulates both the entry of many substances, and their exit. Large-molecular-weight compounds do not readily leave the lumen whereas smaller-molecular weight compounds do. Further evidence for a blood-epididymis barrier is derived from the fact that some sugars and amino acids are also considerably restricted (Cooper, 1982; Hinton et al., 1984) from leaving the epididymal lumen (see Fig. 25.5). Such findings probably reflect the ability of the epididymis to conserve needed compounds for sperm maturation and for its own functions. One of the main functions of the blood-epididymis barrier is to provide a favourable environment for sperm maturation and survival. It is not clear, however, whether some or all of the substances secreted into the epididymal luminal fluid are necessary for this function. Obviously, more basic research is needed to answer this question.

PROTECTIVE ROLE

A further role of the blood-epididymis barrier is the protection of the maturing spermatozoa from outside influences. The antigenic properties of spermatozoa are well known (see review by Hancock, 1981) so it is important that there is separation between the spermatozoa and the immune system. Epididymal luminal fluid has indeed, a very low immunoglobulin content (see Weininger et al., 1982).

Many toxic metabolites and toxic environmental agents are also probably excluded from entering the epididymal lumen. However, this aspect of epididymal function has not received much attention and it is not known how readily such agents are able to cross the blood-epididymis barrier.

BLOOD-EPIDIDYMIS BARRIER AND THE DEVELOPMENT OF A MALE CONTRACEPTIVE AGENT

The epididymis has been considered by many investigators to be a good site of attack for a male contraceptive agent. As spermatozoa progress along the epididymal duct they transform into cells capable of motility and fertilizing an ovum. Potential agents could interfere in either one or both of these processes.

A contraceptive could act directly on epididymal function and thereby cause changes in sperm maturation, or alternatively the agent could enter the epididymis and act directly on the spermatozoa. Some sites on the epididymis where a potential male contraceptive could act are summarized in Table 25.1. Antifertility agents under past and present investigation for their action on the epididymis are shown in Table 25.2.

CONCLUDING REMARKS

The main function of the blood-epididymis barrier is to provide a milieu or microenvironment favourable for sperm maturation and survival. In doing so, the epididymis is able to regulate many substances across its epithelium both for its needs and for the protection of the spermatozoa.

Table 25.1 Transport and synthetic activities of the epididymis which may represent sites of attack for a male contraceptive agent.

Site	Comments
1. Ions	
(a) Na^+, K^+ transport	The Na^+/K^+ ratio in luminal fluid may be important for sperm motility and fertilizing ability
(b) Ca^{2+}, Mg^{2+} transport	Both ions important for sperm motility
(c) H^+, HCO_3^- transport	pH of luminal fluid may be important in sperm motility, development and survival
(d) H_2O transport	Important in increasing sperm concentration
2. Organic solutes	
(a) D-Glucose transport	Important in overall cellular metabolism. Provides inositol, lactate and is a precursor to sialic acids and glycoproteins
(b) L-Carnitine transport	May be important in development of sperm motility
(c) Amino acid transport	Important in synthesis of proteins for epididymal function and sperm maturation, e.g. surface components. Amino acids alone appear to be involved in motility development, capacitation process and protection from osmotic stress.
(d) Inositol transport and synthesis	Important for membrane components in sperm and epididymis. May be important for sperm metabolism and survival in epididymis
(e) Androgen transport and synthesis	Important for normal epididymal functions, sperm maturation and survival
(f) Lipoprotein transport	May be important in delivery of phospholipids, cholesterol and choline for epididymal and sperm metabolism
(g) GPC synthesis (?)	Function not known

Table 25.2 Some male antifertility agents investigated for their action on the epididymis

Compounds	Comments
(a) Methylene dimethanesulphonate	Structure very similar to glycerol and GPC. One of the first chemical agents shown to act on epididymal sperm. Toxic side-effects
(b) Alpha-chlorohydrin	Similar structure to glycerol and GPC. Enters epididymal lumen readily and interferes with sperm metabolism. Sperm motility much reduced. Active metabolite appears to be responsible for antifertility effect. Toxic side-effects
(c) Chlorinated hexoses	e.g. 6-chloro-6-deoxy-D-glucose. Enters epididymal lumen readily. Interferes in sperm metabolism so as to disrupt motility. May also be interfering in epididymal function.
(d) Antiandrogens	e.g. cyproterone acetate, flutamide. Epididymis considered to be very sensitive to androgens. Questionable as to whether these compounds effective in working on epididymis alone.

Further basic research on epididymal physiology will be necessary before we are able to understand the complex interactions between the epididymis, the microenvironment and spermatozoa. A fuller understanding of this interaction will aid many investigators in their quest for a male contraceptive and will hopefully provide information regarding certain forms of male infertility.

Acknowledgements

This work was supported by N.I.H. grants HD 14445 and HD18257.

References

Amann, R.P., Killian, G.J. and Benton, A.W. (1973). Differences in the electrophoretic characteristics of bovine rete testis fluid and plasma from the cauda epididymis. *J. Reprod. Fertil.*, **35**, 321

Barker, L.D.S. and Amann, R.P. (1971). Epididymal physiology II: Immunofluorescent analysis of epithelial secretion and absorption, and of bovine sperm maturation. *J. Reprod. Fertil.*, **26**, 319

Bohmer, T., Sar, M., Stumpf, W.E. and Hansson, V. (1979). Autoradiographic study of the [^{3}H]-carnitine distribution in rat epididymis. *Int. J. Androl.*, **2**, 62

Brandt, H, Acott, T.S., Johnson, D.J. and Hoskins, D.D. (1978). Evidence for an epididymal origin of bovine sperm forward motility protein. *Biol. Reprod.*, **19**, 830

Brooks, D.E. (1979a). Biochemical environment of sperm maturation. In Fawcett, D.W. and Bedford, J.M. (eds.) *The Spermatozoon*, pp. 23–34. (Baltimore-Munich: Urban and Schwarzenberg)

Brooks, D.E. (1979b). Carbohydrate metabolism in the rat epididymis: evidence that glucose is taken up by tissue slices and isolated cells by a process of facilitated diffusion. *Biol. Reprod.*, **21**, 19

Brooks, D.E. (1981). Secretion of proteins and glycoproteins by the rat epididymis: regional differences, androgen-dependence, and effects of protease inhibitors, procaine and tunicamycin. *Biol. Reprod.*, **25**, 1099

Brooks, D.E., Hamilton, D.W. and Mallek, A.H. (1973). The uptake of L-[methyl-^{3}H] carnitine by the rat epididymis. *Biochem. Biophys. Res. Commun.*, **52**, 1354

Brown, C.R., von Glos, K.I., and Jones, R. (1983). Changes in plasma membrane glycoproteins of rat spermatozoa during maturation in the epididymis. *J. Cell Biol.*, **96**, 256

Cooper, T.G. (1982). Secretion of inositol and glucose by the perfused rat cauda epididymis. *J. Reprod. Fertil.*, **64**, 373

Cooper, T.G. and Waites G.M.H. (1979a). Investigation by luminal perfusion of the transfer of compounds into the epididymis of the anesthetised rat. *J. Reprod. Fertil.*, **56**, 159

Cooper, T.G. and Waites, G.M.H. (1979b). Factors affecting the entry of testosterone into the lumen of the cauda epididymis of the anaesthetised rat. *J. Reprod. Fertil.*, **56**, 165

Crabo, B. (1965). Studies on the composition of epididymal content in bulls and boars. *Acta Vet. Scand. Suppl.*, **5**, 1

Friend, D.S. and Gilula, N.B. (1972). Variations in tight and gap junctions in mammalian tissue. *J. Cell Biol.*, **53**, 758

Hamilton, D.W. (1981). Evidence for α-lactalbumin-like activity in reproductive tract fluids of the male rat. *Biol. Reprod.*, **25**, 385

Hammerstedt, R.H. and Rowan, W.A. (1982). Phosphatidylcholine of blood lipoprotein is the precursor of glycerophosphorylcholine found in seminal plasma. *Biochim. Biophys. Acta*, **710**, 370

Hancock, R.J.T. (1981). Immune responses to sperm. In Finn, G.A. (ed.) *Oxford Reviews of Reproductive Biology*. Vol I, pp. 182–208. (Oxford: Clarendon Press)

Hinton, B.T. (1980). The epididymal microenvironment: a site of attack for a male contraceptive? *Invest. Urol.*, **18**, 1

Hinton, B.T., Hernandez, H. and Howards, S.S. (1984). Microperfusion studies of organic solute transport across the epithelium of the rat caput epididymidis. *J. Reprod. Fertil.*, (In press)

Hinton, B.T. and Howards, S.S. (1981). Permeability characteristics of the epithelium in the rat caput epididymidis. *J. Reprod. Fertil.*, **63**, 95

Hinton, B.T. and Howards, S.S. (1982). Rat testis and epididymis can transport [^{3}H]-3-*O*-methyl-D-glucose. [^{3}H]-inositol and [^{3}H]-α-aminoisobutyric acid across its epithelia *in vivo*. *Biol. Reprod.*, **27**, 1181

Hinton, B.T., Pryor, J.P., Hirsch, A.V. and Setchell, B.P. (1981). The concentration of some inorganic ions and organic compounds in the luminal fluid of the human ductus deferens. *Int. J. Androl.*, **4**, 457

Hinton, B.T. and Setchell, B.P. (1980). Concentration and uptake of carnitine in rat epididymis. A micropuncture study. In Frenkel, R.A. and McGarry, J.D. (eds.) *Carnitine Biosynthesis, Metabolism, and Functions*, pp. 237–250. (New York: Academic Press)

Hinton, B.T. Snoswell, A.M. and Setchell, B.P. (1979). The concentration of carnitine in the luminal fluid of the testis and epididymis of the rat and some other mammals. *J. Reprod. Fertil.*, **56**, 105

Hinton, B.T., White, R.W. and Setchell, B.P. (1980). The concentration of free myo-inositol in the luminal fluid of the mammalian testis and epididymis. *J. Reprod. Fertil.*, **58**, 395

Hoffer, A.P. and Hinton, B.T. (1984). Morphological evidence for a blood–epididymis barrier and the effects of gossypol on its integrity. *Biol. Reprod.*, **30**, 991

Hohlbrugger, G. Scheiswfurth, H. and Dahlheim, H. (1982). Angiotensin I converting enzyme in rat testis, epididymis and vas deferens under different conditions. *J. Reprod. Fertil.*, **65**, 97

Howards, S.S., Jessee, S.J. and Johnson, A.L. (1976). Micropuncture studies of the blood-seminiferous tubule barrier. *Biol. Reprod.*, **14**, 264

Howards, S.S., Lechene, C. and Vigersky, R. (1979). The fluid environment of the maturing spermatozoon. In Fawcett, D.W. and Bedford, J.M. (eds.) *The Spermatozoon*, pp. 35–41. (Baltimore–Munich: Urban and Schwarzenberg)

Johansen, L. and Bohmer, T. (1979). Uptake of ^{3}H-L-carnitine by isolated rat epididymal tubules. *Arch. Androl.*, **2**, 117

Jones, R. (1978). Comparative biochemistry of mammalian epididymal plasma. *Comp. Biochem. Physiol.*, **61B**, 365

Jones, R and Brown, C.R. (1982). Association of epididymal secretory proteins showing alpha-lactalbumin-like activity with the plasma membrane of rat spermatozoa. *Biochem. J.*, **206**, 161

Koskimies, A.I. and Kormano, M. (1975). Proteins in fluids from different segments of the rat epididymis. *J. Reprod. Fertil.* **43**, 345

Levine, N. and Marsh, D.J. (1971). Micropuncture studies of the electrochemical aspects of fluid and electrolyte transport in individual seminiferous tubules, the epididymis and the vas deferens in rats. *J. Physiol. (Lond.)*, **213**, 557

Nicolson, G.L., Brodginski, A.B., Beattie, G. and Yanagamachi, R. (1979). Cell surface changes in the proteins of rabbit spermatozoa during epididymal passage. *Gamete Res.*, **2**, 153

Oliphant, G. and Singhas, C.A. (1979). Iodination of rabbit sperm plasma membrane. Relationship of specific surface proteins to epididymal function and sperm capacitation. *Biol. Reprod.*, **21**, 937

Olson, G.E. and Hinton, B.T. (1984). Changes in the protein composition within the luminal fluid of the rat testis and epididymis as revealed by two-dimensional gel electrophoresis. *Biol. Reprod.*, **5**

Setchell, B.P, and Hinton, B.T. (1981). The effects on the spermatozoa of changes in the composition of luminal fluid as it passes along the epididymis. *Prog. Reprod. Biol.*, **8**, 58

Suzuki, F. and Nagano, T. (1978a). Regional differentiation of cell junctions in the excurrent duct epithelium of the rat testis as revealed by freeze-fracture. *Anat. Rec.*, **191**, 503

Suzuki, F. and Nagano, T. (1978b). Development of tight junctions in the caput epididymal epithelium of the mouse. *Dev. Biol.*, **63**, 321

Thomas, T.S., Reynolds, A.B. and Oliphant, G. (1984). Evaluation of the site of synthesis of rabbit sperm acrosome stabilizing factor using immunocytochemical and metabolic labeling techniques. *Biol. Reprod.*, **30**, 693

Turner, T.T. (1979). On the epididymis and its function. *Invest. Urol.*, **16**, 311

Turner, T.T., Cochran, R.C. Howards, S.S. (1981). Transfer of steroids across the hamster blood testis and blood epididymal barriers. *Biol. Reprod.*, **25**, 342

Turner, T.T., D'Addario, D.A. and Howards, S.S. (1979). Effects of vasectomy on the blood-testis barrier of the hamster. *J. Reprod. Fertil.*, **55**, 323

Turner, T.T., Giles, R.D. (1982). Sperm motility-inhibiting factor in rat epididymis. *Am. J. Physiol.*, **242**, R199

Turner, T.T., Plesums, J.L. and Cabot, C.L. (1979). Luminal fluid proteins of the male rat reproductive tract. *Biol. Reprod.*, **21**, 883

Usselman, M.C. and Cone, R.A. (1983). Rat sperm are mechanically immobilized in the caudal epididymis by 'Immobilin', a high molecular weight glycoprotein. *Biol. Reprod*, **29**, 1241

Weininger, R.B., Fisher, S., Rifkin, J. and Bedford, J.M. (1982). Experimental studies on the passage of specific IgG to the lumen of the rabbit epididymis. *J. Reprod. Fertil.*, **66**, 251

Wong, P.Y.D., Au, C.L. and Ngai, H.K. (1978). Electrolyte and water transport in rat epididymis; its possible role in sperm maturation. *Int. J. Androl. Suppl.*, **2**, 608

Young, L.G. and Goodman, S.A. (1980). Characterization of human sperm cell surface components. *Biol. Reprod.*, **23**, 826

26
The tenacity of the blood–testis and blood–epididymal barriers

T.T. TURNER and S.S. HOWARDS

THE BLOOD–TESTIS AND BLOOD–EPIDIDYMAL BARRIERS

The blood–testis barrier (Setchell and Waites, 1975; Howards *et al.*, 1976) and the blood-epididymal barrier (Turner, 1979; Turner *et al.*, 1981) prevents blood-borne substances from freely diffusing into the lumen of the seminiferous and epididymal tubules. The structural component of these barriers are the epithelial cell–cell tight junctions known to be present in the seminiferous (Flickinger and Fawcett, 1967; Dym and Fawcett, 1970) and epididymal (Friend and Gilula, 1972; Suzuki and Nagano, 1978) epithelia. Morphological studies of the testis have shown that the ability of these tight junctions to exclude lanthanum from the seminiferous tubule lumen is not impaired by cryptorchism (Hagenas *et al.*, 1977), short-term efferent duct ligation (Osman and Ploen, 1978), or pre-pubertal treatment with oestrogen (Vitale *et al.*, 1973). It appears from these morphological studies then that the cell–cell tight junctions are quite stable to injury, and disruption of this aspect of the blood-testis barrier cannot be called upon as the contributing reason for the antispermatogenic effects of many physiological insults to the testis.

There is a problem with morphological studies, however, in that they are limited to static observation and are only qualitative in nature. Morphological studies of lanthanum exclusion may be insensitive to subtle changes in the leakiness of the cell–cell tight junctions. *In vivo* micropuncture of the rat and hamster seminiferous and epididymal tubules can be used to study the net transport of [³H]inulin (MW 5000) across the blood-testis and blood-epididymal barriers. This method allows one to quantitate the 'tightness' of the epithelium to inert macromolecules which are smaller than the colloidal lanthanum particles observed in microscopical studies but which are still of sufficient size to be excluded by normal cell–cell tight junctions. The degree of leakiness to [³H]inulin induced in the epithelia by various treatments can also be assessed. *In vivo* micropuncture allows for multiple sampling over time from the same animals and should be more sensitive to changes in epithelial permeability than the previously used electron microscopal procedures. We have reviewed all our results and compiled the data into the present form because of the consistent evidence that has accumulated regarding the tenacity of the blood–testis and blood–epididymal barriers in experimental animals with conditions pertinent to those seen in clinical practice.

OESTROGEN AND THE BLOOD–TESTIS AND BLOOD–EPIDIDYMAL BARRIERS

The experiments

Adult male rats received 0.5 ml injection of oestradiol valerate (20 mg/ml in castor oil–benzylbenzoate) on days 0, 4, 8 and 12 of treatment. The micropuncture procedure was performed on day 14. Thus, the animals received an average of 2.9 mg oestradiol valerate per day over 14 days. Sham-injected animals received vehicle alone and controls received no injection. At the time of micropuncture, animals were anaesthetized with urethane (1 mg/kg), nephrectomized, and prepared for micropuncture as described previously (Howards *et al.*, 1975). Carotid and jugular cannulae were installed for blood sampling and isotope infusion, respectively. [^{3}H]inulin (specific activity 380 mCi/g; New England Nuclear, Boston, MA.) was infused at 1 mCi in 1 ml physiological saline) via the jugular cannula over a 5 min time period. Beginning 20 min after the completion of infusion and continuing at 20 min intervals thereafter for a total of 140 min, blood samples were taken from the carotid cannula and micropuncture samples of the luminal content were obtained from the seminiferous tubules and the cauda epididymidis.

After collection of the microsamples (spermatozoa + fluid), cell-free fluids were obtained by centrifuging the samples at 10 000 *g* for 15 min. at 0°C. Cell-free fluids were placed under water equilibrated mineral oil and triplicate 100 nl samples of each fluid were transferred via a calibrated volumetric pipette into a mini-scintillation vial containing 3 ml scintillation fluid. Radioactivity in the samples was measured in a scintillation spectrophotometer (Beckman 7000, Beckman Instruments Co., Irvine, CA).

Counts per minute (CPM) per unit volume of tubule fluid were divided by the CPM unit volume of blood plasma collected at the same time period. This quotient multiplied by 100 equals the percentage of blood plasma isotope concentrations that appeared in reproductive tract fluids at each collection time. Within each group of animals the mean amount of [^{3}H]inulin entering the seminiferous and epididymal tubule was calculated for each time period. Testicular weights of each animal in each group were obtained. At the end of the micropuncture procedure, blood samples were taken from sham and oestradiol-treated animals for testosterone analysis by conventional radioimmunoassay. Intra- and inter-assay variability were 4% and 7%, respectively. The permeability data and testis weights from each group of animals were compared by analysis of variance. Serum testosterone concentrations were compared by the Student's *t* test. A *p* value of 0.05 or less was considered significant.

The results

Oestradiol treatment did not alter the net transport of [³H]inulin across the rat blood–testis or blood–epididymal barrier (Fig. 26.1). In control animals, seminiferous tubule and cauda epididymal tubule fluid isotope concentrations plateaued at approximately 5% and 1% of blood isotope concentrations, respectively. In oestradiol-treated animals, these values were between 7–8% and 3–4%, respectively, values not significantly different from controls. Sham injections had no effect. This lack of alteration in the barriers to [³H]inulin was in spite of the fact that oestradiol-treated testis weights (0.98 ± 0.03 g) were significantly less than control weights (1.85 ± 0.05 g) and serum testosterone concentrations in treated rats (1.45 ± 0.15 ng/ml) were

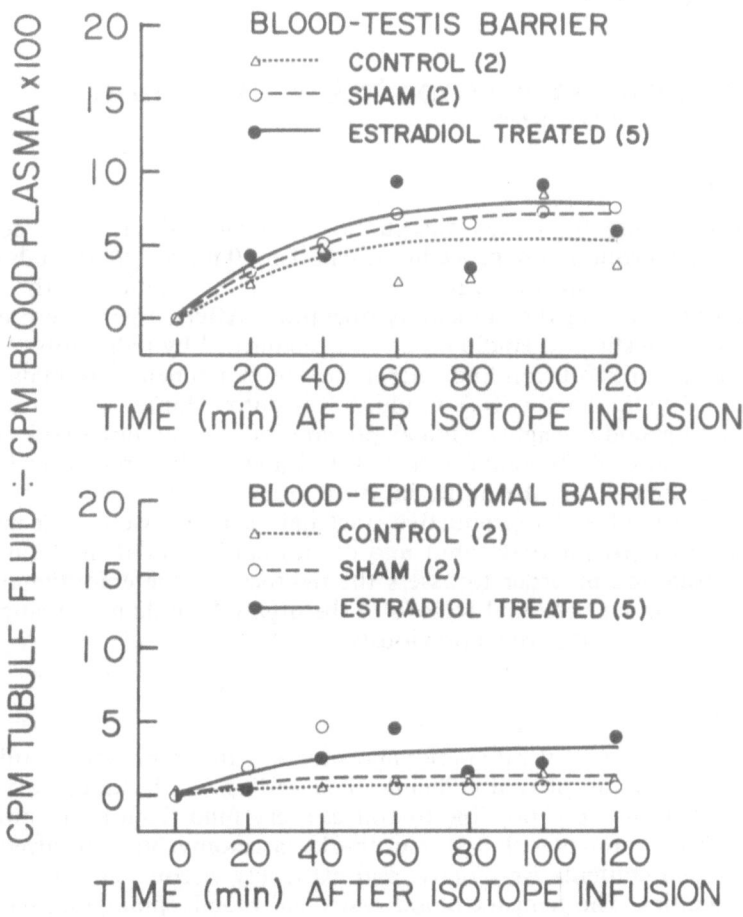

Fig. 26.1 Net transport of [³H]inulin into the seminiferous and epididymal tubules in control (n = 2) and sham-injected (n = 2) rats and those treated with 2.9 mg oestradiol valerate/day (n = 5) for 14 days. Oestradiol treatment reduced testis size by half yet did not significantly alter the net transport of [³H]inulin

significantly less than those in control animals $(4.29 \pm 0.48\,\text{ng/ml})$. Thus, oestradiol treatment of adult male rats suppressed serum testosterone concentrations and reduced testis size by half, yet did not cause a significant alteration in the net transport of [³H]inulin across either the blood–testis or blood–epididymal barriers (Fig. 25.1).

The results of this study complement the work of Vitale et al. (1973) who presented morphological evidence that oestradiol treatment delayed but did not prevent the establishment of the blood–testis barriers in pubertal rats. Additionally, Furuyama et al. (1981) have reported that human patients presenting with post-pubertal pituitary failure have morphologically intact Sertoli–Sertoli cell tight junctions. It appears then, that the established blood–testis and blood-epididymal barriers of adults are not impaired by androgen deprivation.

VASECTOMY AND THE BLOOD–TESTIS AND BLOOD–EPIDIDYMAL BARRIERS

The experiments

Ten hamsters were bilaterally vasectomized 10 months prior to isotope infusion and micropuncture procedures. Another 10 untreated animals were used as concurrent controls. Care was taken to avoid damage of the vasal artery and vein during the vasectomy operation. After surgery, scrotal reposition of the testis and epididymides was confirmed by palpation. At the time of the isotope infusion and micropuncture experiments, animals were anaesthetized with Inactin (Byk Guilden Konstanz, Hamburg, Germany), i.p., 200 mg/kg body weight. Animal preparation was as described above but the total dose of [³H]inulin was $330\,\mu\text{Ci/animal}$. Micropuncture began 15–20 min after the initial isotope infusion and continued over a 210 min time period. Blood and reproductive tract fluid samples were collected as described above except that caput and corpus epididymidal fluid samples were also collected in order to assess the tightness of the epididymal epithelium in the more proximal regions of the organ. Sample processing and data analysis were as described previously.

The results

Sampling fluids from several epididymal sites and the seminiferous tubules of the same animals proved difficult, thus adding to the data variance. Additionally, it was not possible to collect every fluid from every animal, especially those animals with a 10-month-old vasectomy. Vasectomized epididymal lumen contents were dense and extremely viscous, adding further to the difficulties. The hamster blood–testis and blood–epididymal barriers to [³H]inulin were not significantly altered by vasectomy, however. Mean $\pm$ SE isotope concentrations in seminiferous tubule fluid and cauda epididymidal tubule fluid during the last 1.5 h of the 3.5 h experiment were $7.54 \pm 1.77\%$ and $5.56 \pm 2.61\%$ of blood plasma isotope concentrations, respectively (Fig. 26.2). Cauda values from control and vasectomized hamsters were 3.93 ± 1.08 and $4.87 \pm 1.57\%$, respectively (Fig. 26.2). Caput and cauda epididymidal fluid values were not different from cauda values in either control or vasectomized animals.

The results of our studies, do not demonstrate a change in the blood-testis barrier to [³H]inulin in hamsters with long-term vasectomy. These results are consistent with the findings of Neaves (1973) who showed that the rat Sertoli–Sertoli cell tight junctions still excluded lanthanum from the

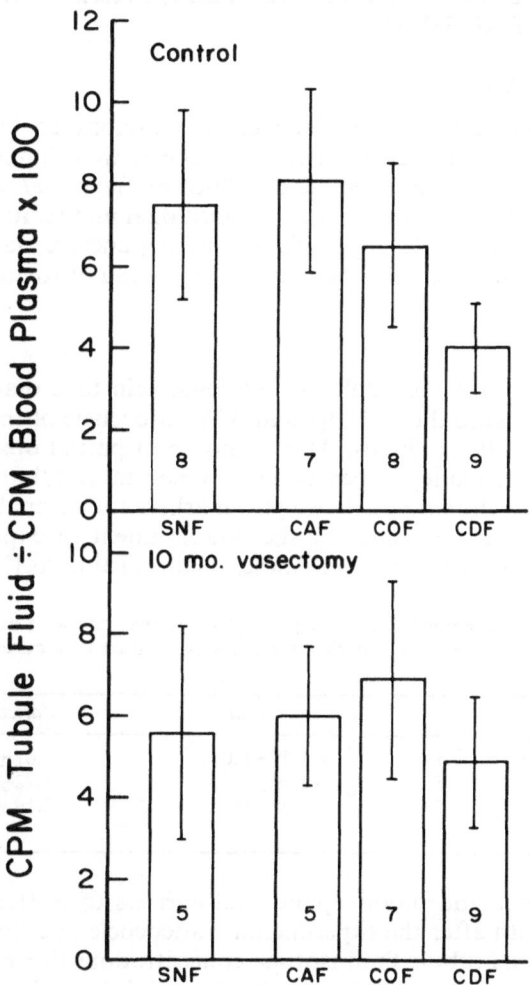

Fig. 26.2 Mean $\pm$SE percentage of blood isotope concentrations appearing in hamster reproductive tract fluids. Data illustrated are those collected during the last 1.5 h of the 3.5 h isotope-infusion experiments. Male tract tubules were sampled by micropuncture to obtain seminiferous tubule fluid (SNF), caput epididymal fluid (CAF), corpus epididymal fluid (COF), and cauda epididymal fluid (CDF). There were no significant differences within or between fluids

seminiferous tubules 4 months after vasectomy. A perhaps more surprising result was that the blood–epididymal barrier was not affected by long-term vasectomy. Despite the physical distention of the cauda epididymal tubule and the increase in intratubular hydrostatic pressure that is known to occur there (Johnson and Howards, 1975), the blood–epididymal barrier is maintained throughout the length of the organ (Fig. 26.2).

VARICOCOELE AND THE BLOOD–TESTIS AND BLOOD–EPIDIDYMAL BARRIERS

The experiments

Experimental, unilateral, left varicocoele was established in five rats one month prior to micropuncture. The varicocoeles were induced by partial obstruction of the left renal vein as described by Saypol *et al.* (1981). Five rats received the sham operation and an additional unoperated rat was used as a concurrent control. Isotope infusion, micropuncture, sample handling and data analysis were as described above for oestradiol-treated rats.

The results

Partial obstruction of the adult rat left renal vein to a diameter of 1 mm was sufficient to cause the development of a varicocoele of the left testicular vein in five out of five animals. After 1 month of partial obstruction of the renal vein, the left kidney appeared grossly normal in all animals. Neither testis weight nor seminal vesicle weight, markers for normal androgen status, were significantly affected by the establishment of experimental varicocoele 1 month prior to obtaining these weights (Table 26.1).

Table 26.1 Testis and seminal vesicle weights (g) of normal rats with experimental varicocoele. Values were obtained one month after the surgery used to induce the unilateral left varicocoele

Organ	n	Normal	Varicocoele
Right testis	5	1.79 ± 0.08	1.81 ± 0.03
Left testis	5	1.79 ± 0.07	1.72 ± 0.06
Seminal vesicle (paired)	5	2.00 ± 0.10	2.19 ± 0.14

The blood–testis and blood–epididymal barriers to [^{3}H]inulin were also still intact 1 month after the experimental varicocoele operation (Fig. 26.3). Mean seminiferous tubule fluid isotope concentrations during the last 1.5 h of the experiments were approximately 4% and 3% of blood isotope concentrations for sham and treatment animals, respectively. Cauda fluid values were approximately 1.6% and 0.4% in sham and treatment animals, respectively. All these values were consistent with concurrent and historical control values. There were no differences in values obtained from right or left testicles.

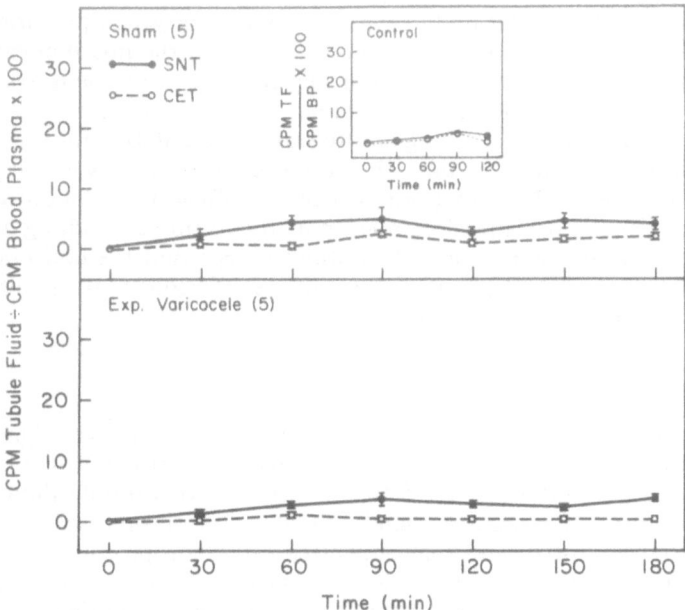

Fig. 26.3 Net transport of [³H]inulin in control, sham-operated, and experimental varicocoele animals. Varicocoele of a duration of 30 days did not disrupt either the blood–testis or blood–epididymal barrier, SNT, seminiferous tubule; CET, cauda epididymidal tubule

Varicocoele is a naturally occurring lesion in humans and is commonly believed to be associated with infertility (see Turner, 1983). The experimental animal model used to study this human lesion is the induction of a unilateral dilatation of the left testicular vein in rats. This unilateral varicocoele appears similar to that observed in human males. The model is known to produce bilateral increases in testicular temperature and blood flow (Saypol et al., 1981) and to cause a decrease in cauda epididymidal sperm concentrations and sperm motility (Turner et al., 1982). The experimental varicocoele established in rats did not cause alterations in either the blood–testis or blood–epididymal barriers to [³H]inulin 1 month after the surgery establishing the varicocoele (Fig. 26.3). This finding is consistent with the study by Cameron et al. (1980) who reported the presence of normal Sertoli–Sertoli cell tight junctions in human males with varicocoele.

CRYPTORCHIDISM AND THE BLOOD–TESTIS AND BLOOD–EPIDIDYMAL BARRIERS

The experiment

Twenty rats were randomly assigned to four groups of five animals each. Five animals served as concurrent controls. The remainder were anaesthetized with sodium pentobarbitol (Nembutol, Abbot Laboratories, Chicago,

IL) at a dose of 40 mg/kg body weight. A laparotomy was performed, the testicles were moved into the abdominal cavity, and the inguinal canal was closed with a purse-string suture of 4-0 silk, thus blocking the movement of the testicles back into the scrotum. Sham-operated animals were treated identically except the purse-string suture was immediately removed and the testicles returned to the scrotum. The cryptorchid testicles were established for either 1 week or 2 weeks prior to isotope infusion and micropuncture procedures. The isotope infusion, micropuncture, sample handling and data analysis were performed as described above except that the collection time periods were 0, 1, 2 and 3 h after the isotope infusion. Only seminiferous tubule fluid samples were collected.

The results

Net transport of [³H]inulin into the rat seminiferous tubule was significantly altered both at 1 and 2 weeks after establishment of cryptorchism (Fig. 26.4). Three hours after isotope infusion, seminiferous tubule fluid isotope concentrations reached approximately 7% of blood plasma isotope concentrations in both control and sham-operated rats. Isotope concentrations in seminiferous tubule fluid of 1 and 2 week cryptorchid rats reached 20-25% of blood plasma isotope concentrations at the same time period (Fig. 26.4).

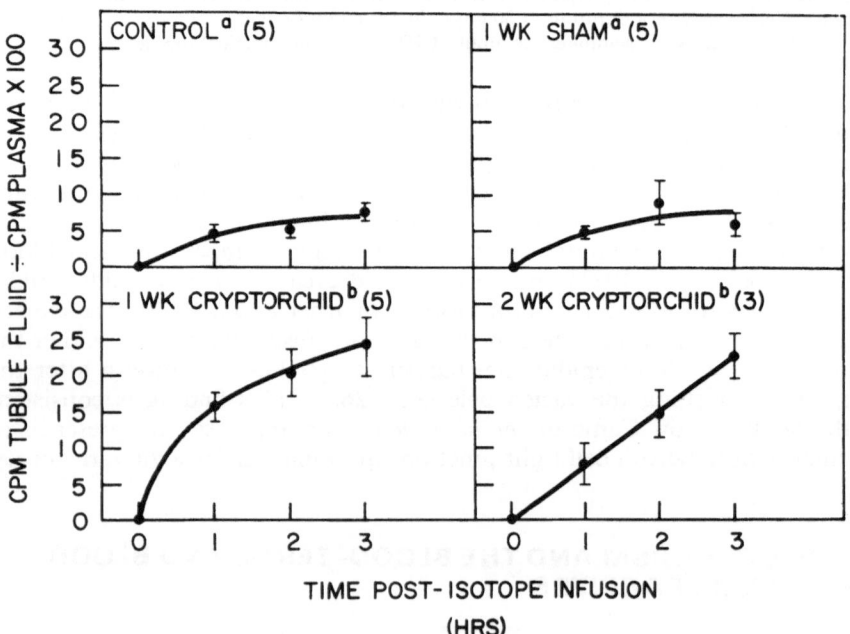

Fig. 26.4 Net transport of [³H]inulin in seminiferous tubules of control, sham-operated and cryptorchid rats. Both one and two weeks of cryptorchism significantly impaired the ability of the blood–testis barrier to exclude inulin. [a,b]Groups having different superscripts are significantly different ($p < 0.05$)

Testis size was subjectively judged to be reduced by one-third after 1 week cryptorchism and by one-half after 2 weeks cryptorchism.

It is apparent that cryptorchidism is a serious physiological insult to the testis. One and 2 weeks after establishment of experimental cryptorchism in adult rats the testes were drastically reduced in size, taking on the gross appearance of the testis of oestradiol-treated animals. In contrast to the oestradiol-treated testis, however, cryptorchid testis did have a significant increase in net [³H]inulin transport across the seminiferous tubule epithelium. While seminiferous tubule fluid isotope concentrations in normal animals of all studies plateaued at about 5% of blood isotope concentrations, isotope concentrations in the seminiferous tubule of cryptorchid testicles was on the order of 25% of blood isotope concentrations at the end of the 3 h micropuncture experiments (Fig. 26.4). While Hagenas *et al.* (1977) found that induced cryptorchism did not destroy the rat blood–testis barrier as judged by the lanthanum exclusion technique, they did note that seminiferous tubule from long-term (7–12 day) cryptorchid rats did seem to allow deeper penetration of lanthanum than did seminiferous tubules from short-term (1–2 day) cryptorchid rats. Thus, it appears that the blood–testis barrier of adult animals is significantly altered by experimental chryptorchism.

It is interesting to note that the cryptorchid testis still retained most of its capacity to restrict the entry of [³H]inulin into seminiferous tubule fluid. The tubules of the cryptorchid rat had effectively collapsed after 1 and 2 weeks cryptorchism, examination of histological sections showed that 75% of the cryptorchid testicles had a clearly disorganized seminiferous epithelium. Still, net [³H]inulin movement across the seminiferous epithelium was restricted to 25% of blood isotope concentrations. The fact that these atrophied, cryptorchid testicles still retained considerable capacity to limit the movement of macromolecules is perhaps as noteworthy as the fact that there was a significant change from controls.

CONCLUDING REMARKS

Over the last 5 years, studies from our laboratory have examined the effects of oestradiol treatment, vasectomy, varicocoele, and cryptorchism on several aspects of the physiology of the seminiferous and epididymal tubules. These treatments were used to induce conditions similar to those seen in some patients presenting with complaint of infertility. One feature common to all these studies was the investigation of the integrity of the blood–testis barrier since a contributing cause for the antispermatogenic effects of these conditions in humans might be increased 'leakiness' of the epithelial cell–cell tight junctions.

It should be noted that these studies only address [³H]inulin permeance of the seminiferous and epididymal tubule, a measure of the integrity of the epithelial cell–cell tight junctions. The physiological aspects of the blood-testis or blood–epididymal barrier, i.e.—synthesis of tubule fluid components, secretion into the lumen, active and facilitated transport phenomena, etc., are not addressed in these studies.

In every study which included examination of both seminiferous and cauda epididymidal tubule fluid, there was less net transport of [^{3}H]inulin into the cauda epididymal tubules than into the seminiferous tubule (Figs 26.1, 26.3 and 26.4). This is also the case for net transport of [^{14}C]urea into rat tubules (Howards et al., 1975) and 3-0-[^{3}H]methyl-D-glucose into hamster tubules (Turner et al., 1983). Thus it appears that the blood–epididymal barrier is in some aspects a more formidable one than the more highly touted blood–testis barrier.

In this chapter I have reviewed a series of different studies from our laboratory. These studies have demonstrated that physiological insults to the testis do not generally alter the ability of the blood–testis or blood–epididymal barriers to exclude the inert [^{3}H]inulin molecule. Even the significant 'leakiness' induced in the blood–testis barrier by cryptorchism was limited in extent. Our findings using in vivo micropuncture to study a dynamic transport process generally support the more static morphological observations of others who have shown the blood–testis barrier to be resistant to damage. The epithelial cell–cell tight junctions that form the structural component of the blood–testis and blood–epididymal barriers are clearly important for maintenance of the microenvironment of developing spermatozoa. The prerequisite of normal spermatogenesis for species perpetuation provides a probable teleological reason for the remarkable tenacity of the blood–testis and blood–epididymal barriers.

Acknowledgements

This work was supported by NIH grants HD90490 and HD18252.

References

Cameron, D.F., Syndle, F.E., Ross, M.H. and Drylie, D.M. (1980). Ultrastructural alterations in the adluminal testicular compartment in men with varicocele. Fertil. Steril., 33, 526

Dym, D. and Fawcett, D.W. (1970). Observations on the blood–testis barrier of the rat and the physiological compartmentation of the blood–testis barrier. Biol. Reprod., 3, 308

Flickinger, C. and Fawcett, D.W. (1967). The junctional specializations of Sertoli cells in the seminiferous epithelium. Anat. Rec., 158, 207

Friend, D.S. and Gilula, N.B. (1972). Variations in tight and gap junctions in mammalian tissues. J. Cell Biol., 53, 758

Furuyama, S., Kumamato, Y. and Akegaki, S. (1981). Blood–testis barrier in men with idiopathic hypogonadotrophic eunuchoidism in post-pubertal pituitary failure. Arch. Androl., 5, 361

Hagenas, L., Ploen, L., Ritzen, E.M. and Ekwall, H. (1977). Blood–testis barrier: Maintained function of the inter-Sertoli cell junctions in experimental cryptorchidism in the rat, as judged by a simple lanthanum-immersion technique. Andrologia, 9, 250

Howards, S.S., Johnson, A.L. and Jessee, S.J. (1975). Micropuncture and microanalytical studies of the rat testis and epididymis. Fertil. Steril., 26, 13

Howards, S.S., Johnson, R.L. and Jessee, S.J. (1976). Micropuncture studies of the blood-seminiferous tubule barrier. Biol. Reprod., 14, 264

Johnson, A.L. and Howards, S.S. (1975). Intratubular hydrostatic pressure in testis and epididymis before and after vasectomy. Am. J. Physiol., 228, 556

Neaves, W.B. (1973). Permeability of Sertoli cell tight junctions to lanthanum after ligation of ductus deferens and ductuli efferentes. *J. Cell Biol.*, **59**, 559

Osman, D.I. and Ploen, L. (1978). The terminal segment of the seminiferous tubules and the blood-testis barrier before and after efferent ductule ligation in the rat. *Int. J. Androl.*, **1**, 235

Saypol, D.C. (1981). Varicocele. *J. Androl.*, **2**, 61

Saypol, D.C., Howards, S.S., Turner, T.T. and Miller, E.D. (1981). The influence of surgically induced varicocele of testicular blood flow, temperature, and histology in adult rats and dogs. *J. Clin. Invest.*, **68**, 39

Setchell, B.P. and Waites, G.M.H. (1975). The blood-testis barrier. In Hamilton, D.W. and Greep, R.O. (eds.) *The Handbook of Physiology*, Section 7: *Endocrinology*, vol. 5, (Washington, DC: American Physiological Society)

Suzuki, F. and Nagano, T. (1978). Development of tight junctions in caput epididymal epthelium of mouse. *Dev. Biol.*, **63**, 321

Turner, T.T. (1979). On the epididymis and its function. *Invest. Urol.*, **16**, 311

Turner, T.T. (1983). Varicocele, still an enigma. *J. Urol.*, **129**, 695-699

Turner, T.T., D'Addario, D.A. and Howards, S.S. (1981). The blood epididymal barrier to [^{3}H]inulin in intact and vasectomized hamsters. *Invest. Urol.*, **19**, 89

Turner, T.T., D'Addario, D.A. and Howards, S.S. (1983). The transepithelial movement of [^{3}H]-3-0-methyl-D-glucose in the hamster seminiferous and cauda epididymidal tubules. *Fertil. Steril.*, **40**, 530

Turner, T.T., Hartmann, P.K. and Howards, S.S. (1979). Urea in the seminiferous tubules: Evidence for active transport. *Biol. Reprod.*, **20**, 511

Turner, T.T., Saypol, D.C. and Howards, S.S. (1982). A successful model for the study of varicocele. Abstracts of the *Annual Meeting of the Society for the Study of Reproduction*

Vitale, R., Fawcett, D.W. and Dym, M. (1973). The normal development of the blood-testis barrier and the effects of clomiphene and estrogen treatment. *Anat. Rec.*, **176**, 333

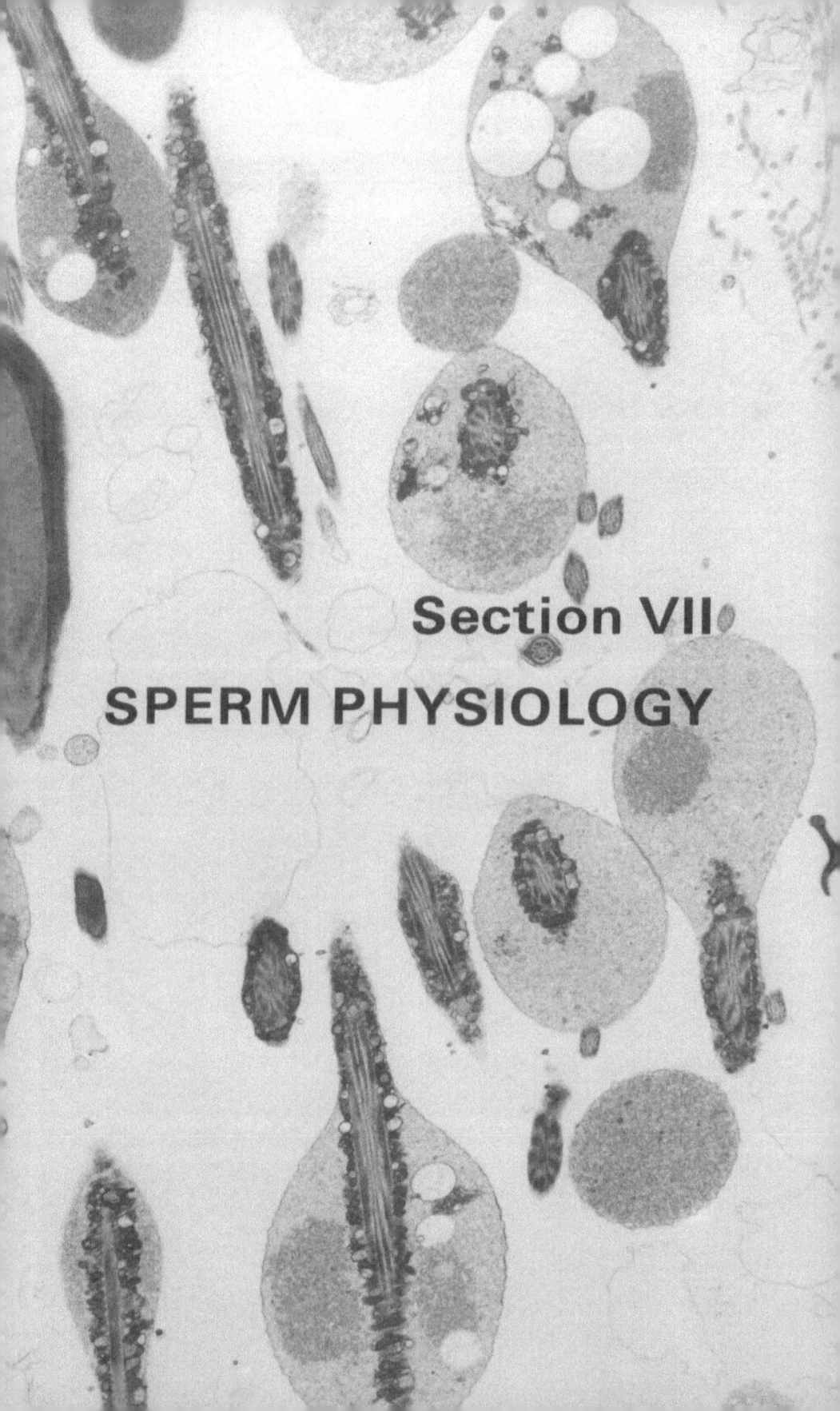

Section VII

SPERM PHYSIOLOGY

27
Sperm maturation and transport

L. C. ELLIS and B. R. NEMETALLAH

Spermatozoa are immotile in the testis and do not acquire vigorous linear motility until they have traversed the epididymis (Youchem, 1930). Transport of the inactive spermatozoa from the seminiferous tubules into the rete testis and through the epididymis results from forces not indigenous to the sperm cells. Ciliary action within the deferent ducts (Zawish-Ossenitz, 1933), active secretion of fluid by the seminiferous tubules (Setchell, 1969), contractile activity of the tunica albugineae (Davis et al., 1969) and contractility of the seminiferous tubules are potential mechanisms of propulsion of the sperm from the tubules to the epidiymis. Ciliary action has been discounted because of inadequate numbers of cilia being present in the male tract (Leeson, 1962) and a lack of potential (Winet, 1977), while fluid secretion (Setchell, 1969) and contractions of the testicular capsule and seminiferous tubules increase sperm efflux from the rete testis (Hafs et al., 1974a, b; Shirai et al., 1975). Peristaltic pumping of the tubules could be the prime method of transport of sperm through the testis into the epididymis, at least in some species (Ellis et al., 1978; Winet, 1980: Free et al., 1980).

Prostaglandins (PGs) were first discovered in human semen and were present there at higher concentrations when compared to other tissues. Recent observations (Gerozissis et al., 1982) indicate that the bulk of PGs in human semen originate in the seminal vesicles. A paucity of information exists as to why the levels of PGs are so high in the semen of humans and sheep. Currently PGs are thought to regulate sperm metabolism in the epididymis including the induction of motility and they also appear to be essential for sperm viability (Srivastava et al., 1981). High concentrations of seminal PGs could be important in activating the female tract to ensure rapid transfer of sperm towards the ovum to facilitate conception, but this only represents postulation and lacks direct evidence.

Initial studies on the characterization of PGs in human seminal fluid showed 13 PGs present including 8 dehydrated PGs of the A and B series, plus the 19-hydroxy derivatives of the A and B series (Hamberg and Samuelson, 1966). Fresh semen, however, contained large quantities of 19-hydroxy PGE, and E_2, in addition to PGE_1, E_2 and E_3. Thus, the occurrence of 19-hydroxy-PGAs and PGBs and PGAs and PGBs as reported in earlier studies, but detected in only small quantities from fresh semen (Taylor and Kelly, 1974) are not present naturally in the semen. They are present as artifacts resulting from temperature-dependent dehydration (Taylor and Kelly, 1974; Cooper and Kelly, 1975; Jonsson *et al.*, 1975).

Kelly *et al.* (1979) and Srivastava *et al.* (1981) have observed reduced amounts of 19-hydroxy-PGEs and PGEs in the semen of men with very high sperm counts when compared with normal men. These reduced levels of PGs could be due to metabolism by the sperm or binding of the PGs to the sperm (Skakkebaek *et al.*, 1976). Recently, sperm have been observed to bind PGEs and Fs (Mercado *et al.*, 1978) and very little PGs can be recovered from centrifuged spermatozoa (Cooper and Kelly, 1975). If PGs do bind to spermatozoa this would tend to support the supposition that PGs normally act to modify sperm metabolism at the time of ejaculation (Kelly, 1977).

SPECIES DIFFERENCES IN CONTRACTILITY OF THE SEMINIFEROUS TUBULES AND TESTICULAR CAPSULE

Contractile cells, found in the testicular capsule of all mammals examined, are most prominent in rabbit, dog and pig capsules and less prevalent in

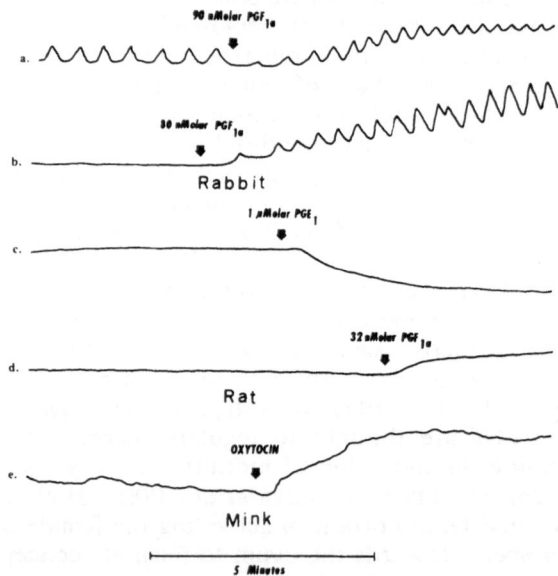

Fig. 27.1 Response of testicular capsular contractions to various pharmacological agents *in vitro:* (a) increased frequency of contractions and decreased magnitude of contractions of an actively contracting rabbit testicular capsule by $PGF_{1\alpha}$; (b) induction of contractility with an increase in tonus of an inactive rabbit testicular capsule by $PGF_{1\alpha}$; (c) decrease in tonus of an inactive rabbit testicular capsule induced by a relatively high concentration of PGE_1; (d) an increase in tonus of a rabbit testicular capsule induced by $PGF_{1\alpha}$; and (e) an increase in tonus of a mink testicular capsule induced by oxytocin—the undulations of the trace represent changes in buoyancy brought about by air bubbles coalescing on the preparation and then being released and by the increased sensitivity needed to record the event (Ellis *et al.*, 1981a)

human and rat testes (Fig. 27.1). There are species differences in the distribution of the contractile cells in the capsule. In the rabbit the contractile cells are distributed fairly uniformly over the testis, but in the human, porcine, canine, murine and feline capsules most of these cells are found in the posterior aspect of the testes where the capsule and mediastinum merge

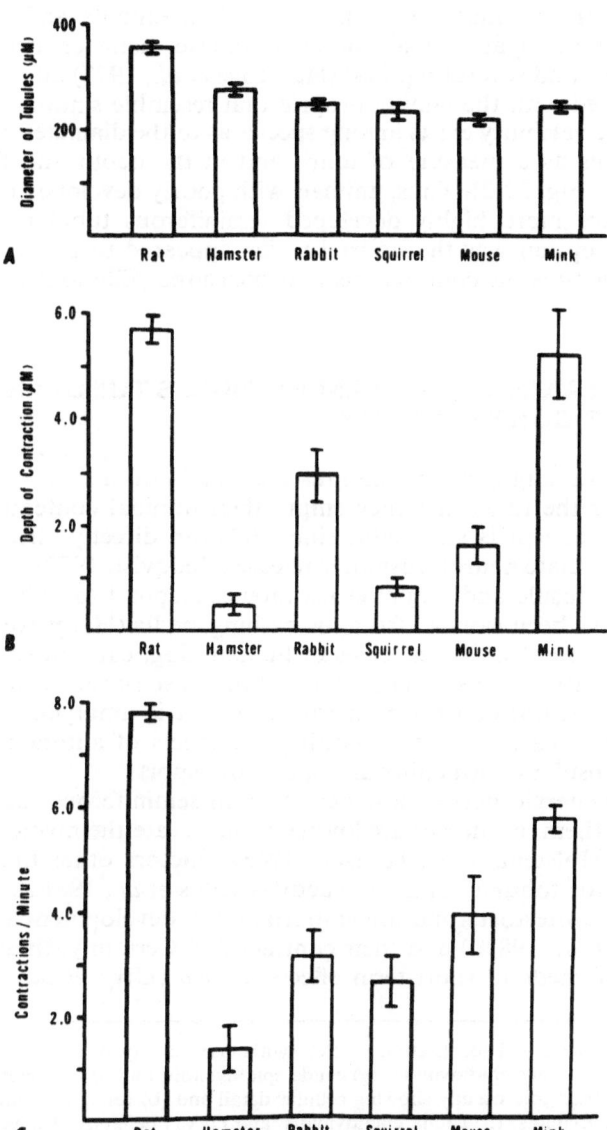

Fig. 27.2 Species differences in the contractility of the seminiferous tubules *in vitro*: (A) average diameters of the seminiferous tubules; (B) depth or magnitude of contractions; and (C) frequency of contractions (Ellis *et al.*, 1981a)

399

(Hargrove *et al.*, 1977). Functional differences are also noted for the contractility of the above species. Rabbit and boar capsules exhibit spontaneous phasic contractile activity. Others such as rats, mink and squirrels exhibit either tonic or no contractions after pharmacological stimulation (see Ellis *et al.*, 1981a). The human capsule exhibits periodic and powerful contractions (Firlit *et al.*, 1975).

Similarly, the seminiferous tubules of all mammals and several non-mammals studied (rat, human, monkey, mouse, hamster, cat, sheep, pig, domestic fowl and several reptiles) (Hargrove *et al.*, 1977) all contain myoid cells associated with the lamina propria that resemble smooth muscle cells. Considerable varibility exists among species as to the diameter of the seminiferous tubules as a measure of tonus and in the depth and frequency of contractions (Fig. 27.2). Thus, animals with poorly developed capsular contractions have more highly developed seminiferous tubular contractions. The only exception was the squirrel which appeared to be past its peak of fertility at the time the contractions were measured (Ellis *et al.*, 1981a).

PROSTAGLANDINS AND SEMINIFEROUS TUBULAR AND CAPSULAR CONTRACTILITY

Prostaglandins might affect the muscular walls of the male reproductive tract to alter the rates that they empty their luminal contents (von Euler, 1936). This concept is still viable since PGs can directly affect the musculature or modulate neurotransmitter release (Hedqvist, 1977).

Both the capsule and seminiferous tubules respond to PGs, and PG-like materials have been isolated from the bathing media (Hargrove *et al.*, 1977). Nerves are present in the capsules of human, dog, cat and rat testes (Hargrove *et al.*, 1977; Ellis *et al.*, 1981a). For most species (except dog) the evidence for neural control of sperm transport is ambiguous. No specific generalizations can be made regarding the effects of autonomic nerves on testicular capsular contractility and sperm transport.

While adrenergic nerves pass near human seminiferous tubules without penetrating them, no nerves are known to innervate the myoid cells (Baumgarten and Holstein, 1967; Hodson, 1965). Factors other than nerves are responsible for tubular contractile activity (Ellis *et al.*, 1981a). Testosterone and 5α-dihydrotestosterone are important for development of the myoid cells (Ellis *et al.*, 1981a) and their contractility. Certainly, these two androgens have immediate short-term effects *in vivo* (Urry *et al.*, 1976) and *in*

Fig. 27.3 Histochemical localization of PG synthetase activity in rat: (a) testis; (c) caput epididymidis; (e) corpus epididymidis; (g) cauda epididymidis; and (i) vas deferens all observed with phase-contrast microscopy showing cellular detail and (b) testis; (d) caput epididymidis; (f) corpus epididymidis, (h) cauda epididymidis; and (j) vas deferens observed under bright-field microscopy with dihomo-gamma-linolenic acid as the substrate showing a lack of staining in the testis and caput epididymidis, slight staining of sperm tails in the corpus epididymidis along with heavy staining of fat-cells in the epididymal fat-pad and moderate staining of sperm tails in the vas deferens with some staining in some cells lining the tubule within the epididymis

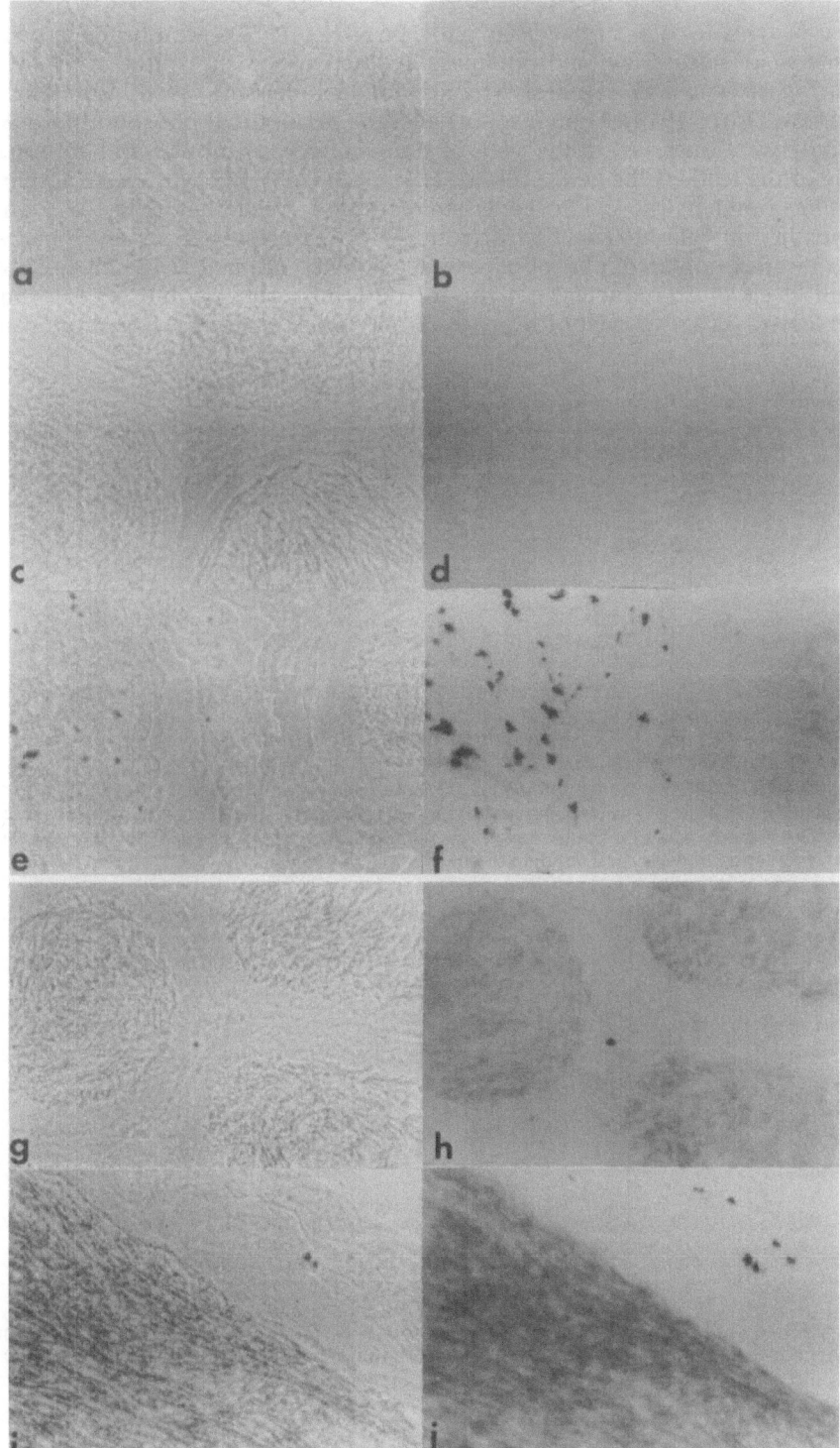

vitro (Farr and Ellis, 1980; Ellis and Hargrove, 1977). Membrane arachidonic acid release by phospholipase A_2 activity is the initial and rate-limiting step in PG synthesis (Lands and Samuelsson, 1968; Vonkeman and von Dorp, 1968). High levels of alkaline pH optimal phospholipase A_2 activity were observed in the walls of the seminiferous tubules and germinal cells of the testis (Ellis *et al.*, 1981a). Histochemically PG synthetase activity was maximal in the cauda epididymidis and vas deferens (Fig. 27.3 and Johnson and Ellis, 1978). Testosterone, 5α-dihydrotestosterone and progesterone all stimulated phospholipase A_2 activity *in vitro* (Figs 27.4–27.6). High levels of 5α-reductase activity for both progesterone and testosterone and 20α-reductase activity for progesterone in the walls of the seminiferous

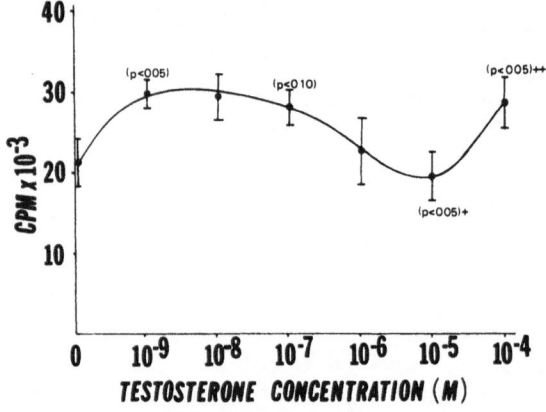

Fig. 27.4 Testosterone activation of rat testicular alkaline pH optimal phospholipase A_2 activity. The 10^{-9} M group was significantly higher ($p<0.05$) than the control group, whereas the 10^{-5} M group was significantly lower ($p<0.05$ than the 10^{-7} M group. The 10^{-4} M group was significantly higher ($p<0.05$) than the 10^{-5} M group

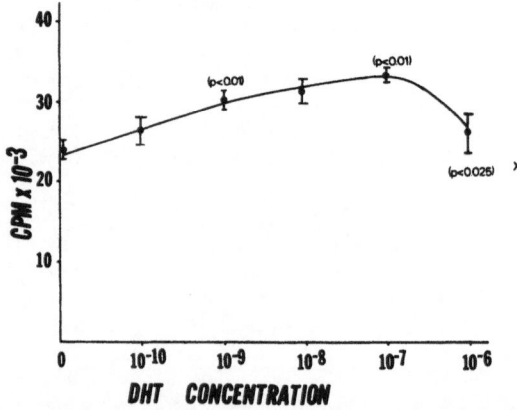

Fig. 27.5 5α-Dihydrotestosterone (DHT) activation of rat testicular alkaline pH optimal phospholipase A_2 activity. The 10^{-9} to 10^{-7} M groups were significantly higher ($p<0.001$) than the control group. The 10^{-6} M group was significantly lower ($p<0.025$) than the 10^{-7} M group

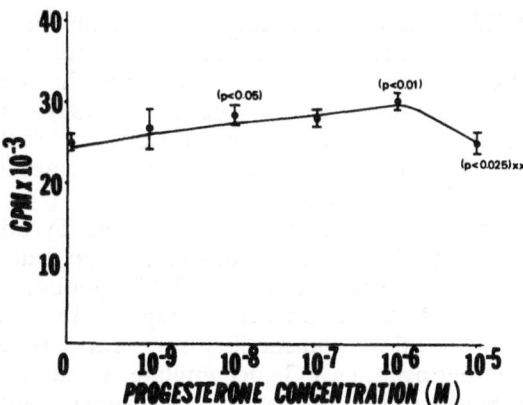

Fig. 27.6 Activation of rat testicular alkaline pH optimal phospholipase A_2 activity by progesterone. The 10^{-8} M and 10^{-6} M groups were significantly higher ($p < 0.025$) than the 10^{-6} M group

tubules (Ellis *et al.*, 1981a) could prevent progesterone and the androgens from prematurely activating phospholipase A_2 activity concomitant with an accumulation of PGs in the seminiferous tubules that could interrupt spermatogenesis. Indeed, androgen binding protein (ABP) appears to be pivotal to this concept because PG synthesis by the germ cells is normally not active because ABP prevents the hormones from activating phospholipase A_2 activity in the testis and caput epididymis (Ellis *et al.*, 1981) to give the pattern of PG synthesis observed histochemically (see Fig. 27.3 and Johnson and Ellis, 1978). Testosterone passing through the walls of the seminiferous tubule could activate the myoepithelial cells inducing contractility, but its action on phospholipase A_2 activity within the seminiferous tubule would be circumvented since it would bind with ABP and thus be unavailable to activate the enzyme. Later, starting in the corpus epididymidis, the ABP would be absorbed leaving the androgen free to activate the phospholipase A_2 enzyme to initiate motility and to participate in capacitation, etc. Preliminary data from our laboratory show that PGE_2 can activate sperm adenyl cyclase activity. The above concepts reaffirm previous research that considerable arachidonic acid is lost from the spermatozoa as they pass through the epididymis (Poulos *et al.*, 1973, 1975; Arora *et al.*, 1975). Spermatozoa synthesize PGs in the epididymis (Fig. 27.3 and Johnson and Ellis, 1978). Amounts of PGs in the semen are directly proportional to sperm density (Sturde, 1968). The vas deferens contain significantly higher concentrations of PGE and PGF than was found in either the epididymis or seminal vesicles (Badr *et al.*, 1975). Our preliminary data show increases of PGE content of the epididymis starting with the caput epididymidis that becomes maximal in the vas deferens.

Histamine stimulates rat and rabbit capsular contractions *in vitro* through H_1 receptors and anti-PGE and anti-PGF attenuate its response (Nemetallah and Ellis, 1983). Moreover, neither PGE nor PGF appear to be involved in the stimulatory effects of either acetylcholine, epinephrine or serotonin

(Nemetallah and Ellis, unpublished data). An increase in testicular temperature from 33 to 35°C increased the strength of testicular capsular contractions *in vitro* but increases from 35 to 37°C diminished contractility and the force of contractions (Nemetallah and Ellis, 1983). This increase in temperature markedly reduced the effectiveness of acetylcholine, serotonin, epinephrine, $PGF_{2\alpha}$, histamine and bradykinin in their ability to stimulate contractility of the testicular capsule.

When a fresh rabbit testis is placed in oxygenated Tyrode's solution *in vitro*, some time is required for contractions to develop, but if enough time is allowed, essentially all preparations will exhibit spontaneous contactility (Nemetallah and Ellis, 1983). If an active preparation is placed in fresh oxygenated Tyrode's solution, contractility stops for a time and then becomes active as the endogenous PGs accumulate. If one of these inactive preparations is placed in the original bathing media, contractility is restored. Adding PGs to the bathing media also activates an inactive preparation. Changing the bathing media of a rabbit testis contracting *in vivo*, however, has little effect on contractility (Ellis *et al.*, 1981a), but changing the bathing media *in vitro* of boar testes does not affect contractility (Ohanian *et al.*, 1979). The failure of contractility to be effaced under the above two conditions suggests that in these two preparations PG synthesis is rapid enough to exceed its metabolism. The rat testicular capsule and interstitial cells both produce PGs and both contain the PG 15-hydroxydehydrogenase and Δ^{13}-reductase enzymes (Ellis and Jorgensen, 1982) for PG inactivation. The concentration of PGs is about 100 times higher in the capsule than in the parenchyma (Gerozissis and Dray, 1977). PG 15-hydroxydehydrogenase activity was also significantly higher in the capsule than in the interstitial cell or seminiferous tubules (due to a greater mass), while 25.4% was found in the interstitial cells and 16.9% in the capsule. When corrected for protein content, 90 756 CPM/mg protein was found in the capsule while only 9123 and 21 099 CPM/mg protein were present in the seminiferous tubules and interstitial cells, respectively. Some activity was present in the seminiferous tubular walls and is important in regulating tubular contractility. The activity of both of these enzymes was stimulated by FSH and LH, but prolactin inhibited the Δ^{13}-reductase activity (Ohuo-Obasiolu *et al.*, 1982).

SPERM TRANSPORT IN EXCURRENT DUCTS

$PGF_{2\alpha}$ injection prior to semen collection increases the number of spermatozoa in ejaculates of bulls (Hafs *et al.*, 1974a) and rabbits (Hafs *et al.*, 1974a,b; Reichard *et al.*, 1978). In stallions (Cornwell *et al.*, 1974) $PGF_{2\alpha}$ appeared to increase the number of spermatozoa in the first ejaculates when administered over a short period, but decreased the numbers during prolonged treatment (Kreider *et al.*, 1981). In the boar $PGF_{2\alpha}$ injections induced a redistribution of spermatozoa during ejaculation so that a greater percentage of cells appeared in the sperm-rich fraction (Hemsworth *et al.*, 1977). The volume of this fraction was increased whereas the sperm-poor fraction volume was reduced. In rabbits long-term treatment of the bucks with $PGF_{2\alpha}$ twice daily for 60 days exhibited no effect on the percentage of motile spermatozoa or total sperm output, but did accelerate the appearance of labelled cells in the ejaculate (Hunt and Nicholson, 1972). In the rat, however, spermatogenesis was diminished when $PGF_{2\alpha}$ was injected daily for 15 days (Abbatiello et al., 1976). The reduction of sperm counts in stallions after prolonged $PGF_{2\alpha}$ injections also is suggestive of interference of spermatogenesis (Kreider et al., 1981). Subcutaneous or interscrotal implants of $PGF_{2\alpha}$ reduced the numbers of spermatozoa in the epididymis and vas deferens of rats in 14 days (Saksena et al., 1978). Similarly, both $PGF_{1\alpha}$ and $PGF_{2\alpha}$ suppressed spermatogenesis in the mouse at the meiotic phase concomitant with degeneration of spermatozonia.

ROLE OF CYCLIC NUCLEOTIDES IN SPERM MATURATION AND TRANSPORT

When mature bovine caudal sperm are mixed with accessory gland secretions a doubling of sperm cyclic AMP occurs (Hoskins et al., 1978). A large increase in hamster interspermic cyclic AMP content occurs (perhaps 10-fold) and this suggests that cyclic AMP content prior to ejaculation may be close to zero. It is well known that cyclic AMP determines the intensity of sperm motility since an increase (some 40%) in cyclic AMP in bovine sperm caused them to become more motile (Garbers et al., 1973). A drop of 25 to 50% in total cyclic AMP content of washed sperm cells of several species resulted in immotile cells (Hoskins et al., 1978; Tash and Mann, 1973). Moreover, Morton et al. (1974) have shown that Ca^{2+} is much higher in seminal plasma than in epididymal fluid and that Ca^{2+} or cyclic AMP activates hamster sperm.

Intracellular cyclic AMP levels are the net result of synthesis (adenyl cyclase activity) and breakdown (phosphodiesterase activity). Recent studies in the rat (Purvis et al., 1982) and sheep (our unpublished preliminary observations plus those of Amann et al., 1982) show that cyclic AMP levels increase as sperm transverse the epididymis and that phosphodiesterase activity diminishes while adenyl cyclase activity increases. Similar observations have been observed for phosphodiesterase activity in bovine spermatozoa (Casillas et al., 1978; Stephens et al., 1979). Of importance is the fact that both adenyl cyclase and phosphodiesterase activity are located predominantly in the tail region where they could be coupled with the contractile mechanism. The loss of phosphodiesterase activity from spermatozoa is consistent with the loss of sperm protein during epididymal transit (preliminary unpublished observations). Of interest is the fact that we observed a decrease in ram spermatozoal cyclic GMP concentration during epididymal transit while others (Purvis et al., 1982) reported that rat cyclic GMP phosphodiesterase activity diminished. Thus, guanyl cyclase activity must diminish as sperm pass through the epididymis.

Recent observations show that dihydrotestosterone binds to ABP and that the highest level of ABP–dihydrotestosterone is in the caput, but lowest in the cauda epididymides (Purvis and Hanson, 1978). Thus, if dihydrotestosterone were progressively freed from ABP, from the corpus to the cauda epididymides the androgen would be free to activate PG synthesis. PGE_2 would then be available to stimulate adenyl cyclase activity to produce cyclic AMP which in turn could be responsible for initiating glycolysis, motility and other maturational changes of sperm.

PHOSPHOLIPASE A_2 ACTIVITY AND THE ACROSOMAL REACTION

Recent evidence suggests that phospholipase A_2 activity and lipids are involved in the acrosomal reaction (Llanos *et al.*, 1982; Fleming & Yanagimachi, 1981). A phospholipase A_2 and an associated phosphatidylcholine hydrolysing activity are components of bovine serum albumin used in the media for capacitating sperm and they induce the acrosomal reaction *in vitro* (Fleming and Yanagimachi, 1981). However purified albumin, devoid of these two activities, was still capable of inducing capacitation and the acrosomal reaction. Bee venom phospholipase A_2 activity could also induce these responses in the absence of epinephrine, but not in the presence of the catecholamine. It was concluded that phospholipase A_2 of bovine serum albumin may contribute to capacitation by mimicking the action of native sperm phospholipase A_2 (Singleton and Killian, 1983).

Acknowledgements

This work was sponsored by grants from the Utah State University Research Project SB-1100 and National Institutes of Health no. 5 R01 HD123-25-02. BRH was supported by a postdoctoral research fellowship sponsored by the Egyptian Cultural and Educational Bureau.

References

Abbatiello, E.R., Kaminsky, M. and Wiesbroth, S. (1976). The effect of prostaglandin $F_{1\alpha}$ and $F_{2\alpha}$ on spermatogenesis. *Int. J. Fertil.*, **21**, 82–8

Amann, R.P., Hay, S.R. and Hammerstedt, R.H. (1982). Yield, characteristics, motility and cAMP content of sperm isolated from seven regions of ram epididymis. *Biol. Reprod.*, **27**, 723–33

Arora, R., Dinaker, N. and Prasad, M.R.N. (1975). Biochemical changes in the spermatozoa and luminal contents of different regions of the epididymis of the Rhesus monkey, *Mucaca mulatta. Contraception*, **6**, 689–700

Badr, F.M., Barcikowski, B. and Bartke, A. (1975). Effect of castration, testosterone treatment and heredity on prostaglandin concentration in the male reproductive system of mice. *Prostaglandin*, **9**, 289–97

Baumgarten, H.G. and Holstein, A.F. (1967). Catecholaminhatige nerven fasern in Hoden des menschen. *Z. Zellforsch. Mikrosk. Anat.*, **79**, 389–95

Casillas, E.R., Elder, C.M. and Hoskins, D.P. (1978). Adenylate cyclase activity in maturing bovine spermatozoa: Activation by GTP and polyamines. *Fed. Proc.*, **37**, 1688 (abstract)

Cooper, I. and Kelly, R.W. (1975). The measurement of E and 19-hydroxy E prostaglandins in human seminal plasma. *Prostaglandins*, **10**, 507–14

Cornwell, J.C., Koonce, K.L. and Kreider, J.L. (1974). Effect of prostaglandin $F_{2\alpha}$ on semen characteristics of the stallion. *J. Anim. Sci.*, **38**, 226 (abstract)

Davis, J.R., Langford, G.A. and Kirby, P.J. (1969). The testicular capsule. In Johnson, A.D., Gomes, W.R. and Vandermark, N.L., (eds.) *The Testis*. Vol. I, pp. 281–337 (New York: Academic Press.)

Ellis, L.C., Boccio, J.R., Cunningham, M.J., Groesbeck, M.D. and Cosentino, M.J. (1981a). Rat testicular phospholipase A_2 activity. *J. Androl.*, **2**, 94–102

Ellis, L.C., Buhrley, L.E. Jr and Hargrove, J.L. (1978). Species differences in contractility of seminiferous tubules and tunica albuginia as related to sperm transport through the testis. *Arch. Androl.*, **1**, 139–46

Ellis, L.C., Groesbeck, M.D., Farr, C.H. and Tesi, R.J. (1981b). Contractility of seminiferous tubules as related to sperm transport in the male. *Arch. Androl.*, **6**, 283–94

Ellis, L.C. and Hargrove, J.L. (1977). Prostaglandins. In Johnson, A.D. and Gomes, W.R. (eds.) *The Testis*, Vol. IV, pp. 289–313 (New York: Academic Press)

Ellis, L.C. and Jorgensen, R.D. (1982). Age changes in rat testicular capsular and parenchymal Δ^{13}-reductase and 15-hydroxyprostaglandin dehydrogenase activities. *Arch. Androl.*, **8**, 121–8

Farr, C.H. and Ellis, L.C. (1980). *In vitro* contractility of rat seminiferous tubules in response to prostaglandins, cyclic GMP, testosterone and 2,4'-dibromoacetophenone. *J. Reprod. Fertil.*, **58**, 37–42

Firlit, C.F., King, L.R. and Davis, J.R. (1975). Comparative response of the isolated human testicular capsule to autonomic drugs. *J. Urol.*, **113**, 500–4

Fleming, A.D. and Yanagimachi, R. (1981). Effects of various lipids on the acrosome reaction and fertilizing capacity of guinea pig spermatozoa with specific reference to the possible involvement of lysophospholipids in the acrosome reaction. *Gamete Res.*, **4**, 253–74

Free, M.J., Jaffe, R.A. and Morford, D.E. (1980). Sperm transport through the rete testis in anesthetized rats: role of the testicular capsule and effect of gonadotropins and prostaglandins. *Biol. Reprod.*, **22**, 1073–8

Garbers, D.L., First, N.L. and Lardy, H.A. (1973). The stimulation of bovine sperm metabolism by cyclic nucleotide phosphodiesterase inhibitors. *Biol. Reprod.*, **8**, 589–98

Gerozissis, K. and Dray, F. (1977). Prostaglandins in the isolated testicular capsule of immature and young adult rats. *Prostaglandins*, **13**, 777–83

Gerozissis, K., Jouannet, P., Soufir, J.C. and Dray, F. (1982). Origin of prostaglandins in human semen. *J. Reprod. Fertil.*, **65**, 401–4

Hafs, H.D., Louis, T.M. and Stelflug, J.N. (1974b). Increased sperm numbers in deferent duct after prostaglandin $F_{2\alpha}$ in rabbits. *Proc. Soc. Exp. Biol. Med.*, **145**, 1120–4

Hafs, H.D., Louis, T.M., Wates, R.J., Stelflug, J.N. and Haynes, N.B. (1974a). Increased sperm output of rabbits and bulls treated with prostaglandin $F_{2\alpha}$. *Prostaglandins*, **8**, 417–22

Hamberg, M. and Samuelson, B. (1966). Prostaglandins in human seminal plasma. *J. Biol. Chem.*, **241**, 257–63

Hargrove, J.L., MacIndoe, J.H. and Ellis, L.C. (1977). Testicular contractile cells and sperm transport. *Fertil. Steril.*, **28**, 1146–57

Hedqvist, P. (1977). Basic mechanisms of prostaglandin action on autonomic neurotransmission. *Ann. Rep. Pharmacol. Toxicol.*, **17**, 259–79

Hemsworth, P.H., Donnelly, J., Findlay, J.K. and Galloway, D.B. (1977). The effects of prostaglandin $F_{2\alpha}$ on sperm output in boars. *Prostaglandins*, **13**, 933–41

Hodson, N. (1965). Sympathetic nerves and reproductive organs in the male rabbit. *J. Reprod. Fertil.*, **10**, 209–20

Hoskins, D.D., Brant, H. and Scott, T.S. (1978). Initiation of sperm motility in the mammalian epididymis. *Fed. Proc.*, **37**, 2534–42

Hunt, W.L. and Nicholson, N. (1972). Studies on semen from rabbits injected with ^{3}H-thymidine and treated with prostaglandin E_2 and prostaglandin $F_{2\alpha}$. *Fertil. Steril.*, **23**, 763–8

Johnson, J.M. and Ellis, L.C. (1978). The histochemical localization of prostaglandin synthetase activity in reproductive tract of the male rat. *J. Reprod. Fertil.*, **51**, 17–22

Jonsson, H.T., Middleditch, B.S. and Desiderio, D.M. (1975). Prostaglandins in human seminal fluid: two novel compounds. *Science*, **187**, 1093–4

Kelly, R.W. (1977). Effect of seminal prostaglandins on the metabolism of human spermatozoa. *J. Reprod. Fert.*, **50**, 217–22

MALE FERTILITY AND ITS REGULATION

Kelly, R.W., Cooper, I. and Templeton, A.A. (1979). Reduced prostaglandin levels in the semen of men with very high sperm concentrations. *J. Reprod. Fert.*, **56**, 195-9

Kreider, J.L., Ogg, W.L. and Turner, J.W. (1981). Influence of prostaglandin $F_{2\alpha}$ on sperm production and seminal characteristics of the stallion. *Prostaglandins*, **22**, 903-13

Lands, W.E.M. and Samuelsson, B. (1968). Phospholipid precursors of prostaglandins. *Biochim. Biophys. Acta*, **164**, 426-9

Leeson, T.S. (1962). Electron microscopy of the rete testis of the rat. *Anat. Rec.*, **144**, 57-67

Llanos, M.N., Lui, C.W. and Meizel, S. (1982). Studies of phospholipase A_2 related to the hamster sperm acrosome reaction. *J. Exp. Zool.*, **221**, 107-17

Mercado, E., Villalobos, M., Dominguez, R. and Rosado, A. (1978). Differential binding of PGE and $PGF_{2\alpha}$ to the human spermatozoa membrane. *Life Sci.*, **22**, 429-36

Morton, B., Harrigan-Lum, J., Albagli, L. and Jooss, T. (1974). The activity of motility in quiescent hamster sperm from the epididymis by calcium and cyclic nucleotides. *Biochem. Biophys. Res. Commun.*, **56**, 372-9

Nemetallah, B.R. and Ellis, L.C. (1983). Temperature induced alterations in rabbit testicular contractility *in vitro*. *Arch. Androl.*, **10**, 161-8

Nemetallah, B.R., Howell, R.E. and Ellis, L.C. (1983). Histamine H_1 receptors and prostaglandin-histamine interactions modulating contractility of rabbit and rat testicular capsules *in vitro*. *Biol. Reprod.*, **28**, 632-5

Ohanian, C., Rodriquez, H., Piriz, H., Martini, I., Rieppi, G., Garofalo, E.G. and Roca, R.A. (1979). Studies on the contractile activity and ultrastructure of the boar testicular capsule. *J. Reprod. Fertil.*, **57**, 79-85

Ohuo-Obasiolu, C.C., Groesbeck, M.D. and Ellis, L.C. (1982). Control of rat testicular prostaglandin dehydrogenase, Δ^{13}-prostaglandin reductase and total prostaglandin dehydrogenase activities. *J. Androl.*, **3**, 329-36

Poulos, A., Brown-Woodman, P.D.C., White, I.G. and Cox, R.I. (1975). Changes in phospholipids of ram spermatozoa during migration through the epididymis and possible origin of prostaglandin $F_{2\alpha}$ in testicular and epididymal fluid. *Biochim. Biophys. Acta*, **388**, 12-18

Poulos, A., Voglmayr, J.K. and White, I.G. (1973). Phospholipid changes in spermatozoa during passage through the genital tract of the bull. *Biochim. Biophys. Acta*, **306**, 194-202

Purvis, K., Cusan, H., Attramadal, A., Ege, A. and Hansson, V. (1982). Rat sperm enzymes during epididymal transit. *J. Reprod. Fertil.*, **65**, 381-7

Purvis, K. and Hansson, V. (1978). Androgens and androgen-binding protein in the rat epididymis. *J. Reprod. Fertil.*, **32**, 59-63

Reichard, L.A., Hafs, H.D., Haynes, N.B., Collier, R.J., Kiser, T.E. and McCarthy, M.S. (1978). Sperm output and serum testosterone in rabbits given prostaglandin $F_{2\alpha}$ or E_2. *Prostaglandins*, **16**, 135-42

Saksena, S.K., Lau, I.F. and Chang, M.C. (1978). Effects of prostaglandin $F_{2\alpha}$ on some reproductive parameters of fertile male rats. *Prostaglandins Med.*, **1**, 107-15

Setchell, B.P. (1969). Testicular blood supply, lymphatic drainage and secretion of fluid. In Johnson, A.D., Gomes, W.R. and Vandemark, N.L. (eds.) *The Testis*. Vol. I, pp. 101-239 (New York: Academic Press)

Shirai, M., Mitsukawa, S. and Matsuda, A. (1975). Impetus to transferring non-motile sperm in the seminiferous tubules into the epididymis. *Tohulu J. Exp. Med.*, **115**, 95-6

Singleton, C.L. and Killian, G.J. (1983). A study of phospholipase in albumin and its role in inducing the acrosome reaction of guinea pig spermatozoa *in vitro*. *Arch. Androl.*, **10**, 161-8

Skakkebaek, N.E., Kelly, R.W. and Corker, C.S. (1976). Prostoglandin concentrations in the semen of hypogonadal men during treatment with testosterone. *J. Reprod. Fertil.*, **47**, 119-21

Srivastava, K.C., Bansal, R.K. and Giwari, K.P. (1981). Prostaglandin E and 19-hydroxyprostaglandin E content in the semen of men with normal sperm characteristics, men with abnormal sperm characteristics, vasectomized men and polyzoospermic men. *Dan. Med. Bull.*, **28**, 201-3

Stephens, D.T., Wang, J.L. and Hoskins, D. (1979). The cyclic AMP phosphodiesterase of bovine spermatozoa: multiple form, kinetic properties and changes during development. *Biol. Reprod.*, **20**, 483-91

Sturde, H.C. (1968). Experimentaelle Untersuchungen zur Frage der Prostaglandine und Ihrer Beziehungen zur Mänlichen Fertilität. *Arzneimittel-Forschung*, **18**, 1158-63

Tash, J.S. and Mann, T. (1973). Adenosine 3':5'-cyclic monophosphate in relation to motility and senescence of spermatozoa. *Proc. R. Soc. London. Ser. B*, **184**, 109–14

Taylor, P.L. and Kelly, R.W. (1974). 19-Hydroxylated E prostaglandins as the major prostaglandins in human semen. *Nature (London)*, **10**, 507–14

Urry, R.L., Assay, R.W. and Cockett, A.T.K. (1976). Hormonal control of seminiferous tubule contractions. A hypothesis of sperm transport from the testicle. *Invert. Urol.*, **14**, 194–7

Von Euler, U.S. (1936). On the specific vasodilating and smooth-muscle stimulating substances from accessory genital glands in man and certain animals (prostaglandin and vesiglandin). *J. Physiol.*, **88**, 213–34

Vonkeman, H. and van Dorp, D.A. (1968). The action of prostaglandin synthetase on 2-arachidonyl-lecithin. *Biochim. Biophys. Acta*, **164**, 430–2

Winet, H. (1977). Can cilia alone propel gametes in the oviductal isthmus and the testicular ductuli efferentes? *Fed. Proc.*, **36**, 372 (Abstract)

Winet, H. (1980). On the mechanism for flow in the efferent ducts. *J. Androl.*, **1**, 304–11

Youchem, D.E. (1930). A study of the motility and resistance of rat spermatozoa at different levels in the reproductive tract. *Physiol. Zool.*, **3**, 309–29

Zaqisch-Ossenitz, C. (1933). Der Flimmerstrom in den Ductuli efferentes des Hodens und die Bewegung der Spermien. *Z. Zellfors. Mikroscop. Anat.*, **32**, 84–106

28
Ionic mechanisms of sperm motility initiation

P.Y.D. WONG and W.M.LEE

Sperm maturation and storage are two important functions of the mammalian epididymis. When spermatozoa are first produced in the testis, they are immature, immotile and incapable of fertilizing the female ovum. It is only after transit through the epididymis that they gradually acquire their potential for forward motility and fertilizing capacity. However, when they reach the cauda epididymidis, they are maintained in the quiescent state. During ejaculation they burst into vigorous motility when mixed with copious secretion from the accessory glands.

Several laboratories have been interested in the mechanisms underlying the transition of the spermatozoa from the immotile to the motile state during ejaculation. Several factors have been proposed to account for this change. They are released from mechanical restraint (Cascieri *et al.*, 1976), provision of oxygen and substrate (Mann, 1964) and calcium (Morton, *et al.*, 1973) by the accessory gland fluids, change in osmolarity of the fluid (Turner and Howards, 1978) etc. However, none of these factors alone is able satisfactorily to explain the initiation of sperm motility. This article reports on the possible involvement of inorganic ions in sperm motility initiation.

Na^+-H^+ EXCHANGE

When spermatozoa are flushed out from the rat or hamster cauda epididymidis with oil, they are immotile, or when flushed out with a sodium-free medium (SFM), they show only transient motility. However, if these immotile spermatozoa are resuspended in a sodium-containing medium (SCM), they initiate or regain their forward motility within 15 min (Fig. 28.1) (Wong *et al.*, 1981). The sodium-induced motility has been used to examine the ionic basis of sperm motility initiation. Sperm motility initiation induced by extracellular sodium ions is associated with release of protons from the sperm. Both sperm motility initiation and acid release are closely dependent on the extracellular sodium concentration and partially inhibited by amiloride which blocks Na^+ entry into cells. Other monovalent

411

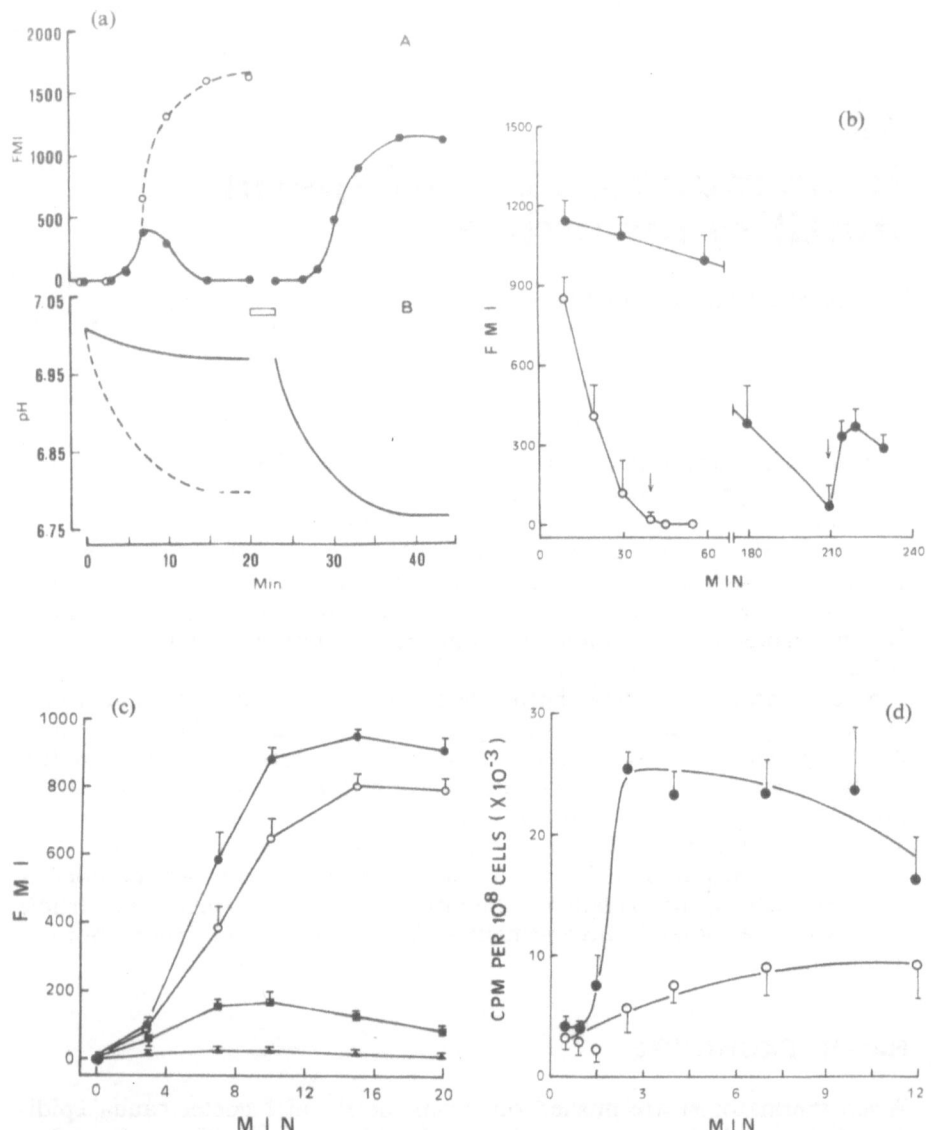

Fig. 28.1 (a) Effect of dilution on (A) forward motility and (B) acid release of the rat caudal epididymal sperm. Spermatozoa were flushed out of the cauda epididymidis with oil and diluted with a sodium containing medium (SCM) (o) or a sodium free medium (SFM) (●) to produce a sperm concentration of 10^7 sperm/ml. At the bar, the SFM incubated sperm were resuspended in SCM. (b) Effect of A23187 on motility of the rat caudal epididymal sperm. Spermatozoa were flushed out from the cauda epididymidis with oil and incubated in either SCM (●) or SFM (O) until forward motility ceased. At the arrows A23187 was added to give a final concentration of 50 nmol/l. A23187 was first dissolved in dimethylformamide/ethanol (3:1) to 10 mmol/l. Subsequent dilutions in distilled water was made before addition to spermatozoa. Each point shows the mean ± SEM of four experiments. (c) Effect of verapamil on sperm motility initiation. Rat cauda epididymal sperm were flushed out from

cations, except ammonium ions, cannot substitute sodium in initiating motility (Wong et al., 1981).

K+ EFFLUX FROM SPERM

Although sodium ions are required for motility initiation in rat cauda epididymal sperm, high K^+ has been shown to inhibit motility. At a K^+ concentration of 50 mmol/l (the concentration found in the rat cauda epididymidis), sperm motility is inhibited by 80% (Wong and Lee, 1983). K^+ movement across the sperm membrane has been followed by using Rb^+ as a marker of K^+. When the $^{86}Rb^+$ preloaded sperm are resuspended in a sodium-free medium, there is a little efflux of $^{86}Rb^+$. However, if they are suspended in a sodium-containing medium, the efflux rate is greatly increased. The increase in $^{86}Rb^+$ efflux is associated with an initiation of sperm motility. Both $^{86}Rb^+$ efflux and motility initiation are triggered by a K^+ ionophore 18-crown-6 (2 mmol/l). However, the ionophore-induced $^{86}Rb^+$ efflux and motility initiation only occurred in the presence of extracellular sodium. Tetraethylammonium (TEA) chloride, which blocks K^+ channels, inhibits motility initiation in a dose-dependent manner (Wong and Lee, 1983). Because of the high dependence of H^+ efflux and sperm motility initiation on extracellular sodium, sperm motility initiation may involve a complex ionic event. There is an exchange of extracellular sodium for intracellular H^+ and K^+. These permeability changes of the sperm membrane are associated with a change in sperm membrane potential (Wong and Lee, 1983).

ROLE OF CALCIUM

Calcium ions are important in sperm motility initiation. In the absence of extracellular calcium, the initiation of sperm motility is abolished (Lee et al., 1981). This requirement for calcium may be attributed to an influx of calcium ions essential for activation of flagellar movement in the rat caudal spermatozoa. This phenomenon is analogous to influx of calcium into smooth muscle and cardiac muscle cells prior to muscle contraction. Calcium ionophore A23187 can increase sperm metabolism and motility by

the epididymis with a sodium free medium (SFM) to suppress motility. They were then suspended in SCM containing $\bigcirc$ ($\bullet$), 0.5 ($\bigcirc$), 1 ($\blacksquare$) or 2 ($\blacktriangle$) mmol/l verapamil. Each point shows the mean $\pm$ SEM of three experiments. (d) $^{45}Ca^{2+}$ influx into spermatozoa during motility initiation. Spermatozoa were flushed out from the rat caudal epididymidis with a sodium free medium (SFM) to suppress motility. They were then incubated in SCM ($\bullet$) or SFM ($\bigcirc$) containing $2 \mu Ci/ml$ $^{45}Ca^{2+}$ (sperm concentration $10^8/ml$). At intervals, 0.5 ml of sperm suspension was applied to Whatman GF/A filters under aspiration and washed 5 times with 3 ml ice-cold SCM. Trapped cells on the filters were digested with 0.5 ml KOH (0.1 mol/l) and counted for radioactivity. Each point shows the mean $\pm$ SEM of 4 (SCM) and 3 (SFM) experiments. See Wong et al. (1981) for the determination of Forward Motility Index (FMI) and the composition of solutions used inducing calcium influx into sperm (Storey, 1975). Ionophore A23187 (50 nmol/l) stimulated motility in spermatozoa suspended in a sodium containing medium but not in a medium in which sodium ions had been depleted (Fig. 28.1b). In contrast, calcium antagonist like verapamil inhibited the sodium-induced sperm motility in a dose-dependent manner (Fig. 28.1c). Lastly sperm motility initiation was associated with $^{45}Ca^{2+}$ influx into sperm (Fig. 28.1d).

RELATION TO CYCLIC AMP

Sperm motility initiation is accompanied by an increase in Na^+-linked H^+ and K^+ efflux from sperm cells. Concomitant with these is the Ca^{2+} influx into sperm. How do these membrane effects relate to the biochemical events

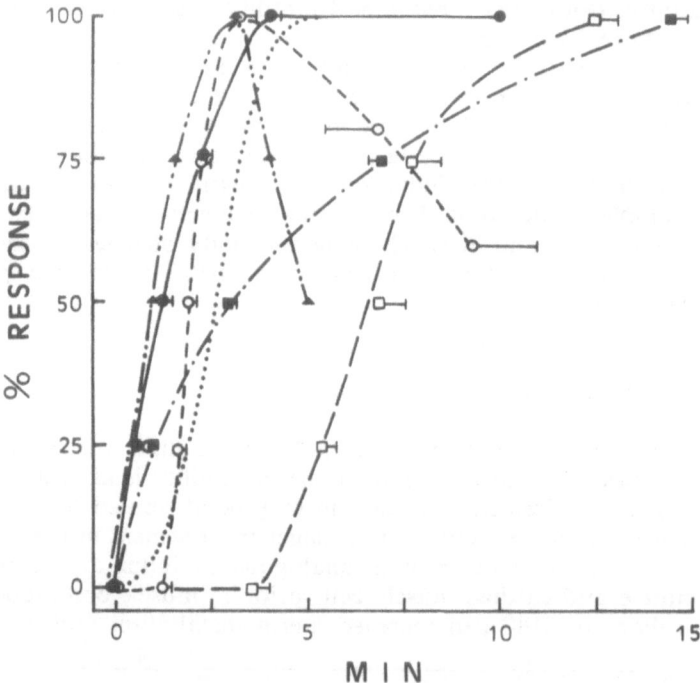

Fig. 28.2 Shows the time course of events during motility initiation in the hamster and rat epididymal spermatozoa. (A) increase in intracellular cyclic AMP concentration in the hamster epididymal spermatozoa subjected to motility initiation by Ca^{2+} solutions (▲) (adapted from Morton *et al.*, 1974). (B) development of forward motility of the hamster epididymal sperm after suspending them in a sodium containing medium (SCM) (dotted line). (C) K^+ efflux (●) (Wong and Lee, 1983), (D) Ca^{2+} influx (○) (Fig. 28.1d), (E) H^+ ion efflux (■) (Wong *et al.*, 1981) from the rat cauda epididymal spermatozoa subjected to motility initiation after suspension in SCM. (F) forward motility of the rat caudal epididymal sperm under conditions as in (C), (D) and (E) (□). In all instances induction of motility by suspension of sperm in various solutions started at time zero. The maximal values obtained are called 100% and the values measured at time zero are called 0%

414

of motility initiation? Cyclic adenosine-3':5' monophosphate has been proposed as the intracellular messenger involved in mammalian sperm motility (Hoskins and Casillas, 1975). In support of this contention is the observation that cyclic AMP accumulates rapidly in hamster (Morton et al., 1974) and bull sperm (Lee et al., 1981) undergoing induced motility initiation. If the rise of cyclic AMP in the hamster sperm is plotted on the same time scale as the permeability changes in rat cauda sperm subjected to motility activation, the cyclic AMP rise is as rapid as the permeability change (Fig. 28.2). Although direct comparison of the results obtained from different species is difficult, it can be seen that the accumulation of intracellular cyclic AMP and ion fluxes well precede the mechanical stimulation of motility. Whether cyclic AMP rise results in a change of membrane permeability to ions, or whether it is the calcium influx that activates adenyl cyclase remains an open question. The role that calcium and cyclic nucleotides play in mediating many sperm cell functions has recently received much attention (Garbers et al., 1980; Lambert and Lambert, 1981).

SPERM MOTILITY INITIATION *IN VIVO*

Whilst it is difficult to study sperm motility in intact animals *in vivo*, our system does offer a possibility for elucidating the ionic mechanism of sperm motility initiation. The rat caudal epididymal fluid has been shown to contain a low concentration of Na^+ (20 mmol/l) and Ca^{2+} (0.2 mmol/l) but a high concentration of K^+ (55 mmol/l) (Levine and Marsh, 1971; Howards et al., 1979). This ionic composition greatly inhibits motility initiation *in vitro* (Wong and Lee, 1983). In many mammalian species including man, the seminal fluid is plasma-like in ionic composition; the sodium ions being contributed by the accessory glands (Salisbury, 1962; Mann, 1964). In the rat, the Na^+ and K^+ concentrations of the seminal vesicular fluid, determined on 16 animals, averaged 10.32 ± 0.63 (mean $\pm$ SEM) and 0.21 ± 0.04 (mean $\pm$ SEM) mmol/l respectively. These levels of Na^+ and K^+ are known to favour motility initiation *in vitro* (Wong et al., 1981). These results show that the high K^+ and low Na^+ fluid in the cauda epididymidis maintains the spermatozoa in a quiescent state during storage. During ejaculation the spermatozoa encounter a high Na^+ but low K^+ secretion from the accessory glands. This addition of Na^+ and dilution of K^+ and other unknown inhibitory factors activate the already mature sperm to full progressive motility. The whole process is rendered possible by the specific peptides and proteins in the tract (Wong et al., 1982).

CONCLUDING REMARKS

Motility initiation of the rat caudal epididymal spermatozoa requires the presence of extracellular sodium and calcium but is inhibited by a high concentration of potassium. At the potassium concentration of 50 mmol/l (concentration found in the rat caudal fluid), motility initiation is greatly suppressed. Motility initiation of the rat caudal epididymal spermatozoa is accompanied by a release of hydrogen and potassium ions but an influx of calcium. These ion movements and motility initiation are highly dependent on extracellular sodium. It is proposed that motility initiation is associated with an exchange of extracellular sodium for intracellular H^+ and K^+. Calcium influx into sperm may be essential for the activation of flagellar movement. Since blockers of Na^+, K^+ and Ca^{2+} channels inhibit the respective ion movements and motility initiation it is suggested that these ion fluxes may be important effectors of the underlying process. Although these ionic events precede the mechanical activation of motility. Cyclic AMP may be the intracellular messenger in initiating mammalian sperm motility. The interrelationship among various ion movements, and between these various ion movements and the generation of cyclic AMP remain unknown.

References

Cascieri, M., Amann, R.P. and Hammerstedt, R.H. (1976). Adenine nucleotide changes at initiation of bull sperm motility. *J. Biol. Chem.*, **10**, 787-93

Garbers, D.L., Tubb, D.J. and Kopf, G.S. (1980). Regulation of sea urchin sperm cyclic AMP-dependent protein kinases by an egg associated factor. *Biol. Reprod.*, **228**, 526-32

Hoskins, D.D. and Casillas, E.R. (1975). Function of cyclic nucleotides in mammalian spermatozoa. In Geiger, S. (ed.) *Handbook of Physiology, Section 7*, vol. 5, pp. 453-60 (Baltimore: Williams and Wilkins)

Howards, S., Lachene, C. and Vigersky, R. (1979). The fluid environment of the maturing spermatozoa. In Fawcett, D.W. and Bedford, J.M. (eds.) *The Spermatozoon*, pp. 35-42 (Baltimore-Munich: Urban and Schwarzenberg)

Lambert, C.C. and Lambert, G. (1981). The ascidian sperm reaction: Ca^{2+} uptake in relation to H^+ efflux. *Dev. Biol.*, **88**, 312-17

Lee, W.M., Tsang, A.Y.F. and Wong, P.Y.D. (1981). Effects of divalent ions and lanthanide ions on motility initiation in rat caudal epididymal spermatozoa. *Br. J. Pharmacol.*, **73**, 633-8

Levine, N. and Marsh, D.J. (1971). Micropuncture studies of the electrochemical aspects of fluid and electrolyte transport in individual seminiferous tubules, the epididymis and the vas deferens in rats. *J. Physiol.*, **213**, 557-70

Mann, T. (1964). *The Biochemistry of Semen and of the Male Reproductive Tract*, pp. 354-5 (New York: J. Wiley)

Morton, B., Harrigan, J. and Joose, T. (1973). The activation of motility in quiescent hamster sperm from the epididymis. *Biol. Reprod.*, **9**, 71-2

Morton, B., Harrigan-Lum, J., Albahli, L. and Jooss, T. (1974). The activation of motility in quiescent hamster sperm from the epididymis by calcium and cyclic nucleotides. *Biochem. Biophys. Res. Commun.*, **56**, 372-9

Salisbury, G.W. (1962). Ionic and osmotic conditions in relation to metabolic control. In Bishop, D.W. (ed.) *Spermatozoon Motility*, pp. 59 (Washington: AAAS)

Storey, B.T. (1975). Energy metabolism of spermatozoa. IV. Effects of calcium on respiration of mature epididymal sperm of the rabbit. *Biol. Reprod.*, **13**, 1-9

Turner, T.T. and Howards, S.S. (1978). Factors involved in the initiation of sperm motility. *Biol. Reprod.*, **18**, 571-8

Wong, P.Y.D. and Lee, W.M. (1983). Potassium movement during sodium-induced motility initiation in the rat caudal epididymal spermatozoa. *Biol. Reprod.*, **28**, 206-12

Wong, P.Y.D., Lee, W.M. and Tsang, A.Y.F. (1981). The effects of extracellular sodium on acid release and motility initiation in rat caudal epididymal spermatozoa *in vitro*. *Exp. Cell Res.*, **131**, 97-104

Wong, P.Y.D., Tsang, A.Y.F. and Lee, W.M. (1982). Secretion of marcomolecules by the rat epididymis. *Int. J. Androl. Suppl.*, **5**, 34-47

29
Reproductive effects of sperm surface antibodies

R. BRONSON, G. COOPER and D. ROSENFELD

Only recently has convincing evidence accumulated that immunity to spermatozoa can impair reproductive function. Although it had been known by the late 19th century that antibodies to spermatozoa could be experimentally induced (Landsteiner, 1899; Metchnikoff, 1899), the spontaneous appearance of sperm-directed antibodies in the serum of fertile members of many species raised the question of whether such antibodies played a role in the aetiology of infertility in man. Whereas nearly two decades ago, experimental induction of immunity to spermatozoa was shown to impair reproductive performance in laboratory animals, numerous serological studies of women comparing the incidence of antisperm antibodies in fertile and subfertile populations have failed to substantiate an association between immunity to spermatozoa and infertility.

In this chapter we review the prior experimental evidence that immunization to spermatozoa alters reproduction and describe the possible loci of this effect on reproductive processes. The pitfalls of the previous epidemiological approaches will be discussed and recent evidence providing proof that spontaneously occurring sperm-directed antibodies in men and women can cause infertility will be summarized.

Given this knowledge criteria will be presented that must be met for the successful development of a contraceptive vaccine based upon immunization against spermatozoa.

EXPERIMENTAL INDUCTION OF INFERTILITY BY IMMUNIZATION WITH SPERMATOZOA

In 1964, McLaren was able to show that repeated intraperitoneal injection of spermatozoa, in the absence of adjuvants, resulted in the formation of agglutinating antibodies which diminished the fertility of female mice. There was a wide individual variation between animals in titres of circulating antibodies. Females demonstrating high titres of antisperm agglutinins showed a marked reduction in both size of the first litter and total breeding performance over a six month period. While these immunized females ovulated a normal number of eggs, a reduced number of oviductal sperm was found on the morning following mating, as compared with controls. This observation correlated with a diminished percentage of fertilized eggs when oviducts were examined 48 h following mating (Table 29.1). Edwards (1964), using Freund's adjuvant and a shorter period of immunization, confirmed McLaren's findings that immunity to spermatozoa leads to a reduction in litter size. In his work, and a subsequent study by McLaren (1968), no association was found between the degree of impairment of fertility and antisperm antibody titre. It then seemed unlikely that the secretion of antisperm antibodies *per se* within the uterine lumen could alone account for the failure of spermatozoa to reach the oviduct. Edwards postulated that cellular immunity to spermatozoa perhaps led to a more rapid

Table 29.1 Relation between sperm agglutinin titre, number of spermatozoa found in the ampulla of one oviduct of an immunized or control female about 11 h after mating and the percentage of eggs fertilized in the other oviduct two days later

Sperm agglutinin titre	Mean no. of sperm in oviduct	Eggs fertilized (%)
Controls*	8.6 (14)†	82
1:8	3.0 (1)	22
1:256	0.0 (3)	38
1:512	1.5 (2)	28
1:1024	0.5 (4)	25
1:2048	0.0 (2)	0
All immunized females	0.75 (12)	24.7

Adapted from McLaren (1964)
* Unimmunized control mice
† Number of mice are shown in parentheses

removal of sperm in the uterus, thus accounting for the failure of fertilization.

Bell (1968) and more recently Seki and Mettler (1982), have found a correlation between sperm antibody titre and reproductive impairment. Embryotoxicity of sera containing autologous antisperm antibodies was also documented as an additional factor leading to immune infertility.

In other species, injection of female guinea pigs with homologous spermatozoa in adjuvants has led to temporary sterility (Katsh, 1959). Immunization by intravaginal administration of sperm has been reported in guinea pig (Behrman and Otani, 1963) and the rabbit (Pommeranke, 1928) as well. Using *in vitro* techniques, heterologous antisperm antibodies have been found to impair fertilization in rabbits (Menge, 1971; Metz and Anika, 1970). Auto-antibodies induced in male guinea pigs have been shown to impair the acrosome reaction (Tung *et al.*, 1980), when added to a medium that supports egg penetration *in vitro* and prevents zona penetration of acrosome reacted guinea-pig spermatozoa (Yanagimachi *et al.*, 1981).

DO ANTISPERM ANTIBODIES CAUSE INFERTILITY IN HUMANS?

By the mid-1960s, at the time when the experimental basis of immune infertility was established in animals, Franklin and Dukes (1964) had shown that a significant proportion of women whose failure to conceive was otherwise unexplained possessed sperm agglutinins in their sera. They raised the question whether these spontaneously occurring iso-antibodies might play a role in the pathogenesis of human infertility. Subsequent attempts to show that infertility can have an immune basis in humans have essentially employed epidemiological methods which unfortunately have produced conflicting data. Why has the epidemiological approach failed to establish this premise? It was apparent from the earliest experimental studies that there is a wide variation in the extent of reproductive failure between individual animals sensitized to sperm. Immunity to spermatozoa is not an all or nothing phenomenon. This is also true in humans, where the presence of

Table 29.2 Comparison of sperm-directed antibodies by immunoglobulin class in serum and semen

Semen	Serum			
	IgA	IgA	Both	None
IgA	0		0	0
IgG	0	3	0	0
Both	0	5	19	3
None	4	11	9	0

In 24 of 51 cases antisperm antibodies were detected in serum but not on sperm. In 3 cases, immunoglobulins were detected on the sperm surface but not in serum

antisperm antibodies within the reproductive tract has been shown to be dependent upon their serum concentration (Rumke, 1974). The extent to which antisperm antibodies are present in reproductive tract secretions would be expected to influence the degree of fertility impairment.

There are two potential sources of immunoglobulins found in the reproductive tract. Antibodies may appear as transudates from the blood (Rumke, 1974) and/or by direct local secretion by submucosal plasma cells (Uehling, 1971; Murdoch et al., 1982). As a consequence, antisperm antibodies may be present in serum but undetectable on either ejaculated spermatozoa (Table 29.2) or in oviductal, uterine or vaginal secretions (Bronson et al., 1983a). Conversely, local immunity to sperm has been demonstrated by detection of IgA immunoglobulins within the reproductive tract in the absence of detectable humoral antibodies, in both men and women (Menge et al., 1982). A dichotomy of immune states may then exist between the systemic circulation and the reproductive tract. These observations suggest the difficulty that would be encountered in simple epidemiological investigations which rely solely on serological detection of humoral antibodies, as an index of immunity to spermatozoa.

An additional factor leading to the inability of epidemiological methods to provide proof of an immune cause of infertility in humans was reliance on agglutination techniques as the sole criterion for antibody detection. Bacterial contamination of sperm (Bell, 1968) as well as beta-globulins (Rose *et al.*, 1976) can cause agglutination of spermatozoa, especially in minimally diluted (less than 1:4) serum, in the absence of antisperm antibodies. Such non-specific agglutination has falsely identified a population that would be included in the immune infertile group. If conception occurred, these individual would be classed as fertile in spite of their 'immunity' to sperm.

NEW APPROACHES TO THE PROBLEM

The necessity of documenting, in men and women suspected of having immunity to spermatozoa, the presence of antisperm antibodies in the reproductive tract is apparent. As antibody responses most often are polyclonal, immunoglobulins of varying specificities to the sperm surface would be expected. One must then define those regions of the sperm surface to which antibodies are detected, as well as the class of immunoglobulins bound to each region. The use of polyacrylamide beads coupled to immunoglobulin class-specific rabbit anti-human antibodies (Immunobeads, Bio-Rad) accomplishes this by serving as antibody detectors, through bead rosetting patterns (Bronson *et al.*, 1981a) (Fig. 29.1). This allows one to detect immunoglobulins directly on the surface of living spermatozoa.

Validation of the specificity of immunobead binding to the surface of

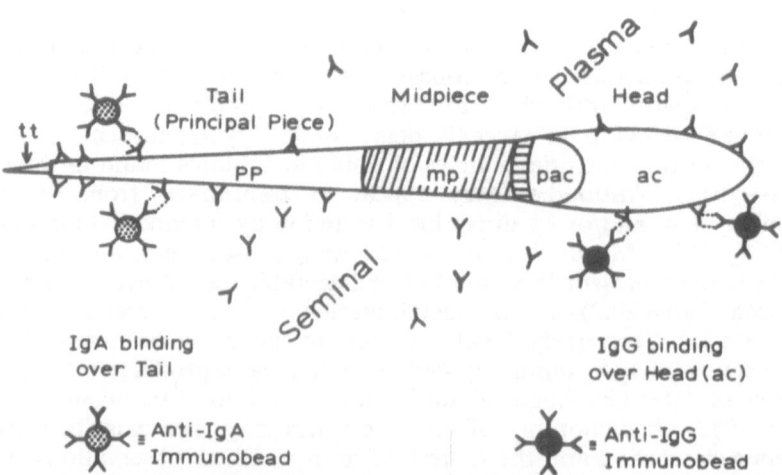

IMMUNOBEADS DETECT MEMBRANE-BOUND ANTIBODIES

Fig. 29.1 Rabbit anti-human IgA, G or M antibodies linked covalently to polyacrylamide beads (Immunobeads, Bio-Rad) were used to detect immunoglobulins bound to the sperm surface. Illustrated here, bead rosetting would have detected IgAs bound to the principal piece of the tail and IgGs bound to the sperm head

420

motile spermatozoa was achieved in several ways: (1) incubation of sperm from known fertile semen donors, as a control population, with immuno-bead suspensions revealed complete absence of bead binding to the sperm surface, except for the tail end-piece (0–4% of sperm exhibit a single bead bound to this region). (2) Immunobead rosetting patterns following passive antibody transfer to antibody-negative sperm, utilizing the same serum, were consistently reproducible from test to test. (3) Comparisons were made of the localization of immunobead binding upon the sperm surface by use of fluorescein-labelled protein A, as well as the rosetting by protein A-positive staphylococci. (4) Absorption of antibody-positive sera with antibody-free spermatozoa resulted in a significant loss of antisperm antibody within the test serum, as judged by subsequent immunobead binding.

PROOF THAT SPONTANEOUSLY OCCURRING IMMUNITY TO SPERMATOZOA CAN CAUSE INFERTILITY

Given the failure of prior studies convincingly to document different incid-ences of antisperm antibodies in fertile and infertile populations, our approach has been to study the function of antibody-bound spermatozoa directly, through experimental methods that allow fertilization *in vitro*. Utilizing immunobead—sperm rosetting, it was possible rigorously to ca-tegorize those antibodies present in the sera of individual men and women sensitized to sperm. Such antisperm antibodies were shown to be present not only in blood, but also directly on the surface of spermatozoa in eja-culates of men with autoimmunity to sperm. The detailed characterization of the bloods of men and women sensitized to spermatozoa has allowed us to establish a 'library' of sera containing antibodies of unique specificities to the sperm surface, for each immunoglobulin class. By selecting individual sera for passive antibody transfer to sperm, antisperm antibodies of IgA, G or M classes could each be transferred to different regions of the sperma-tozoan surface. Spermatozoa of proven fertile men concurrently participat-ing in an AID programme were washed free of seminal plasma, and sus-pended in dilute antibody-positive sera. The ability of such antibody-bound sperm to interact with eggs *in vitro* was compared with populations of antibody-free sperm of the same individuals. The zona-free hamster egg was utilized to study the ability of these antibody-bound sperm to acrosome react, fuse with the oolemma, and penetrate the vitellus. Whether such antibody-bound sperm could attach to the zona pellucida, a prerequisite to its subsequent penetration, was also studied using non-viable human eggs, as human spermatozoa are narrowly selective in their ability to attach to the zona pellucida of other species.

When antibodies were transferred to the sperm surface *prior* to their exposure in a medium that allows capacitation and acrosome reaction *in vitro* (a modified Biggers, Whittingham, Whitten medium), such immuno-globulin binding to the acrosomal and post-acrosomal regions of the sperm head failed to inhibit the subsequent ability of such sperm to penetrate zona-free eggs (Bronson *et al.*, 1981a). To the contrary, antibody-bound sperm exhibit an *increased* ability to penetrate zona-free hamster eggs (Table 29.3). Could such antibodies promote the acrosome reaction by cross-linking integral proteins of the plasma membrane, a phenomenon similar to antibody-induced patching and capping of leukocyte membrane proteins?

These experimental conditions mimic the circumstances that sperm encounter in men demonstrating auto-immunity to spermatozoa; a short-term exposure to anti-sperm antibodies within the seminal fluid with a limited number of immunoglobulin molecules bound to their surfaces at the time of their entry into the female reproductive tract. The amount of antibody to which the sperm plasma membrane is exposed in this instance is limited to that acquired during exposure to semen immunoglobulins while in the

Table 29.3 Ability of human spermatozoa antibody bound over their heads to penetrate zona-free hamster eggs *in vitro*

Serum category	eggs penetrated (%)	No. penetrating sperm per egg
Antibody negative	76.2 (84)*	1.4±0.27†
Antibody positive		
N	100 (17)	2.5±0.6
P	100 (17)	5.1±1.3
M	89.5 (19)	3.5±9.6
Th	100 (35)	9.3±2.4
R	96.8 (32)	4.3±0.7
K	79.6 (49)	1.5±0.3

* Number eggs inseminated
† Mean ± SEM
Spermatozoa exposed to antibody positive sera, in the absence of complement, exhibited an improved ability to penetrate zona-free eggs. Sera were selected that contained immunoglobulins that bind to acrosomal and postacrosomal regions of the sperm head, as detected by immunobead rosetting

vagina after coitus, in addition to that bound within the epididymis prior to ejaculation (Weininger *et al.*, 1982).

In women sensitized to sperm, spermatozoa are continually exposed to antisperm antibodies within the female reproductive tract, including the time of fertilization. Hence, the conditions that spermatozoa encounter in men and women immune to sperm are not comparable. When spermatozoa are exposed to sera contining antisperm antibodies during their capacitation and acrosome reaction, varying results are obtained for individual sera. The egg-penetrating ability of sperm may be inhibited in the absence of any loss of sperm motility in some cases suggesting impairment of the acrosome reaction. The timing of exposure of spermatozoa to antisperm antibodies is then critical in determining their effect on subsequent sperm function.

The ability of sperm-directed antibodies to mediate complement-dependent membrane damage and its effect on the fertilizing ability of sperm has been studied. As seminal plasma contains complement inhibitors (Petersen *et al.*, 1980) spermatozoa of sensitized men retain their viability within the ejaculate despite the presence of sperm-directed immunoglobulins within seminal fluid. On entry of the female reproductive tract, however, such sperm become liable to complement-mediated membrane damage.

Sera containing antibodies directed primarily against the sperm tail or sperm head (as judged by rosetting of immunobeads) were chosen for study. Spermatozoa were co-incubated with heat-inactivated human sera and guinea-pig serum, as a source of complement. Pre-absorption of the guinea-pig serum with human spermatozoa eliminated heterologous antibodies that cross-react with the human sperm tail (Witkin et al., 1980b) minimizing subsequent sperm motility loss.

As anticipated from studies of immune haemolysis (Humphrey and Dourmashkin, 1965), antibodies of the IgA class, which do not interact with the early components of the complement cascade (Cl-3) fail to impair sperm motility (Bronson et al., 1982b). The Isojima test (Isojima et al., 1972), a commonly utilized complement-dependent method of detecting immunity to spermatozoa, would fail to detect sperm-directed immunoglobulins of the IgA class. In contrast, IgMs, large multivalent molecules which promote rapid complement activation (Colton et al., 1969) cause extensive sperm motility loss, even when directed against antigens limited to the sperm tail end piece. IgGs must bind to at least 40% of the sperm tail principal piece to impair sperm motility, a not unexpected finding, given the relative inefficiency of this immunoglobulin class to effect sheep red blood cell lysis, when compared with IgMs (Humphrey and Dourmashkin, 1965). Antibodies of IgA and G classes, when present on the sperm head and in the absence of tail binding, failed significantly to impair sperm motility (usually less than 30% less) in the presence of guinea-pig serum as a source of complement. Complement-dependent cytotoxicity tests would fail to detect such antibodies.

It had previously been shown with both heterologous (Russo and Metz, 1974) and homologous sera (LeBouteiller et al., 1975) that antisperm antibodies promote extensive disruption of the acrosomal and plasma membranes of rabbit and guinea-pig sperm, in the presence of complement. Would the motile human sperm previously exposed to complement-fixing antibodies, which had appeared to be morphologically normal under phase contrast microscopy, lose their ability to penetrate eggs? A selected population of highly motile sperm obtained by a swim up technique (Rumke, 1980) were exposed to these same sera (containing head-directed antibodies) either in the presence or absence of complement and thereafter used to inseminate zona-free hamster eggs. The ability of these sperm to contact the egg, as judged by numbers of sperm adherent to the oolemma, was comparable for all immunoglobulin classes, irrespective of whether complement was active or not. The small loss of sperm motility associated with exposure to sera containing IgM antisperm antibodies did not affect gamete contact. There was however a marked difference in the ability of spermatozoa exposed to these antibodies to penetrate zona-free hamster eggs. There was no impairment in egg penetrating ability of sperm exposed to IgA molecules, despite their exposure to active complement prior to capacitation in vitro. Extensive loss of penetrating ability occurred, on the other hand, after co-incubation with complement (guinea-pig serum) and human

Table 29.4 Effect of antisperm antibodies in the presence or absence of complement on ability of human sperm to penetrate zona-free hamster eggs

Immunoglobulin class of antisperm antibody[b] present in test serum	Complement[a] present		Heat-Inactivated Complement	
	% Eggs penetrated (no. eggs Inseminated)	No. penetrating sperm/inseminated egg	% Eggs penetrated (range) (no. eggs inseminated)	No. penetrating sperm/inseminated egg
IgM	40.3 ± 14.8^c (60)	0.48 ± 0.14	73.4 ± 9.0 (51)	1.3 ± 0.19
IgG or A/G	54.6 ± 28.1 (95)	0.89 ± 0.55	76.1 ± 17.6 (97)	1.8 ± 0.67
IgA	93.8 ± 9.4 (80)	2.7 ± 1.7	87.6 ± 14.4 (58)	2.6 ± 2.0

[a] Guinea-pig serum from a single animal was used as a source of complement

[b] Antisperm antibodies directed solely against the sperm head (post acrosomal and/or acrosomal regions) as determined by immunobead binding

[c] Mean of % penetration for each serum ± SD

424

serum containing primarily head-directed antisperm antibodies of the IgM class, with a similar effect, though less marked, seen for IgGs (Table 29.4).

There can be no doubt that spontaneously occurring sperm surface antigens are capable of damaging spermatozoa. A limiting factor that would determine in part the extent of loss of sperm function would be the level of complement activity within the female reproductive tract. Secretions of the cervix, uterus and oviducts, as well as follicular and peritoneal fluids, would all be potential sources of complement.

ANTIGENIC HETEROGENEITY OF HUMAN SPERMATOZOA

The proportion of spermatozoa with detectable immunoglobulins on their surfaces varies widely between subfertile men (Table 29.5). Variations in

Table 29.5 Proportion of antibody-bound spermatozoa in ejaculates following three days' sexual abstinence of 78 men with auto-immunity to sperm

Antibody-bound sperm in semen* (IgA and/or G) (%)	No. ejaculates in each percentile
11–20	3
21–40	8
41–60	8
61–80	16
81–100	43

* As detected by immunobead rosetting

the proportion of antibody-bound sperm were found to depend on the ejaculatory frequency, a not unexpected finding, as immunoglobulins accumulate within the accessory gland secretions during longer periods of abstinence (Table 29.6). Sperm antibody levels within the ejaculate may also wax or wane over the course of many months (Table 29.7).

Table 29.6 Comparison of the proportion of antibody bound spermatozoa as determined by immunobead binding in first and second ejaculates* of three men with auto-immunity to sperm

Ejaculate no.	Ig class and binding specificity† IgA			IgG		
	Head	Tail	Tail Tip	Head	Tail	Tail Tip
First	7	80	95	95	100	100
Second	6	52	84	68	100	100
First	11	73	100	62	98	100
Second	5	46	90	63	96	100
First	3	—	1	71	—	68
Second	2	—	2	38	—	36

* 1 h interval between ejaculates
† % sperm exhibiting antibody binding over each region of the sperm surface

Table 29.7 Comparison of antisperm antibodies in two men with auto-immunity to sperm on different occasions in the absence of treatment

Date of testing	Sperm in ejaculate that were antibody bound (%)	
	IgA	IgG
8 Jan. 1981	100	100
13 July 1981*	60	20
29 Oct 1981	53	100
26 Apr 1982	2	1

* Post-coital tests showed improved sperm swimming behaviour and conception occurred, following spontaneous remission of auto-immunity

While it was initially assumed that the variation in antibody binding to spermatozoa between men reflected the limiting concentration of antibody in seminal fluid, relative to the number of antigenic sites in aggregate on the sperm surfaces, this proved not to be an adequate explanation. If antibody concentration were limiting in those instances where less than 100% of spermatozoa were antibody bound, there should be no residual antisperm antibody remaining in the seminal fluid following removal of sperm from semen by centrifugation. To the contrary it became clear that there were cases in which antibody-free sperm were indeed detected in the ejaculate, despite the presence of unbound antisperm antibody of similar immunoglobulin class and specificity remaining within the residual seminal fluid. An explanation for this observation would be that antigenic heterogeneity exists between spermatozoa.

Such antigenic heterogeneity could occur on the basis of haploid expression of histocompatibility antigens. Snell (1944) has claimed to have detected antigens on spermatozoa of certain inbred mice (C 57 Black) lacking in others (Balb C). Cytotoxicity tests have provided circumstantial evidence that two populations of HLA-bearing human spermatozoa exist in ejaculates, suggestive of haploid expression of these antigens.

Spermatozoa have been shown to acquire surface coating of glycoproteins in their passage through the epididymis and at the time of ejaculation (Nicolson *et al.*, 1977; Olson and Orgebin-Crist, 1982). Tissue-specific antigens are secreted by the seminal vesicles at the time of ejaculation (Dravland and Joshi, 1981). Antigenic heterogeneity of ejaculate sperm could then be on the basis of a variation in the acquisition of coating proteins during the transit of sperm through the male reproductive tract. O'Rand has noted (1982, personal communication) in the rabbit, utilizing monoclonal antibodies to specific regions of the sperm plasma membrane, variations in expression of a surface antigen on individual sperm. While all spermatozoa obtained from the cauda epididymis expressed this antigen, a significant and variable number of ejaculated sperm failed to display the antigen. After placement of these sperm within the uterus, on subsequent retrieval, the surface antigen was detected uniformly. This observation suggests that masking of surface antigens occurs during ejaculation, in a nonuniform way.

AETIOLOGY OF IMMUNITY TO SPERMATOZOA

In pubertal males, at the onset of spermatogenesis, new antigens make their appearances on the sperm surface (Millette and Bellve, 1977). Spermatozoa in the latter stages of meiosis and subsequent spermiation are sequestered within the lumen of the seminiferous tubule by a blood-testis barrier which has its anatomic correlate in the tight junction situated between Sertoli cells (Dym and Caviacchia, 1977; Fawcett *et al.*, 1970). These sperm antigens are to a large extent sequestered from the immune system.

Roughly 50% of men who have undergone vasectomy have been found to have humoral antisperm antibodies. An inverse relationship has also been found (Linnett and Hjort, 1981) between the presence of these antibodies within the reproductive tract secretions, documented at the time of vasovasostomy, and the chance of subsequent fertility. Men with bilateral congenital absence of segments of the male reproductive tract (e.g. congenital absence of the vas deferens, epididymis or seminal vesicles) as seen in cystic fibrosis (Holsclaw *et al.*, 1971) have also been found to be at risk for immunity to spermatozoa (Girgis *et al.*, 1982). Both congenital and acquired obstructions of sperm egress appear to play a role in auto-immunity to spermatozoa, perhaps by allowing entry of sperm antigens into general circulation. Can cryptic unilateral intra-testicular obstruction, at the level of the seminiferous tubules, lead to antisperm antibody formation? In such cases semen quality might well appear normal, given the wide fertile range.

It is unlikely that lymphoid elements of the immune system gain access to spermatozoa within the testis. There is no clinical evidence of immune orchitis in men exhibiting high levels of humoral or local antisperm antibodies. In addition, the sperm output of these men is most often found to be no different from non-immune men, as reflected in their semen analyses. Using rapid semen dilution and/or competitive *in vitro* immunoabsorption with a suspension of antibody-negative, freeze-thawed human donor sperm, we have been able to lower the available antisperm antibody in liquefying seminal fluid that is free to bind within minutes post-ejaculation to the motile ejaculate sperm of men with auto-immunity to sperm. By titrating the number of freeze-thawed non-viable sperm added to suspensions as immunoabsorbant (into which the sensitized individual ejaculates) we have been able to obtain spermatozoa completely free of surface-bound immunoglobulins. This would indicate that the epididymal sperm of these men are not antibody-bound. Rather, these immunoglobulins bind to spermatozoa after ejaculation, at the time of their contact with the seminal plasma (Bronson *et al.*, 1982e). Such evidence indicates that at least in some individuals, antisperm antibodies have not gained access to the seminiferous tubules, reti testis or epididymis. Indeed, Zanchetta (1982, personal communication) has failed to detect in sera of men with azoospermia or severe oligospermia antisperm antibodies directed against sperm elements of the seminiferous tubules.

An alternative explanation for the absence of orchitis and subsequent suppression of spermatogenesis would be that those antigens associated with auto-immunity to sperm do not make their appearance on spermatozoa within the testis, but rather, at later stages of sperm development, such as during epididymal maturation. In theory, some antigens might not be intrinsic to the sperm plasma membrane but rather, surface-coating proteins derived from secretions of the accessory glands at the time of ejaculation. A tissue-specific antigen secreted by the seminal vesicles has been identified in the rat which binds to spermatozoa at the time of ejaculation (Dravland and Joshi, 1981). In a small series of experiments performed in our laboratory, epididymal sperm were retrieved from a man undergoing orchidectomy for prostatic malignancy. When these spermatozoa were incubated with sera of three different individuals, each containing high levels of antisperm antibodies, as judged previously using ejaculated sperm, there was no difference in the binding patterns of antisperm antibodies to epididymal sperm as compared with the ejaculated sperm. Hence, those sperm antigens to which the antibodies are directed are expressed on spermatozoa prior to ejaculation and would appear to be integral components of the plasma membrane.

Spontaneous remission of auto-immunity to spermatozoa may occur. The aetiology of sperm antibody production in such cases is clearly different from that of men with apparent or occult obstruction of sperm egress from the reproductive tract (where sperm antibody levels would be expected to be chronically elevated) and would suggest a transient rather than chronic exposure to those antigens (cross-reacting bacterial or food antigens?) that elicit the antibody response. Following the inciting episode (genitourinary tract infection?) antisperm antibody levels would be expected to peak and then subsequently fall due to transient exposure of the immune system to the antigen.

The presence of antisperm antibodies in women is not surprising. In fact, naturally occurring sperm-directed antibodies can be demonstrated in the sera of several species (Edwards, 1960). The lack of immunity to spermatozoa in the majority of women is the more puzzling situation, given that sperm constitute an inoculum of millions of cells from a foreign individual of a different haplotype and sex. In 1977, a high-molecular-weight immunosuppressive factor was identified in seminal plasma (Lord *et al.*, 1977) which was shown to impair lymphocyte activation in both mixed lymphocyte cultures and in response to mitogens. Epididymal sperm themselves have also been shown, in mice, to be immunosuppressive (Marcus, *et al.*, 1978). The ejaculate then contains factors which blunt the immune response of women, making coitus without subsequent immunization against sperm possible. Do husbands of women who are highly sensitized to sperm lack this immunosuppressive seminal fluid factor?

Spermatozoa have been found on the fimbrial surfaces of the oviduct as well as in peritoneal fluid of women after coitus (Templeton and Mortimer, 1982). The isthmus of the oviduct is known to regulate the number of sperm within the ampulla (Harper, 1973). While millions of sperm are present within seminal plasma, only tens to hundreds are present in any one instance within the ampulla of the oviduct, the site of fertilization (Ahlgren, 1969). As described earlier intraperitoneal administration of intact spermatozoa, in the absence of adjuvants, has been shown to lead on repeated inoculation to the production of antisperm antibodies in mice. Could abnormal transport of large numbers of spermatozoa to the peritoneum lead to sensitization to sperm, with the appearance of antisperm antibodies in certain women? Intrauterine insemination, in which large numbers of spermatozoa gain rapid access to the upper portion of the reproductive tract, has been associated with an increase in antibody titres in women previously sensitized to spermatozoa (Kremer et al., 1978). Does intrauterine insemination in the absence of prior sensitization, carry with it a risk of subsequent immunity to spermatozoa?

WHAT IS THE ANTIGEN?

Plasma membrane preparations of epididymal sperm contain antigens which on repeated inoculation result in impaired reproductive performance (Bell and McLaren 1970). At least three distinct sperm surface antigens to which spontaneously occurring antisperm antibodies are directed in humans have been partially purified (D'Almeida et al., 1981). Monoclonal antibodies have been developed to specific plasma membrane antigens of both rabbit (O'Rand, 1981) and human (Sokoloski et al., 1982) spermatozoa. At least one of these antigens, in the rabbit, appears to be located near the sperm-zona receptor as antibodies raised against it have been found to block binding of sperm to the zona pellucida and subsequent fertilization. Certain human sera of infertile men and women who possess antisperm antibodies would similarly block binding of human sperm to the human zona pellucida (Bronson et al., 1982d), suggesting that these spontaneously occurring antibodies are also directed against the sperm-zona receptor of human sperm or regions of the plasma membrane in close proximity to it.

It is important to distinguish these cell surface antigens from the subsurface antigens within spermatozoa. Naturally occurring antibodies to internal cellular components of sperm are relatively ubiquitous in men and women and can be demonstrated using methanol fixed spermatozoa where the sperm plasma membrane has been removed (Tung et al. 1971b). Such antibodies have not been associated with alterations in reproductive function. The ability to absorb these naturally occurring antisperm antibodies with bacteria suggests that these immunoglobulins cross-react with antigens of sperm rather than being directed primarily against spermatozoa. The prepubertal appearance of these antibodies, prior to the onset of active spermatogenesis, provides additional evidence for this postulate.

TESTS CURRENTLY UTILIZED FOR THE DETECTION OF SPERM ANTIBODIES—THEIR PITFALLS

It is generally thought that complement-mediated immobilization of sperm is a highly reliable method of detecting antisperm antibodies, in contrast to agglutination tests (e.g. Franklin-Dukes and Kibrick) in which aggregation of spermatozoa may occur on a non-immune basis (Rose et al., 1976). We correlated the location of the antibodies bound to different regions of the sperm surface and the immunoglobulin class of antibody bound to each region with the ability of such antibodies to promote complement-mediated motility loss. Complement-dependent immobilization tests will not detect antisperm antibodies of the IgA class, which do not fix the early components of the complement cascade. In addition, at least two-fifths of the sperm tail principal piece must be antibody-bound by IgG to result in a significant loss of motility (greater than 50%—Fig. 29.2). Binding of antibodies of either A, G or M clases to the sperm head is also not associated with significant motility loss in the presence of active complement.

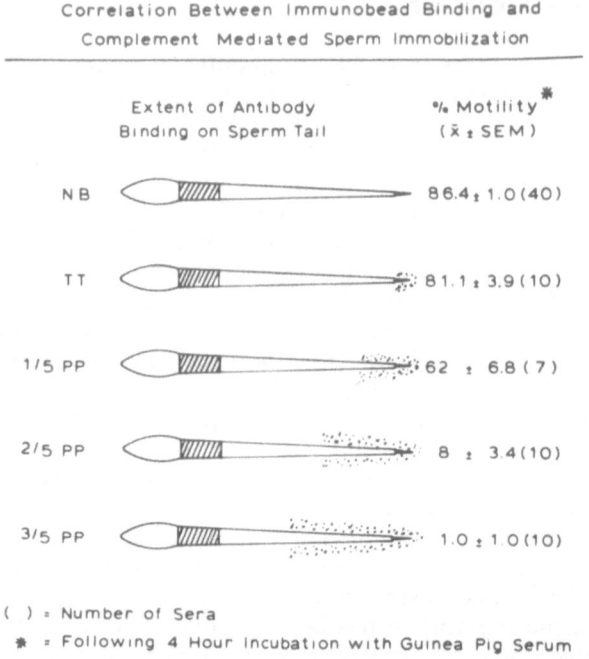

Correlation Between Immunobead Binding and
Complement Mediated Sperm Immobilization

	Extent of Antibody Binding on Sperm Tail	% Motility* ($\bar{x} \pm$ SEM)
N B		86.4 ± 1.0 (40)
T T		81.1 ± 3.9 (10)
1/5 PP		62 ± 6.8 (7)
2/5 PP		8 ± 3.4 (10)
3/5 PP		1.0 ± 1.0 (10)

( ) = Number of Sera

∗ = Following 4 Hour Incubation with Guinea Pig Serum

Fig. 29.2 Correlation between immunobead binding and complement-mediated sperm immobilization. At least 2/5 of the sperm tail principal piece must be IgG bound for immobilization

Investigations utilizing fluorescein labelled antiglobulins suffer from a high incidence of non-specific binding (Rose et al., 1976) perhaps due to naturally occurring antibodies to internal sperm components. This high level of background binding of immunoglobulins could also be due to the presence of receptors to the Fc region of the immunoglobulin molecule on the sperm plasma membrane (Witkin et al., 1980a). Tests which utilize sonicated sperm as an antigen source to detect sperm antibodies (Mather et al., 1980) probably suffer from a high incidence of falsely positive results, due to exposure of sub-surface intracellular components during the cell disruption (Bronson et al., 1981b).

Table 29.8 Comparison of sperm-bound antibody and residual antisperm antibodies detected within the seminal fluid of 14 men with auto-immunity to spermatozoa

Patient identification	Sperm surface-bound antibody with regional antibody specificities	Residual antisperm antibodies	
		Detected	*Missing*
LC	Head and tail-directed IgA/G	Head and tail IgA	IgG classes
C	Tail and tail end piece IgA/G	End piece IgA/G	Tail-directed antibodies
F	Head and tail IgA/G	Head-directed IgA/G	Tail-directed antibodies
Fr	Head and tail IgA/G	Head-directed IgA/G	None
B	Head and tail IgA/G	Head-directed IgA/G	None
J	Head and tail IgA/G	Head-directed IgA/G	None
K	Tail end piece IgA/G	Tail end piece IgG	IgA classes
L	Head IgA/G, tail end piece IgG	Tail end piece IgG	Head IgG; IgA classes
Lv	Head and tail IgA/G	Head IgA/G	Tail-directed antibodies
Mc	Head and tail IgA/G	Head and tail IgA	IgG classes
M	Head, tail and end piece IgA/G	Head and end piece IgA/G	Tail-directed antibodies
O	Head and tail IgG, end piece IgA	End piece IgA	Head and tail-directed antibodies
Q	Head and end piece IgA/G	End piece IgA	End piece IgG
R	Head IgG and end piece IgA/G	None	IgA/G classes

431

Although ELISA techniques (Witkin *et al.*, 1980b) or use of radiolabelled antiglobulins (Haas *et al.*, 1980) provide high levels of specificity and sensitivity in the detection of antisperm antibodies, these tests as currently utilized do not allow one to determine regional specificity of such antibodies nor the proportion of spermatozoa in the ejaculate that are antibody bound. Differing expressions of sperm surface antigens between men have also been demonstrated (Bronson *et al.*, 1983). These tests are useful, however, in screening large numbers of sera for the presence of antisperm antibodies or in quantitating antibody responses to treatment.

Although analysis of seminal plasma for antisperm antibodies represents a significant step forward in defining the immune status of an individual, when contrasted to reliance solely upon serum antibody tests, this approach is not sufficient to characterize the sperm-directed immunoglobulins within the reproductive tract. Residual antibodies remaining within seminal plasma usually need not reflect those antibodies bound directly on the sperm plasma membrane (Table 29.8). In instances where antibody concentration is limiting relative to sperm antigens, all specific antibody would be bound on sperm surfaces, and hence none remains to be detected within seminal plasma.

CAN AN ANTISERUM TO SPERMATOZOA BE DEVELOPED AS A CONTRACEPTIVE VACCINE?

Prerequisites to the development of an antisperm antiserum are that: (1) the antigen be unique to sperm, such that there would be no risk of cross-reaction with other tissues; (2) the antigen be effective in blocking fertilization at one or more loci (sperm-zona binding, the acrosome reaction, gamete membrane fusion); (3) there be no risk of alteration in general immune responses due to the possible shared antigenicity between spermatozoa and certain classes of T lymphocytes (Mather *et al.*, 1980); (4) circulating immune complexes must not be present in sufficient amounts to damage the vascular system and lead into subsequent glomerular or arterial disease.

The frequency of immunization required to maintain the contraceptive effectiveness of this approach is unclear. Would the repeated exposure to spermatozoa through coitus be sufficient to maintain such immunity in women? Given the wide genetic diversity between the response of individuals to antigenic stimuli, would the response to immunization be sufficiently uniform to allow the use of a generalized, simple regimen that could be administered by gynaecologists, whose immunological experience is limited? What would be the risk of developing IgE immunoglobulins during immunization, which might lead to unwanted side-effects, such as bronchospasm and vaginal oedema. Would atopy or allergy be a relative contraindication to immunization?

The administration of whole spermatozoa, especially in association with the adjuvant, used to boost the immune response, might lead to the production of unwanted antibodies (e.g. antinuclear antibodies) and might in themselves lead to long-term health risks. Antibodies to sperm nuclear proteins have been demonstrated in men and women with spontaneously occurring sperm antibodies (Rumke, 1974). Those immunoglobulins, should they gain access to the sperm nucleus, might potentially increase the risk of congenital anomalies.

Spontaneously occurring iso- and auto-antibodies to spermatozoa have been shown to promote the ability of human sperm to penetrate zona-free hamster eggs, leading to the entry of more than one sperm into the ooplasm under conditions *in vitro* that are usually associated with monospermic fertilization (Bronson *et al.*, 1981a). If preparations of whole sperm plasma membrane are utilized as an antigen for immunization, antibodies might form which by promoting the acrosome reaction at the zona surface increase the likelihood of polyspermic fertilization and subsequent spontaneous abortion. These considerations illustrate the need for immunization with highly characterized, purified sperm membrane antigens.

Passive immunization with monoclonal antibodies of known specificity to antigens of the sperm plasma membrane might circumvent these concerns. Unfortunately, this approach would necessitate repeated parenteral administration to maintain levels of antisperm antibodies commensurate with effective fertility control. Given the large blood volume in humans, the amount of antibody needed to be injected might cause discomfort at the time of parenteral administration, and hence would not be well tolerated. The use of ascitic fluid from a non-human species (e.g. mouse ascites tumours) as is commonly used for research purposes, would not be acceptable, due to the risk of antibody formation to these foreign proteins. A human monoclonal antibody source would appear to be necessary.

While at first glance, the creation of immune infertility by immunization with sperm holds promise as a means of contraception, numerous considerations must be addressed and solved before this approach becomes a practical and safe option.

References

Alhgren, M. (1969). Migration of spermatozoa to the fallopian tubes and abdominal cavity of women, including some immunological aspects. *Med. Diss*, Lund (Lund Student Literature)

Anderson, D.J. and Alexander, N.J. (1979). Consequences of autoimmunity to sperm antigens in vasectomized men. In *Immunological Aspects of Reproduction, Clinics in Obstet Gynecol.*, **6,** 425

Behrman, S.J. and Otani, Y. (1963). Transvaginal immunization of the guinea pig with homologous testis and epididymal sperm. *J. Fertil.*, **81,** 329

Bell, E.B. (1968). An immune-type agglutination of mouse spermatozoa by *Pseudomonas maltophilia. J. Reprod. Fertil.*, **17,** 275

Bell, E.B. and McLaren, A. (1970). Reduction of fertility in female mice iso-immunized with a subcellular sperm fraction. *J. Reprod. Fertil.*, **22,** 345

Bronson, R.A., Cooper, G.W., Gold, J., Kaplan, M., Brody, N. and Rosenfeld, D.L. (1983c). Comparison of antisperm antibodies in homosexual and infertile men with auto-immunity to spermatozoa. *Society for Gynecologic Investigation*, 17–20 March Washington, DC

Bronson, R.A., Cooper, G.W. and Rosenfeld, D.L. (1981a). Ability of antibody-bound human sperm to penetrate zona-free hamster ova *in vitro. Fertil. Steril.*, **36,** 778

Bronson, R.A., Cooper, G.W. and, Rosenfeld, D.L. (1981b). Detection of antibody-bound sperm by immunobead binding. *Second S.B. Gusberg Symposium on Reproductive Immunology*, Mount Sinai Medical Center, New York, New York, 18–19 June

Bronson, R.A., Cooper, G.W. and Rosenfeld, D.L. (1982a). Ability of antibody bound human sperm to penetrate zona-free hamster ova *in vitro. Fertil. Steril.*, **36**, 778–83

Bronson, R.A., Cooper, G.W. and Rosenfeld, D.L. (1982b). Letter to the Editor. *Fertil. Steril.*, **37**, 449

Bronson, R.A., Cooper, G.W. and Rosenfeld, D.L. (1982c). Correlation between regional specificity of antisperm antibodies to the spermatozoan surface and complement-mediated sperm immobilization. *Am. J. Reprod. Immunol.*, **2**, 222

Bronson, R.A., Cooper, G.W. and Rosenfeld, D.L. (1982d). Sperm-specific iso- and auto-antibodies inhibit binding of human sperm to the human zona pellucida. *Fertil. Steril.*, **38**, 724–29

Bronson, R.A., Cooper, G.W. and Rosenfeld, D.L. (1982e). Use of freeze-thawed sonicated human sperm as an *in vitro* immunoabsorbant. *Third Annual International Symposium on the Immunology of Reproduction*. Bowman Gray School of Medicine, 24–26 June Winston-Salem, NC

Bronson, R.A., Cooper, G.W. and Rosenfeld, D.L. (1983d). Investigations of complement-mediated sperm membrane damage: II Effects of head-directed human iso- and auto-antibodies on the ability of human sperm to penetrate zona-free hamster eggs. *Fertil Steril* (in press)

Bronson, R.A., Cooper, G.W., Rosenfeld, D.L., Birnbach, S.J. and Scholl, G.M. (1983b). Correlation between the proportion of antibody-bound sperm in ejaculates and their penetration of cervical mucus. *39th Annual meeting, American Fertility Society*, 16–20 April San Francisco, CA

Bronson, R.A., Cooper, G.W., Rosenfeld, D.L. and Scholl, G.M. (1983a). Correlation between the presence of antisperm antibodies detectable in serum and within vagino-cervical secretions. *39th Annual Meeting, American Fertility Society*, 16–20 April San Francisco, CA

Colton, H.R., Borsos, T. and Rapp, H.J. (1969). Titration of the first component of complement on a molecular basis: suitability of IgM and unsuitability of IgG hemolysins as a sensitizer. *Immunochem.*, **6**, 461

D'Almeida, M., Lefroit-Jolly, M. and Voixin, G.A. (1981). Studies on human spermatozoa autoantigens I. Fractionation of sperm membrane antigens: evidence of three antigenic systems. *Clin. Exp. Immunol.*, **44**, 359

Dravland, E. and Joshi, M.S. (1981). Sperm-coating antigens secreted by the epididymis and seminal vesicle of the rat. *Biol. Reprod.*, **25**, 649

Dym, M. and Caviacchia, J.C. (1977). Further observations on the blood testis barrier in monkeys. *Biol. Reprod.*, **17**, 390–407

Edwards, R.G. (1960). Antigenicity of rabbit semen, bull semen and egg yolk after intravaginal or intramuscular injection in female rabbits. *J. Reprod. Fertil.*, **1**, 385

Edwards, R.G. (1964). Immunological control of fertility in female mice. *Nature*, **203**, 50

Fawcett, D.W., Lear, L.V. and Heidger, P.N. (1970). Electron microscopic observations on the structural components of the blood testis barier. *J. Reprod. Fertil. Supply.*, **10**, 105–22

Franklin, R.R. and Dukes, C.D. (1964). Antispermatozoal antibody and unexplained infertility. *Am. J. Obstet. Gynecol.*, **89**, 6–9

Girgis, S.M., Eklandioas, E.M., Iskander, R., El-Dakhly, R. and Girgis, R.N. (1982). Sperm antibodies in serum and semen in men with bilateral congenital absence of the vas deferens. *Arch. Androl.*, **8**, 301–5

Hass, G.G., Cines, D.B. and Schreiber, A.D. (1980). Immunologic infertility: identification of patients with antisperm antibody. *N. Engl. J. Med.* **303**, 722–7

Harper, M.J.R. (1973). Stimulation of sperm movement from the isthmus to the site of fertilization in the rabbit oviduct. *Biol. Reprod.*, **8**, 369–77

Hellema, H.W.J. and Rumke, P. (1978). The micro-sperm immunization test: the use of only motile spermatozoa and studies of complement. *Clin. Exp. Immunol.*, **31**, 1–11

Holsclaw, D.S., Perlmutter, A.D., Jockin, H. and Shwachman, H. (1971). Genital abnormalities in male patients with cystic fibrosis. *J. Urol.*, **106**, 568

Humphrey, J.H. and Dourmashkin, R.R. (1965). Electron microscope studies on immune cell lysis. In *CIBA Foundation Symposium on Complement*, pp. 175–189. (Boston: Little, Brown and Co)

Isojima, S., Tsuchiya, K., Koyama, K., Tanaka, C., Noka, O. and Adachi, H. (1972). Further studies on sperm-immobilizing antibody found in sera of unexplained cases of sterility in women. *Am. J. Obstet. Gynecol.*, **112**, 199

Katsh, S. (1959). Infertility in female guinea pigs induced by injection of homologous sperm. *Am. J. Obstet. Gynecol.*, **78**, 276

Kremer, J., Jager, S., Kniken, J. and Van Slochteren-Draaisma, T. (1978). Recent advances in diagnosis and treatment of infertility to antisperm antibodies. In Cohen, J. and Hendry, W.F.H. (eds) *Spermatozoan Antibodies and Infertility*, p. 114 (Oxford: Black)

Landsteiner, R. (1899). *Zentr. Bakteriol Parasites*, **25**, 549

LeBouteiller, P., Toillet, F. and Voisin, G.A. (1975). Ultrastructural lesions induced *in vitro* in guinea pig spermatozoa by a specific auto-antibody (Anti-T) and complement. *Immunology*, **23**, 983

Linnet, L. and Hjort, T. (1981). Association between failure to impregnate after vasovasostomy and sperm agglutinins in semen. *Lancet*, **1**, 117-19

Lord, E.M., Sensabaugh, G.S. and Stites, D.P. (1977). Immunosuppresive activity of human seminal plasma. I. Inhibition of *in vitro* lymphocyte activation. *J. Immunol.*, **118**, 1704

Marcus, A.H., Herman, J.H. and Hess, E.V. (1978). The effect of human spermatozoa on antigen and mitogen induced blastogenesis. *Arch. Androl.*, **89**,

Mather, S., Goust, J.M., Williamson, H.O. and Fudenberg, H.H. (1980). Antigenic cross-reactivity of sperm and T lymphocytes. *Fertil. Steril.*, **34**, 469-76

McLaren, A. (1964). Immunological control of fertility in female mice. *Nature*, **201**, 582-5

McLaren, A. (1968). Studies on the isoimmunization of mice with spermatozoa. *Fertil. Steril.*, **17**, 492

Menge, A.C. (1971). Antiserum inhibition of rabbit spermatozoal adherence to ova. *Proc. J. Exp. Biol. Med.*, **138**, 98-102

Menge, A.C., Medley, N.E., Mangione, C.M. and Dietrich, J.W. (1982). The incidence and influence of antisperm antibodies in infertile human couples on sperm-cervical mucus inter-action and subsequent fertility. *Fertil. Steril.*, **38**, 439-46

Metchnikoff, E. (1899). Etudes sur la resorption de cellulles. *Ann. Inst. Pasteur (Paris)*, **13**, 737

Metz, C.B. and Anika, J. (1970). Failure of conception in rabbits inseminated with an agglu-tinating, univalent antibody treated semen. *Biol. Reprod.*, **2**, 284

Murdoch, A.J.M., Buckley, C.H. and Fox, H. (1982). Hormonal control of the secretory immune system of the human uterine cervix. *J. Reprod. Immunol.*, **4**, 23

Nicolson, G.L., Ushi, N., Yanagimachi, R., Yanagimachi, H. and Smith, J.R. (1977). Lectin-binding sites on the plasma membrane of rabbit spermatozoa: changes in surface receptors during epididymal maturation and after ejaculation. *J. Cell. Biol.*, **74**, 950

Olson, G.E. and Orgebin-Crist, M.C. (1982). Sperm surface changes during epididymal ma-turation. *Ann. N.Y. Acad. Sci.*, **383**, 92

O'Rand, M.D. (1981). Inhibition of fertility and sperm-zona binding by antiserum to the rabbit sperm membrane autoantigen RSA-1. *Biol. Reprod.*, **25**, 621-8

Pommeranke, W.T. (1928). Effects of sperm injection into female rabbits. *Phys. Zool.*, **1**, 97

Petersen, B.H., Lammel, C.J., Stites, D.P. and Brooks, G.F. (1980). Human seminal plasma inhibition of complement. *J. Lab. Clin. Med.*, **96**, 582

Rose, N.R., Hjort, T., Rumke, P., Harper, M.J.K. and Vyazov, O. (1976). Techniques for detection of iso- and auto-antibodies to human spermatozoa. *Clin. Exp. Immunol.*, **23**, 175

Rumke, P.H. (1974). The origin of immunoglobulins in semen. *Clin. Exp. Immunol.*, **12**, 287-97

Russo, J. and Metz, C.B. (1974). The ultrastructural lesions induced by antibody and comple-ment in rabbit spermatozoa. *Biol. Reprod.*, **10**, 293

Seki, M. and Mettler, L. (1982). Influence of spermatozoal antibodies in the reproduction of mice. *Am. J. Reprod. Immunol.*, **2**, 225

Snell, G.D. (1944). Antigenic differences between sperm of different inbred strains of mice. *Science*, **100**, 272

Sokoloski, J. Wolf, D. and Bechtol, R. (1982). Mapping the human sperm surface: molecular characterization of an individual antigen. *Society for the Study of Reproduction, 15th Annual Meeting*, University of Wisconsin, Madison, Wisconsin, 19-22 July

Templeton, A.A. and Mortimer, D. (1982). The development of a clinical test of sperm migration to the site of fertilization. *Fertil. Steril.*, **37**, 410

Tung, K.S.K., Cooke, W.D. Jr., McCarty, T.A. and Robitaille, P. (1976). Human sperm antigens and antisperm antibodies. II. Age-related incidence of antisperm antibodies. *Clin. Exp. Immunol.*, **25**, 73-9

Tung, K.S.K., Okada, A. and Yanagimachi, R. (1980). Sperm autoantigens and fertilization. 1. Effects of antisperm antibodies on rouleaux formation, viability and acrosome reaction of guinea pig sperm. *Biol. Reprod.*, **23**, 877-88

Uehling, D.T. (1971). Secretory IgA in seminal fluid. *Fertil. Steril.*, **22**, 769-73

Weininger, R.B., Fisher, S., Rifkin, J. and Bedford, J.M. (1982). Experimental studies on the passage of specific IgG to the lumen of the rabbit epididymis. *J. Reprod. Fertil.*, **65**, 251-8

Witkin, S.S., Brown, C.A., Good, R.A. and Day, N.K. (1980a). Sperm immobilization by sera from unimmunized guinea pigs: Requirements for immunoglobulins and complement. *J. Reprod. Immunol.*, **2**, 65

Witkin, S.S., Shohnai, S.K., Gupta, S., Good, R.A. and Day, N.K. (1980b). Demonstration of IgG Fc receptors on spermatozoa and their utilization for the detection of circulating immune complexes in human serum. *Clin. Exp. Immunol.*, **41**, 441

Yanagimachi, R., Okada, A. and Tung, K.S.K. (1981). II. Effects of anti-guinea pig sperm antibodies on sperm-ovum interactions. *Biol. Reprod.*, **24**, 512

30
Sperm calcium homeostasis during maturation

M.P. BRADLEY and I.T. FORRESTER

THE ROLE OF Ca²⁺ IN SPERM METABOLISM MOTILITY

Intracellular Ca^{2+} ions play an extremely critical role in many cellular events (Bygrave, 1978; Carafoli and Crompton, 1978; Kretsinger, 1980). Calcium is involved in the activation and inhibition of many enzymes as well as the modulation of certain contractile and motile systems, hormonal regulation and diverse membrane-linked functions such as the excitation-secretion coupling of nerve endings and exocytotic functions in general. Thus Ca^{2+} appears to have an ubiquitous role in the regulation of a diverse range of cellular events. It is now appreciated that the intracellular concentration of free Ca^{2+} is the vital parameter which must be considered in assessing Ca^{2+} as a metabolic messenger. The cytoplasmic concentration of free Ca^{2+} in most cells is in the range $10^{-6}-10^{-7}$ mol/l (Baker, 1978). The two major factors which determine the maintenance of this low intracellular free Ca^{2+} concentration are the current status of the internal Ca^{2+} concentration and the modulation of the plasma membrane Ca^{2+} transport systems. The precise involvement of Ca^{2+} in modulating mammalian sperm functions is still uncertain although it has been shown to influence motility (Hoskins et al., 1978; Davis, 1978); capacitation (Singh et al., 1978; Saling et al., 1978); the acrosome reaction (Talbot and Franklin, 1976); respiration (Storey and Keyhani, 1974) and glycolysis plus sperm cell volume (Bredderman and Foote, 1971; McGrady et al., 1974).

The role of Ca^{2+} in sperm motility is controversial for it has been observed that Ca^{2+} may have either an inhibitory or excitatory effect. These seemingly contradictory data may be the results of experiments where the effect of exogenously added total calcium was examined with no regard for the free ionized Ca^{2+} concentrations in solution. Total extracellular Ca^{2+} concentrations do not necessarily relate to the intrasperm free Ca^{2+} levels. Although there is a relationship between Ca^{2+} and motility in mammalian spermatozoa, more definitive experiments have been done with invertebrate spermatozoa. What follows is a brief review of the literature concerned with both mammalian and invertebrate studies.

Mammalian sperm studies

Peterson and Freund (1976) reported that the plasma membrane of human spermatozoa is impermeable to Ca^{2+}. When intact spermatozoa were exposed to low concentrations of the divalent cation ionophore A23187 there was an increase in the plasma membrane permeability and a resultant mitochondrial Ca^{2+} accumulation. They proposed that in human spermatozoa the selective exclusion of extracellular Ca^{2+} may be critical to the survival of the sperm cell and that increases in the intrasperm Ca^{2+} concentration could lead to inhibtion of motility.

Davis (1978), examined the effects of Ca^{2+} on the motility and fertilization rate of rat spermatozoa *in vivo*. He noted that at a Ca^{2+} concentration of 1.7 mmol/l, sperm motility was inhibited, but when these spermatozoa were placed in a medium containing 3.4 mmol/l Ca^2, vigorous motility continued for about 2 h. The sperm fertilizing capacity was also found to be Ca^{2+}-sensitive. At Ca^{2+} concentrations of 2.6 and 3.4 mmol/l, fertilization rates were 83% and 91% respectively. In a medium containing 1.7 and 5.8 mmol/l Ca^{2+} fertilization rates were 31% and 13% respectively. Morton *et al.*, (1978) set out to try and clarify the many varied findings concerned with Ca^{2+} concentrations and optimum sperm motility. It was demonstrated that in several species, including man, the motility of spermatozoa within the epididymis (i.e. prior to ejaculation) appears to be strictly related to the levels of free Ca^{2+} in the epididymal plasma.

Invertebrate sperm studies

The mobility of sea urchin spermatozoa also depends critically on the concentration of environmental Ca^{2+} ions. These spermatozoa exhibit a monophasic response to increases in the Ca^{2+} concentration above the usual environmental concentration (Young and Nelson, 1974). Motility was found to be maximal in 9 mmol/l Ca^{2+} and then it declined as the Ca^{2+} concentration was further increased. Calcium also modulates sperm flagellar beat symmetry. Brokaw *et al.* (1974) were able to demonstrate in demembranated sea urchin spermatozoa, that high concentrations of Ca^{2+} (5 mmol/l) induced an asymmetrical beating pattern and the spermatozoa would swim in circular paths. However, symmetrical flagellar beat patterns could be induced if the Ca^{2+} concentration was reduced to 1 nmol/l free Ca^{2+}. This observation confirmed by other workers (Gibbons and Gibbons, 1980; Gibbons, 1980) using demembranated sea urchin spermatozoa. In these experiments it was found that sperm quiescence could be induced at Ca^{2+} concentrations ranging from 0.04 to 2 mmol/l. Quiescence could be reversed by the reduction of free Ca^{2+} in the medium by the addition of EGTA. They concluded that sperm quiescence was induced by a rise in the intrasperm free Ca^{2+} concentration perhaps as a consequence of membrane depolarization.

In biological systems which are akin to spermatozoa (such as motile bacteria or protozoa) changes in the internal Ca^{2+} concentration of the organism also appear to be responsible for changes in the ciliary-beat patterns. Bessen *et al.*, (1980) demonstrated that at free Ca^{2+} concentrations at 1 μmol/l or less, demembranated flagella from *Chlamydomonas*, exhibited a beat pattern with an asymmetrical wave form resembling that of intact cells at the same free Ca^{2+} concentrations. In the presence of 100 μmol/l Ca^{2+} the axonemes beat with a symmetrical wave form similar to that of flagella during backward swimming *in situ*. These changes in flagellar motility were due solely to alterations of the free Ca^{2+} concentrations and were not a reflection of changes in the Ca-ATP levels of the medium. The importance of regulating very precisely the intraflagellar Ca^{2+} concentrations in *Chlamydomonas* is emphasized by these results. Bessen subsequently proposed without evidence that Ca^{2+} regulation in the flagellar plasma of *Chlamydomonas* occurs at the level of the flagellar plasma membrane possibly via a Ca^{2+}-pump mechanism.

In summary the regulation of the flagellar-beat activity, and hence sperm motility by Ca^{2+}, is strictly dependent upon the maintainance of precisely defined intraflagellar Ca^{2+} levels.

CALCIUM HOMEOSTASIS WITHIN THE FLAGELLUM OF THE MAMMALIAN SPERMATOZOON

A simple experiment which demonstrates the necessity for ram spermatozoa to maintain a low intraflagellar free Ca^{2+} concentration can be performed as follows. Incubation of freshly ejaculated motile ram spermatozoa in a Ca^{2+} containing buffer does not significantly alter either the pattern or vigour of their motility. However, the subsequent addition of the Ca^{2+} ionophore A23187 (3 μmol/l) leads to the complete abolition of sperm motility (I.T. Forrester, unpublished results). Since the Ca^{2+} ionophore selectively affects only the plasma membrane at this concentration, this treatment would induce a large influx of Ca^{2+} into the spermatozoa. Some of the Ca^{2+} will be immediately accumulated by the mitochondria. However, the excess Ca^{2+} present which is not accumulated by the mitochondria is inhibitory to sperm motility. Similar observations on the effects of Ca^{2+} ions on sperm motility have recently been made by Gibbons (1980) using demembranated sea urchin spermatozoa. It is therefore important to under-

Table 30.1 Comparison of Ca^{2+}-transporting membranes in some representative cell types

Cell type	Plasma membrane		Mitochondria		Endo(sarco)plasmic Reticulum
	Ca^{2+}-ATPase	Na^+/Ca^{2+}	Ca^{2+} porter	Na^+/Ca^{2+} porter	Ca^{2+}-ATPase
Erythrocyte	+	−	−	−	−
Hepatocyte	+	−	+	−	+
Myocardial	+	+	+	+	+
Spermatozoa	+	+	+	+	− (Absent)

stand the nature of the Ca^{2+} control mechanisms in mammalian spermatozoa plus their subcellular location and function.

In most mammalian cells the concentrations of intracellular free Ca^{2+} are regulated at two levels. Within the cell, increases in the cytoplasmic free Ca^{2+} levels are compensated for by a rapid Ca^{2+} uptake into the mitochondria and endoplasmic reticulum. Secondly, at the plasma membrane, Ca^{2+} is actively excluded from the cell by outwardly directed Ca^{2+} pumps (Ca^{2+}-ATPases) (Table 30.1). The mitochrondrion is an important intracellular organelle in mammalian spermatozoa, because mature sperm do not contain an endoplasmic reticulum.

Sperm mitochondrial Ca²⁺ transport

Sperm Ca^{2+} transport has been investigated in spermatozoa from several species including rabbit epididymal (Storey and Keyhani, 1974), bovine epididymal (Babcock et al., 1975), human ejaculated (Peterson and Freund, 1976) and both ram ejaculated and epididymal spermatozoa (Bradley et al., 1979; Stewart and Forrester, 1979; van Eerten and Forrester, 1980). In all cases energy-dependent Ca^{2+} fluxes occur across the sperm plasma and mitochondrial membranes. The intrasperm Ca^{2+} concentrations may be controlled by the mitochondrial complex which acts like a 'sponge' to take up or release Ca^{2+} under the appropriate conditions. In the absence of an endoplasmic reticulum, the function of mitochondria in spermatozoa may be similar to the function of the sarcoplasmic reticulum in striated muscle; that is, they act as a Ca^{2+} reservoir. If this is the case in mammalian spermatozoa, then sperm motility would be very dependent upon fully functional mitochondria in a coupled state.

Although Ca^{2+} efflux from the mitochondria of mammalian spermatozoa can be induced by uncoupling agents (Bradley et al., 1979), these findings would normally have little relevance in vivo. However, if the mitochondria of mammalian spermatozoa do actually contribute to intrasperm Ca^{2+} homeostasis, naturally occurring Ca^{2+} efflux mechanisms should occur in vivo in response to the correct intracellular signal. For example, Na^+ and acetylcholine may be effectors of sperm mitochondrial Ca^{2+} efflux (Stewart and Forrester, 1979).

It is unlikely however that the mitochondrial Ca^{2+} uptake/efflux mechanisms within spermatozoan flagella are the major Ca^{2+} homeostatic pathways for two reasons. First, the mitochondrial Ca^{2+} uptake process is inhibited by 1–5 mmol/l Mg^{2+} (van Eerten and Forrester, 1980b). Since the cytoplasmic levels of Mg^{2+} in most mammalian cells are the order of 1–3 mmol/l, it is possible that under normal metabolic conditions the mitochondrial Ca^{2+} uptake pathway in mammalian spermatozoa is completely inhibited. Secondly, in many mammalian cells the bulk of Ca^{2+} fluxes are carefully regulated at the plasma membrane and presumably similar modes of Ca^{2+}-regulation exist in the spermatozoan flagellum.

Sperm Plasma Membrane Ca²⁺ Transport

Extensive research in a wide variety of eukaryotic cells has shown that intracellular Ca^{2+} is regulated by the concerted operation of specific membrane-associated pumps located in the plasma membrane, endoplasmic reticulum and the inner mitochondrial membrane (Table 30.1) (Bygrave, 1978; Carafoli and Crompton, 1978). In spermatozoa, which lack an endoplasmic reticulum the major Ca^{2+} transporting mechanisms are found in the plasma membrane. Here the Ca^{2+} control machinery are in direct contact with their external environment. For example, the seminal plasma has a high concentration of exogenous free Ca^{2+} (Mann, 1964). Thus a considerable concentration gradient of Ca^{2+} exists between the extra- and intracellular environments. However, several separate groups have noted that intact, viable mammalian spermatozoa are impermeable to Ca^{2+} (Babcock *et al.*, 1976; Peterson and Freund, 1976; Storey, 1978; Stewart and Forrester, 1976).

The Plasma Membrane Ca²⁺-ATPase

A Ca^{2+} efflux system commonly observed in the plasma membranes of eukaryotic cells in the Ca^{2+}-pump (Ca^{2+}-ATPase). The prime function of this enzyme is to pump Ca^{2+} out of the cell at the expense of ATP hydrolysis. As a result, intracellular Ca^{2+} levels can be carefully regulated.

Evidence for a Ca^{2+}-ATPase in the plasma membranes of mammalian spermatozoa was reported by Voglmayr *et al.* (1969a,b) who described both Ca^{2+}-ATPase and Mg^{2+}-ATPase activities in ram testicular and epididymal spermatozoa. Using fractionated spermatozoa it was found that the ATPase activities were highest in the flagellum. There was also an increase in sperm ATPase activity as sperm post-testicular maturation progressed. Guinea-pig spermatozoa contain a Ca^{2+}-ATPase on the periacrosomal segment of the plasmalemma and on the outer acrosomal membrane as demonstrated by qualitative techniques (Gordon *et al.*, 1978).

Calcium-ATPase activity in the total plasma membrane of bull spermatozoa has been described (Vijayasarathy *et al.*, 1980). The sperm plasma membranes used in this study were a mixed population derived from the flagellar, head, and acrosome and therefore the contribution of the enzyme to sperm function cannot be specifically defined.

In ram spermatozoa, the flagellar plasma membrane has been shown to contain a variety of ATPase activities (Bradley and Forrester, 1980). Of importance was the finding that a Ca^{2+}-ATPase was also present (Table 30.2). In the presence of Ca^{2+}, the Mg^{2+}-ATPase of ram sperm flagellar plasma membranes increased to approximately 18.5 μmol/l ADP produced mg protein^{-1} h^{-1}. The additional 2.5 μmol ADP produced mg protein^{-1} h^{-1} in the presence of Ca^{2+} was defined as the Ca^{2+}-dependent-ATPase activity. Furthermore, Ca^{2+}-ATPase assays of the flagellar plasma membranes derived from both ram caput and caudal spermatozoa revealed that caput sperm membranes have no detectable Ca^{2+}-ATPase activity. A reduced level of Ca^{2+}-ATPase activity in the flagellar plasma membranes of caudal spermatozoa (1.8 μmol ADP produced mg protein^{-1} h^{-1}

Table 30.2 ATPase activities in isolated flagellar plasma membranes from ram ejaculated spermatozoa

Additions[a,c]	ATPase[b] specific activity
Mg^{2+}	15.78 ± 0.2
$Ca^{2+} + Mg^{2+}$	18.50 ± 0.3
$Na^+ + K^+ + Mg^{2+}$	5.00 ± 0.3

[a] Mg^{2+}-ATPase measured in the presence of 0.1 mmol/l EGTA and 3 mmol/$MgCl_2$. Ca^{2+}-ATPase measured in the presence of 0.1 mmol/l/EGTA, 3 mmol/l $MgCl_2$ and 4.85 mmol/l $CaCl_2$. The difference between the Mg^{2+}-ATPase activity and the $Ca^{2+} + Mg^{2+}$-ATPase activity is defined as the Ca^{2+}-ATPase activity. $(Na^+ + K^+)$-ATPase measured in the presence of 0.1 mmol/l EGTA but omitting ouabain and Ca^{2+}.
[b] Expressed as μmol ADP produced mg membrane protein^{-1} h^{-1}. The figures are the mean SD of at least four separate determinations.
[c] ATPase activities were not inhibited by 50 μmol/l oligomycin

was also shown relative to ejaculated spermatogen (3.9 μmol). The isolated flagellar plasma membrane vesicles from ram caudal and ejaculated spermatozoa were also capable of ATP-dependent Ca^{2+} accumulation (Bradley and Forrester, 1980). Consistent with the enzymatic data above it was found that both the rate and extent of Ca^{2+} uptake was reduced in flagella plasma membranes isolated from caudal spermatozoa. This reduced level of Ca^{2+} transport in caudal sperm could be a consequence of the maturational status of caudal sperm, which are unable to maintain Ca^{2+} homeostasis to the same degree as ejaculated spermatozoa. This condition may be responsible for the different patterns of motility observed between caudal and ejaculated spermatozoa. We have looked for modulators of the Ca^{2+}-ATPase which may be responsible for changing the properties of the Ca^{2+} transport system during post-testicular maturation.

Na^+-Ca^{2+} exchange transporter

Na^+-Ca^{2+} exchange is a carrier-mediated transport process in which the transmembrane movement of Ca^{2+} is directly coupled to the movement of Na^+ in the opposite direction. The Na^+-Ca^{2+} exchange transporter is present in the giant squid axon (Dipola and Beague, 1980), brain (Stahl and Swanson, 1969), and secretory tissues such as the adrenal medulla, pancreas and neurohyphophysis (Douglas, 1968; Rubin, 1970) and cardiac sarcolemmal vesicles (Reeves and Sutko, 1979). The physiological role of this transport system in heart is uncertain. However, the system could be responsible for removing Ca^{2+} from the cell, or alternatively for bringing Ca^{2+} into the cell during membrane depolarization, inducing an elevation of intracellular Na^+. The stoichiometry for the Na^+-Ca^{2+} exchange system in cardiac cells has been determined as 3 mol Na^+ exchanged for 1 mol of Ca^{2+} (Pitts *et al.*, 1980).

The plasma membrane Na^+-Ca^{2+} transporter has many different properties from the Ca^{2+}-pump. First, transport does not require ATP. Inhibitors of Ca^{2+} transport, lanthanum and vanadate, do not effect Na^+-

induced Ca^{2+} transport when present at the same concentrations which inhibit the Ca^{2+}-pump. Calmodulin has no effect on the Na^+-Ca^{2+} transporter. Interestingly the Na^+-Ca^{2+} exchange systems appear to be found only in cells which originate predominantly from excitable tissues. Mammalian spermatozoa have many characteristics in common with cells from excitable tissues. For example, sperm mitochondrial Ca^{2+} transport responds to ruthenium red, Na^+ and Mg^{2+} in a similar manner to that reported for heart mitochondria (Bradley et al., 1979b; Carafoli and Crompton, 1978).

The ram sperm flagellar plasma membrane also contains a Na^+-Ca^{2+} antiporter system (Bradley and Forrester, 1980b). Further it was shown that the Na^+-Ca^{2+} exchange system in caudal sperm membranes was operating at a significantly reduced rate, compared to that found in membranes from ejaculated spermatozoa.

The regulation of intracellular Ca^{2+} by many cells is thought to occur primarily by plasma membrane-located Ca^{2+}-pumps (Racker, 1980). In cells which also contain a plasma membrane Na^+-Ca^{2+} exchange system, the two Ca^{2+} efflux processes may work in concert to control cytosolic Ca^{2+}. It has been proposed that in these situations the high-capacity, low-affinity Na^+-Ca^{2+} antiporter is the predominant plasma membrane Ca^{2+}-extruding system (Caroni and Carafoli, 1980). The low-capacity, high-affinity plasma membrane Ca^{2+}-pump functions as a fine control of intracellular Ca^{2+}. If this is also the arrangement in mammalian sperm then it is possible to postulate a model for intrasperm Ca^{2+} regulation. Spermatozoa are normally subject to a continuous Na^+ influx, in response to the high levels (70-100 mmol/l) of seminal plasma Na^+ (Mann, 1964). This condition would generate, via the Na^+-Ca^{2+} antiporter, an opposite and continuous efflux of Ca^{2+} from the spermatozoa to lower intrasperm Ca^{2+}. The plasma membrane Ca^{2+}-ATPase may further facilitate this process by pumping out Ca^{2+} in excess of that normally handled by the Na^+-Ca^{2+} antiporter. Accordingly it is the Ca^{2+} pump which is more responsible for the precise modulation of the intracellular free Ca^{2+} concentration of the spermatozoon. Such a concept is strengthened by the observation that the Ca^{2+}-ATPase activity and Ca^{2+} uptake rates in isolated flagellar plasma membrane vesicles from ram caudal spermatozoa are of a lower activity compared to the activities found in the flagellar plasma membranes of ram ejaculated sperm.

Since ram caudal sperm motility is uncoordinated and generally lacks significant forward motility, compared to ram ejaculated spermatozoa, it is felt that caudal sperm motility is altered prior to or at ejaculation, via modulation of the flagellar plasma membrane Ca^{2+}-ATPase. Such an event would lead to a lowering of intracellular free Ca^{2+} and hence a change to coordinated forward motility. The question which has to be asked of course is: What specifically activates the Ca^{2+} pump prior to, or at, ejaculation?

CALSEMIN: A POSSIBLE BIOLOGICAL MODULATOR OF THE MAMMALIAN SPERM CALCIUM HOMEOSTASIS

In 1980, Forrester and Bradley, first reported the existence of a heat-stable protein fraction in human seminal plasma which was able to activate the red blood cell ghost membrane Ca^{2+}-ATPase. Subsequently it was found that this protein fraction would also activate the flagellar plasma membrane Ca^{2+}-ATPase and caudal ram spermatozoa to a level found in ram ejaculated spermatozoa. Using a phenothiazine affinity column followed by DEAE-Sephadex chromotagraphy, it has been possible to purify this protein to apparent homogeneity. It has an estimated molecular weight of 20 000.

This protein, named calsemin, is a unique Ca^{2+}-dependent regulator protein. Its amino acid composition differs from that of the regulatory protein calmodulin. Further, calsemin is a glycoprotein whereas calmodulin does not contain carbohydrate sugars. Calsemin demonstrates a peculiar property of protein–protein aggregation into higher molecular weight species in the presence of sodium dodecyl sulphate. This aggregation phenomenon which has also been reported to occur with glycophorin A, is not a widely reported one (Furthmayr and Marchesi, 1976) and may be an important fact to consider in the interpretation of sodium dodecyl sulphate gels of certain proteins.

In some respects calsemin is similar to calmodulin. For example, (i) they both stimulate activator-requiring PDE and Ca^{2+}-ATPase activity, (ii) enzyme activation was Ca^{2+}-dependent, (iii) activation was abolished by phenothiazines, and (iv) both calmodulin and calsemin are acidic, heatstable, low-molecular-weight proteins (Means and Dedman, 1980). A comparison of the properties of these two proteins are summarized in Table 30.3.

Table 30.3 Comparison of the properties of calsemin and calmodulin

	Calsemin (CaSem)	*Calmodulin* (CaM)
Structural		
Calcium binding	3–4 sites (two affinities)	4 sites
Molecular weight	16 500–20 000	15 000–18 500
Charge	pI ~ 4	pI ~ 4
UV analysis	no phe fine spectrum	phe fine spectrum
N-terminal	free glycine	blocked glycine
Carbohydrate present	+	−
Trimethyl-lysine present	−	+
Mobility shift ($\pm Ca^{2+}$)	−	+
Activates		
3':5'-cyclic nucleotide phosphodiesterase	+	+
Ca^{2+}-ATPase, RBC and sperm	+	+
Cellular location	extracellular	intracellular
CaM immunoreactivity	+	+
CaSem immunoreactivity	+	−
phenothiazine sensitivity	+	+

The Ca^2-binding properties of calsemin were determined by the method of equilibrium dialysis. Two classes of Ca^{2+} binding sites were found; a low-affinity site with a Kd 4.03 μmol/l and high-affinity site with a K_d of 7.4 μmol/l. The high-affinity site apparently binds 3 Ca^{2+} ions/mol and the low-affinity site 0.27 Ca^{2+} ions/mol. In comparison, calmodulin contains four Ca^{2+}-binding sites with a dissociation constant of 2.4 μmol/l (Dedman et al., 1977), although Watterson et al. (1976) had previously reported that bovine brain calmodulin had two distinct classes of Ca^{2+} binding sites. High-affinity binding ($K_d = 1 \times 10^{-5}$ mol/l) of 2 mol Ca^{2+} bound per mol calmodulin, and a low-affinity site (K_d 8.6 $\times 10^{-7}$ mol/l) which also bound 2 mol of Ca^{2+}/mol calmodulin.

The amino acid analysis of calsemin revealed that it contains at least 20% glycine. Glutamine and proline are all present in calsemin in higher amounts

Table 30.4 Amino acid composition of calsemin: comparison with ovine brain calmodulin

Amino acid	Calsemin (Ram)	Calsemin (Human)	Calmodulin (Ovine)
Lys	11	14	9
His	7	9	5
Arg	9	13	7
Asp	13	13	20
Thr	10	9	9
Ser	15	14	7
Glu	13	16	29
Pro	12	11	9
Gly	17	49	11
Ala	11	11	11
Cys	0	4	0
Val	9	9	8
Met	4	5	8
Isol	7	8	8
Leu	9	11	10
Tyr	6	8	5
Phe	7	9	8

Results are expressed as mol%

than in calmodulin. In particular, calsemin contains cysteine which is absent in calmodulin. There are also several more tyrosine residues in calsemin than calmodulin (Table 30.4). Dansyl chloride N-terminal analysis shows that human calsemin has a glycine at the N-terminus. The calsemin carbohydrate content was composed of 35% galactose, 18% glucose, 14% fucose, 13% mannose, 3% galactosamine, 6% glucosamine and 11% ribose sugars.

Calsemin will also stimulate the flagellar-beat activity of caudal epididymal spermatozoa in a Ca^{2+}-dependent manner by 300%, although a total induction of forward sperm motility by calsemin has not been demonstrated (Bradley and Forrester, 1982). On the basis of these experimental observations, a model is proposed to describe the development of forward motility during the final stages of post-testicular sperm maturation (Fig. 30.1). An important part of this model incorporates the fact that epididymal spermatozoa are known to be more permeable to Ca^{2+} than ejaculated sper-

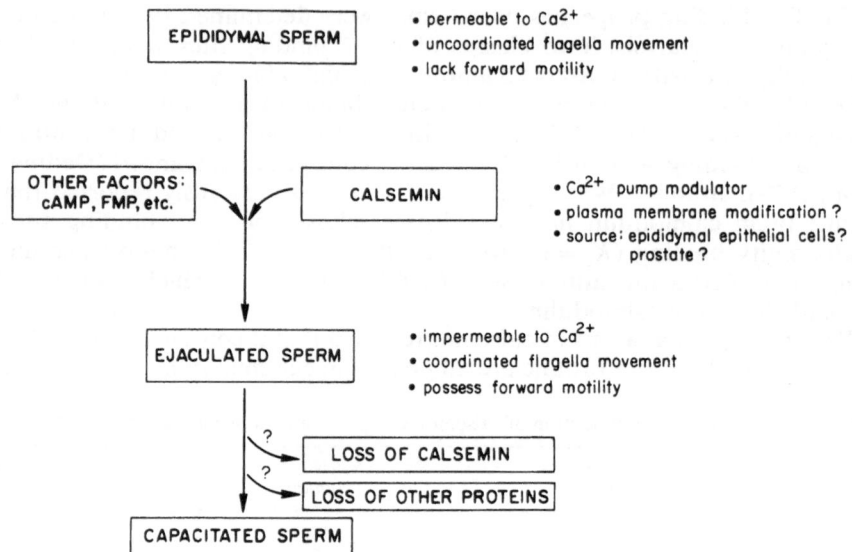

Fig. 30.1 Proposed model of how Ca^{2+}, calsemin and sperm motility may be related during post-testicular maturation

matozoa (Singh *et al.*, 1978), to lack forward motility (Acott and Hoskins, 1978) and to have an uncoordinated flagellar beat. It is proposed that at ejaculation, or immediately prior to that event, calsemin is secreted from either the prostate gland or the epididymal epithelial cells to interact with caudal spermatozoa. This interaction results in the activation of the flagellar plasma membrane Ca^{2+} pump (and possibly other Ca^{2+}-dependent enzymes) which in turn results in a decrease of intracellular free Ca^{2+}. This allows the coordinated beating of the flagellum to be initiated.

Although there is evidence that several of these interactions do take place, the induction of forward motility in caudal sperm in the presence of calsemin has not been demonstrated. Calsemin may not be the only factor required to initiate full motility. Indeed, there is abundant evidence which demonstrates that cyclic nucleotides, especially cAMP, also play an important role in modulating this function (Garbers and Kopf, 1980).

Another protein factor which appears to be important in the development of sperm motility which needs to be considered, is forward motility protein (FMP) (Acott and Hoskins, 1978). FMP is a heat-stable, acidic, glycoprotein fraction of molecular weight 37 000, found in bovine seminal plasma, that initiates forward motility in bovine caput spermatozoa (provided high concentrations of theophylline are also present). Interestingly calsemin and FMP are both heat-stable, acidic glycoproteins and appear to exist as multiple protein aggregates.

There are however several major differences between forward FMP and calsemin. Firstly, calsemin specifically requires the addition of exogenous Ca^{2+} to mediate its biological function. Secondly, FMP appears to function only in the presence of cyclic nucleotides. No such requirement for calsemin has been found. As yet, the specific metabolic processes that FMP alters have not been clearly defined. Whether or not calsemin and forward motility protein are identical will not be resolved until homogenous preparations of FMP are obtained for comparison.

It is recognized that the interaction of calsemin with the plasma membrane Ca^{2+}-ATPase may be only one of a series of metabolic reactions which occur at ejaculation. For example, Rufo et al. (1982) have recently reported the purification of a Ca^{2+}-transport inhibitor from bovine seminal plasma which blocks Ca^{2+} uptake into ejaculated sperm by altering components of the sperm plasma membrane. It is conceivable that both this

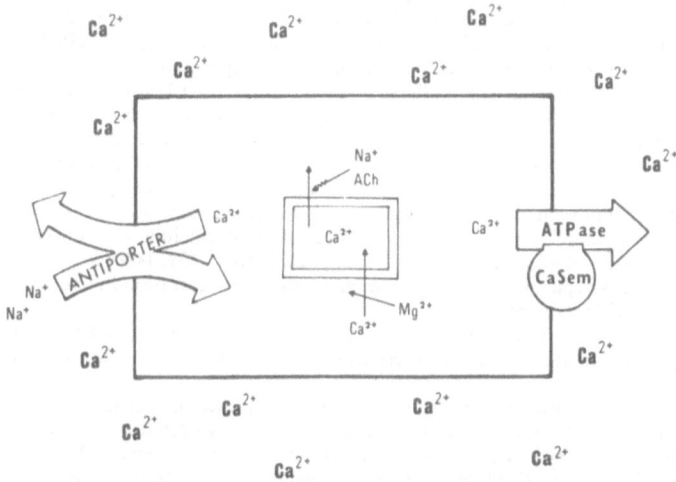

Fig. 30.2 A summary of the major Ca^{2+} transport mechanisms present in mammalian spermatozoa

protein and calsemin could work in concert with each other to reduce intrasperm free Ca^{2+}. However, our findings do provide a partial biochemical explanation of the transitional change in sperm motility associated with post-testicular maturation and Ca^{2+} homeostasis.

In summary, data have been presented which demonstrate that the mammalian spermatozoon has the ability to maintain precisely Ca^{2+} homeostasis within its flagellum, through the concerted action of a flagellar plasma membrane Na^+/Ca^{2+} antiporter, and a Ca^{2+} pump (Fig. 30.2). The Ca^{2+} pump can be activated by an extracellular protein, named calsemin, which may be important in modulating Ca^{2+} homeostasis in spermatozoa after ejaculation.

Acknowledgements

This work was supported by the Medical Research Council of New Zealand and the Ford Foundation of New York. We thank Diane Smithson for the typing of this manuscript.

References

Acott, T.S. and Hoskins, D.D. (1978). Bovine sperm forward motility protein. *J. Biol. Chem.*, **253**, 6744–50

Babcock, D.F., First, N.L. and Lardy, H.A. (1975). Transport mechanism for succinate and phosphate localized in the plasma membrane of bovine spermatozoa. *J. Biol. Chem.*, **250**, 6488–95

Babcock, D.F., First, N.L. and Lardy, H.A. (1976). Action of ionophore A23187 at the cellular level. *J. Biol. Chem.*, **251**, 3881–6

Baker, P.F. (1978). The regulation of intracellular calcium in giant axons of *Loligo* and *Myxicola. Ann. NY Acad. Sci.*, **307**, 250–68

Besson, M., Fay, R.B. and Witman, G.B. (1980). Calcium control of waveform in isolated flagellar axonemes of *Chlamydomonas. J. Cell. Biol.*, **86**, 446–55

Bradley, M.P., van Eerten, M.T.W.. and Forrester, I.T. (1979a). The energy-dependent uptake of Ca^{2+} by mammalian spermatozoa. *Proc. Univ. Otago Med. School*, **57**, 5–6

Bradley, M.P., van Eerton, M.T.W., Rayns, D.G. and Forrester, I.T. (1979b). Membrane integrity and the regulation of calcium in mammalian spermatozoa. *Biol. Reprod.*, **20**, 61A

Bradley, M.P. and Forrester, I.T. (1980a). A $(Ca^{2+}+Mg^{2+})$-ATPase and active Ca^{2+} transport in the plasma membranes isolated from ram sperm flagella. *Cell Calcium*, **1**, 381–90

Bradley, M.P. and Forrester, I.T. (1980b). A sodium–calcium exchange mechanism in plasma membrane vesicles isolated from ram sperm flagella. *FEBS Lett.*, **121**, 15–18

Bradley, M.P. and Forrester, I.T. (1982). Human and ram seminal plasma both contain a calcium-dependent regulator protein calsemin. *J. Androl.*, **3**, 289–96

Bredderman, P.J. and Foote, R.H. (1971). The effect of calcium ions on cell volume and motility of bovine spermatozoa. *Proc. Soc. Exp. Biol. Med.*, **137**, 1440–3

Brinley, F.J. and Scarpa, A. (1975). Ionized magnesium concentration in axoplasm of dialyzed squid axons. *FEBS Lett*, **50**, 82–5

Brokaw, C.J., Josslin, R. and Bobrow, L. (1974). Calcium-ion regulation of flagellar beat symmetry in reactivated sea urchin spermatozoa. *Biochem. Biophys. Res. Commun.*, **58**, 795–800

Bygrave, F.L. (1978). Mitochondria and the control of intracellular calcium *Biol. Rev.*, **53**, 43–79

Carafoli, E. and Crompton, M. (1978). The regulation of intracellular calcium. In Bronner, F. and Kleinzeller, A. (eds.) *Current Topics in Membranes and Transport*, Vol. 10, pp. 151–216.

Caroni, P. and Carafoli, E. (1980). An ATP-dependent Ca^{2+}-pumping system in dog heart sarcolemma. *Nature*, **283**, 765–7

Davis, B.K. (1978). Effect of calcium on motility and fertilization by rat spermatozoa *in vitro*. *Proc. Soc. Exp. Biol. Med.*, **157**, 54–6

Dipolo, R. and Beauge, L. (1980). Mechanisms of calcium transport in the giant axon of the squid and their physiological role. *Cell Calcium*, **1**, 147–69

Douglas, W.W. (1968). Stimulus-secretion coupling: the concept and clues from *chromaffina* and other cells. *Br. J. Pharmacol.*, **34**, 451–74

Forrester, I.T. and Bradley, M.P. (1980). A $(Ca^{2+}+Mg^{2+})$ ATPase in epididymal and ejaculated sperm flagellar plasma membranes. *Ann. NY Acad. Sci.*, **356**, 382–4

Furthmayr, H. and Marchesi, U.T. (1976). Subunit structure of human erythrocyte glycophorvin A. *Biochemistry*, **15**, 1137–44

Garbers, D.L. and Kopf, G.G. (1980). The regulation of spermatozoa by calcium and cyclic nucleotides. *Adv. Cyclic Nucleotide Res.* **13**, 251–306

Gibbons, B.H. (1980). Intermittent swimming in live sea urchin sperm. *J. Cell. Biol.*, **84**, 1–12

Gibbons, B.H. and Gibbons, T.R. (1980). Calcium-induced quiescence in reactivated sea urchin sperm. *J. Cell. Biol.*, **84**, 13–27

Gordon, M., Dandekar, P.V. and Eager, P.R. (1978). Identification of phosphatases on the membranes of guinea pig sperm. *Anat. Rec.*, **191**, 123–34

Hoskins, D.D., Brandt, H. and Acott, T.S. (1978). Initiation of sperm motility in the mammalian epididymis. *Fed. Proc.*, **37**, 2534–42

Kretsinger, R.H. (1980). Structure and evolution of calcium-modulated proteins. *CRC Crit. Rev. Biochem.*, **8**, 119–74

McGrady, A.V., Nelson, L. and Ireland, M. (1974). Ionic effects on the motility of bull and chimpanzee spermatozoa. *J. Reprod. Fertil.*, **40**, 71–6

Mann, T. (1964). *The Biochemistry of Semen and of the Male Reproductive Tract.* 2nd Edn. (London: Methuen)

Means, A.K. and Dedman, J.R. (1980). Calmodulin - an intracellular calcium receptor. *Nature*, **285**, 73–77

Morton, B.E., Sagadraca, R. and Fraser, C. (1978). Sperm motility within the mammalian epididymis: species variations and correlation with free calcium levels in epididymal plasma. *Fertil. Steril.*, **29**, 695–8

Peterson, R.N. and Freund, M. (1976). Relationship between motility and the transport and binding of divalent cations to the plasma membrane of human spermatozoa. *Fertil. Steril.*, **27**, 1303–7

Pitts, B.J.R., Okhuyson, C.H. and Entman, M.L. (1980). Stoichiometry and kinetics of sodium/calcium exchange. In Siegel, F.L., Carafoli, E., Kretsinger, R.H., Maclennan, D.H. and Wasserman, R.H. (eds.) *Calcium-binding Proteins: Structure and Function* pp. 39–46 (Amsterdam Elsevier/North Holland)

Racker, E. (1980). Fluxes of Ca^{2+} and concepts. *Fed. Proc.*, **239**, 2422–6

Reeves, J.P. and Sutko, J.L. (1979). Sodium-calcium ion exchange in cardiac membrane vesicles. *Proc. Natl. Acad. Sci. (USA)*, **76**, 590–4

Rubin, R.P. (1970). The role of calcium in the release of neutrotransmitter substances and hormones. *Pharmacol. Rev.*, **22**, 389–428

Rufo, G.A., Singh, J.P., Babcock, D.F. and Lardy, H.A. (1982). Purification and characterization of a calcium transport inhibitor from bovine seminal plasma. *J. Biol. Chem.*, **257**, 4527–632

Saling, P.M., Storey, B.T. and Wolf, D.P. (1978). Calcium-dependent binding of mouse epididymal spermatozoa to the zona pellucida. *Dev. Biol.*, **65**, 515–25

Singh, J.P., Babcock, D.F. and Lardy, H.A. (1978). Increased Ca^{2+} influx is a component of capacitation of spermatozoa. *Biochem. J.*, **172**, 549–56

Stahl, W.L. and Swanson, P.D. (1969). Uptake of Ca^{2+} by subcellular fractions isolated from brain. *J. Neurochem.*, **16**, 1553–63

Storey, B.T. and Keyhani, E. (1974). Energy metabolism of spermatozoa: III - Energy-linked uptake of Ca^{2+} by the mitochondria of rabbit epididymal spermatozoa. *Fertil. Steril.*, **25**, 976–84

Storey, B.T. (1978). Effects of ionophores and inhibitors and uncouplers of oxidative phosphorylation on sperm respiration. *Arch. Androl.*, **1**, 169–77

Talbot, P. and Franklin, L.E. (1976). Morphology and kinetics of the hamster sperm acrosome reaction. *J. Exp. Zool.*, **198**, 163–176

Vijayasarathy, S., Shivaji, S. and Balaram, P. (1980). Plasma membrane bound Ca^{2+}-ATPase activity in bull sperm. *FEBS Lett.*, **114**, 45–7

Voglmayr, J.K., White, I.G. and Quinn, P.J. (1969a). Comparison of adenosinetriphosphatase activity in testicular and ejaculated spermatozoa of the ram. *Biol. Reprod.*, **1**, 121–9

Voglmayr, J.K., Quinn, P.J. and White, I.G. (1969b). Characteristics of adenosinetriphosphatase of ram ejaculated and isolated sperm tails. *Biol. Reprod.*, **1**, 215–22

Young, L.G. and Nelson, L. (1974). Calcium ions and control of the motility of sea urchin spermatozoa. *J. Reprod. Fertil.*, **41**, 371–8

31
The zona-free hamster egg sperm penetration assay

N.J. SPIRTOS, S.A. HAMDI, M.E. HULL and N.J. COSSLER

Infertility is generally defined as the absence of conception following one year of unprotected sexual intercourse. The aetiology of infertility can be attributed to either male or female factors. Each partner of the infertile unit assumes equal risk and responsibility for the problem at the beginning of the infertility investigation. The goal of diagnostic testing of the infertile couple is to identify those male and female factors that may be responsible for the infertility. Once properly diagnosed, the couple may then be offered logical treatment in hopes of improving their fertility potential.

Many times, the standard tests, do not provide insight into the exact nature of the disorder. These infertile couples then become labelled as 'unexplained' and subjected to empirical treatment modalities. Such therapies are occasionally associated with the spontaneous occurrence of pregnancy, but the majority fail.

It becomes paramount, therefore, to develop scientific methods that investigate the process of fertilization. Unexplained infertile couples could then be offered rational therapeutic options. One such scientific method is the zona-free hamster egg sperm penetration test. This test of male fertility is the only method currently available, short of human *in vitro* fertilization and embryo transfer, that objectively measures the fertilizing capability of human spermatozoa.

Other than a previous history of fatherhood, the most commonly used method of evaluating male fertility is gross examination of spermatozoa using light microscopy. The objective parameters studied, such as sperm concentration, motility and morphology, are subject to wide variation depending upon observer experience. The results of a routine semen analysis do not provide information concerning the fertilizing capacity of human spermatozoa. The sperm penetration assay (SPA) provides much needed information concerning the fertility potential of the male in infertile couples.

GAMETE PHYSIOLOGY

Gamete physiology will be briefly reviewed first to facilitate an understanding of zona-free hamster egg and human sperm interaction. Human ova are surrounded by a non-cellular proteinaceous layer called the zona pellucida. Normal fertilization requires a species-specific attachment of motile human spermatozoa to the zona pellucida. Prior to sperm–egg fusion the spermatozoa must undergo capacitation and the acrosome reaction. Capacitation and the acrosome reaction are poorly understood events that occur in the female reproductive tract. The process involves destabilization of the sperm's outer membrane, which then fuses with the outer membrane of the acrosome during the acrosome reaction (Thadani, 1982). The inner membrane of the acrosome thus becomes the outer membrane of the sperm itself, which subsequently allows the release of proteolytic enzymes necessary for fertilization (Thadani, 1982). Once a motile sperm has penetrated the zona pellucida it rapidly traverses the perivitelline space and quickly penetrates the vitelline membrane of the ovum. As this process occurs, a series of events begins, collectively known as the cortical granule reaction. With penetration, proteolytic enzymes are released from the cortical granules, and a biophysical alteration of the zona pellucida occurs which prevents polyspermy. After fertilization, the haploid number of chromosomes contained within the ovum and sperm become organized into a female and male pronucleus, respectively. Fusion of the two pronuclei then allows replication of genetic material with the resultant formation of an embryo.

Since the zona pellucida of the hamster ovum is species–specific, spermatozoa of other mammalian species will not fertilize a hamster oocyte until the zona pellucida has been removed by trypsin treatment (Yanagimachi, 1972). Zona-free hamster oocytes have been shown to be susceptible to penetration by capacitated human spermatozoa (Yanagimachi et al., 1976). However, since a major barrier to fertilization has been chemically extirpated, positive results of the SPA may merely indicate the intrinsic ability of human spermatozoa to undergo capacitation and the acrosome reaction and subsequent fusion with the ova (Yanagimachi et al., 1976). Negative results of the SPA, however, may indicate that the spermatozoa tested are unable to accomplish all or some of these physiological processes and would probably be unable to effect fertilization in vivo (Yanagimachi et al., 1976).

The following discussion will focus on the methodology of the sperm penetration assay as it is performed at the C.S. Mott Center for Human Growth and Development. Subsequently, the ultrastructural observations of sperm binding to zona-free hamster oocytes and the various factors affecting sperm penetration (capacitation time, media composition, sperm concentration, preservation of semen and hamster eggs, and sperm antibodies) will be discussed. Finally, a review of the clinical applications of the SPA will be undertaken.

METHODOLOGY OF ZONA-FREE HAMSTER EGG SPERM PENETRATION

The first day of the oestrous cycle is determined by testing the vaginal secretion of 8–10 week old female golden hamsters. The secretion on day one is usually yellow in colour and stretches as an elastic thread between the vaginal orifice and the examiner's finger. On day one of the oestrous cycle, the hamster is injected intraperitoneally with 50 iu of pregnant mare serum (PMS). In the evening of day three of the oestrous cycle (54–56 h after the PMS injection), the hamster is then injected intramuscularly with 40 iu of human chorionic gonadotropin (HCG) (Yanagimachi *et al.*, 1976).

Collection of ova

On the morning of day four of the oestrous cycle (16–18 h after the HCG injection) the hamster is killed and the ovaries and oviducts surgically removed. Using the dissecting microscope, the oviduct is flushed with BWW medium to segregate the cumulus mass. The ova are then freed from the cumulus cells with 1% hyaluronidase in BWW solution. Prior to insemination, the zona pellucida of each ovum is chemically dissolved through the use of 0.03% trypsin in BWW.

Preparation of semen

The human semen sample to be tested by the sperm penetration assay (SPA) is collected one day prior to the scheduled insemination day (day three of the oestrous cycle). Following a routine semen analysis, 1 ml of semen is transferred to a sterile centrifuge tube to which 9 ml of BWW medium containing 1 mg/ml of human serum albumin (HSA) is added. After thoroughly mixing the contents of the tube with a Pasteur pipette, the sample is centrifuged at 600 g for 6–8 min. The supernatant is then carefully removed and the pellet containing the spermatozoa washed again in the same manner. Following the second wash, the pellet is resuspended in 1 ml of BWW medium containing 35 mg/ml of HSA and incubated for 30–45 min in 5% CO_2 at 37°C in 95% humidity. The sample is then adjusted to contain 10 million motile sperm/ml. The sample is then placed in a loosely capped plastic tube (12 by 75 ml) and reincubated overnight under the same atmospheric conditions for an additional 18–20 h.

Insemination

Immediately prior to insemination, the percentage of motile spermatozoa is estimated. Exactly 0.3 ml of the sample is placed into a clean watch glass and covered by a thin layer of mineral oil. Between 25 and 40 zona-free hamster ova are added to the semen and the insemination dish is incubated for 4–5 h in 5% CO_2 at 37°C in 95% humidity. Following the incubation, the ova are removed from the insemination dish and transferred through three consecutive washes in BWW medium containing 1 mg/ml of human serum albumin to remove loosely adherent spermatozoa. The ova are placed onto clean glass slides and gently pressed under coverslips mounted on four drops of a mixture of vaseline-paraffin wax. The ova are examined under a phase-contrast microscope for the presence of swollen sperm heads and accompanying tails in the cytoplasm.

Interpretation of SPA

A minimum of 25 ova should be examined for sperm penetration. Sperm penetration is said to be present when a swollen sperm head (pronucleus formation) is seen within the cytoplasm. The ovum penetration rate is determined by dividing the number of penetrated ova by the number of ova inseminated times 100. For quality control, a semen sample from a previously tested fertile male should be run concurrently with each group of semen samples. Owing to the remarkable fluctuation in semen parameters, the SPA should be repeated within 6 weeks.

Preparation of BWW (Biggers, Whitten and Whittingham) medium

To prepare 1 litre of BWW medium, add to 800 ml of distilled water the following:

Sodium chloride (NaCl)	5.54 g
Potassium chloride (KC1)	0.36 g
Calcium lactate	0.53 g
Potassium phosphate (monobasic)	0.16 g
Sodium bicarbonate (NaHCO$_3$)	2.11 g
Pyruvic acid sodium salt	0.03 g
Magnesium sulphate (MgSO$_4$)	0.29 g
Dextrose (hydrous)	1.00 g
Sodium lactate	3.68 ml
Human serum albumin	1.00 g
Antibiotic solution	1.00 ml

(Penicillin 0.12 g + streptomycin 0.1 g + 2.0 ml of distilled water: 1ml of this solution is added to 1000 ml of already prepared BWW)

The beaker is filled to a volume of 1000 ml. It is important to allow the albumin to dissolve slowly and without stirring in order to prevent frothing. After mixing the medium for 15–30 min, sterilization is accomplished by filtering through a millipore filter under positive pressure. In order to maintain the pH between 7.2 and 7.4, 30% of the volume of the bottle is left empty. Five percent CO_2 can then be added to the bottle each time it is opened and prior to its next refrigeration.

SPERM BINDING TO ZONA-FREE HAMSTER OOCYTES

Observations of human spermatozoa and zona-free hamster (ZFH) oocytes using a dissecting microscope reveal that spermatozoa either bounce off or become attached to oocytes (Talbot and Chacon, 1982). The number of spermatozoa which bind to a single ovum may range from 1 to 200 but, generally, 20–50 are found to be attached. Thus, it has been suggested that those sperm that bounce off oocytes have not undergone capacitation or completed the normal acrosome reaction. This is consistent with the fact that only 10-20% of spermatozoa complete the normal acrosome reaction under culture conditions (Talbot and Chacon, 1982). Scanning electron microscopy reveals that bound spermatozoa loose their acrosomal caps and are intimately attached to the oolemma, a fact that suggests that the inner acrosomal membrane is essential for binding. This is to be distinguished from the acrosomal loss occurring as a consequence of cell death (false acrosome reaction). In this case, electron microscopy reveals vesiculating equatorial segments or disrupted plasma membranes (Talbot and Chacon, 1982).

Under electron microscopy, fusion of human spermatozoa with ZFH oocytes show that the oolemma of the microvilli fuse with the plasma membrane of spermatozoa at the postacrosomal region. After fusion, the nuclear envelope of the sperm begins to break down and dispersion of chromatin occurs near the fusion site. Ooplasma appears to flow in and engulf the dispersing nucleus (Talbot and Chacon, 1982).

These findings indicate that if no sperm bind to ZFH oocytes during a SPA, it might be concluded that the spermatozoa had not undergone normal acrosome reactions in culture. These results may also be useful in evaluating and enumerating the number of sperm bound per oocyte, as this number would be related to the number of reacted sperm. Thus, this assay may be used not only in evaluating the number of penetrated oocytes, but also in determining the numbers of bound sperm. One could then discriminate between males whose sperm failed to undergo acrosome reactions (none or little binding) and those whose sperm reacted but failed to fuse with the oolemma (oocytes with sperm bound to them but not penetrating them) (Talbot and Chacon, 1982).

FACTORS AFFECTING PENETRATION OF ZONA-FREE HAMSTER OOCYTES

Media composition and capacitation time

Factors that affect sperm penetration of ZFH oocytes include the medium in which the spermatozoa are incubated and in which capacitation presumably occurs. The influence of medium composition, osmolarity and albumin concentration on the ability of human spermatozoa to undergo the acrosome reaction and penetrate ZFH ova has been investigated (Aitken et al., 1983). Raising the osmolarity but not the albumin concentration of the media has been found significantly to increase the proportion of spermatozoa exhibiting an acrosome reaction with a subsequent increase in the penetration of hamster ova, without influencing motility. Hyperosmolar media, therefore, seem to correlate positively with capacitation, the acrosome reaction and sperm penetration of ZFH oocytes.

Other parameters that are important in the performance and standardization of the SPA are the albumin concentration of the media utilized and the length of capacitation time of the spermatozoa prior to the addition of ZFH oocytes. Human serum albumin (HSA) or bovine serum albumin

(BSA) are generally used in the culture media for the SPA. Human spermatozoa may be capacitated in media containing high concentrations (3.5%) of HSA or low concentrations (0.3%) of BSA (Gould *et al.*, 1983). Overnight preincubation (18–24 h) of spermatozoa in media containing 3.5% HSA enhance sperm fusion with living ZFH egg vitelli, but the capacity for zona penetration is lost when spermatozoa are mixed with non-living human oocytes. Preincubation of sperm suspensions for 18–24 h in media containing 0.3% BSA, however, do not result in this same increase in the percentage of penetrated hamster vitelli. These differences can be attributed to the concentration of HSA rather than a general effect of albumin concentration, because overnight preincubation in 3.5% BSA does not interfere with zona penetration. Using 3.5% HSA, the percentage of spermatozoa that undergo the acrosome reaction increase from 8% after 4 h of incubation to 62% after 22–28 h. The percentage of motile sperm remain high after overnight incubation in 3.5% HSA, but both the mean swimming speed and flagellar activity decline. These spermatozoa give the appearance of quivering on the zona surface rather than thrusting against it, thus, the ability for strong zona binding seems to be lost (Gould *et al.*, 1983).

High-HSA media may, thus, induce rapid sperm capacitation but a long preincubation period prior to the introduction of oocytes allows postcapacitation sperm aging to occur with the resultant loss of zona binding and penetration (Gould *et al.*, 1983). Most clinical laboratories, therefore, use low-albumin media over long preincubation periods (18–24 h) (Rogers *et al.*, 1979; Hall, 1981; Karp *et al.*, 1981; Stenchever *et al.*, 1981; Tyler *et al.*, 1981) or high albumin media over short (4 h) preincubation periods (Overstreet *et al.*, 1980).

Sperm motility and sperm penetration of ZFH oocytes has also been shown to increase significantly when spermatozoa are incubated with 10% human preovulatory serum (Berger *et al.*, 1983). It is postulated that human preovulatory serum may contain substances that facilitate the acrosome reaction, thereby, leading to increased sperm binding and penetration of ZFH oocytes.

Sperm concentration

In addition to the media composition, osmolarity and incubation time, sperm concentration is also an important consideration that affects the results of the SPA. The concentration of motile sperm is linearly related to the mean number of sperm that penetrate ZFH ova (Binor *et al.*, 1980). No penetration is usually observed at concentrations less than 600 000 motile cells/ml, whereas above this concentration, penetration increases to a maximal value of approximately 3.6 sperm/egg. Other investigators, however, have shown that at sperm concentrations below 500 000 sperm/ml, more than 50% of donor spermatozoa do not penetrate ZFH ova (Martin and Taylor, 1983). The mean penetration rate demonstrates a linear increase with increasing sperm concentrations (Fig. 31.1). At 50 000 sperm/ml, the mean penetration rate is 2.7%; at 100 000 sperm/ml, 3.9%; at 500 000 sperm/ml, 12.5%; at 1 000 000 sperm/ml, 20.5%; at 5 000 000 sperm/ml, 24.0%; and

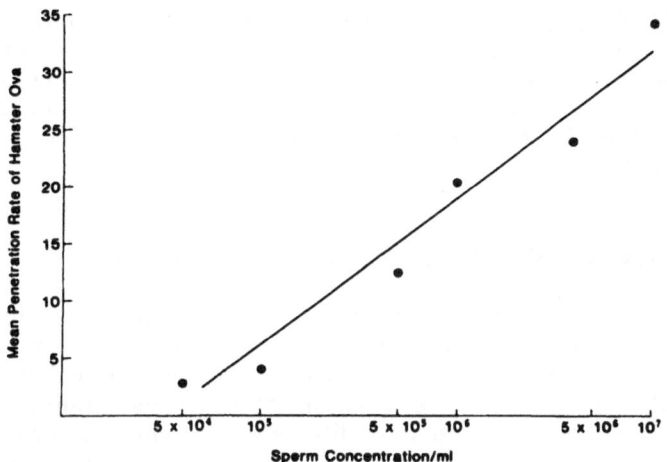

Fig. 31.1 Effect of sperm concentration on mean hamster ovum penetration rates (Martin and Taylor, 1983)

at 10 000 000 sperm/ml, 34.3%. The optimum concentration for ovum penetration, therefore, seems to be 10 000 000 sperm/ml. The interpretation of the SPA and comparison between individual rates may, thus, be only valid when consistent sperm concentrations are used (Martin and Taylor, 1983).

Cryopreservation of human spermatozoa and hamster oocytes

Since the SPA is available only at a limited number of referal centres, the use of fresh semen becomes a limiting factor in the practicality of the test. However, if semen could be adequately frozen without loss of its penetrating potential, the SPA would then be available to many more infertile couples. Frozen-thawed human spermatozoa do exhibit the ability to penetrate ZFH oocytes (Binor *et al.*, 1980), but there is some disagreement as to whether the freezing process does (Binor *et al.*, 1980) or does not (Cohen *et al.*, 1981) affect the fertilizing capability of human spermatozoa. Freeze-thawed sperm, although capable of penetrating ZFH oocytes, may do so with lesser frequency than do fresh sperm at equal concentrations of motile spermatozoa (Binor *et al.*, 1980). Although the penetration rates of cryopreserved spermatozoa are significantly less than the penetration rate utilizing fresh spermatozoa, sperm penetration testing of cryopreserved sperm yields the same fertility classification as fresh sperm. In other words, patients retain their fertile or subfertile (below 20% penetration) classification in the SPA when frozen sperm is used instead of fresh. With these limitations and advantages in mind, the use of cryopreserved sperm should simplify the SPA procedure, thereby allowing more availability of the test.

Just as human spermatozoa may be cryopreserved for future use, large numbers of ZFH ova may be preserved at specialized centres and distributed to laboratories lacking proper animal facilities (Aitken, 1983). The frozen ova may then be thawed at any time and used in the SPA. Approxi-

457

mately 90% of cryopreserved hamster oocytes appear morphologically normal after thawing and sperm penetration rates seem to be similar to those obtained with fresh ova on the same semen specimen (Fleming and Yanagimachi, 1979). As the cryopreservation process becomes more and more refined and reproducible, the SPA utilizing frozen specimens may ultimately make this test a routine laboratory procedure.

IMMUNOLOGY OF SPERM PENETRATION ASSAY

There is mounting clinical and experimental evidence that immunological responses to spermatozoa and other reproductive tract antigens may be a contributing aetiological factor in couples now designated as having 'unexplained' infertility. The exact mechanisms by which these immunologically mediated responses may cause infertility, however, remain to be elucidated. Antisperm antibodies have been proposed as one such mechanism and, while their existence is not disputed, a causal role in infertility has yet to be clearly demonstrated. The presence of these antibodies in both fertile and subfertile/infertile couples has made the differentiation between what may constitute a pathological condition and what may be considered normal population variance difficult. As discussed below, alterations in the SPA has been proposed by some authors as a potential diagnostic marker for the pathological presence of antisperm antibodies.

Possible mechanisms for interference with reproductive function by antisperm antibodies include the following (Haas *et al.*, 1980):

(1) Arming of macrophages and subsequent enhancement of phagocytic clearing of spermatozoa from the genital tract
(2) Sperm cytotoxicity, given the presence of adequate levels of complement
(3) Prevention of cervical mucus penetration
(4) Adverse peristalsis interfering with sperm migration through the uterus or tubes
(5) Perturbation of implantation
(6) Decrease in sperm number or motility
(7) Interference with capacitation or the acrosome reaction
(8) Impairment of spermatozoal/egg interaction

The SPA has, to date, been suggested as a potential measure of only the last of these purported mechanisms, i.e. impairment of spermatozoal/egg interaction secondary to the presence of antisperm antibodies. Thus, even if the reliability and validity of the SPA for discriminating the pathological presence of these antibodies is established, considerable caution must be maintained in interpreting negative results.

In assessing perturbations in the SPA as a function of antisperm antibodies, at least two criteria need first be met. The first is that normal values for the SPA from fertile populations must be known. The SPA, a delicate test, requires strict control of multiple variables in its performance. These variables (capacitation time, insemination mixtures, sperm and ova preparation and concentration) will all influence the range of normality established by each laboratory. With standardization of the assay, however, recent reports (Aitken *et al.*, 1982a) indicate that the threshold of normality for the SPA, given a minimum concentration of 400 000 to 600 000 motile spermatozoa/ml in insemination mixtures, is approximately 10% penetrance. These reports further suggest that if negative results (less than 10% penetrance) are obtained with motile concentrations of spermatozoa above this minimum level, then this is an indication of subnormal fertility not associated with the conventional parameters of semen analysis such as density, total count, morphology, volume and per cent motility. Thus the search for other potential causes of subnormal fertility including antisperm antibodies can begin.

This suggestion of decreased fertility with less than optimum ZFH egg penetrance leads to the second required criteria, i.e. that the inability adequately to penetrate ZFH oocytes is predictive of the inability to fertilize human ova *in vivo*. One recent *in vitro* observation (Margalioth *et al.*, 1983b) has indicated that results of the SPA may discriminate for the ability of spermatozoa to fertilize human eggs. In this study, spermatozoa from 7 patients that demonstrated less than 20% ZFH egg penetrance also failed to induce cleavage in 17 human ova inseminated for purposes of *in vitro* fertilization. Of the 13 patients whose spermatozoa reached greater than 20% penetrance of ZFH oocytes, 10 showed cleavage of at least one ovum.

Given a reasonable credence in the reliability and valididy of the SPA, changes in its outcome associated with antisperm antibodies can then be examined. Initial animal studies indicate that sperm penetration of ZFH eggs may be inhibited in the presence of antisperm antibodies. In one set of experiments (Teartos, 1979), univalent (FaB) anti-hamster sperm antibodies were raised in rabbits and then mixed with hamster spermatozoa. These spermatozoa showed a consistently decreased penetration of ZFH oocytes when compared with spermatozoa mixed with preimmune FaB fragments. The presence of antibodies, however, did not totally block ZFH egg penetration and the percentage penetrance progressively increased as the time between spermatozoa-antibody mixing and subsequent ZFH egg addition decreased.

Indications of decreased ZFH egg penetrance in the presence of antibodies in pure animal research led to investigation of outcome using antibodies raised to human antigens. Decreased penetrance has been observed using sperm from fertile human donors after exposure to antibodies raised in rabbits to human epididymal sperm, epididymal sperm-FaB, sperm extract and sperm extract-FaB after absorption with spleen, liver and kidney cells with or without seminal plasma (Menge and Black, 1979). Exposure to these antibody preparations all resulted in a significant decrease from control values, however the range of penetrance was 0% to 34±9% making a clear prognostic interpretation difficult. Interestingly, direct treatment of ZFH ova with rabbit anti-human epididymal sperm antibodies prior to SPA testing also depressed the penetration rate (10%) in comparison with normal sera or BWW. This depressed penetrance rate was not noted following prior treatment of ova with anti-epididymal sperm-FaB. These results suggest that there may be hindrance to sperm penetration secondary to non-specific antibody binding on the vitelline membrane itself or to binding of antisperm antibody by the Fc portion to the vitellus.

Examination of SPA changes using natural, human iso- and autoantibodies from infertile couples has produced mixed outcomes. In one study (Haas *et al.*, 1980), IgG antisperm antibodies were obtained from plasma of infertile men and tested with sperm from known fertile donors where penetration characteristics were defined separately and served as internal controls. A trend towards decreased ZFH egg penetrance was observed in the presence of plasma positive for IgG antibodies in comparison with negative plasma and control (buffer) solutions. However, while four of six positive plasmas significantly and reproducibly inhibited sperm penetration in comparison to controls, the penetrance range, in the presence of IgG positive plasma, extended from 0% to 54%. Thus, if the minimum threshold for normality in the SPA is accepted as greater than 10% penetrance, the statistically significant decrease in antibody-associated penetrance may not have clinical significance. Further, since the plasmas were tested by direct addition to the sperm/egg mixture, inhibitory effects directed solely against the ZFH egg vitelline membrane cannot be excluded.

Although the majority of reports concerning antibody-associated sperm penetrance have found evidence of inhibition in the SPA, there is some evidence that ZFH egg penetrance may be enhanced in the presence of sperm-specific antibodies bound to the head region (Bronson *et al.*, 1981). These head-specific IgG and IgA antisperm antibodies were obtained from sera of men and women involved in infertility investigations and were bound to known fertile donor sperm prior to sperm/egg mixture to lessen the possibility of a direct antibody/egg interaction. To test whether some factor other than sperm-directed immunoglobulins may have enhanced the SPA, the antibodies were removed from the positive sera by serial absorption and, following incubation in the absorbed sera, a decreased egg penetrance was noted. These results indicate that sperm-specific immunoglobulins may not necessarily impair the acrosomal reaction or sperm/egg membrane fusion. Finally, using passive antibody transfer to fertile donor sperm prior to capacitation, these same sera that allowed facilitated ZFH egg penetrance were associated with nearly complete inhibition of sperm attachment to human zona pellucida (Bronson *et al.*, 1982). Thus the suggestion that some antisperm antibodies may block fertilization at the level of the zona pellucida and not the vitelline membrane giving false-positive results in the SPA.

The results of changes in the SPA in association with antisperm antibodies are inconclusive. The apparent heterogeneous polyclonal nature of spontaneously occurring sperm-specific antibodies implies that individual serum will vary in its ability to impair, enhance, or not influence sperm-vitelline membrane and sperm-zona pellucida interaction (Bronson *et al.*, 1982). Although the SPA shows much clinical promise in predicting decreased fertilizing ability in spermatozoa, its ability to predict immunologically mediated impairment of reproductive function remains to be demonstrated.

CLINICAL APPLICATIONS OF SPERM PENETRATION ASSAY

Although the routine semen analysis is the most commonly used estimate of male fertility, it fails to provide evidence concerning the ability of spermatozoa to complete the process of fertilization. Comparing the sensitivity, specificity and the false–positive and false–negative rates of the SPA with conventional semen analysis, the SPA has been found to be superior in every parameter (Shy et al., 1982). In this study, for example, 100% (29/29) of the infertile men tested were properly classified by the SPA (negative penetration), whereas 41% (12/29) were incorrectly classified as normal by routine semen analysis. Even though the SPA is a reproducible method of predicting male fertility, its cost and limited availability restrict its usefulness. A logical protocol (Shy et al., 1982) to assess a couple's fertility is as follows. Assuming the initial semen analysis is normal, the standard infertility evaluation (ovulation assessment, endometrial biopsy, serum progesterone, hysterosalpingography, postcoital test) is completed. A SPA is then indicated when a couple is unable to achieve pregnancy after 3 years in the presence of a normal semen analysis. A SPA is also useful before embarking on intensive, expensive and risky medical and surgical therapy for female factors when the semen analysis is normal (Shy et al., 1982). The SPA regimens may also be performed following failure of standard therapeutic regimens for diagnosed female factors. Finally, a SPA may be indicated if at least one parameter of the semen analysis is near or just below the lower limits of normal. The SPA, thus, helps determine the significance of this abnormality (Shy et al., 1982). Routine semen analysis and the SPA are, therefore, important clinical tools which complement each other in the evaluation of an infertile couple.

The clinical interpretation of a 'positive' or 'negative' result of the SPA is controversial. The assay has not previously been standardized between laboratories, and mean penetration rates of human sperm from fertile males between 34 and 81% with a range of 0 to 100% have been observed (Table 31.1). The minimum penetration rate that is associated with normal male fertility appears to be approximately 11% (Karp et al., 1981; Cohen et al.,

Table 31.1 SPA Results in fertile males

Study	Mean Penetration (%)	Range of penetration (%)
Martin and Taylor (1982)	34	0–60
Chan et al. (1983)	36	—
Aitken et al. (1982a)	44	14–90
Cohen et al. (1982)	54	11–100
Rogers et al. (1979)	56	14–100
Tyler et al. (1981)	60	24–89
Hall et al. (1980)	64	20–100
Hall (1981)	66	20–100
Margalioth et al. (1983a)	69	20–100
Hammond et al. (1982)	73	20–100
Zausner–Guelman et al. (1981)	81	—

1982; Stenchever *et al.*, 1982). In couples exhibiting unexplained infertility, the mean penetration rate is only 31%, a figure significantly less than the penetration rates in normal fertile controls (Aitken *et al.*, 1982b). Fewer males with penetration rates of 0-10% produce offspring when compared to males exhibiting penetration rates of 11-100% (Aitken, 1983). Males with penetration rates of 1-10% may father children, whereas males exhibiting zero penetration probably will not (Aitken, 1983). An occasional male of proven fertility will consistently demonstrate a zero penetration rate (Martin and Taylor, 1982). This observation alone suggests that the SPA cannot discriminate between fertile and infertile males with 100% accuracy. Clearly, penetration scores below the normal fertile range are not incompatible with pregnancy, although the fertility of such patients appears to be significantly decreased (Aitken, 1983). That a cohort of subfertile males will not be identified by routine semen analysis emphasizes the diagnostic value of the ZFH egg sperm penetration test in couples with unexplained infertility (Aitken, 1983; Tyler *et al.*, 1981; Hammond *et al.*, 1982).

Besides the obvious importance of the SPA in helping males with unexplained infertility, this test may also be used in evaluating patients with oligozoospermia. In a study of 27 such oligozoospermic males, a mean penetration rate of only 3% was observed (Aitken *et al.*, 1982c), as compared to the 44% mean penetration rate in males exhibiting normal fertility (Aitken *et al.*, 1982a). Spermatozoa from two of these oligozoospermic men demonstrated greater than 10% penetrance, while spermatozoa from 19 patients exhibited no penetration. A zero penetration rate observed in the SPA may, therefore, be clinically significant in identifying those oligozoospermic patients for whom there is very little chance of fertilizing a human egg *in vivo*. This realization may, thus, spare the infertile couple many years of fruitless attempts at conception and allow artificial donor insemination or adoption procedures to be considered. Since eight of these 27 (30%) men did exhibit some minimal fertilizing capability, human *in vitro* fertilization and embryo transfer (IVF-ET) may be a viable alternative in this subgroup of infertile couples given that the sperm concentration required is generally less than 1 million motile sperm/ovum. To be effective, however, these spermatozoa must be actively motile with normal morphology. With the advent of human IVF-ET, oligospermia may now be a very treatable infertility disorder, whereas in the past, the prognosis was poor.

Another clinical application of the SPA concerns its use in the proper selection of couples for *in vitro* fertilization and embryo transfer. The fertilizing assessment with this bioassay correlates highly with the fertilization of human eggs *in vitro* (Wolf *et al.*, 1983). Sixteen of 18 (89%) husbands whose sperm fertilized their wives' eggs also demonstrated a positive fertility assessment (greater than 10% penetration) using the SPA. Two husbands, however, did not meet the minimum penetration criteria of at least 10% (0% and 6%, respectively) but were still able to fertilize their spouse's eggs *in vitro*. Although this false-negative assessment occurred, a high correlation between the SPA and human IVF still exists. The SPA, therefore, should precede IVF-ET, so as to select only those males who demonstrate at least a minimal fertilizing capacity. Couples eliminated in this manner could either resort to the utilization of donor semen in conjunction with IVF-ET or forego the procedure all together.

As stated previously, spermatozoa must undergo a series of biochemical and biophysical changes before they are capable of fertilization (Lipshultz, 1983). Capacitation and the acrosome reaction are prerequisities for *in vitro* and *in vivo* fertilization. It is certainly possible that some males are infertile because of abnormal or delayed capacitation. Spermatozoa incubated with egg yolk buffer (Lipshultz, 1983), oestradiol (Chan *et al.*, 1983), or caffeine and theophylline (Perreault and Rogers, 1980) demonstrate increased ability to penetrate zona-free hamster eggs during a SPA. Pretreatment of spermatozoa with one of these substances may correct the problem of delayed capacitation and allow conception to occur following homologous artificial insemination (AIH). The SPA will evaluate the effects of treatment in those patients exhibiting abnormal capacitation.

Other potential uses of the SPA include: (1) evaluation of males exposed to diethylstilboestrol (DES) *in utero* (Stenchever *et al.*, 1981); (2) evaluation of males exposed to environmental pollutants; and (3) evaluation of men treated with chemotherapeutic drugs and/or irradiation for various forms of cancer (Shy *et al.*, 1982). The SPA may, thus, be used in many situations where male infertility is of primary concern.

In conclusion, the aspects of sperm function assessed by the zona-free hamster egg sperm penetration test include the ability of spermatozoa to capacitate, acrosome-react, fuse with the vitelline membrane and become incorporated into the ooplasm and undergo nuclear condensation (Aitken, 1983). The SPA technique also affords an excellent opportunity to inspect directly the chromosomes of the decondensed sperm head (Paulsen, 1983), thus providing a new area for scientific investigation. Although an imperfect surrogate for the human ovum, the sperm penetration assay is an important clinical tool that can adequately assess the functional capacity of human spermatozoa from infertile males.

References

Aitken, J. (1983). The zona-free hamster egg penetration test. In Hargreave, T.B. (ed.) *Male Infertility*, pp. 75–86 (Berlin, Heidelberg, New York, Tokyo: Springer-Verlag)

Aitken, R.J., Best, F.S.M., Richardson, D.W., Djahanbakhch, O. and Lees, M.M. (1982a). The correlates of fertilizing capacity in normal fertile men. *Fertil. Steril.*, **38**, 68–76

Aitken, R.J., Best, F.S.M., Richardson, D.W., Djahanbakhch, O., Mortimer, D., Templeton, A.A. and Lees, M.M. (1982b). An analysis of sperm function in cases of unexplained infertility: conventional criteria, movement characteristics, and fertilizing capacity. *Fertil. Steril.*, **38**, 212–21

Aitken, R.J., Best, F.S.M., Richardson, D.W., Djahanbakhch, O., Templeton, A. and Lees, M.M. (1982c). An analysis of semen quality and sperm function in cases of oliogozoospermia. *Fertil. Steril.*, **38**, 705–11

Aitken, R.J., Wang, Y.F., Liu, J., Best, F. and Richardson, D.W. (1983). The influence of medium composition, osmolarity and albumin content on the acrosome reaction and fertilizing capacity of human spermatozoa: development of an improved zona-free hamster egg penetration test. *Int. J. Androl.*, **6**, 180–93

Berger, T., Marrs, R.P., Saito, H. and Kletzky, O.A. (1983). Factors affecting human sperm penetration of zona-free hamster ova. *Am J. Obstet. Gynecol.*, **145**, 397–401

Binor, Z., Sokoloski, J.E. and Wolf, D.P. (1980). Penetration of the zona-free hamster egg by human sperm. *Fertil. Steril.*, **33**, 321–7

Bronson, R.A., Cooper, G.W. and Rosenfeld, D.L. (1981). Ability of antibody-bound human sperm to penetrate zona-free hamster ova *in vitro*. *Fertil. Steril.*, **36**, 778–83

Bronson, R.A., Cooper, G.W. and Rosenfeld, D.L. (1982). Sperm-specific isoantibodies and autoantibodies inhibit the binding of human sperm to the human zona pellucida. *Fertil. Steril.*, **38**, 724–9

Chan, S.Y.W., Tang, L.C.H. and Ma, H. (1983). Stimulation of the zona-free hamster ova penetration efficiency by human spermatozoa after 17β-estradiol treatment. *Fertil. Steril.*, **39**, 80–4

Cohen, J., Felten, P. and Zeilmaker, G.H. (1981). *In vitro* fertilizing capacity of fresh and cyopreserved human spermatozoa: a comparative study of different freezing and thawing procedures. *Fertil. Steril.*, **36**, 356–62

Cohen, J., Weber, R.F.A., van der Vijver, J.C.M. and Zeilmaker, G.H. (1982). *In vitro* fertilizing capacity of human spermatozoa with the use of zona-free hamster ova: interassay variation and prognostic value. *Fertil. Steril.*, **37**, 565–72

Fleming, A.D. and Yanagimachi, R. (1979). Cryopreserved zona-free hamster ova: their potential use for assessing the fertilizing capacity of human spermatozoa. *Biol. Reprod.*, **20**, 41A (abstr)

Gould, J.E., Overstreet, J.W., Yanagimachi, H., Yanagimachi, R., Katz, D.F. and Hanson, F.W. (1983). What functions of the sperm cell are measured by *in vitro* fertilization of zona-free hamster eggs. *Fertil. Steril.*, **40**, 344–52

Haas, G.G., Sokoloski, J.E. and Wolf, D.P. (1980). The interfering effect of human IgG antisperm antibodies on human sperm penetration of zona-free hamster eggs. *Am. J. Reprod. Immunol.*, **1**, 40–3

Hall, J.L. (1981). Relationship between semen quality and human sperm penetration of zona-free hamster ova. *Fertil. Steril.*, **35**, 457–63

Hall, J.L., Sloan, C.S. and Hammond, M.G. (1980). Correlation of heterologous *in vitro* fertilization using human sperm and hamster ova with clinical evaluation of male infertility. *Fertil. Steril.*, **33** (abstr), 238

Hammond, M.G., Sloan, C.S. and Hall, J.L. (1982). Application of interspecies *in vitro* fertilization in the initial assessment of the infertile couple. *Am. J. Obstet. Gynecol.*, **142**, 340–3

Karp, L.E., Williamson, R.A., Moore, D.E., Shy, K.K., Plymate, S.R. and Smith, W.D. (1981). Sperm penetration assay: useful test in evaluation of male fertility. *Obstet. Gynecol.*, **57**, 620–3

Lipshultz, L.I. (1983). Update: new aspects in the diagnosis of male infertility. *Fertility News.*, **17**, 3–5

Margalioth, E.J., Laufer, N., Navot, D., Voss, R. and Schenker, J.G. (1983a). Reduced fertilization ability of zona-free hamster ova by spermatozoa from male partners of normal infertile couples. *Arch. Androl.*, **10**, 67–71

Margalioth, E.J., Navot, D., Laufer, N., Yosef, S.M. Rabinowitz, R., Yarkoni, S. and Schenker, J.G. (1983b). Zona-free hamster ovum penetration assay as a screening procedure for *in vitro* fertilization. *Fertil. Steril.*, **40**, 386–8

Martin, R.H. and Taylor, P.J. (1982). Reliability and accuracy of the zona-free hamster ova assay in the assessment of male fertility. *Br. J. Obstet. Gynaecol.*, **89**, 951–6

Martin, R.H. and Taylor, P.J. (1983). Effect of sperm concentration in the zona-free hamster ova penetration assay. *Fertil. Steril.*, **39**, 379–81

Menge, A.C. and Black, C.S. (1979). Effects of antisera on human sperm penetration of zona-free hamster ova. *Fertil. Steril.*, **32**, 214–18

Overstreet, J.W., Yanagimachi, R., Katz, D.F., Hayashi, K. and Hanson, F.W. (1980). Penetration of human spermatozoa into the human zona pellucida and the zona-free hamster egg: a study of fertile donors and infertile patients. *Fertil. Steril.*, **33**, 534–42

Paulsen, C.A. (1983). Another look at the sperm penetration assay. *Fertil. Steril.*, **40**, 302–4

Perreault, S.D. and Rogers, B.J. (1980). Stimulation of human spermatozoal fertilizing ability by caffeine and theophylline. *Proceedings of the Annual Meeting of the Society for the Study of Reproduction*, 11–14 August, Ann Arbor, Michigan, p. 44

Rogers, B.J., Campen, H.V., Ueno, M., Lambert, H., Bronson, R. and Hale, R. (1979). Analysis of human spermatozoal fertilizing ability using zona-free ova. *Fertil. Steril.*, **32**, 664–70

Shy, K.K., Soules, M.R. and Karp, L.E. (1982). The SPA-a new test of male fertility. *Contemporary OB/GYN*, **19**, 210-23

Stenchever, M.A., Spadoni, L.R., Smith, W.D., Karp, L.E., Shy, K.K., Moore, D.E. and Berger, R. (1982). Benefits of the sperm (hamster ova) penetration assay in the evaluation of the infertile couple. *Am. J. Obstet. Gynecol.*, **143**, 91-6

Stenchever, M.A., Williamson, R.A., Leonard, J., Karp, L.E., Ley, B., Shy, K. and Smith, D. (1981). Possible relationship between *in utero* diethylstilbestrol exposure and male fertility. *Am. J. Obstet. Gynecol.*, **140**, 186-93

Talbot, P. and Chacon, R.S. (1982). Ultrastructural observations on binding and membrane fusion between human sperm and zona pellucida-free hamster oocytes. *Fertil. Steril.*, **37**, 240-8

Teartos, S.J. (1979). Inhibition of *in vitro* fertilization of intact and denuded hamster eggs by univalent anti-sperm antobodies. *J. Reprod. Fertil.*, **55**, 447-55

Thadani, V.M. (1982). Clues from research into cross-species fertilization. *Contemporary OB/GYN*, **20**, 203-9

Tyler, J.P.P., Pryor, J.P. and Collins, W.P. (1981). Heterologous ovum penetration by human spermatozoa. *J. Reprod. Fertil.*, **63**, 499-508

Urry, R.L., Carrell, D.T., Hull, D.B., Middleton, R.G. and Wiltbank, M.C. (1983). Penetration of zona-free hamster ova and bovine cervical mucus by fresh and frozen human spermatozoa. *Fertil. Steril.*, **39**, 690-4

Wolf, D.P., Sokoloski, J.E. and Quigley, M.M. (1983). Correlation of human *in vitro* fertilization with the hamster egg bioassay. *Fertil. Steril.*, **40**, 53-9

Yanagimachi, R. (1972). Penetration of guinea pig spermatozoa into hamster eggs *in vitro*. *J. Reprod. Fertil.*, **28**, 477-80

Yanagimachi, R., Yanagimachi, H. and Rogers, B.J. (1976). The use of zona-free animal ova as a test-system for the assessment of the fertilizing capacity of human spermatozoa. *Biol. Reprod.*, **15**, 471-6

Zausner-Guelman, B., Blasco, L. and Wolf, D.P. (1981). Zona-free hamster eggs and human sperm penetration capacity: a comparative study of proven fertile donors and infertility patients. *Fertil. Steril.*, **36**, 771-7

Aitken, R. J., Best, F. S. M. and Richardson, D. W. (1982). The correlates of fertilizing capacity in normal fertile men, *Fertil. Steril.*, **38**, 68

Barros, C., Gonzalez, J., Herrera, E. and Bustos-Obregon, E. (1979). Human sperm penetration into zona-free hamster oocytes as a test to evaluate the sperm fertilizing ability, *Andrologia*, **11**, 197

Binor, Z., Sokoloski, J. E. and Wolf, D. P. (1980). Penetration of the zona-free hamster egg by human sperm, *Fertil. Steril.*, **33**, 321

Hall, J. L. (1981). Relationship between semen quality and human sperm penetration of zona-free hamster ova, *Fertil. Steril.*, **35**, 457

Rogers, B. J. (1985). The sperm penetration assay: its usefulness reevaluated, *Fertil. Steril.*, **43**, 821

Index

467